Healing Power Of Medicine

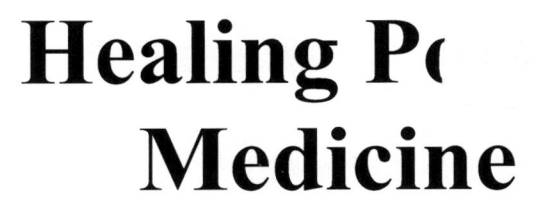

Medicine To Heal Or Medicine To Kill
Book 2 Revised Edition

Reed T. Sainsbury, N.D.

Copyright © **Reed T. Sainsbury, N.D. 2019**

All rights reserved. No part of this book may be used or reproduced by any means, graphic, electronic or mechanical, including photocopying, recording or taping or by any information storage retrieval system without the written permission of the publisher except in the case of brief quotations embodied in critical articles and reviews.

Books may be ordered through booksellers or by contacting:
Life Essentials Natural Healing Clinic at www.healingthecause.com or calling 256 543-3801

Because of the dynamic nature of the internet, any web addresses or links contained in this book may have changed since publication and may no longer be valid.

ISBN: 9798603483672
Library of Congress Control Number: Applied For
Printed in the United States of America

TABLE OF CONTENTS

Acknowledgement	9
Dedication	10
Foreword by Rashid A. Buttar, D.O.	11
Introduction	13
Disclaimer	15

Chapter 1   THE PULSATION OF LIFE   16

You Are A Self-Healing Organism	16
The Cell Is Immortal	17
Cyanide From Seeds — Mother Nature's Cure For Cancer	23
Herbs	24
Graviola	25
Identifying The Root Cause Of Your Disease	26
Energetic Frequencies	30
Heavy Metals	32
Kirlian Photography	35
Electrical Medical Devices	36
Acupuncture Points & Meridians	37
Electro Dermal Screening (EDS)	37
Homeopathy	41
Common Homeopathic Remedies	42

Chapter 2   HEALTH CARE OR DISEASE MAINTENANCE?   47

America's Disease Maintenance System	47
Eliminating Competition	49
A Cure For Cancer — Outlawed In The USA	50
Americans Have The Most Expensive Health Care, But Not The Best	52
Horse Urine For Health?	60
Dr. Semmelweis — Killed For Teaching The Truth	65
Murder By Prescription	66
Vioxx — A Killer Drug — Deemed Safe & Effective By The FDA	69
Hippocratic Or Hypocritical?	70
Medical Myths Of The Past	71
Removing The Nails In The Tire	72
The Paradox Of Modern Medicine	74
Prescription Drugs — A Vicious Disease Cycle	75
Heroes In The Emergency Room	77
The Cancer Industry	78
Cancer Is Not A Genetic Disease, It's A Metabolic Disease	80
Mammograms Cause Cancer	81

	Is The PSA Test For Prostate Cancer Reliable Or Necessary?	84
	Healing Cancer	88
	Is Cancer A Fungus?	92
	Chemotherapy — Deadly Mustard Gas — Causes Cancer	96
	Poison For Health?	97

Chapter 3 HEALING THE CAUSE OF DIS-EASE — 101

The Lymphatic System	101
Firemen Put Out Fires & Lymph Nodes Fight Infection	103
Rebounding (Lymphasizing)	107
Do Drugs Heal Disease?	108
Mother Nature's Food Chain	109
The Germ Is Nothing — The Terrain Is Everything	110
Fever (Leukocytosis) — How Your Body Destroys Pathogens	113
Colds	115
Own Your Dis-ease & Be Healed	119
Exercise For Weight Loss & Healthy Blood Sugar	121
The Facts About Fats	123
Coconut Oil — Fuel For Life	125
Intermittent Fasting	125
Breast Milk	126
Blood Sugar	127
Cereal Killers & Gluten – Food Or Poison?	127
Molecular Mimicry	129
You Crave What You Are Allergic To	130
Do You Have Allergies Or A Digestion Imbalance?	131
Stomach Acid — Your Friend For Life	132
Your Gut Flora (Microbiome)	137
Diabetes — Insulin Resistance	140
Glycemic Index Chart	144
Healthy Meals & Snacks	146
Seven Remedies Dr. Chappell Has Identified To Reverse Diabetes	148
Why Can't I Lose Weight?	150
Fermented Vegetables — Balance Your Microbiome	152
Bone Broth	153
Diet Drinks Sabotage Weight Loss	154
Aspartame: An Addictive Excitoneurotoxic Carcinogenic Drug	155
Soft Drinks	157
Caffeine	158
All Calories Are Not Created Equal	158
Weight Loss Without Trying	159
Hypothyroid Symptoms	161
Goiters	162
Losing Weight & Keeping It Off	164
What's The Healthiest Water To Drink?	165
Stevia — Mother Nature's Sugar Substitute	167

		Healing Skin Issues	167
		Don't Ignore Your Body's Warning Signs	169
Chapter	**4**	**HEALERS OR DRUG DEALERS?**	**171**
		Epilepsy Healed	171
		Toxic Chemicals In The Environment	173
		Healing Cancer With Whole, Living Foods	179
		The Healing Energy Of Plants	181
		Mother Nature's Intelligence	183
		Is It God's Will Or Are You Justifying Eating Junk Foods?	184
		A Headache Healed	186
		Remodeling Your House	187
		DNA & Your Divine Intelligence	188
Chapter	**5**	**MEDICAL MYTHS EXPOSED**	**190**
		Your Gallbladder — Crucial For Healthy Digestion	190
		Table Salt Vs. Organic Sodium	191
		Liver/Gallbladder Flush For Stones	196
		The Cholesterol Myth — Busted For Fraud	199
		Sugar, Grains & Carbs Cause Heart Attacks — Not Fat	210
		Eggs	210
		Deadly Hydrogenated Oils — The True Villains of Heart Disease	211
		Deadly Genetically Modified Organisms (GMOs)	213
		The Appendix	214
		There Are No Incurable Diseases	214
		Dis-ease: Your Body's Way Of Filing Bankruptcy	216
		Antibiotics Weaken Your Immune System & Increase Diabetes	218
		Acidosis – The Terrain That Favors Dis-ease	221
		The Terrain, Not The Germ, Causes Dis-ease	222
		Healing The Cause Of Kidney Stones, Bone Spurs & Arthritis	227
		Eat Right For Your Blood Type Diet	230
		Mother Nature's Foods — Healing Light Energy	231
		Chakras	232
		Toxic Silver Dental Fillings	235
		Mercury Facts	241
		Are Your Root Canals & Cavitations Harboring Toxic Bacteria?	242
		Dr. Weston Price Proved How Toxic Root Canals Are	243
		Cavitations — A Breeding Ground For Infection	244
		Tooth / Meridian Relationship Chart	247
		Locate A Biological Dentist — Science-Based Dentistry	248
		Autism — Symptom Of Heavy Metal Poisoning	248

Chapter 6 VACCINATIONS – WOLVES IN SHEEP'S CLOTHING 250

VAERS (Vaccine Adverse Event Reporting System)	254
Disease Mortality Rates	259
Unhealthy Living Conditions Cause Disease Epidemics	260
Better Sanitation — The Eradicator of Disease, Not Vaccinations	261
Diseases Declined 90% Before Vaccines Were Introduced	262
The Origin Of Vaccinations — Two Dead Boys	264
Strict Vaccination Laws = Increased Disease Outbreaks	265
Polio Facts, Lies & The Rest Of The Story	267
Iron Lung Or Transverse Myelitis?	270
Making The Polio Vaccine With SV-40 Virus	271
The Contaminated Polio Vaccine Infects 220,000 People	272
SV-40, A Cancer-Causing Virus In The Polio Vaccine	273
DDT — The Toxic Polio-Mimicking Insecticide	275
Polio Vaccine Maker Admits Failure — Media Claims Success?	278
Measles	281
Wild Measles Protects Against Diseases In Adulthood	285
Pertussis (Whooping Cough)	285
Silence Of The Scarlet Fever Streptococcus Vaccine Killer	287
Flawed Vaccine Efficacy	288
Vaccines Weaken Your Immune System	292
Vaccinations — The Missing Link to Food Allergies	295
Molecular Mimicry Again	297
Mercury (Thimerosal) In Vaccines	298
Aluminum In Vaccines	304
Flu Shots — Proven To Be Toxic & Worthless	307
Gardasil	311
Autism	313
CDC Whistleblower Admits MMR - Autism Cover-Up	313
Chickenpox Vaccines — Creates Shingles	318
Vaccinations Increase The Risk Of Diabetes	319
Wild Measles, Mumps & Chickenpox Protect Against Cancer	320
Tetanus	322
Dr. Carrel Produces Cancer In Chickens With Vaccine Ingredients	323
CDC Corruption	325
Dr. Mikovits Discovers Disease-Causing Retroviruses In Vaccines	326
Vaccine Ingredients	329
Nature's Infectious Disease Busters	332
Homeopathy — An Alternative To Vaccines	333
What To Do For Pertussis (Whooping Cough)	334
What To Do For Measles	335
Malaria	336
Traveler's Diarrhea	336
Vaccines Made From Aborted Fetal Tissue	338
Vaccine Exemption Affidavit	339
Mandatory Vaccinations — A Violation Of The Nuremburg Code	342

		Travel Vaccines	343
		The Vaccine Friendly Plan — For Those Who Vaccinate	344

Chapter 7   HEALTHY LIVING   347

Chiropractic Adjustments	347
Competitive Athletes — What To Eat?	348
Where Do Cows Get Protein?	351
High-Protein Diets — Not So Healthy	351
Mother Nature's Healers	354
Who Are The Healthiest People In The World?	355
U.S. Senate Document No. 264	357
Poison In Our Drinking Water	357
Chlorine	358
Fluoride	358
Antidepressant Drugs Cause Abnormal Behavior	363
Headaches	365
Aspirin	365
Natural Birth = Healthy Baby	366

Chapter 8   MASTER OF PUPPETS   369

How Much Do Your Drugs Actually Cost?	369
Rockefeller Oil Interests & I.G. Farben	370
The Big Drug Deal	371
Restructuring Medicine In The USA	371
Why Don't Insurance Companies Cover Natural Health Care?	372
The FDA — A Pawn In The Game	374
Money Handlers	374
Medical Ghost Writing	376
Paying To Squash Competition	377
Miasms	378

Chapter 9   HEALTH SECRETS YOUR DOCTOR NEVER TOLD YOU   380

Health Tips	477
Herbal Formulas For Children	477
Dr. Sainsbury's Health Plan	478
Health Evaluation	485
Homemade Natural Remedies	488
The Chinese Meridian Clock	489
Stress — Fight Or Flight	490
4-7-8 Breathing Technique For Anxiety, Stress, Cravings & Sleep	492

Chapter 10   EMOTIONS – ENERGY IN MOTION   493

Healing The Cause Of Cancer	493
Healing My Allergies	496
When The Student Is Ready, The Teacher Appears	497
Kinesiology	498
The Power Of The Mind	499
Allergies — Caused By A Traumatic Emotional Event	504
The Now	508
Anxiety & Panic Attacks — Caused From Childhood Trauma	509
The Needy Mind – Wanting Things - More, Better & Different	510
What We Hate in Others Is What We Condemn In Ourselves	513
Most Of Us Would Rather Be Right Than Happy	514
Double-Minded — Thinking One Way & Feeling The Other	514
Dyslexia	515
Healing Our Emotional Conflicts	516
Placebos: A Factor In Your Healing	517
What Are You Getting To Be Right About In Life?	518
Writing A Letter To Bring Closure & Healing	519
Resolving Conflicts	520
The World We Create With Thoughts	522
Being Grateful	523
Weight Gain — Self-Protection	523
Love	525
Agape Love	527
Why Relationships Fail	529
Validating Children's Feelings	531
Transforming Your Life — The Landmark Forum	532
The Power Of The Spoken Word	535
Winning	537
Conclusion	540

EDITOR'S NOTE: Unless otherwise credited, all photographs, illustrations, charts and other artwork are the creation and sole property of Reed Sainsbury. Others are used with permission from their creators or owners as noted.

Acknowledgements

I would like to thank the following people who have helped me write this book. God being the Creator of all has given me everything I am and everything I have. To the Almighty, I am eternally grateful for the abundance with which He blesses me.

I'd like to thank the three beautiful children God has entrusted me with: Dallas (Dally Wally), Brooklyn (Brooky Wooky) and Rockman (Rocko — The Magnificent). They are my greatest teachers. Thank you for teaching me that the greatest treasures in life aren't bought with money but are a happy smile and a contagious, joyful laugh.

I want to thank my parents, especially my father, who has taught me to always seek the truth and to remember that there are always two sides to every story. A special thanks goes to my mother for always being the most unselfish person I have ever known. Her silent example of serving has taught me a priceless secret to happiness.

I'd like to thank my teachers, friends and mentors. I especially want to thank the late Dr. James J. Hawver for teaching me to always look for the cause and to ask the body, because it never lies. I'd like to thank Dr. Marijah McCain, Dr. Larry Bristow, Dr. Rashid Buttar, Dr. Ben Johnson, Dr. Joseph Mercola, Dr. Mark Hyman, Dr. Tom O'Bryan, Dr. David Pearlmutter, Dr. Bernard Jensen, Dr. Richard Anderson, Dr. Joel Wallach, Dr. James Duke, Dr. Josh Axe, Dr. Jordan Rubin, Dr. Humbart Santillo, Dr. Robert Mendelsohn, Dr. James Wilson, Dr. David Hawkins, Dr. Richard Gerber, Dr. Robert Becker, Dr. Patrick Flynn, Dr. Patrick Quillin, Dr. Keesha Ewers, Dr. John Bergman, Dr. Leonard Coldwell, Dr. David Brownstein, Dr. Wayne Dyer, Dr. Sherri Tenpenny, Dr. Suzanne Humphries, Dr. Boyd Haley, Dr. Judy Mikovits, Dr. Lorraine Day, Dr. Mark Breiner, Dr. Hal Huggins, Dr. Weston Price, Dr. Bruce Lipton, Dr. Masaru Emoto, Dr. Leonard Horowitz, Dr. Joseph Christiano, Dr. David Watts, Dr. Gary Null, Dr. Russell Blaylock, Dr. Candace Pert, Dr. William Davis, Amazon John Easterling, Mike Adams, Robert Kennedy Jr., Ty Bollinger, Del Bigtree, Burton Goldberg, Edward Griffin, Eustace Mullins, Louise Hay, Karol Truman, Collin Tipping, Jas Malcolm, Scott Forsyth, Max Skousen and my brother Scott Sainsbury. Thank you for your words of wisdom, motivation and inspiration to do the right thing.

I'd like to thank Cyndi Owens Nelson, B.A., M.S. Ed., for all of her editing services to make this book a success. I want to thank Clint Kisor for his awesome cartoon illustrations in this book. I want to thank Brandy Vaughan, founder of LearnTheRisk.org, for permission to use her vaccine graphs and photos. I also want to thank Roman Bystrianyk and Dr. Suzanne Humphries for permission to use their vaccine graphs and pictures as well. A special thanks goes to Dr. Mamta Dalwani for permission to use her tooth/organ relationship chart. I want to thank my daughter Dallas for all of her help in completing this work.

Dedication

I dedicate this book to everyone who is sick and tired of being sick and tired. This is for medical doctors, health-care professionals and, most importantly, to you, the person who is fed up with our current medical system that suppresses symptoms with toxic, harmful drugs that maintain disease but never heals. When it's your health, you want the best. You want something that works, because you deserve it. This book is for you. May the innate intelligence within heal you, as you provide your body, mind and spirit with the proper environment and tools necessary to experience optimum health.

In memory of Dr. James J. Hawver – A man who was committed to Healing the Cause

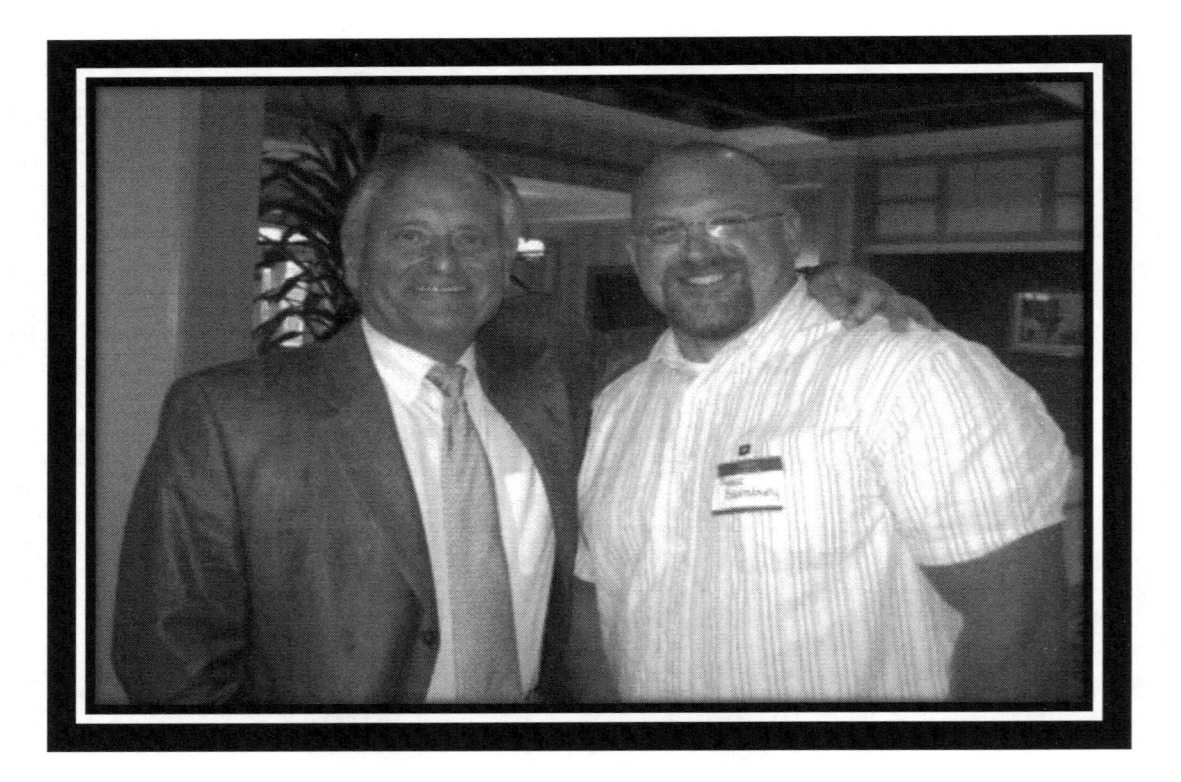

"What we do for ourselves dies with us. What we do for others and the world remains and is immortal." General Albert Pike, 1809-1891

Foreword

With the impending failure of the current medical system in place, along with the increase in chronic disease the aging population is facing, it is no wonder that the public at large is no longer tolerating the inadequacies of traditional medicine. As a result, there are many books about natural health and holistic healing on the market today. Some of these books give the readers information that they have been searching for, while others provide a sense of reinforcement for belief systems the reader may already possess or intuitively are guided towards. However, it has been my experience that many of the books on the market today that have an integrative or holistic slant lack a certain component necessary to make a connection with the reader.

Many of the people seeking a book on integrative medicine or holistic healing are doing so because of a personal challenge or the condition of a loved one that has been refractory to conventional treatment. The reason for them reading such a book is a "real" reason and not merely a curiosity. Some of these people may even be considered "desperate" due to their impending situation or condition. It is truth that the reader seeks and help the reader desires. And so the search goes on for the right book containing the right information that may shed some light on the dilemma the reader is facing.

Despite many of these books containing important information and even information that the reader may be searching for in particular, most of these books lack the passion and conviction behind the words that have been written. I would venture to say that some might even be "dry" and boring. They certainly lack the quality of capturing the interest of the reader to the point that one doesn't want to put down the book. In fact, it is rare to find a nonfiction, scientifically-based health information book that has not been watered-down, edited, re-edited, changed, amended or otherwise completely ruined to the point where the original intention of the author has been completely lost and the emotion and passion have been virtually dissected out.

It would be analogous to the white bread we see in the food markets that have had all the nutrient value removed from the flour used to make the bread, and then re-fortified with vitamins and minerals that are considered to be good for the body. The question is, why remove these nutrients from the flour in the first place? Similarly, the good information is removed or changed when edited or amended for the final printing of most books and, in the process, the passion of the author and the conviction of his or her beliefs is lost to the reader.

This is a frustration that I have personally experienced while writing my own books. The editors have changed the content to such a degree that the meaning and intention behind my words was changed so much that sometimes I didn't even recognize the words as ever having been mine. The only solution seemed to be either not to write the book or self-publish the manuscript to retain the original intention.

So it was with great pleasure that I read the manuscript I was asked to review when requested to write this forward. I found myself becoming engrossed in the personal story of Dr. Sainsbury, how he began his journey and what led him on the path that eventually found him writing a book on natural health. The varied topics presented in a strong and zealous manner with tangible examples and engrossing stories made for a book that is as entertaining as it is informative. Some may find it "too extreme" to one side, but I would disagree. It is the nature of most health books to avert being too extreme, when in reality, it is exactly what is needed. Remember that truth is on one side and a lie is on the other extreme. For those who feel that ANY book on health that is biased to one side lacks a balanced perspective, I would counter that those who write in this manner have seen the light and cannot step back into the darkness, for being "balanced" would require keeping one foot in the darkness.

For the novice, this book is a raw look at the reality of what many of us know to be the truth regarding medicine and healing. It is an unapologetic and passionate presentation that will help initiate those who are first learning of this subject. For the veteran, it provides a refreshing point of view that will often put a smile on your face because you know exactly the emotion that the author was experiencing as he wrote the words. This book will help open many eyes and will be a contribution to the cause of awakening the collective consciousness that no longer will tolerate the inadequacies and failure of traditional medicine.

Rashid A. Buttar, DO
FAAPM, FACAM, FAAIM

> **"The two most important days in your life are the day you are born and the day you find out why."** Mark Twain 1835-1910

Introduction

Most of us have spent a miserable night hunched over the toilet throwing up all night. We've experienced having "the flu," and it is hell. There is nothing in this world that is worth as much as your health. After being sick, to be able to sleep peacefully and then to wake up feeling refreshed and full of energy so that you can work and play pain free causes a humble man to fall on his knees and thank God for blessing him with good health, which is worth more than any amount of money.

> **"The health of the people is really the foundation upon which all their happiness and all their powers as a state depend."** Benjamin Disraeli, Former Prime Minister of the United Kingdom 1804-1881

Are you sick and tired of being sick and tired? This book is for all the people who want to understand the mysteries of health and how the body truly heals. So many people want to understand why they are sick and what they need to do in order to get well, but their medical doctor has failed to teach them what is causing their disease, and what is needed to heal. If you don't find out what's causing the disease, how are you going to heal it? Most know deep down that the solution to solving their health problems is not a list of more adverse-reaction-causing prescription drugs.

When you are fed up with your doctor playing the symptom-chasing game with your health, and each year the prescription list gets a little longer and your health gets a little worse, then it is time to put a stop to the insanity. It is time for a change. THIS IS YOUR WAKE-UP CALL. This book will empower you with wisdom so that you can give your body what it needs to heal. Nature's medicine doesn't harm your liver and ruin your kidneys so you spend the rest of your life going in for dialysis treatments every other day.

When your medical doctor starts prescribing new drugs to combat adverse side effects from the first one, then that should be a big flashing warning sign to wake up from your dream drug, fairy tale, health fantasy. When the medicine that is supposed to be helping you is backfiring and causing more harm than good, why would anyone stay on that path? My health isn't worth the risk of taking toxic drugs and playing Russian roulette in hopes that the side effects are not worse than the symptoms I'm attempting to cover up.

> **"Every drug stresses and hurts your body in some way."** Robert Mendelsohn, M.D. 1926-1988, Former President of the National Health Federation and Author of *Confessions of a Medical Heretic*

Anyone who doesn't have sense enough or intuition to feel and know that this feeble attempt to achieve optimum health is a laughable joke should put this book down now and stop reading. If your brain is so indoctrinated that you can no longer reason with good common logical sense, then you are wasting your time.

Corrupt statistics and slick attorneys can prove just about anything, especially if large sums of money for their personal gain are involved. We live in a world that is greatly influenced by money and not necessarily what is in your health's best interest. As you turn the pages you'll be met with common sense, health wisdom and natural remedies that have been proven effective. Healing comes on different levels for different people. There is no cure-all for everyone. In our clinic, we work with what each individual needs, not what works for 51 percent.

> **If you have been diagnosed with a disease you have two choices:**
> 1. **Prepare To Suffer OR**
> 2. **Prepare To Heal**

When a medical doctor diagnoses someone with a supposedly incurable disease and the doctor's plan is to maintain the disease with toxic drugs that suppress the symptoms without ever finding the cause and providing the individual with an opportunity to heal, that is when many Americans demand an alternative. When patients take drugs for many years and begin suffering adverse side effects from the toxic drugs, they become disgusted with modern medicine and demand a different approach. Within the pages of this book, you'll find the wisdom to put a stop to that foolish nonsense.

> **"Do you understand that all the things that are killing us today are sanctioned by our government and kept hush by the medical system? We need to wake up."** Dr. Darrell Wolfe

Disclaimer

The author is in no way attempting to treat, diagnose, prevent or cure disease with any of the information contained in this book and accepts no liability for you choosing to follow any recommendations. Consult your physician before following any recommendations in this book.

It is important to understand that the laws in the USA forbid me from being able to treat, diagnose, cure or prevent disease. The AMA has a patent on those words and only a licensed medical doctor can do that. And although it is legal for a licensed medical doctor to violate the Hippocratic oath and prescribe toxic drugs that cause harm and sometimes even kill patients, it is illegal for me to claim I can cure you using natural, nontoxic remedies, even though thousands of people can testify how they have been healed using natural remedies.

I am not a medical doctor. I don't want to be a medical doctor. I am a naturopathic doctor. The word "doctor" means to teach. When you come in to our office, we focus on finding the cause of disease. We do not "treat" symptoms or "maintain" disease with drugs.

After we identify the cause of your disease, we support the organs, glands and systems with natural nutritional formulas and detoxification therapies that balance the body. When your body is balanced, healing occurs and symptoms go away naturally, just as ants and flies go away when there's nothing for them to feed on in a clean trashcan. If your symptoms go away, it's not our fault. We didn't cure you, your intelligent body responded naturally, just how God created it to by the environment you chose to provide it. This is called health, and it is your God-given birthright to heal any and every disease you may have developed according to the environment you provided for your body, mind, and spirit to dwell within.

> **"I believe that it is second-degree murder if a patient dies after a doctor sends him home telling him that he will die because there is no cure. What the doctor should say is that he (the doctor) does not know what to do; therefore, the patient should go to someone who does know. Or, the doctor could say, 'Based upon what I know about your disease and what I know about my treatments, you will die in xx months, if you follow my program."** Richard Anderson, N.M.D.

Chapter 1
THE PULSATION OF LIFE

> "All truth passes through three stages. First, it is ridiculed. Second, it is violently opposed. Third, it is accepted as being self-evident." Arthur Schopenhauer, German Philosopher 1788-1860

We are surrounded by intelligent life activity. Just south of Mount Rainier in Washington state is the Columbia River. Each year, millions of salmon swim from the Pacific Ocean up the Columbia, hundreds of miles to high mountain streams. Some make their journey up to the Snake River and then turn up the Salmon River, where they miraculously find their way back to the very creeks and exact location where they were born. After the long journey back to their birthplace, they lay their eggs to renew the cycle of life. How do they know where to go to get back to their exact birthplace? Science doesn't have an exact answer. Obviously, there is a governing energy field with salmon and all of life that we don't fully understand. The universe in which we live is governed by intelligent order. It is through this intelligence that we are living along with every other form of life, including these amazing salmon.

> "We don't know a millionth of 1 percent about anything." Thomas Edison 1847-1931

You Are A Self-Healing Organism

Your body is so intelligent that if you cut out 50 percent of your liver, it will grow back. As a matter of fact, if we keep cutting out half of it, the cells in the remaining half will grow and divide again and again until your liver returns to normal size. Just as your liver knows how to grow back, your body knows how to heal.

> "Intelligence is present everywhere in our bodies ... our own inner intelligence is far superior to any we can try to substitute from the outside." Deepak Chopra, M.D.

God created and engineered your body to be self-healing when given correct nutrition and detoxification support. The stressors in the body, which we call toxins, must be removed in order for cells to heal. You can't feed your body sugary cereal, diet sodas, chips, snack cakes and cookies and expect healing miracles. That is as absurd as putting fruity drink mix in your gas tank and complaining that your car doesn't seem to be running right. Just as your car requires a decent grade of gasoline to burn in the engine, your body requires living cell food to be healthy. The human body was designed to run on mostly vegetables, healthy fats, fruits and berries in moderation and healthy protein.

> **"... a kind of super intelligence exists in each of us, infinitely smarter and possessed of technical know-how far beyond our present understanding."** Lewis Thomas, M.D.

When we bring the body back into balance with whole living foods, addressing the cause with natural plant-derived supplements, then we see God's miracles in action and it is called healing. This is how you were created and engineered to function by the Almighty Creator. The power is within you. You have a choice to suppress that intelligent power with drugs or give your cells some tools to work with so they can perform the miracle of life by regenerating and healing.

> **"Each cell is an intelligent being that can survive on its own, as scientists demonstrate when they remove individual cells from the body and grow them in a culture. ... these smart cells are imbued with intent and purpose; they actively seek environments that support their survival while simultaneously avoiding toxic or hostile ones."** Bruce Lipton, Ph.D., Cell Biologist, Stanford University School of Medicine

The Cell Is Immortal

Dr. Alexis Carrel of the Rockefeller Institute performed an interesting experiment. He proved the cell is immortal. He was able to keep tissue cells alive indefinitely by nutritious feedings and by washing away tissue wastes. As long as the tissue excretions were removed regularly, these cells thrived. Unsanitary conditions resulted in lower vitality, deterioration, and death.

> **"Each cell of the blood stream, each corpuscle, is a whole universe in itself."** Edgar Cayce 1877-1945

Dr. Carrel proved how important it is for proper waste elimination by keeping a chicken heart alive for 29 years until someone failed to cleanse its excretions. He concludes, *"The cell is immortal. It is merely the fluid in which it floats which degenerates. Renew this fluid at intervals, give the cell something upon which to feed, and as far as we know, the pulsation of life may go on forever."*

> **"Where there is perfect drainage, there is no death."** P.L. Clark, M.D.

Dr. Carrel was awarded the Nobel Prize for proving the cell is immortal. Why doesn't our current medical system focus on removing waste material from cells through the lymphatic system? Because drugs do not help the lymphatic system drain toxins, they cause the opposite! Doctors focus on the heart and circulatory system but ignore the lymphatic waste-removal system. If we truly had a health-care system in this country, medical doctors would be focusing their efforts on the lymphatic system so toxins could drain from the body, allowing our immortal cells to be healthier and live longer.

> **"Until man duplicates a blade of grass, Nature can laugh at his so-called scientific knowledge. Remedies from chemicals will never stand in favorable comparison with the products of Nature — the living cell of the plant, the final result of the rays of the sun, the mother of all life. When correctly used, herbs promote the elimination of waste matter and poisons from the system by simple, natural means. They support Nature in its fight against disease, while chemicals (drugs), not being assimilable, add to the accumulation of morbid matter and only simulate improvement by SUPPRESSING the SYMPTOMS."**
> Thomas A. Edison

Being an engineering and scientific genius, Thomas Edison understood what it takes to make things work. Viewing the complexity of cells and how awesome the human body is, he knew that no scientist or doctor would ever be able to produce a chemical substance superior to what Mother Nature ingeniously produces in living herbs to nourish and detoxify cells of the human body.

> **"The doctor of the future will give no medicine, but will interest his patients in the care of the human frame, in diet, and cause and prevention of disease."**
> Thomas A. Edison

Advancing in health care means having an open mind and seeing what produces results and what does not, regardless of the past. Without an open mind, we fail to learn, and without learning there is no progress. If we want to heal cancer, we must step outside the box.

> **"Truth wears no mask, seeks neither place nor applause, bows to no human shrine; she only asks a hearing."** Eleanor McBean, Ph.D., N.D. 1905-1989

Education is the process of receiving or giving systematic instruction, but what happens if that instruction is flawed? Throughout time, humanity has taken what the greatest minds of each generation believes to be true until someone comes along and proves something better, enlightening us all. But many of those theories in time prove to be false as new discoveries open our minds to how "wrong" we were; nonetheless, we embraced it as the "the truth," at that time. For example, Galileo was imprisoned for claiming that the sun, not the earth, was the center of the solar system. Christopher Columbus set out to prove "the truth" wrong as he sailed across the ocean and didn't fall off, proving the world was round. The truth all of a sudden was no longer believed.

> **"If we worked on the assumption that what is accepted as true really is true, then there would be little hope for advance."** Orville Wright, First Pilot in History

What "truth" do we hold onto now that will be proven false in 50 years? I once believed Santa flew through the sky in a sleigh and visited everyone in the world every Christmas Eve. Medical doctors used bloodletting to bleed their patients of bad blood. We came to realize that bloodletting is completely ridiculous, just like the sun revolving around the earth. After attempting to bleed bad blood from patients, doctors would then give them a compound of mercury and chlorine called "calomel." Further investigation proved mercury to be a poison. Ironically, it is still used in dental fillings, vaccines and other so-called medicines. We believed and did some pretty atrocious and foolish things in the past. At the time, we thought we knew what was best, just like we do now. Fifty years from now we will be saying, "Oh, you're from the generation that injected children with 72 doses of vaccines, took chemotherapy, used cholesterol-lowering drugs and had your gallbladders removed." Time and experience will hopefully teach us wisdom so that we can let go of foolish practices that keep producing the same disastrous results. Think about it, if drugs really worked, diseases would be on the decline, not incline, right? Cancer would be on its way out, not increasing like kids with cell phones. Consider the simple fact that 60 percent of all Nobel prizes awarded in medicine and biology were awarded for newly proven insights, which insights were subsequently disproven. Beware of any organization, especially if it's government-funded, or doctors that claim "the science is settled." Any honest researcher knows the science or "truth" is never settled as long as we have a brain and desire to use it; otherwise, there would be no hope for the advancement of humanity.

> **"Drugs do not — and cannot — heal, because a body that depends on outside control cannot be considered healthy."** Dean Black, Ph.D., President - BioResearch Foundation

In the future, we'll look back and laugh at our foolishness for what we attempted to do now with man-made prescription drugs as we strive to achieve optimal health. Unfortunately, science and medicine progress funeral-by-funeral. You get to choose if you want to be part of their experimental "practice" or to empower your body with cell-building nutritional support and life-saving detoxification sustenance to heal the cause and experience vibrant health, free of drugs.

> **"What is attraction? What is repulsion? What makes planets run on scheduled time? Why cannot our scientists even run a train on two rails without accidents and destruction of life and property? What is man at best but a blunderbuss and a terrible sinner? Who knows the secret of the atom? Who has yet penetrated the secrets of a grain of sand? Who has solved the mysteries of a dewdrop? Ask a scientist these questions and in despair he is forced to answer what a kitchen maid would answer, 'I don't know.'"** Dr. V.G. Rocine, Norwegian Homeopath

Every second, your body creates about 2 million red blood cells. In the time it took you to read the last paragraph, about 300 million cells were created and about 10 million red blood cells died. Every four days, you have a new stomach lining. Skin cells live about four months, and sperm cells peter out after three days. Your body is constantly dying and renewing itself. Ninety-eight percent of the atoms in your body will be replaced within a year. No doctor has to tell the intelligence within how or when to do this; it just knows and does it automatically. There is an unseen commander in chief in charge of the whole operation, always working for your greatest good and way smarter than any doctor with a stethoscope and prescription pad that some bow down and worship.

In Paul Bragg's book, *Toxicless Diet,* he explains that every three months you get an entirely new blood stream. Every 11 months, every cell in the body has renewed itself, so you practically have a new body every 11 months. Every two years, you get an entirely new bone structure, so in three years you really are born again … the renewal process has taken place.

> **"We are all elements of spirit, indestructible and eternal, and multiplexed in the divine."** William A. Tiller, Ph.D., Stanford University

If every cell within your body dies and is replaced with a new one within a year or two, doesn't it make sense that those cells are only going to rebuild with the nutrition found in the food you are eating? You are only as good as the food you eat. In other words, you are what you eat. More accurately put, you are what you digest. And most Americans have toxic livers as well as clogged colons with severe gut flora imbalances and mucoid plaque from taking antibiotics, using birth control pills and eating way too much sugar, too many grains (gluten) and too many acidic foods.

Your cells are like carpenters remodeling a house. Can they remodel if their materials are just as weak as the ones they are trying to replace? Can your arthritic joints become pain free if they never receive the raw ingredients necessary to build healthy tendons, ligaments, muscles and bones? Of course not. Only a fool would remodel his house using termite-infested wood, crumbly old wiring and a cheap, substandard cement for the foundation.

Your body needs a continual supply of nutrition every day, and the elimination channels must remain open for the waste material to empty. Imagine if you told your construction crew that no garbage or waste material could be removed from the house for a month while they labored. Within a short time, there would be so much trash built up (scrap wood, drywall, etc.), it would start interfering with their work. Most of our cells are working, but they are loaded with garbage that prevents them from functioning properly. As a result, they become inflamed, and this puts pressure on other parts of the body, which creates pain. The solution for pain is not more ibuprofen, but to get the lymphatic system draining so the toxins can be expelled, thus decreasing the inflammation and pain.

> **"Drugs never cure disease — at best they only suppress or alleviate the symptoms. Lasting results can be attained only when a wise doctor assists and supports the body's own healing forces, which institute the health-restoring process and accomplish the actual cure."** Paavo Airola, Ph.D., N.D. 1918-1983

A city here in America has a zoo filled with beautiful, healthy animals. As Dr. Joel Wallach explains, veterinarians are forced to understand health because if their animals aren't healthy, they lose their jobs. Veterinarians simply can't afford to perform bypass surgery and other expensive surgical procedures on animals like we humans do. They don't have a health-care system, and they certainly can't tell the veterinarian what's bothering them. So, how do they keep animals healthy in the zoo? They feed the animals a strict diet. A sign posted near a junk-food vending machine warns: ***"Do not feed this food to the animals or they may get sick and die."*** Do you think that if this artificial food is not safe for chimpanzees and gorillas, then maybe we should not consume it either?

> **"If you need a good doctor get a veterinarian; animals can't tell him what's wrong, he's just got to know!"** Will Rogers 1879-1935

We humans require living foods to live. We do not obtain the life force needed for health from artificial food colorings, preservatives, flour and sugar. Every other form of life on earth depends upon their diet for health and strength, and we humans are no different. Eating a largely processed-food diet leads to an unnatural lifestyle filled with disease, sickness and death.

Disease is a natural result of an unnatural lifestyle. Dr. Reuben exhorts, *"You lock your doors against thieves, don't you? But a thief will only steal your property. Shouldn't you lock your body against bad foods that will steal your life?"*

> **"We are part of the earth and it is part of us ... for all things are connected."** Chief Seattle, Suquamish Chief 1786-1866

Acetone, acetaldehyde, methyl burrate, ethyl coproate, hexyl acetate, methanol, acrolein and croton aldehyde are all highly-toxic, poisonous substances by themselves. Next time you eat a strawberry, it may surprise you to know that you are ingesting all of these poisonous substances. So why don't they kill you? Because, all of these substances, taken in a natural, organic, balanced form created by Mother Nature, renders them harmless. The synergy created through nature's intelligence transforms these poisonous isolates into highly nutritious foods. Only when we start isolating certain substances from nature do they become poisons. Isolating ingredients from plants to produce drug compounds that have adverse side effects is Mother Nature's way of shaking her head and cautiously reminding us that she put those ingredients together for a reason. Just because man hasn't evolved enough to comprehend that doesn't justify us tearing apart what she has created and intensifying the potency of a certain ingredient 400 times.

Taking too much Vitamin A from a synthetic pill can cause you to overdose. Pregnant women are warned that too much Vitamin A can cause birth defects.

Carrot juice is high in Vitamin A. If you drink a gallon of it, you will not overdose on Vitamin A; however, take a whole bottle of synthetic Vitamin A tablets and you might. Why? One is natural and the other isn't. The body is capable of dealing with an excess of natural plant-food nutrients, but synthesized chemicals can be extremely toxic. For example, take the drug Accutane, a synthetic form of Vitamin A, used in treating acne. Side effects from this drug include Irritable Bowel Syndrome (IBS), Crohn's disease, colitis, pancreatitis and hypertension, to name just a few. What man makes in a chemistry lab is usually toxic, whereas herbs found in nature are balanced synergistically with nutrients created for healing. Choose plant-derived nutritional supplements over synthetic vitamin/mineral tablets, and your cells will thank you.

Everything doesn't always necessarily have to be natural to be healthy. There are exceptions. Chelation therapy (EDTA), for example, is not natural. However, it is an effective way to pull heavy metals out of the body and eliminate plaque from the arteries. It is time to use what works as long as we do not harm the body in the process.

Cyanide From Seeds — Mother Nature's Cure For Cancer

"Amygdalin, Vitamin B17 (Laetrile), appears to neutralize the oxidative cancer-promoting compounds such as free radicals. It's just one more key component for keeping cancer from growing or spreading. Contrary to what people have said about laetrile, amygdalin's former name, it should be considered an effective, entirely safe treatment for all types of cancer." Robert C. Atkins, M.D., Founder of the Atkins Diet 1930-2003

Inside most seeds, especially apricots and peaches, is a highly poisonous substance called hydrogen cyanide. The FDA says cyanide is a poison and has banned its use in most states. They are absolutely right. It is a poison. However, we are only being told half of the story. What they fail to report is that the natural cyanide found in apricot and peach pits is safe for us to ingest and poisonous only to cancer cells in the body. In other words, God created a natural cancer cure that is safe and harmless to healthy cells, but attacks and kills cancer cells.

Many doctors around the world use Laetrile (Vitamin B17) to treat cancer. The late Dr. Ernesto Contreras at the Oasis of Hope Hospital in Tijuana, Mexico, taught that Laetrile containing cyanide poses no threat to healthy cells. Dr. Lloyd Schloen, a biochemist at Sloan-Kettering, experimented with Laetrile combined with proteolytic enzymes on cancerous mice. He had a 100 percent cure rate among the mice!

If you can go out to the apricot tree and collect the pits and cure yourself of cancer, can you imagine what a nightmare that would be for the pharmaceutical industry that earned $107 billion from cancer medicine in 2015? The FDA is heavily influenced by Big Pharma to discredit anything natural. Laetrile is no exception; they have done a hatchet job on it to ensure that you will keep on using their expensive chemotherapy and let the apricot pits go in the garbage can since they can't be patented and sold for $35,000 a month like some of the cancer-treatment drugs.

How does the cyanide in the pits know to leave healthy cells alone and only go after cancer? The same way the sun knows how to rise every morning and something is telling your heart to beat this very moment to keep you alive. Just as salmon know where to go to spawn, bees know how to make honey and our skin knows how to knit itself back together after being cut, divine intelligence governs the universe whether we believe and understand it or not. We might make progress in our cancer-healing efforts if we used what God has already perfectly created in nature.

> **"It is still my belief that amygdalin (Laetrile) cures metastases."** Dr. Kanematsu Sugiura 1890-1979, Sloan-Kettering Institute for Cancer Research

Laetrile has been proven most effective at a dose of 6 grams, intravenous once a day, for three weeks at a time. It's a good idea to supplement with zinc, since it helps transports the Laetrile to cancerous areas. Supplementing with enzymes also helps Laetrile work more effectively. Being on a strict, mostly raw food diet has also produced better results.

Pakistan's Hunza people are some of the healthiest people on the planet, living well into their hundreds and still conceiving children past age 60. There's very little disease and virtually no cancer. The Hunza eat 30 to 50 apricot seeds a day. Is this a secret to their vibrant health?

Herbs

Herbal remedies were designed by nature to be taken just as they are found. Once they are chemically altered in a lab, they become toxic and dangerous. Herbs are nature's medicine cabinet. God's intelligence governing Mother Nature gives precise instructions on how to create the perfect combination of vitamins, minerals, amino acids, essential fatty acids and enzymes to put in carrots, celery, gingko biloba, wheatgrass, barley greens, alfalfa, bee pollen, blue green algae, spirulina, dandelion root and echinacea. Naturally grown foods and herbs have been ingeniously put together to cleanse, nourish and heal the body. Drugs have no life force, no nutrition and no enzymes, but herbs have them all. Nature's balancing system is very accurate and when man takes it upon himself to improve upon God's creations, the results can be disastrous. According to the CDC, over 1 million Americans are rushed to the emergency room every year because of adverse reactions to doctor-prescribed drugs.

> "The medicinal plants, or parts of them, must be used as they are found in nature. Extracts or active elements contained in them should not be isolated and then used, because secondary negative effects may result." Dr. Ernesto Comminotto

Graviola

A good example of how herbs work best when unaltered in a chemistry lab is Graviola, also called soursop, from South America's rainforest. Through a series of confidential communications involving a researcher from one of America's largest pharmaceutical companies, the Graviola tree has been studied in more than 20 laboratory tests since the 1970s and has been proven to effectively target and kill malignant cells in 12 different types of cancer. It has tested extremely effective in destroying prostate, lung, breast, colon and pancreatic cancers. Jerry McLaughlin, Ph.D., at Purdue University informs that lab tests showed Graviola to be 10,000 times stronger than Adriamycin, a common chemotherapy drug, in killing colon cancer cells. Unlike chemotherapy, Graviola does not harm healthy cells. The National Cancer Institute (NCI) included Graviola in a plant-screening program that showed its leaves and stems were effective in attacking and destroying malignant cells.

One of America's largest drug companies tried for nearly seven years to synthesize two of the Graviola tree's most powerful anticancer chemicals. This company was investing a lot of time and money in searching for a cure for cancer while guarding their opportunity to patent it and make a fortune. The research was proving Graviola to be a cancer-killing dynamo. Dollar signs flashed in their eyes with this potential gold mine, however, their research came to a screeching halt when they failed to create man-made duplicates of two of the tree's most powerful chemicals. Because federal law mandates that natural substances can't be patented, they would never be able to maximize profits without cornering the market on a drug. Subsequently, the company shelved their research and hid it from the world. One of the researchers couldn't keep quiet about the miraculous anti-cancer herb, Graviola. Understanding the company's goals to make big profits with a patent and their decision to hide the research from the world, he risked his career by reporting the pharmaceutical lab's findings to a company dedicated to harvesting plants from the Amazon rainforest.

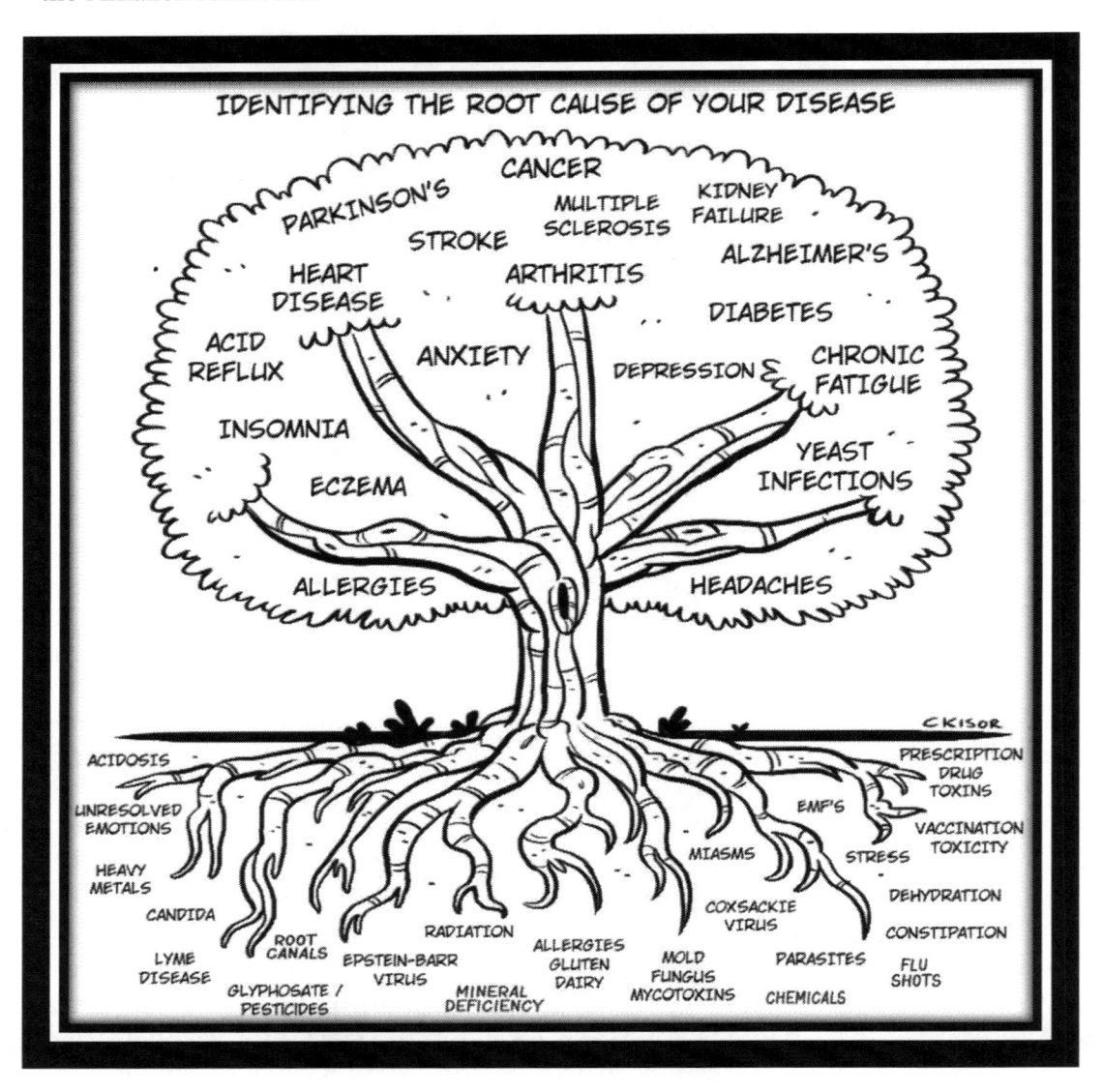

IDENTIFYING THE ROOT CAUSE OF YOUR DISEASE

Branches (diseases): CANCER, PARKINSON'S, MULTIPLE SCLEROSIS, KIDNEY FAILURE, STROKE, ALZHEIMER'S, HEART DISEASE, ARTHRITIS, DIABETES, ACID REFLUX, ANXIETY, DEPRESSION, CHRONIC FATIGUE, INSOMNIA, YEAST INFECTIONS, ECZEMA, ALLERGIES, HEADACHES

Roots (causes): ACIDOSIS, PRESCRIPTION DRUG TOXINS, UNRESOLVED EMOTIONS, EMF'S, VACCINATION TOXICITY, MIASMS, STRESS, HEAVY METALS, DEHYDRATION, CANDIDA, COXSACKIE VIRUS, CONSTIPATION, LYME DISEASE, ROOT CANALS, RADIATION, ALLERGIES GLUTEN DAIRY, MOLD FUNGUS MYCOTOXINS, PARASITES, FLU SHOTS, GLYPHOSATE / PESTICIDES, EPSTEIN-BARR VIRUS, MINERAL DEFICIENCY, CHEMICALS

"For the past 50 years, I have been demonstrating that the use of natural nutritional treatment is and must be the most effective form of medicine and that when it is not used and the profession depends solely on the use of toxic drugs the results are abysmal." Abram Hoffer, M.D., Ph.D., FRCP(C)

26

Just as a skilled mechanic with the proper tools can identify the problem with a car and fix it, so can a doctor identify the cause of your disease and teach you what is needed to heal. Your health doesn't have to be a mystery. So many medical doctors run test after test, and the results come back inconclusive. We have people bring in over $100,000 in medical tests, with no answers. The disease-maintenance system that you pay for is failing to find the cause of your illness because they are not looking for it. Why? There's no money in cellular detoxification and nutritional therapy! Most medical doctors are trained in drugs and surgery, so, when you go into their facility, they will only find something wrong with you that they can treat with a drug or remove surgically.

The following story is a prime example of how modern medicine maintains disease with drugs versus focusing on healing the cause. Kim sent the following letter to me after I had been working with her for two months.

Case Study

After going to doctor after doctor, I was diagnosed with Multiple Sclerosis in 1997. Most of the doctors I saw in the beginning didn't have any answers and pushed my problems and symptoms aside. After the final diagnosis, I was immediately put on Prozac. When I asked why, they stated that all MS patients are put on an antidepressant medication. I was also prescribed a daily injection of Copaxone (MS medication). I had allergic reactions to this and was taken off the Copaxone and given Avonex (a once-a-week injection). It had many side effects, the worst being flu-like symptoms, leaving me unable to function for 24 full hours. Although it was a once-a-week injection, I had one neurologist have me take it twice a week. For a period of about two years on this injection, I was having one MS exacerbation after another. For each exacerbation, I was put on Solu-Medrol and Prednisone. More side effects followed.

This wasn't working, so I was put on another injection, Betaseron. Along with the Betaseron, I was also taking eight other prescriptions to counteract the adverse side effects and also as precautions for any other symptoms. I slowly took myself off these medications because they weren't helping. They were causing more problems and every time I mentioned those problems, the doctor's answer was just more prescriptions. I eventually built up antibodies to the Betaseron. During all this time, I was also having migraine headaches. Every doctor I went to was willing to write me at least three prescriptions just for migraines. When I asked to be tested to find the cause of the migraines, their responses were, "That will take too long.

Just take the medicine prescribed and it will help you sleep off the migraine." No real answers except, "The cause of the migraines could be many things."

I was tired of getting no results and a bunch of prescriptions that would make me feel worse and not help the problem. It was then that I spoke with a friend who told me about Dr. Sainsbury. I set up an appointment immediately.

I had my first appointment with Dr. Sainsbury on September 23, 2006. I was amazed at what he found and the explanations given to me about everything. It all made sense finally.

When I was a child and went for the required school physicals, I was told that I may have a sluggish thyroid, but not to worry, it was nothing. Dr. Sainsbury found an energetic disturbance with my thyroid, without me telling him about it. It was something that I had forgotten about but he found it to be part of the cause of my problems.

The EDS (Electro Dermal Scan) results showed the migraines, my Raynaud's Phenomenon, female problems, constant metallic taste in mouth, etc., were caused from toxins and nutritional deficiencies in my body. Dr. Sainsbury gave me a plan to balance and heal my body, which included nutritional supplements, herbs and homeopathic remedies to detoxify the mercury, copper, nickel, candida yeast and parasites out that were showing up as the cause of my symptoms. Dr. Sainsbury recommended I have my metal dental fillings removed and replaced with composites.

When I left the exam, I was in tears. For the first time in years, I actually had answers as to what was going on with my body.

Since I've been on Dr. Sainsbury's program and had the silver dental fillings removed, the metallic taste in my mouth has disappeared. Within just a couple of days of taking the supplements the difference I felt was amazing. ***The heaviness in my legs was gone, the tingling in my hands and feet was gone, my leg spasms seemed to be gone and I was able to sleep through the night for the first time in years. And no migraines! All this without prescription-drug side effects.***

A couple of weeks after seeing Dr. Sainsbury, I had an appointment with my neurologist, who had taken me off the Betaseron because the side effects were getting worse. I was getting physically ill after each injection. His suggestion was another type of injection, one that was just recently put back on the market after having been removed because it was causing more damage than helping. Two people died from taking it.

When I refused to take it because of that fact, he was upset with me. I explained to him that I was doing a detox/cleanse program recommended by a naturopathic doctor. He said I was wasting my money and I needed these prescriptions. When I told him how good I was feeling from being on the natural program he shook his head, dropped my chart down, threw his hands in the air and said, "I'm done. There's nothing I can do for you. You'll have to find another doctor." I walked out of that office without a handful of prescriptions and knew I did the right thing.

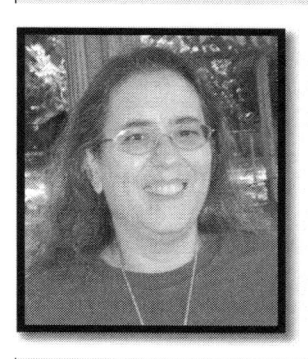

Another benefit from doing the detox and cleansing that I didn't expect was that my hair was coming back. Years ago, my hair had slowly been falling out, and I was told there was nothing that could be done about it, it was just a fact of life. But now, little by little, it's coming back.

For the first time in years, I have a doctor who hears what I'm saying and has answers and solutions for me. I feel like I'm living now and not merely existing. I'm not just another prescription.

Thank you, Dr. Sainsbury!

Kim Powell
Newnan, Georgia

Kim is one of many disgusted with her medical doctor's drugs because they didn't work for her and the side effects were devastating. What kind of doctor would get mad enough to throw her chart down and quit when she was feeling so much better? What kind of doctor isn't interested in seeing his patients get well so they don't have to be a slave to expensive toxic drugs? One of her prescriptions, Betaseron injection was costing her $1,700 a month and causing her to be nauseated for the next 24 hours after each dose.

"There isn't a single medication on the market that couldn't be replaced by a botanical remedy." James Duke, Ph.D., Ethnobotanist, Author of *The Green Pharmacy*

For those who are sick and tired of taking drugs and feeling better for a short time only to crash again and start another vicious yo-yo cycle of more drugs, I invite you to practice what I teach. If it fails to empower you with health, then call me a liar and go back to dulling your God-given senses with man-made chemical drugs.

> **"Do not be angry with me if I tell you the truth."** Socrates 470-399 B.C.

Most of us did not get in our condition overnight and most likely will not heal overnight. When the train called disease is going down the tracks at 50 mph, it takes time to bring it to a stop and get it going in the opposite direction towards health. Be patient and consistent. A champion athlete doesn't win the gold medal by skipping workouts, eating junk food and abusing his body. You get what you pay for and you get what you put in, or as the Bible says, you reap what you sow. There is no such thing as a magic cure for optimum health. Good nutrition, clean water, exercise, sunshine, proper rest and a joyful heart are required for health.

Doctors will cut out your gallbladder, uterus, tonsils, adenoids and appendix. Common sense ought to tell you that your Creator might have put those things in you for a reason. Just because you are done having babies doesn't mean your uterus needs to go in the trashcan. The reality is, drugs and surgery are a business no different than selling cars and cell phones. The goal is to make money, not necessarily to do what is best for your health.

> **"When the dollar sign enters the field of health or religion, the sincerity and the love fade away."** T.O. McCoye

Energetic Frequencies

Our solar system is held in place through magnetic polarities. There are magnetic fields that go around the earth from North to South. Just as the earth has north and south magnetic poles, so does every cell in our body.

> **"The thought wave is electrical. The energy coming from the eyes is electrical. Muscles work by electrical impulses from the brain. In essence, the human body is an electrical being, and our health, strength and endurance depend upon the energy currents that run through the body."** C. Samuel West, D.N., N.D. 1932-2004, Author of *The Golden Seven Plus One*

We are electrical beings. Mother Earth and our physical bodies vibrate at roughly the same frequency, about 8 hertz. Every cell functions through very minute electrical currents generated along the cell membrane by the sodium-potassium pump. Our cells have zeta potential, which means they have the ability to retain an electrical charge ranging from 70 to 90 millivolts. When we are sick, the electrical potential goes down. Cancer patients have been known to drop to 15 or lower. Once we lose our electrical potential, the lights go out and we die.

In 1994, the Nobel Prize was given to Dr. Alfred G. Gillman of the University of Texas Southwestern Medical Center and Dr. Martin Rodbell of the National Institute of Environmental Health Sciences for discovering that cells communicate with each other by sending and receiving "radio" signals.

"Signal transduction is the single-most important unifying concept in modern-day biology and medicine." Dr. Robert Bell, Head of the Department of Molecular Cancer Biology, Duke University

Have you ever been listening to the radio in your car or talking on your phone and drive under power lines and get static? Heavy metals and other toxins in the body cause cellular static. When cells do not receive the right signals, they begin to mutate. This is cancer. Cancer isn't a disease. It's a symptom of your cells not receiving the right signals. This is why it is so important to detoxify the body. If the cells can't communicate effectively, we cannot heal. Any military general knows that the key to winning a battle is to destroy your enemy's ability to communicate. Without proper cellular communication, there is chaos. Your immune system doesn't receive orders on who to kill and who to leave alone. This is how autoimmune disorders occur.

The intelligence that governs our bodies would never attack our own cells. When your immune system begins to attack your own cells, it's because there is a toxicity issue and your body knows it has to dispel the toxins. Some of the toxins that trigger autoimmunity are foreign proteins like gluten, heavy metals, pesticides and viruses. Why?

Toxins Causing Dis-ease	
Heavy Metals	Epstein-Barr
Silver Fillings	Radiation
Fluoride	Vaccinations
Lyme Disease	Pesticides
Chemicals	Acidosis
Allergies	Gluten

Because they are foreigners (non-self), and the body does its best to remove illegal aliens from within, no different than a country removing potential terrorists or illegals that do not have permission to be in the country.

Every disease has a cause, especially autoimmune disorders and cancer. There is always a toxin setting off the smoke alarm, rallying the troops. Would you trust a firefighter who arrives on the scene and turns the smoke alarms off and walks away without extinguishing the fire? Of course not, that would be absurd; nevertheless, doctors who put you on immunosuppressant drugs without finding the cause of the fire and putting it out are just treating the symptoms, or the smoke, by taking the batteries out of the smoke alarms. If you want to get well, we have to find what's causing the fire and put it out. Are you going to let your house burn down and your body deteriorate on immunosuppressant drugs or find someone to put the fires out?

> **"The physician should look for the force and nature of illness at its source. He is not to look to that which can be seen, for we are not called to extinguish the smoke, but the fire itself."** Theophrastus Paracelsus 1493-1541

Like a military unit caught in battle without a means of communication, it is easy to mistake your own men for the enemy. When cells do not get the right signals, like confused soldiers, they can begin attacking themselves, triggering autoimmune disorders. Some examples of this chaos occurring are ALS (Lou Gehrig's disease), multiple sclerosis, lupus, rheumatoid arthritis and Hashimoto's disease. We almost always see heavy metal poisoning and Lyme disease as culprits interfering with cellular communication lines in these types of illnesses. When heavy metals accumulate in your body and interfere with cellular activity, doctors label you with a disease. The name of the disease depends upon where the toxins settle and the manner in which they manifest themselves. In order to heal, the metals have to be removed. Where do we get heavy metals?

HEAVY METALS	SOURCES OF EXPOSURE
Aluminum	Vaccines, cookware, cosmetics, deodorants, tomato paste, baking powder, antacids, aluminum foil, soft drinks/aluminum cans, water treatment plants, medications
Antimony	Fireproof clothing, battery electrodes, ceramics, pigments, gunpowder
Arsenic	Pesticides, herbicides, insecticides, animal foods (disease prevention/antibiotics), rice, chicken, wine, apple juice, batteries, outdoor products (treated lumber, decks, picnic tables, play structures), women's makeup, tattoo inks, auto exhaust, seafood
Beryllium	Coal-burning industry, manufacturing, ceramics, welding, machine shops, metal recycling, electronics, dental supplies, automotive parts, prosthesis manufacturing
Bismuth	Paints, pigments, ceramics, glass, cosmetics, lipstick, batteries
Cadmium	Mining, smelters, paints, pigments, electroplating, nuts, bolts, batteries, plastics, rubber, engraving, soldering, brazing, dentures, cigarette smoke,

	women's makeup, tattoo ink, processed foods (especially white flour), rice, fertilizers, sewer sludge, auto exhaust
Copper	Copper water lines, drinking water, cookware, insecticides, contraceptives, cigarette smoking
Lead	Paints, batteries, alloying, soldering, Chinese toys, ceramics, fuels, bullets, fishing sinkers, leaded pipes/joints, women's makeup, cosmetics, tattoo ink, hair dyes, glass production
Mercury	Vaccinations, flu shots, dental amalgams, barometers, thermometers, lab equipment, batteries, electrodes, fungicides, pesticides in paper, coal-burning power plants, wildfires, hospital incinerators, tattoo ink, fluorescent lights, fish, seafood, corn syrup, water-based paints
Nickel	Cigarettes, diesel exhaust, cocoa, chocolate, soya products, hydrogenated oils, batteries, dental materials, electroplated jewelry, pigments, arc welding, tattoo ink
Tin	Canned foods/drinks, solders, bronze, brass & pewter, dye pigments, bleaching agents, anticorrosion plating of steel, toothpaste (stannous fluoride), insecticides, rubber, silicone
Uranium	Drinking water from wells, ceramics, colored glass (yellow)

> **"I have found heavy metal toxicity in a large percentage (80 percent) of patients suffering from chronic illnesses, including thyroid disorders. In the case of autoimmune disorders, nearly 100 percent of my patients have laboratory signs of heavy metal toxicity."** David Brownstein, M.D.

According to Dr. David Watts, toxic metals are minerals that do not have any known biological functions and are considered poisonous to the body. These metals interfere with our mineral functions. For example, toxic lead accumulates in the mitochondria membrane of cells, an area where magnesium is most needed. Adequate amounts of magnesium can greatly help reduce lead absorption from the intestinal tract. Lead also displaces calcium, and is deposited in the bones and joints. It can destroy normal cartilage tissue, causing arthritis. Hyperactive children usually have more dental cavities, which may be caused by lead poisoning. Toxic cadmium will stimulate the adrenal glands, causing magnesium loss, which increases sodium retention, contributing to high blood pressure. Supplementing with magnesium can help prevent and control cadmium-induced high blood pressure. Smokers and being around secondhand cigarette smoke is a toxic source of cadmium poisoning. Burning rubbish, old tires

Dr. David Brownstein's Detoxification Support
- Cilantro drops: 4/day
- Garlic: 500 mg/day
- L-Glutamine: 3-6 g/day
- Selenium: 400 mcg/day
- Vitamin C: 3000 mg/day
- Vitamin E: 800 IU/day

and plastics can be a major source of cadmium poisoning. Paper and lumber products contain mercury to inhibit fungal growth. Burning newspapers in the fireplace can give off a toxic mercury vapor, causing many health challenges. Arsenic is put in chicken feed to inhibit mold growth. Those who consume a lot of chicken are found to have high levels of arsenic.

The great Roman Empire used lead pipes to carry their drinking water. Many cities with older buildings still use lead water pipes. It has been speculated that the famous artist Van Gogh was poisoned by lead used in his paints that caused the deterioration of his mental state. Until 1995, we still burned leaded gasoline in automobiles, which polluted the atmosphere to the point that it has been detected in polar ice caps. Older homes are covered in lead-painted walls. When demolition crews tear down old buildings, lead paint dust settles on schoolyards, parks and playgrounds. Public water supplies contain harmful metals. Most cosmetics, such as lipstick, eye shadow and blush, contain metals. Pesticides and herbicides sprayed on the foods you eat contain metals. Furniture manufactured with flame-retardant chemicals is loaded with metals. Prescription drugs contain metals as binding agents. E-cigarettes contain cadmium. What most people aren't aware of is the fact that we are exposed to toxic heavy metals every day, regardless of how organic and green your diet is. And if you have silver dental fillings or have received vaccinations, then your system has had an enormous exposure.

When's the last time your doctor checked you for heavy metal toxicity? The sad reality is most don't because they do not have drugs to clear heavy metals from the body. Some of your functional or integrative medical clinics incorporate EDTA and DMPS IV therapies to help detoxify heavy metals, and these can be very beneficial. The bottom line is, we are bombarded with heavy metal toxins everywhere we turn. A wise person does a detox program periodically to stay healthy, before symptoms manifest and diseases are diagnosed.

"All matter is energy." Albert Einstein 1879-1955

Energy has always been mysterious because you can't see it. The most powerful things in the universe are unseen, such as love. Through the ages, energy has been called many things. Some refer to it as life force or vital force. Christ called it light. The yogis in Eastern India call it prana, and the Chinese refer to it as chi. Hippocrates called it "vis medicatrix naturae" (nature's life force). The reality is, energy exists whether you believe it or not. Many things in our universe are an illusion. It's not that they aren't real, but that they are much different than they appear.

> **"Body chemistry is governed by quantum cellular fields."** Dr. Murray Gell-Mann, Nobel Prize Laureate

All matter in the universe is energy, and energy is made up of atoms. Atoms are made up of electrons, protons and neutrons. Negatively charged electrons spin 600 miles per second around the nucleus containing neutrons and positively charged protons. As they spin, they generate an electromagnetic field. That field will either attract or repel other molecules. And everything in the universe is made up of molecules. We only see about 1 percent of who we are, the other 99 percent of who we are is unseen.

Science acknowledges that some sort of "energy" is what holds the electron in orbit around the nucleus. The faster those atoms move, the more solid the physical object seems. For example, your desk isn't really solid, but it appears to you as a solid object because the atoms are spinning so fast. The way you see matter is an illusion. Your hands that are holding this book, the chair you are sitting on, the floor and walls around you, all seem so solid, practical and non-mystical. Yet, scientists have found that each of these is made up almost completely of empty space. For example, think of just one of the atoms that is spinning in the period at the end of this sentence. Yes, right there. Think of just one of the millions of atoms in the ink that made that dot. If we were to enlarge the nucleus of that atom to the size of an average orange, the electrons circling around it would be about 400 miles away, with nothing but space in between. No other atoms are in there. And what is the nucleus? It is a universe in itself and is mostly space. Ultimately, we find all of these particles turn out to be no more than energy charges.

> **"Everything is energy. Nothing is solid. Everything vibrates at its own level of reality, and while form appears to be solid, a simple examination under a microscope reveals that that solid object is actually alive with dancing molecules vibrating at a little less than the speed of light and thus appearing to us to be solid."** Wayne W. Dyer, Ph.D. 1940-2015

Kirlian Photography

Semyon D. Kirlian, a Russian scientist, helped us understand that each of us has an electromagnetic field, sometimes referred to as an aura, surrounding our bodies. Kirlian photography is a way to capture these energy fields. Through special photographs, he demonstrated that disease could be detected in the body's electrical field. Diseased areas of the body will show dark spots, while healthy areas of the body will manifest different colors.

It is interesting to note that when Kirlian photography is used with individuals who are missing limbs, the electrical body still protrudes from where the limb used to be, and many will say they still sense something when moving the missing limb in the space of a solid object.

> **"All living organisms emit an energy field."** Semyon D. Kirlian, USSR 1900-1980

If you take a potato and take a picture of it with Kirlian photography, you can see a beautiful energy pattern surrounding the living food. Put that living energy food into a microwave and heat it for several minutes, then take another picture of it. After it has been radiated, the energy field surrounding the potato has been radically destroyed. It is chaotic, jagged and out of balance.

Dr. Harold Burr at Yale University studied energy fields around plants and animals back in the 1940s. He found that we all have this energy field that surrounds us. He taught that an electrical blueprint of the adult body exists at the earliest development, even at the stage of an egg. This electrical blueprint acts as a template that the physical body is destined to follow.

> **"Everything is energy, and that's all there is to it. Match the frequency of the reality you want and you cannot help but get that reality. It can be no other way. This is not philosophy. This is physics."** Albert Einstein

Electrical Medical Devices

Energy medicine is practiced and used by most medical doctors. The electrical current of the heart is measured with an EKG (Electrocardiogram), while electrical activity flowing along the nerves is measured with EMG (Electromyography). Energy resonating in the brain is measured with an Electroencephalogram (EEG). Most of us are familiar with X-rays and (Magnetic Resonance Imaging) MRI, but very few actually understand how they work. The electromagnetic energy in the X-ray frequency is concentrated in a specific area of the body and then collected on a photographic plate. The radiation is absorbed by various bodily tissues that create shadows on the plate, allowing us to identify fractures and abnormalities.

MRI works by placing a human or animal in a tunnel surrounded by a strong magnetic field that aligns the nuclei of the body's hydrogen atoms. Then FM radio beams focused on specific desired areas cause a "resonance" of the aligned nuclei.

When the radio beams are turned off, energy is emitted and the nuclei return to their normal state. Special sensors measure this energy and send it to a computer that produces three-dimensional images of the body, allowing us to view soft tissue damage and abnormalities.

> **"Diseases are to be diagnosed and prevented via energy field assessment."**
> George Crile Sr., M.D., Founder of the Cleveland Clinic 1864-1943

Acupuncture Points & Meridians

An amazing experiment was done to prove the electrical energy flow in a living body. Chinese scientists attached wires to a person's body and generated enough current to light a small light bulb, demonstrating how much electricity is in the human body. Chinese medicine has been teaching for more than 5,000 years that the whole body is connected through a system of energy pathways called meridians. At specific locations on these meridians you have acupuncture points that are sensitive to energy. Just as the blood vessels carry blood through the body, the acupuncture meridians carry energy to every organ and gland. Improper flow of energy through the acupuncture meridians causes energy imbalances in the body that can lead to disease.

Acupuncture points are like lights on a Christmas tree. The electricity (energy) flows through a wire to illuminate each bulb and so does energy within our body flow through our meridians illuminating our organs and glands with life-force energy. There are 12 main meridians in the human body. In acupuncture, inserted needles in the skin at these points on specific meridians act as antennas which have the ability to bring energy into the body or help release it, thus restoring proper energy balance so healing can occur.

> **"The magnetic electrical research field will come to prove that the human body is an electrical being and our health depends on the energy currents which run through the body."** George S. White, M.D.

Electro Dermal Screening (EDS)

Dr. Reinhard Voll was a German medical doctor, anatomy professor, acupuncturist, homeopath and ham radio operator in the late 1940s who was studying Chinese acupuncture meridians. Dr. Voll reasoned that if the Chinese really did have the energy meridians down to a science then you should be able to measure the electrical conductivity of the acupuncture points on the skin using a stylus-shaped electrode made of brass. What Dr. Voll discovered was revolutionary. His experiments proved that you could measure the body's ability to conduct energy and test how the body responds to different substances when placed in the body's energy field. He discovered that by testing healthy individuals, the electrical readings on acupuncture points would measure within a normal range while readings from diseased individuals revealed extremely high in acute, inflammatory situations or extremely low in chronic diseased situations.

Dr. Voll discovered that medicines placed in the energy field of each patient would influence the acupuncture readings either in a positive or negative response. Dr. Voll explains in his own words, *"I diagnosed one colleague as having chronic prostatitis and advised him to take a homeopathic preparation called Echinacea 4X. He replied that he had this medication in his office and went to get it. When he returned with the bottle of Echinacea in his hand, I tested the prostate measurement point again and made the discovery that the point reading, which was up to 90, had decreased to 64, an enormous improvement of the prostate value. I had the colleague put the bottle aside and the previous measurement value returned. After holding the medication in his hand, the measurement value went down to 64 again, and this pattern repeated itself as often as desired."*

> **"If we are beings of energy, then it follows that we can be affected by energy."**
> Richard Gerber, M.D., Author of *Vibrational Medicine*

Bio-Energetic Testing or EDS (Electro Dermal Screening) is a computerized electrical device containing digitally-encoded information relating to a huge library of thousands of possible factors that could be causing imbalances in the organs, glands, and major systems of the body.

EDS (Electro Dermal Screening)	
Homeopathy	Enzymes
Herbs	Hormones
Vitamins	Neurotransmitters
Minerals	Bach Flowers
Amino Acids	Vertebral Stress
Essential Oils	Color Therapy
Phenolics (Allergies)	Sarcodes

Using a simple low-voltage circuit, energetic frequencies are input in the computer to identify the response of the body to those signals. Toxins and pathogens such as viruses, bacteria, fungus, mold, parasites, heavy metals, chemicals, pesticides, Lyme and co-infections resonate at specific vibrational frequencies and are catalogued into the database. When performing an EDS scan, thousands of toxins are checked to identify which frequencies are resonating in your body causing an energetic disturbance. Once these toxic frequencies are identified, their vibrational signature is imprinted or charged into a homeopathic remedy, custom made for that individual's needs.

A homeopathic remedy consists of roughly 10 percent alcohol and 90 percent distilled or structured water. The carbon bonds in the alcohol are able to suspend or hold an electrical charge. A homeopathic remedy may be imprinted with pathogens and toxins such as mercury, streptococcus bacteria and Epstein-Barr virus or nutritional support like vitamins, minerals and hormones. We also imprint what we call sarcodes or energetic healthy blueprints for the body to help restore balance to organs, glands and systems.

How does it work? EDS works by sending very small (unnoticeable) electrical frequencies into your body by holding a brass electrode. We are all familiar with radio stations. When tuned in to a specific frequency such as 105.1 FM you pick up a country music station, while tuning in to 570 AM picks up news and talk radio. Just as each radio station has a specific frequency at which it broadcasts, every nutritional supplement and pathogen resonates at a specific frequency as well. Each of these energetic signatures or frequencies is programmed into the software of the computer. For example, calcium resonates at 320 Hz, potassium at 304 Hz, zinc at 480 Hz, tuberculosis at 769,000 Hz and staphylococcus aureus 378,381 Hz. Once we identify what toxins are resonating in your body, and what nutritional support remedies are needed, all of the specific frequencies are imprinted or charged into a homeopathic remedy.

TOXIN	FREQUENCY (KHz)
Adenovirus	393 KHz
Borrelia Burgdorferi	380 KHz
Candida Albicans	386 KHz
Chlamydia	381 KHz
Coxsackie Virus	364.9 KHz
Epstein-Barr Virus	380,375 KHz
Escherichia coli (E. Coli)	356,393 KHz
Herpes Simplex 1	292,345.5 KHz
Klebsiella Pneumoniae	401,419 KHz
Staphylococcus Aureus	378,381 KHz
Streptococcus Pyogenes	373 KHz

If you have ever downloaded pictures or music from a computer to a jump drive or CD, then you are familiar with what is called a "digital download." Homeopathic imprinting is simply a custom digital download for the frequencies your body needs to get well.

A supplement scan is done to see what formulas are best. Vitamins, minerals, amino acids, enzymes, herbs, phenolics, neurotransmitters, hormones, Bach flower remedies and essential oils are all tested to see what resonates best for you. We don't guess, we test to see what your body needs for balance. EDS is not a diagnostic device. It is only used to identify energetic imbalances within the body.

> **"Electricity will become as ubiquitous in medical practice as surgery or drugs are; in many instances, it will replace them."** Dr. Andrew Bassett, Columbia-Presbyterian Medical Center

One of the advantages to EDS technology is that it can identify energetic disturbances in the body before they become physical problems. It is estimated by some researchers that breast cancer takes seven to 12 years before it manifests physically to the size of a pinhead. So, if we want to be healthy, a wise person doesn't wait until he or she has symptoms or for his or her doctor to make a diagnosis. Now is the time to take care of yourself. Remember the wisdom of Thomas Edison, *"An ounce of prevention is worth a pound of cure."*

> **"Treating humans without concept of energy is treating dead matter."** Albert Szent-Gyorgyi, M.D. Hungary, Nobel Prize Laureate 1893-1986

At Harvard Medical School, a relationship was shown to exist between physical health and energy fields. A cell was held in homeostasis at a certain electromagnetic frequency. When that frequency was altered either positively or negatively, and not returned to equilibrium within 72 hours, the cell died. Every health problem is primarily, therefore, an energetic one, which can be detected and influenced prior to physical manifestations of the condition. EDS provides us with vital information needed to make wise and informed decisions about our health.

EDS – Identifying The Toxins Causing Your Symptoms

Heavy Metals	Pesticides	Parasites	Calcium Plaquing
Chemical Poisoning	Food Allergies	Inhalant Allergies	Prescription Drug Toxins
Viruses	Bacteria	Fungus/Yeast	Glyphosate
Candida Yeast	Mold	Vaccination Toxicity	Suppressed Emotions
Radiation Poisoning	Miasms	Fear	Free Radicals
Aspartame Poisoning	Unloved	Electromagnetic Stress	Arterial Plaquing
Herpes	Lyme Disease	Guilt	Grudge
Silicone Poisoning	Ulcers	Resentment	Nicotine Poisoning
Epstein-Barr Virus	EMF's	Mucor Racemosus	Chakra Imbalances
Aspergillus Niger	Mercury	Lead	Coxsackie Virus
MSG Poisoning	Aluminum	Acidosis	Gluten/Dairy Allergies

> **"Nothing exists except atoms and empty space; everything else is opinion."** Democritus of Abdera

Physics teaches us that every object on earth has a certain vibrational frequency that can destroy itself completely. Opera singers can shatter wineglasses when high notes are hit with the perfect tone. A plucked string on a guitar can cause another string on a different guitar in the same room to start vibrating. Would it not make sense that every disease resonates at a specific vibrational frequency?

> **"Future medicine will be based on controlling energy in the body."** William A. Tiller, Ph.D., Nobel Prize Laureate, Stanford University

Standard orthodox medicine only fixes what has already happened. They can cut out a tumor after it has grown or prescribe a drug after you have been diagnosed with arthritis. EDS has the ability to detect energetic disturbances in the body that may cause the tumor growth. This is the future of medicine. There will come a time when we'll look back and shake our heads at the fact that for generations, we let people get sick before we took action.

> **"Do you remember how electrical currents and 'unseen waves' were laughed at? The knowledge about man is still in its infancy."** Albert Einstein

Homeopathy

Over 500 million people worldwide and 80 different nations use homeopathic medicine. Homeopathy is highly popular in most European countries, especially France, Germany and England. There are five homeopathic hospitals in the United Kingdom, and the royal families of England, including Queen Elizabeth II, rely upon homeopathic medicine for health care. India has over 200,000 licensed homeopaths, and over 100 million people in India rely solely on homeopathy for their medical care. Why don't most Americans use homeopathy? The pharmaceutical industry doesn't want you to know about safe, effective and inexpensive homeopathic treatments. And who do you think controls the media?

> **"In every atom, there are worlds within worlds."** Yoga Vasishtha

Dr. Samuel Hahnemann was a German physician, scientist, chemist, mineralogist and botanist who practiced medicine in the late 1700s and early 1800s, also known as the founder of homeopathy. Medical doctors today do allergy testing by exposing you to tree pollen, mold, dust mites, animal dander, etc., to see what you are allergic to. Whatever you react to is given to you in a remedy as medicine.

In other words, a small dose of what you are allergic to will help alleviate your allergy. This is founded on the law of similars, meaning "like cures like." A substance that will cause illness in a healthy person will cure it in a sick person.

Famous People Who Use (Used) Homeopathy	
Jennifer Aniston	Paul McCartney
John D. Rockefeller	Mahatma Gandhi
Cindy Crawford	Usain Bolt – Gold Medalist
Prince Charles	Cher
David Beckham	Kim Cattrall
Ralph Waldo Emerson	Mark Twain
Catherine Zeta-Jones	Pamela Anderson

Unlike allergy shots, homeopathic remedies only contain a trace amount, and in many situations, just an energetic frequency of the substance. One drop of the original substance is put in distilled water and alcohol and succussed or shaken and diluted until not one trace of the original substance exists. What you are left with is an energetic frequency of that substance. The more diluted the solution, the more powerful the healing agent becomes. So, if you have poison ivy, the homeopathic remedy will contain energetic frequencies of poison ivy. This is why homeopathy is called energy medicine.

> **"No individual has done more good to the medical profession than Samuel Hahnemann (the father of homeopathy)."** C. Everett Koop, M.D., Surgeon General for the United States, 1982-1989

Common Homeopathic Remedies

REMEDIES	SOURCE	USED FOR
Arnica	Fallkraut – plant	Aches, pains, bruises & injuries
Allium cepa	Derived from onions	Allergies, colds, runny nose
Chamomilla	Chamomile – plant	Colic, teething, irritability, ear pain, fevers
Magnesia phosphorica	Magnesium phosphate	Menstrual cramps, neuralgia, sciatica & bloating
Ignatia	St. Ignatius' bean	Grief, anxiety, depression, shock, insomnia, headaches
Nux Vomica	Strychnine tree	Digestive troubles, hangovers, motion sickness, stress
Sulphur	Sublimated Sulphur	Itchiness, acne, eczema, bloating, sore throats
Arsenica Album	Arsenic trioxide	Food poisoning, anxiety, loneliness, feeling cold
Zincum Metallicum	Mineral – zinc	Restless leg syndrome, weakness, numbness, twitching
Gelsemium	Yellow jasmine	The flu, fever, chills, headaches, fatigue, aching muscles
Apis	Crushed honey bee	Bites, stings, swelling, pain, redness, sore throat
Ledum	Marsh tea, wild rosemary	Puncture wounds (tetanus), animal bites, Lyme disease
Belladonna	Nightshade – plant	High fever
Aconite	Wolfsbane – plant	Onset of a cold, fright or shock
Pulsatilla	Wind flower, Pasque	Childhood ear infections, colds, runny/stuffy nose
Calendula	English marigold	Wounds, scrapes, burns, skin redness, diaper rash

> **"I have learned that the human being possesses a marvelous healing power that can be greatly augmented by homeopathy, and that severe illnesses, both physical and mental, can be overcome."** William E. Shevin, M.D.

Dr. Hahnemann performed what he called "provings." His research revealed that an overdose of Cinchona tree bark would cause symptoms of malaria after he took several doses of cinchona and came down with malaria-like symptoms. He later found out that this would work in the reverse, "like cures like" or "the cause is the cure." As he did his provings on hundreds of remedies, his findings were published in what is known as the Materia Medica. For example, the poisonous nightshade plant causes flushing of the skin and a fever. Belladonna, the homeopathic remedy derived from nightshade, will help resolve a fever. Dr. Hahnemann taught the fundamental truth that suppressing symptoms does not cure the underlying disease but actually drives it deeper into the body so that it manifests in another form.

> **"Homeopathy cures a larger percentage of cases than any other form of treatment and is beyond all doubt safer, more economical, and the most complete medical science ..."** Mahatma Gandhi 1869-1948

We all know that if your car battery is dead, you hook jumper cables to your dead battery and connect the cables to the battery of a running car. You then turn the key and your car magically starts. Energy travels through those cables and allows the dead to come to life. Imagine going back in time 500 years and explaining this procedure. You might be hanged for saying such nonsense. Jump-starting a car battery or charging one is similar to imprinting homeopathic frequencies, we are just working with much smaller, very subtle frequencies, but still transferring energy frequencies from one item to another.

> **"The mind is like a parachute. It must be opened to work."** James Chappell D.C., N.D., Ph.D.

Energy is mysterious because you can't hear, see or touch it, but we all know it exists. How about air? When's the last time you saw the air? When's the last time you grabbed a handful? Compress it into a rubber tire and it will lift a 6,000-pound automobile.

> **"The superior doctor prevents sickness; the mediocre doctor attends to impending sickness; the inferior doctor treats actual sickness."** Chinese Proverb

Case Study

In 1989, I started working for the State of Alabama with the Department of Human Resources. My desk was right beside the air conditioning vent and the carpet was always wet. I worked in an office with 80 other women and with them came an enormous array of perfumes, air fresheners, soaps, etc. I soon began having headaches. I went to my medical doctor, who tested me and found nothing wrong. He prescribed antidepressant medication? I then went to an Ear, Nose and Throat Doctor who said I needed nose surgery. A couple of years later, that doctor was arrested for fraud. I then went to see an allergist and he put me on allergy pills and nasal spray. I continued to get worse.

I started having serious female problems. I would start hemorrhaging and have a period every two weeks. My doctor put me on serious painkillers that would knock me out for days. He put me on birth control pills, monthly shots and then gave me a hysterectomy.

My health went downhill fast. My joints started to ache to the point that I could hardly walk. I was diagnosed with arthritis. Then I started alternating between cramping with diarrhea, and bloating with constipation. I would throw up almost every day. The doctor diagnosed me with IBS (Irritable Bowel Syndrome). My blood pressure shot up high, so he put me on blood pressure medication. Then I started getting a metal taste in my mouth right before I would have a reaction of joint pain, stomach pains, etc.

By January 2006, my doctor had me on six different medications. I was taking a drug for blood pressure, arthritis, cholesterol, IBS, birth control and anti-depressants. I kept getting worse and worse and gained 35 pounds in three months. I felt so bad that many days I couldn't make it into work.

I did some research and found the only chemical allergy doctor in Alabama up in Gadsden. So, I went to have all the allergy tests done. He found me to be allergic to almost everything inside buildings but nothing outside. I was diagnosed with MCS (Multiple Chemical Sensitivity). He told me that I was allergic to my environment and that I would probably be on disability within a year. He said there were people that were better off than me who were already on disability so I needed to get myself prepared. **He said there was no cure and it would only get worse!**

He put me on three different allergy drops (more drugs!) and told me to wear a mask and long sleeves. I had to get rid of all my chemicals in the house, quit wearing makeup and never dye my hair again. I did all this and kept having reactions.

In May, my son graduated from high school. I went to the graduation and they had scented candles and flowers. All the chemicals in the air were more than I could handle. After 15 minutes, I was so sick that I couldn't see or walk. My husband had to carry me out. I missed my only child's graduation!

I couldn't walk for three days. I went back to the doctor and told him what happened and he looked at me and said, "Well, Kay, you've got to stay away from those types of situations." I couldn't believe it! I was 41 years old and I felt like my life was being taken away from me! One day my child would get married. Am I supposed to miss that too?

As I was leaving Gadsden, I was crying and praying for help. I saw a sign that said, "Natural Healing Clinic." I figured that I had nothing left to lose so I pulled in and made an appointment.

A week later, I met my hero, Dr. Reed Sainsbury. This man saved my life! I feel like I've gained 10 years to my life! There are only a few people who have had an impact on my life. Dr. Sainsbury is very high on that list.

When I came in for my appointment, I had a reaction from perfume worn by another patient. I couldn't see to fill out the paper work and by the time I went into his office I was crying out of frustration. My hands and ankles hurt. I could hardly think. I was so tired of going to doctors and not getting well. I thought to myself, "This doctor is a quack, I'm wasting my money."

Dr. Sainsbury tested different points on my hands and feet with a probe and the computer would give different readings as to which areas of my body were balanced and out of balance. He found that my liver was very toxic and had an extremely low energy reading. He found that I was allergic to dairy products. He put me on a detoxifying and nutritional program with an emphasis on flushing out my liver. The next thing I knew, I was feeling better.

It's been a year and I'm able to do just about anything now. I'm off all of my prescription medications and feel great. I've started living life again. I've started dancing, which was something I thought I'd never be able to do again. I'm even taking some night classes at the local college. It feels so great to be around the living again!

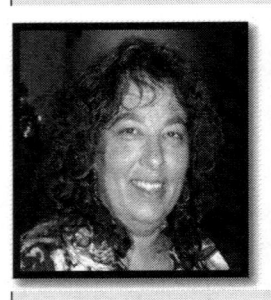

I went back to my old doctor, just one more time, for a physical. He asked me what I was doing because all my lab work came back good. No high blood pressure, no high cholesterol and I have lost 30 pounds. I told him about Dr. Sainsbury and showed him what herbs and other nutritional formulas I was taking. He looked at them and said, "Well, if you believe something works, it will." I told him, "Well — I believed that you and the drugs you kept giving me were going to work too!"

Kay Dement
Montgomery, Alabama

Kay's symptoms were not caused from a deficiency of drugs. Are you like Kay, sick and tired of being prescribed more and more toxic drugs without ever finding the cause?

When Kay came into our clinic sick and frustrated, we found the cause of her illnesses. Her allergy doctor told her there was no cure for her allergies (Multiple Chemical Sensitivity). Any doctor who claims there is no cure for a disease does not understand the magnificence of the human body and The Intelligence that created it. If your doctor claims that there is no cure for your problem then maybe it's time to find a new doctor? If you took your car to a mechanic who could never fix it, would you continue to go to the same mechanic?

Most allergies are caused from a toxic liver and an imbalance with the microbiome in the gut. Most headaches are caused from liver/gallbladder issues as well. Kay needed a liver cleanse and when we gave her body what it needed, it responded just as it was engineered to do. After a liver flush and some nutritional support, she got well. She proved her medical doctor wrong. She is not on disability and she has her life back because we found the cause of her allergies. Are you satisfied playing your doctor's disease maintenance game with toxic drugs?

"There is a divine current within you that carries healing power." Catherine Ponder, Author of *The Healing Secrets of the Ages*

Chapter 2
HEALTH CARE OR DISEASE MAINTENANCE?

> "As a retired physician, I can honestly say that unless you are in a serious accident, your best chance of living to a ripe old age is to avoid doctors and hospitals and learn nutrition, herbal medicine and other forms of natural medicine unless you are fortunate enough to have a naturopathic physician available. Almost all drugs are toxic and are designed only to treat symptoms and not to cure anyone." Alan Greenburg, M.D.

A large percentage of Americans are tired of the prescription drug game. They want to fix the problem, not just suppress the symptom with drugs. It has been estimated by David Eisenberg at Harvard University that 1 out of 3 Americans has used some form of alternative medicine within the last year. Similar statistics reveal that 37 percent of Americans use alternative medicine, and 41.9 percent of households earning over $100,000 per year with post-graduate degrees use alternative integrative medicine.

According to The New York Times, Americans spend $30.2 billion a year on alternative and complementary medicine. What's even more convincing proof that Americans are fed up with taking drugs is the fact that over $30 billion was spent out of their own pockets because insurance didn't cover it! Wise doctors, who truly are interested in seeing their patients get well, address the cause of disease with natural remedies, diet and exercise and use drugs only as a last resort. Responsible Americans will not tolerate disease maintenance quackery. Drugless solutions to their illnesses are sought out and employed because their health is worth it.

America's Disease Maintenance System

> "Perhaps the words 'health care' give us the illusion that medicine is about health. Modern medicine is not a purveyor of health care but of disease-care." Carolyn Dean, M.D., N.D.

According to Time magazine, Americans spend over $374 billion on drugs each year! That's a staggering number. Most medical doctors treat symptoms with drugs. They wait until something breaks down and symptoms occur and then they cut, burn, radiate or poison you with drugs or chemotherapy. Treating the symptoms and failing to correct the cause of disease results in more symptoms, more illness and eventually kidney failure and death.

Our country does not have a health-care system, we have a "disease maintenance system." It is controlled and influenced by money, power, greed and massive corruption. The majority if not all major medical universities are heavily funded by the pharmaceutical industry to ensure that young new doctors are taught to treat the symptoms with prescription drugs. And if you don't believe it, try taking something natural, let's say an herb, and start advertising that it can cure a certain medical condition. It won't be long before you come to understand that the AMA, FDA and pharmaceutical industry have a monopoly on maintaining disease in this country and have patents on the words diagnose, treat, cure or prevent disease. Any competition claiming to cure disease from a non-patented drug will find you in violation of their law. If they feel it's a threat to their multi-billion-dollar empire, then action will be taken to squash all competition.

> "The intrusion of money into science means 'medicine' will never arrive at what truly works, unless they can patent it for maximum profits!" Joel Wallach, D.V.M., N.D.

If you want to see how corrupt the system is, I recommend you watching a documentary on how Dr. Stanislaw Burzynski of Houston, Texas, has successfully helped terminal cancer patients get well using his non-toxic antineoplaston therapy. The FDA continues to harass him while moms, dads and children plead in court how this doctor saved their life. After watching how some of the FDA officials behave, it's very evident what their motives are. The corruption in this country is unbelievable.

The fact that they can shut down competition (anything natural besides patented, expensive and toxic drugs) is their fear-based attempt to maintain disease through prescription drugs with no intention of ever healing the cause. Who cares what is prescribed as long as it works right? If a group of doctors claim they can cure arthritis by using a combination of herbs, vitamins, minerals and enzymes and they are having a 90 percent success rate in doing it, then shouldn't the FDA and insurance companies be in favor of it? Why aren't they? Who do you think owns the insurance companies? You guessed it, your old favorite pharmaceutical gang.

> "A free society, if it is to remain free, cannot permit itself to be dominated by one strain of thought." William J. Baroody Sr.

Doctors who are truly committed to helping their patients heal recommend natural remedies that cleanse and nourish the cells, unlike drugs that add more toxins to the body and cause cellular acidosis, thus providing the body with the terrain that favors even more disease. These doctors have their hands tied in this country. They must prescribe drugs or else the "big boys" put the kibosh on those who step out of line. When doctors decide to stop poisoning their patients with toxic drug therapies, then the noose is cinched and they either "play by the rules," stop working with insurance companies, escape to a different country, or give up their license. I personally know several good medical doctors who have been bullied and persecuted to the point of giving up their licenses or leaving the country. It is a sad reality that you would hope would never happen in the great land of the free, home of the brave. How free are we?

> **"None are more hopelessly enslaved than those who falsely believe they are free!"** Johann Wolfgang von Goethe 1749-1832

If you visit some of the alternative cancer clinics in Mexico, you'll see how many doctors from the U.S. have left the great "home of the free" because they are not free to treat their patients using natural remedies that don't have toxic side effects like drugs do. Health-care practitioners are not free to do what allows people to heal themselves of disease. There is simply too much money involved in dealing drugs and maintaining disease by suppressing symptoms.

> **"Unless we put medical freedom into the Constitution, the time will come when medicine will organize into an underground dictatorship ...To restrict the art of healing to one class of men and deny equal privileges to others will constitute the Bastille of medical science. All such laws are un-American and despotic and have no place in a republic ... The constitution of this republic should make special privilege for medical freedom as well as religious freedom."** Benjamin Rush, M.D., Signer of the Declaration of Independence and personal physician to George Washington

Eliminating Competition

William F. Koch, M.D., Ph.D., was a famous professor at the University of Michigan, Detroit College of Medicine, who had great success in curing cancer, especially leukemia. He had a 46 percent success rate curing advanced cases of cancer and averaged 72 percent success rate curing patients not yet in a terminal stage of cancer. He was using a formula he called "Glyoxylide," a nontoxic, oxidative catalyst that has the capacity to reverse neoplasms and viral parasitism. It works by restoring oxygen to non-oxygenating cells. The FDA and pharmaceutical industry found out about his formula and decided it was an infringement upon their multibillion-dollar cancer monopoly. He was arrested and put on trial. He had over 4,000 other doctors using this cure also. Two of those doctors came to the trial to testify in Dr. Koch's behalf. Both of them were mysteriously murdered. One was hit by a car and the other poisoned. Coincidence?

When something other than radiation and chemotherapy becomes a threat to their multibillion-dollar monopoly, they eliminate the competition. Dr. Koch won the court case but in the process was nearly assassinated 13 times. He realized that he would soon be dead if he didn't flee the good ole' USA, land of the free (as long as you don't cure people of disease and take business away from the drug lords).

Dr. Koch found refuge in South America and continued helping sick cancer patients heal. In Brazil he was offered the highest position in the Brazilian medical services. Shortly after accepting that position, he was mysteriously murdered. Coincidence?

Those who don't want cures finally won and the Glyoxylide formula was lost. This was a blatant attack on freedom and health. Where were all the protesters? Of course, since the same group of people who had Dr. Koch murdered control the media, no mention was ever made about it. You hear the news they want you to hear, not what's necessarily true.

A Cure For Cancer – Outlawed In The USA

> **"The opposite of fact is falsehood, but the opposite of one profound truth may very well be another profound truth."** Niels Bohr, Nobel Prize Winner, Physicist 1885-1962

American medical inventor Royal Raymond Rife in 1929 invented the first microscope capable of staining live viruses with light to make them visible, while keeping them alive, also known as bioluminescence. Some of his technology is still used today in electronics, radiochemistry, biochemistry and optics. By 1933, he constructed the Rife Universal microscope that could magnify objects 60,000 times their original size. He later created the Rife Frequency Generator, a device that transmits specific electronic frequencies to destroy typhus bacteria, polio and herpes viruses and certain cancers. How does it work? Every disease microbe has its own unique electronic signature or frequency at which it resonates. When a pathogen's specific frequency is matched with an electronically transmitted frequency, it causes the cancer cell or pathogen to explode from an excess of energy.

Rife found that by using his Frequency Generator on people who were infected with different bacteria like osteomyelitis (recurrent bone infection), viruses and other chronic infections, he could get them well just like he had done with cancer by destroying the pathogens when tuning in to the right frequency, just as an opera singer shatters a wine glass by producing its resonate note.

Milbank Johnson, M.D., began an investigation of the Rife Frequency Generator to determine whether or not it was a hoax. In 1934, he and his Medical Research Committee at the University of Southern California conducted the first and only study on it for a possible cancer treatment device. Dr. Milbank took 16 patients with terminal or "incurable" cancer and for the next three months treated them with the Rife Frequency Generator daily for 3-minute durations. After three months of treatment, 14 of the 16 terminal cancer patients were declared clinically cured and in good health by a staff consisting of five medical doctors and Alvin Ford, M.D., group pathologist. A few weeks later, the other two patients were declared "cancer-free." Rife's technology proved 100 percent effective for healing cancer!

Who in their right mind would put a stop to this success? It doesn't take a rocket scientist to figure out that if you are in the cancer industry, earning billions of dollars a year, and you don't want a cure, then you don't find one. Uncovering a medical rat's nest, we have found that authorities under the direction of Morris Fishbein, a highly influential editor of JAMA (the Journal of the American Medical Association), attempted to control the Rife technology by purchasing ownership. After being declined, Fishbein made it his mission to destroy Rife's cancer cure technology. It was no accident that a special laboratory built to study Rife's technology was mysteriously burned down and his microscope stolen, after Fishbein's offer was refused. Rife was harassed and even taken to court on phony, trumped-up charges. Many of his records were vandalized and stolen. Fishbein's dirty deeds finally caught up with him and he was eventually convicted of racketeering charges.

Many of the doctors who supported Rife were harassed as well, clinics raided, and two of them were mysteriously murdered. Years later, Dr. Milbank Johnson was about to make a public announcement using the Rife technology to cure cancer. He was found dead and all of his research was mysteriously lost. They tried to claim it was suicide, but years later when they insisted on exhuming the body, they detected poison as the cause of death. So instead of using nontoxic, safe and effective cancer treatments in this country, we cling to the kill, kill, kill approach with toxic chemotherapy. Why? Because the average cancer patient spends between $100,000 and $280,000 over the four years following diagnosis and $350,000 before they die. Treating cancer with chemotherapy is a money-making business. Healing cancer with energy frequencies doesn't meet the pharmaceutical industry's financial goals. If interested in learning more about the Rife technology, read *The Cancer Cure That Worked* by Barry Lynes.

> "This collection of serial killers with reckless disregard for human life extinguishes the hopes and lives of over 100,000 Americans every year. In the past decade they have been responsible for over 1 million innocent deaths, yet not only have they not faced justice, they have enriched themselves with profits that would make Bill Gates envious. These parasitic killers come not from some cave in Afghanistan, but from plush office suites ..." Jay R. Cavanaugh, Ph.D., California State Board of Pharmacy (talking about prescription drug manufacturers)

Different forms of the Rife Frequency Generator technology are still used today, especially in other countries where our government isn't there to harass natural treatments while ignoring the thousands who are harmed and killed each year by FDA "proven safe" drugs. Geronimo Rubio, M.D., medical director of American Metabolic Institute in La Mesa, Mexico, uses the Rife technology and other nontoxic natural healing modalities in his clinic. He has an 80 percent success rate in reversing stage I and II cancers. For more information, go online to www.rubiocancercenter.com

> "The American public has no idea how politics secretly control the practice of medicine." James P. Carter, M.D., Tulane University, Author of *Racketeering in Medicine The Suppression of Alternatives*

Americans Have The Most Expensive Health Care, But Not The Best

We in the U.S. are ranked 43rd in life expectancy. Monaco, Japan and Singapore are ranked the highest. It is interesting to note that their health-care costs are 50 to 75 percent less than the U.S. Why is that? Could it be that they focus on prevention rather than disease maintenance?

Cancer is the second largest revenue producing business in the world next to the petroleum industry. Unhealthy, sick Americans, relying upon drugs to suppress symptoms, keep the disease maintenance system booming. If America suddenly adopted the 10,000-year-old system of traditional Chinese medicine and only paid the doctor when you were well and stopped paying him when you became sick, doctors would learn really fast about herbs, homeopathy, minerals and basic nutritional support.

Americans have the wealthiest, highest priced, most technologically advanced health-care system in the world, yet we rank 43rd in longevity and come in dead last in a comparison of 17 affluent nations. We spend over $3 trillion on health care a year (that's $10,345 per person) and our doctors write over 4 billion prescriptions each year. If we have the best, why aren't we No.1?

> **"America's health-care system is second only to Japan, Canada, Sweden, Great Britain ... well, all of Europe. But you can thank your lucky stars we don't live in Paraguay!"** Homer Simpson

Statistics are now reporting that 50 percent of Americans will develop cancer at some point in their lives. We have the most expensive health-care system in the world, but not the best. According to the CDC, more than 1 million individuals are seen in hospital emergency departments every year due to adverse drug reactions. The fire alarm has been pulled for us to wake up. Would you be concerned if homeopathic and herbal formulas naturopaths recommended people take to get well sent over a million people per year to the emergency room due to adverse reactions?

> **"Only 15 percent of all medical procedures are scientifically validated."** David Eddy, M.D., Ph.D., Duke University

In the South, when tornadoes are a possibility, sirens go off to warn people to take cover and seek safe shelter. When your doctor prescribes a new drug, you may be wise to look at the warning sirens that have been sounded in the Physicians Desk Reference (PDR) about possible adverse side effects. In order to list them all, it takes about 3,500 pages! Is not the fact that drugs have adverse side effects evidence enough that they are poisons and should only be used in emergency situations?

> **"There is no such thing as a safe, harmless drug. All drugs, including common aspirin, are potentially dangerous."** Paavo Airola, Ph.D., N.D.

In a disturbing article written by Barbara Starfield, M.D., MPH, professor at Johns Hopkins School of Public Health, in the Journal of the American Medical

Association (JAMA) — vol. 284. No. 4 483-5 — July 26, 2000, the research reveals that our mainstream medical system kills 225,000 Americans per year. Ironically, Dr. Starfield spent time researching medical errors and became a victim of her own statistics when she died suddenly in 2011 after taking the blood thinner Plavix in combination with aspirin. Her husband, Dr. Neil Holtzman, wrote in sorrow and anger that she died while swimming alone, but the underlying condition was a cerebral hemorrhage caused from the Plavix-aspirin combination.

A study released from Johns Hopkins in May 2016 and published in The British Medical Journal reports that 250,000 deaths per year are due to medical errors and that 10 percent of all U.S. deaths are now caused from medical errors. Considering those 250,000 deaths a year do not include adverse side effects from drugs, only death figures, this is a shocking, red-flag wakeup call that something is terribly wrong with our attempt to get people well in this country.

"If prescription drugs really worked, we would already be a disease-free society!" James F. Balch, M.D., Author of *Prescription For Nutritional Healing*

American medical doctors write an average of 10 prescriptions per person every year in this country, and it's killing us. In 1991, a Harvard University School of Public Health

JAMA **Journal of the American Medical Association Vol. 284 No. 4**

Incidents Per Year

- **12,000 – Unnecessary Surgeries**
- **7,000 – Medication Errors in Hospitals**
- **20,000 – Other Errors in Hospitals**
- **80,000 – Nosocomial Infections in Hospitals**
- **106,000 – Adverse Effects of Medications**

study reported that 1.3 million injuries and 198,000 deaths occur in American hospitals each year as a result of "iatrogenic," or doctor-caused, problems and adverse reactions. Dr. Sydney Wolfe (director of the Ralph Nader-founded watchdog group Public Citizen Health Research Group, Washington, D.C.) in a 1993 news release said, *"300,000 Americans are killed each year in hospitals alone as a result of medical negligence."* In 2001, the California Sun newspaper reported, *"Allopathic doctors kill more people than guns and traffic accidents."*

> "Modern medicine is now better geared for killing people than it is for healing them. The greatest threat to one's health is the physician who practices modern medicine. The treatments doctors use are often more harmful to their patients than the diseases themselves might be." Robert S. Mendelsohn, M.D.

Carolyn Dean, M.D., and Gary Null, Ph.D., in Death by Medicine, Journal of Orthomolecular Medicine, 2005, report that 783,936 iatrogenic deaths occurred in America in 2005. When the prescriptions that are supposed to help you get well end up backfiring and killing people, it's time for change. It's time for a safer solution.

> "When the No. 1 killer in a society is the health-care system, then that system must take responsibility for its shortcomings. It's a failed system in need of immediate attention." Carolyn Dean, M.D., N.D.

The New England Journal of Medicine reports that adverse drug reactions occur in one out of every four individuals who visit their family medical doctor. Even more shocking is that USA Today states adverse drug reactions are the fourth leading cause of hospital admissions. They estimate that 2.2 million Americans are so severely injured from doctor-prescribed drugs that they are either hospitalized for an extended period or permanently disabled. Go to the hospital to get well and the medicine they give you backfires and makes you worse. If you're a betting man, you might be better off playing the odds and just staying home and dealing with your illness rather than playing Russian roulette with their poisonous drugs that have a good chance of making you sicker and possibly even killing you.

> "If you choose to go to a hospital, go into hospitals with your eyes wide open. Medical care, like so many other things, is problematic; it's not a sure thing. Patients must understand hospitals are hazardous and medical care is a dangerous enterprise — you must be willing to put a considerable amount of energy into self-protection." Lowell Levin, M.D., Yale School of Medicine

Would you put your trust in an institution that accidentally killed 250,000 people every year? If Delta Airlines killed 250,000 people each year from airplane accidents, would you risk flying with them? Unfortunately, most Americans get suckered into the prescription drug trap like a desperate, non-thinking mouse who is pinned down by a metal hinge with its snoot on a piece of cheese. It got the cheese, but now the metal hinge is suffocating the life right out of it. For some prescription drug-takers, you got your cholesterol down, but now you have Alzheimer's so bad you can't remember anything, and your kidneys are failing, so you are on dialysis. Is this health care?

    Are we Americans any different than greedy mice going after a piece of cheese on the trap when we treat our symptoms with drugs without ever finding the cause? Do we not care about tomorrow as long as we feel good today? Suppressing symptoms with toxic drugs and never addressing the cause of illness is going to have a price to be paid. The illusion created by a quick-fix drug that the problem has been resolved is similar to the metal hinge crushing the mouse's neck. The metal hinge was never a threat to the hungry mouse until it snapped across its fuzzy neck when he took the bait. The man-made chemical drugs we take may at the time help us feel better, but the acidic terrain, clogged lymphatic system and toxic liver and kidney residue left behind may well prove to be the metal hinge we never see coming that put us 6 feet under.

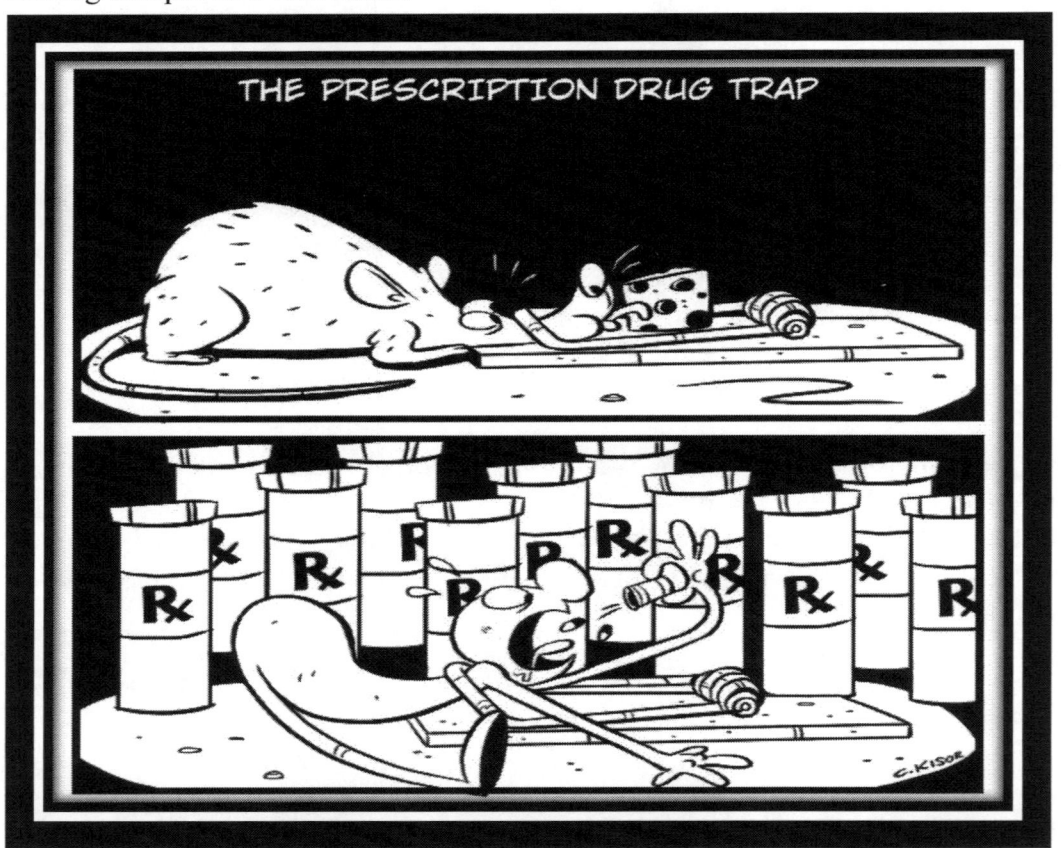

THE PRESCRIPTION DRUG TRAP

> "Basically you die earlier and spend more time disabled if you're an American rather than a member of most other advanced countries."
> Christopher Murray, M.D., Ph.D., World Health Organization

You can't watch TV at night without seeing clever ads promoting drugs as the magic answer to your health problems. Pharmaceutical companies whose business relies upon obedient Americans to take whatever new pill their doctor prescribes promote these laughable myths. One can't help chuckling when they start naming all the possible side effects which, in some cases, are worse than the symptom you are taking the drug for in the first place. Why risk ruining your liver or kidneys with a particular drug to lower your cholesterol? Yes, I know, your doctor has promoted the myth that cholesterol higher than 200 will cause a heart attack or stroke and kill you. More on those lies later.

> "There are some remedies worse than the disease." Pubilius Syrus

QUESTION:	Why are prescription drugs being advertised on TV?
ANSWER:	They want you to tell your doctor what you need.
COMMENT:	Why would the patient need to tell their doctor what drug to use?

If medical doctors prescribed the right drug for each patient to be healthy, then why advertise prescription drugs? After years of medical school, wouldn't you think your doctor would know what you need without some slick pharmaceutical advertisement persuading Americans to, "Ask your doctor if drug X is right for you?"

> "Strive to preserve your health; and in this you will better succeed in proportion as you keep clear of the physicians." Leonardo Da Vinci 1452-1519

When someone comes in our clinic, we perform an EDS Analysis to identify which nutritional deficiencies and toxins are causing their symptoms. We check each organ, gland and system to find out which areas of the body are most compromised. We only recommend individuals taking what their body needs to be balanced.

We have people bring in their bags of supplements, and 95 percent of the stuff they are taking is unneeded for balance. Why? If it were working, they wouldn't be in our office with symptoms, seeking our help. The supplements that do usually test well are plant-derived minerals; digestive enzymes; circulation support; immune support; liver and kidney support; and adrenal and thyroid support.

> "The cause of most disease is in the poisonous drugs physicians superstitiously give in order to effect a cure." Charles E. Page, M.D.

Pharmaceutical companies spend over $6 billion every year on advertising alone. This is why drug commercials are blasted all over the TV. The fact that the FDA has made it a law that, "Only a drug can cure, prevent and treat disease," is evidence enough of a conspiracy to maintain disease by suppressing symptoms and never addressing the cause. This is what Dr. Benjamin Rush warned us about. Americans will never be healthy and free as long as we are addicted to chemical drugs, legal or illegal.

> "During 1991, it is estimated that approximately $5 billion was spent by the pharmaceutical industry on advertising alone to encourage us all to use these chemical agents in spite of the massive amounts of medical documentation and governmental investigation indicating the serious and very dangerous side effects they possess, in addition to their devastating addictive potential." George Berkley (Harvard University associated review — Nieman Reports)

The National Center for Health Statistics (CDC) revealed the leading causes of death in the USA for 2016. It is interesting how they conveniently left out prescription drugs as a major cause of death. According to a study done by Johns Hopkins, more

LEADING CAUSE OF DEATH IN USA (2016)	
1. Heart Disease	635,260
2. Cancer	598,038
3. Medical Drugs	250,000
4. Accidents (unintentional injuries)	161,374
5. Chronic Lower Respiratory	154,596
6. Stroke	142,142
7. Alzheimer's Disease	116,103
8. Diabetes	80,058
9. Influenza & Pneumonia	51,537
10. Nephritis (Kidney Disease)	50,046

than 250,000 people die every year because of medical mistakes, making it the third leading cause of death.

The most shocking fact in medical history is that the leading cause of death in the U.S. is heart disease, cancer and **PRESCRIPTION DRUGS. Prescription drugs are the third leading cause of death in the United States of America.**

> **"The conventional approach of treating specific symptoms with specific drugs or remedies, without taking into consideration the patient's total condition of health and correcting the underlying causes of his ill health, is as unscientific as it is ineffective."** Paavo Airola, Ph.D., N.D.

If the medicine you choose to take that is prescribed by your medical doctor is supposed to help you get well, but in actuality ends up killing 250,000 people every year who trust it and it tops the chart as the third leading cause of death, then something is terribly wrong. Common sense screams the fact that drugs are not safe and they should be used with extreme caution mostly in emergency situations.

> **"If the medical system were a bank, you wouldn't deposit your money here, because there would be an error every one-in-two to one-in-three times you made a transaction."** Stephen Persell, M.D., Northwestern University's Feinburg School of Medicine

Case Study

I was 16 years of age and had yet to begin my period. Out of concern, my mother insisted that I see a gynecologist. Upon my arrival to the doctor's office, I explained my situation and without question or hesitation, the doctor wrote me a prescription for birth control pills. Although I was somewhat concerned about taking the pills, the gynecologist insisted that my problem was "normal" and that the pills would be the solution. So, I started the pills and started having a period. I went to the gynecologist annually and was written another birth control prescription at every visit.

Four years later, and still on the pills, I began to get concerned for my health. My concern was not so much for my immediate health but, rather, for my future health. As I got older, I realized that being on the birth control pills year after year could not be good for the future of my body. After bringing my concern to the attention of my gynecologist, she said I could try coming off the pills and I would, perhaps, be able to have a period without the aid of the pills. I did as she said and came off the pills. I did not, however, have a period. At the age of 20, after being off the pill and without a period for several months, I decided I had better begin taking the pills again.

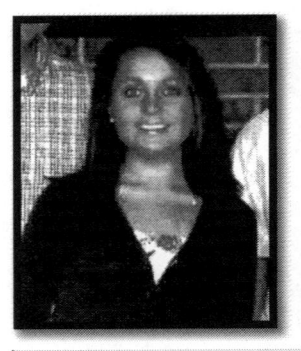

Approximately one year later, I became aware of Dr. Sainsbury and his naturopathic approach to health. I went in for an appointment and he performed an EDS test on me. He explained in detail the natural products he was giving me were to balance and support my endocrine system. After discontinuing the use of my birth control pills and using the natural products from Dr. Sainsbury, I began having a period. Once I finished Dr. Sainsbury's program, I continued to have my period. I am now over a year out of the program, I am on no herbs, pills or products of any sort, and I continue to have my period (like clockwork) every month.

I cannot say enough about Dr. Sainsbury and the way that he has helped teach me the way my body is designed to work. The products he gave me helped my body heal itself, rather than simply concealing the problem with prescription medication. I highly recommend Dr. Sainsbury to anyone. I am a living example of the fact that it works!

Lauren Grier
Rainbow City, Alabama

Horse Urine For Health?

"There is absolutely no reason to use synthetic versions of hormones when there are natural versions available. A natural product will work better in the body and have fewer adverse effects than a synthetic product every time."
David Brownstein, M.D.

The hormone replacement drug Prempro made from pregnant mare's urine is a combination of estrogen and progestin that is reported by JAMA to cause patients to develop Alzheimer's at twice the rate of those taking a placebo. (JAMA 2003;289:2651-2662) The Framingham Heart Study published in the 1985 New England Journal of Medicine showed that women who had taken estrogen were 50 percent more likely to develop heart disease. According to JAMA, a woman increases her risk of breast cancer by 8 percent for each year that she takes combined hormone replacement therapy. (JAMA 283(4):485-491, 2000) And the National Institutes of Health have warned how Prempro increases a woman's risk of breast cancer, heart disease and stroke.

> **"89 percent of doctors rely on drug company salesmen for their information."**
> The Australian Doctor

Prescription medications work by either blocking a receptor site on a cell or poisoning an enzyme. This is why there are side effects. Stanford University's pioneer in cell biology and former professor at the University of Wisconsin's School of Medicine, Bruce Lipton, Ph.D., explains how doctors prescribe synthetic estrogen that does not focus the drug's effects on the intended target tissues. He explains, *"The drug also impacts and disturbs the estrogen receptors of the heart, the blood vessels and the nervous system. Synthetic hormone replacement therapy has been shown to have disturbing side effects that result in cardiovascular disease and neural dysfunctions such as strokes."* He points out why iatrogenic (doctor-caused) illness is a leading cause of death in this country, as we foolishly take drugs to suppress symptoms with no regard as to what the long-term consequences may be. Dr. Otto Sartorius, Director of the Cancer Control Clinic warns, *"Estrogen (and its derivatives) is the fodder on which cancer grows."*

> **"Given that hormone replacement therapy is known to be associated with serious increases in breast cancer, and may pose other risks as well, this trend is disturbing. Why aren't doctors making available the natural, plant-derived forms of estrogen and progesterone, substances that are known to have fewer side effects than their laboratory-produced analogs? The answer reflects the economics of medicine: Since the natural substances are not patentable, there is no incentive for drug companies to study their benefits, and so the vast majority of M.D.s, who get their information about drugs from the drug companies, don't even know about them."** Candace B. Pert, Ph.D., Professor, Georgetown University Medical Center & Author of *Molecules of Emotion*

Some years ago, a book written by Dr. Robert Wilson, *Feminine Forever*, was used as a marketing strategy to promote the use of Hormone Replacement Therapy (HRT) as a cure-all for depressed and menopausal women. Dr. Wilson and his wife Thelma, who was a registered nurse, taught that menopausal symptoms were caused from a woman's ovaries not producing estrogen; therefore, taking synthetic estrogen was the answer. Menopause is a natural change of life when a woman stops menstruating. Dr. Wilson and the pharmaceutical empire would have us believe it is a disease that must be treated with HRT. Entangled in this web of lies was the false theory that cancer, osteoporosis and other dreaded diseases were the result of a lack of estrogen. These scare tactics resulted in massive numbers of women beginning HRT.

> "... much of what is called 'scientific evidence' is really disease-mongering designed to sell more drugs." John Abramson, M.D., Harvard Medical School; Author of *Overdosed America The Broken Promise Of American Medicine*

Study firmly ties hormone use to breast cancer

BY MARILYNN MARCHIONE
Associated Press

SAN ANTONIO — Taking menopause hormones for five years doubles the risk for breast cancer, according to a new analysis of a big federal study that reveals the most dramatic evidence yet of the dangers of these still-popular pills.

Even women who took estrogen and progestin pills for as little as a couple of years had a greater chance of getting cancer.

And when they stopped taking them, their odds quickly improved, returning to a normal risk level roughly two years after quitting.

Collectively, these new findings are likely to end any doubt that the risks outweigh the benefits for most women.

It is clear that breast cancer rates plunged in recent years mainly because millions of women quit hormone therapy and fewer newly menopausal women started on it, said the study's leader, Dr. Rowan Chlebowski of Harbor-UCLA Medical Center in Los Angeles.

SUMMARY

WHAT'S NEW: A new analysis of a big federal women's study more firmly cements the link between menopausal hormones and breast cancer.

FINDINGS: Breast cancer risk doubled when women took estrogen and progestin pills for five years.

Time has an interesting way of proving our ignorance. The truth about hormone replacement therapy began to surface and the Wilsons' teachings began to crumble underneath their feet. Thelma Wilson, who was on HRT, developed breast cancer. After further investigation, Dr. Wilson was paid big bucks by Wyeth Drug Company to market his hormone replacement book. When it was all said and done, Dr. Wilson had received $1.3 million from drug companies for his book encouraging HRT. After the pharmaceutical industry got what they wanted from Dr. Wilson, he was hung out to dry. His own son, Ron, tells how his dad was sued by several drug firms and eventually turned to drugs and alcohol. In 1981, Dr. Wilson committed suicide. JUST SAY NO TO DRUGS.

In the meantime, many women continue their hormone replacement therapy and gain weight as if they were pregnant and ignorantly increase their chances of cancer, Alzheimer's, strokes, blood clots and cardiovascular disease because that's what their doctor prescribed.

When we feed the endocrine system with nutritional support so that the glands can work like they were designed to, symptoms clear up naturally. Many women are deficient in essential fatty acids, which affects the hormones. Evening primrose oil helps balance out hormonal issues

Female Hormone Balancing Support
- Her Formula (suma & maca)
- Endo Glan Plus (endocrine support)
- FHS Formula (homeopathic hormones)
- Ashwagandha
- Holy Basil
- Evening Primrose oil
- Natural Progesterone cream

naturally. It is great for circulation, falling hair, dry skin and loaded with antioxidants. Doesn't that sound like a healthier choice compared to an unnatural drug that has unwanted side effects? Another big culprit causing female problems can be low magnesium and zinc levels. A few natural super-foods that support the adrenals, thyroid and pituitary that help balance the endocrine system are kelp, licorice root, yarrow, dong quai, black cohosh, damiana, ginger, ashwagandha, holy basil, wild yam (natural progesterone cream), suma and maca. An EDS scan will identify which remedies are best for your body chemistry to be balanced and symptom-free.

> "Doctors are always warning their patients about the dangers of consulting 'medical quacks' or resorting to 'unscientific, unproven remedies.' Meanwhile, they have made a living dispensing therapy from their own bag of unproven, unscientific, and often worthless 'cures.'" Robert Mendelsohn, M.D.

Case Study

In March of 2007, my health began to deteriorate. My hair began to fall out and I started having miserable hot flashes around the clock every hour or two, even while sleeping, which made it extremely hard to rest well. I would wake up at 2:15 a.m. every night, and it would take hours for me to get back to sleep.

When I first came to Dr. Sainsbury, I had not had a menstrual cycle in over three months. Prior to my appointment with Dr. Sainsbury, I went in to see my gynecologist to check my hormone levels to see if I was experiencing menopause. The lab work came back completely normal with no signs of menopause.

My beautician, Ava Berry, told me about Reed Sainsbury, a naturopathic doctor who could help with these types of problems. I was somewhat reluctant to try this holistic health care, but decided to give it a shot since my regular doctor had no solution for my problems.

My first visit with Dr. Sainsbury was on May 10, 2007. After an EDS exam, we found that I had several issues. He recommended a few herbal and nutritional formulas (including borage oil, Lunazon & Sumacazon) to bring my body back into balance. I began my nutritional program that same day and have not had one hot flash since!!! It worked that quickly for me. I started having my period again and since being on this program have had one each month. I began sleeping all night within a week. I do not wake up at 2:15 a.m. anymore like I used to. I feel so much better and more rested during the day now. My hair not only stopped falling out but also is so shiny and healthy-looking now. Not only did the problems that I went in for improve, but also my joints that used to ache are better. My skin is no longer dry; it feels like I have lotion on even when I do not. My fingernails do not split and crack anymore; in fact, I have to trim them and I have never had to do this before! Constipation is no longer a problem either.

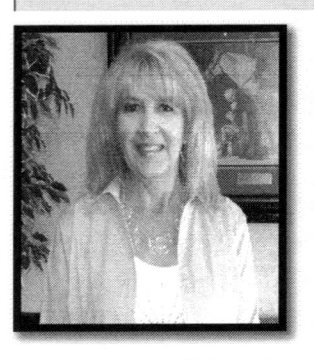

I had previously had a bone density test in 2004 that showed that I had Osteopenia. My GYN doctor prescribed calcium for me but I didn't take it because it caused constipation. In August, I went in for my gynecological visit and another bone density test. When my bone density test came back this year (August 2007), it showed improvement. My doctor was very impressed because he said hardly anyone my age shows improvement. He wanted to know what I had been doing that caused such remarkable improvement. I told him about the Liga-Plus formula and some other natural formulas for bones and joints that Dr. Sainsbury put me on.

After being on Dr. Sainsbury's seven-week program I went back in for another EDS evaluation. Every point that was out of balance at my first appointment checked balanced, near perfect. I am so grateful for the opportunity to have met Dr. Sainsbury and heal my body naturally. Not only do I feel better physically and have more energy but I feel better mentally as well. I feel that my life is in balance. I am on a maintenance schedule now, but if I ever have a feeling of being 'out of balance' again, I know where to go. Thank you, Dr. Sainsbury and Karen, for your help and kindness.

Leigh Reynolds   Hokes Bluff, Alabama

> "Those who have lived the longest seem to be those remote from medical practice." Ruth Wegg, M.D., University of Southern California

Dr. Semmelweis — Killed For Teaching The Truth

Back in the 1800s, before the development of the microscope to see the "unseen microscopic world of germs," there was a doctor named Ignaz Semmelweis. He believed that infection was caused primarily from decaying particles of flesh carried on the hands of the physicians who failed to disinfect their hands after working with cadavers and then touched live patients. He discovered that just soap and water would not kill bacteria causing childbed fever. Dr. Semmelweis insisted that physicians (obstetricians) in his section wash their hands with his special formula he developed, a chlorinated lime solution, to disinfect their hands after working on a cadaver and then moving to a pelvic exam on live patients. After doctors began washing their hands in his sanitizing solution, the mortality rate in his section dropped from 18.3 percent to almost 0.

Simply wash your hands with this special lime solution that kills germs and save lives. What did the medical profession do to show their appreciation for such progress in saving lives? They mocked and ridiculed Dr. Semmelweis for such foolish nonsense. He was cast out and labeled a lunatic because the "science was settled." Taking prescription drugs without addressing the cause and killing 250,000 Americans each year is as absurd as not washing your hands to disinfect them after working on a cadaver and then working on a live patient.

> "History shows us that people who end up changing the world — the great political, social, scientific, technological, artistic, even sports revolutionaries — are always nuts, until they are right, and then they are geniuses." John Elliot

Although Dr. Semmelweis could not prove his theory true because microscopes had not been invented yet and despite the fact that mortality rates dropped considerably when physicians washed their hands in his special chlorinated lime solution, mainstream medicine rejected him for "going against the grain." He was hauled off and put in a Viennese insane asylum, where he was tortured and beaten. On August 13, 1865, 47-year-old, Dr. Semmelweis died from internal injuries sustained from the guards at the asylum.

> "Each progressive spirit is opposed by a thousand mediocre minds appointed to guard the past." Maurice Maeterlinck

Most of his colleagues in medicine and even his own wife and children did not attend his funeral. They killed this doctor because he stood up for what he believed in and even had the success record to prove it, but doctors didn't want to hear the truth. How many ignorant and arrogant doctors today do not want to hear the truth?

It has been said that science and medicine progress funeral by funeral. With the invention of the microscope, we can see why one must disinfect their hands after working with cadavers. Today, Dr. Semmelweis is honored as a medical pioneer and a hospital bears his name. They even turned his childhood home into a museum. This story is tragic, but my purpose for writing this book is to sound another alarm of tragedy that is occurring right now out of arrogance and greed. Just as Dr. Semmelweis was ignored and ridiculed, so is natural health care laughed at and discredited by the pharmaceutical empire, despite people being healed of cancer, arthritis, diabetes, multiple sclerosis and all kinds of diseases by using natural, nontoxic remedies.

Murder By Prescription

FDA Approved Drugs – Recalled – For Harming & Killing People

#	DRUG	CAUSES	#	DRUG	CAUSES
1.	Accutane	birth defects	16.	Omniflox	kidney disfunction
2.	Baycol	kidney failure	17.	Pallodone	stops breathing
3.	Bextra	strokes	18.	Permax	heart valve problems
4.	Cylert	liver damage	19.	Fen-Phen	heart valve disease
5.	Darvocet	toxicity	20.	Posicor	risk of shock
6.	DBI	lactic acidosis	21.	Propulsid	cardiac arrythmias
7.	DES	cancer	22.	PTZ	uncontrollable seizures
8.	Duract	liver damage	23.	Quaalude	seizures
9.	Ergamisol	blood clots	24.	Raplon	bronchospasms
10.	Hismanal	heart complications	25.	Raptiva	brain inflammation
11.	Lotronex	colitis	26.	Raxar	cardiac repolarization
12.	Meridia	heart attack/stroke	27.	Redux	heart valve disease
13.	Merital	anemia	28.	Rezulin	liver failure
14.	Micturin	cardiotoxicity	29.	Seldane	heart problems
15.	Mylotarg	obstruction of veins	30.	Vioxx	heart attack/stroke

"There is nothing so powerful as truth, and often nothing so strange." Daniel Webster, 1782-1852

When the FDA approves a drug, it is supposed to be fully convinced that the drug is both effective and safe, but after seeing how many drugs they claim are safe and then proving otherwise, it appears that we have been paying the fox to guard the hen house. Thousands of people have suffered tremendously and many died after trusting their doctor and taking the drug he or she prescribes. This is just a few of the drugs taken off the market after causing serious harm and death. Be informed before you trust your doctor's latest chemical concoction that the young new pharmaceutical rep told him or her to start prescribing.

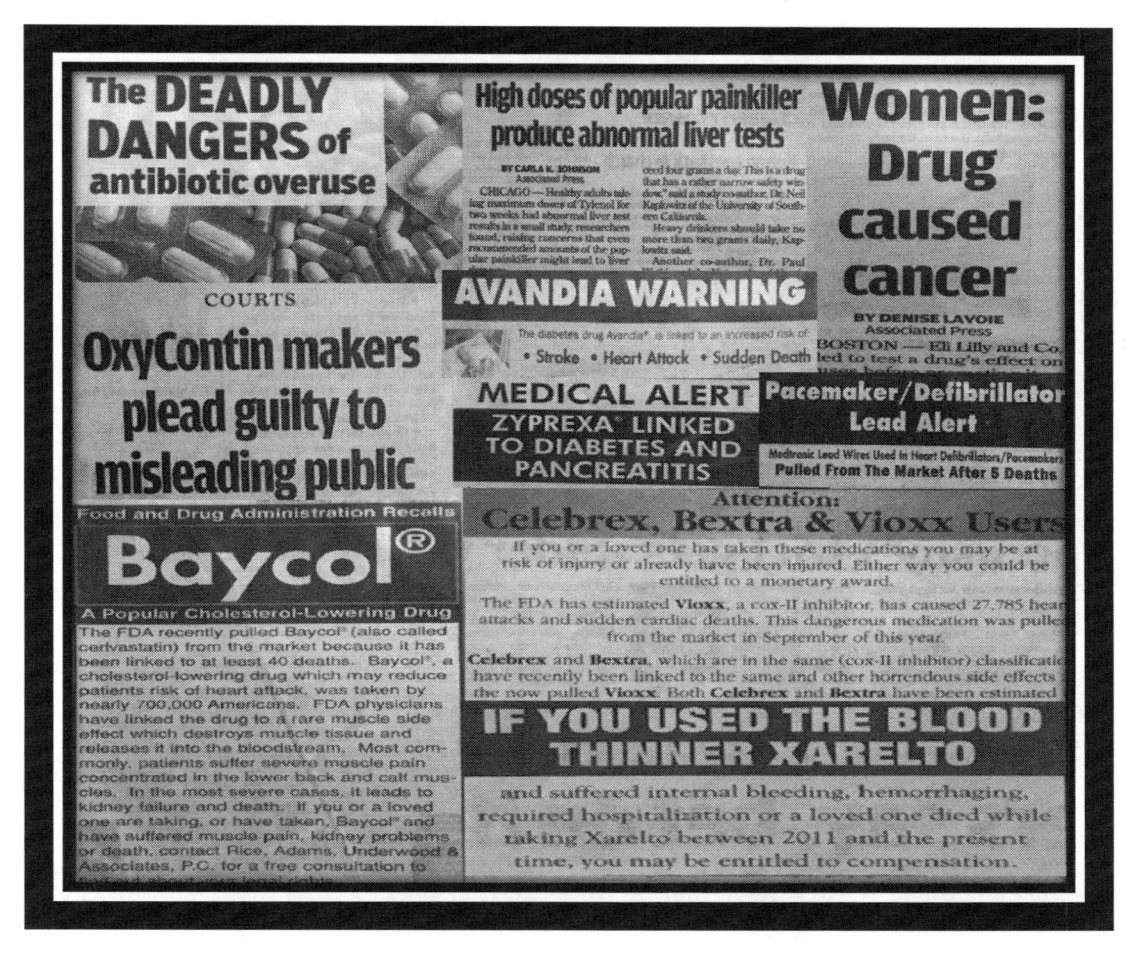

> **"More men die of their medicines than their diseases."** Moliere

These prescriptions were deemed safe at one time until these ticking time bombs exploded and doctors were given orders to stop prescribing the poisonous wonders to their patients. What drugs are you taking now that will be recalled in the future because they harm and kill, even though the FDA has claimed that they are safe?

> "We are made in the image of God ... popping a pill every time we are mentally or physically out of tune is not the answer. Drugs and surgery are powerful tools, when they are not overused, but the notion of simple drug fixes is fundamentally flawed. Every time a drug is introduced into the body to correct function A, it inevitably throws off function B, C or D." Bruce Lipton, Ph.D.

Dr. John Gueriguian of the FDA recommended not allowing the diabetic drug **Rezulin** to be put on the market because it showed no significant advantage over other diabetic drugs and it caused inflammation of the liver. When some key executives complained to senior FDA officials, Dr. Gueriguain was mysteriously removed from the approval process for this drug, and it was allowed to go on the market in 1997. After doctors prescribed over $1.8 billion worth of this liver-destroying drug and it caused more than 400 cases of liver failure along with killing 391 people, the FDA finally took Rezulin off the market in 2004. Dr. Janet McGill told the Los Angeles Times that Warner-Lambert pharmaceutical company, *"Clearly places profits before the lives of patients with diabetes."* It was also reported by the Los Angeles Times that no fewer than 12 of the 22 researchers overseeing the diabetes study were receiving financial grants from Warner-Lambert.

> "For the love of money is the root of all evil..." 1 Timothy 6:10

Do you think researchers that are paid by a drug company to conduct safety trials are going to be completely honest? Big money motivates and manipulates. For more corruption-exposing scandals performed by those dearly trusted researchers, read David Willman's article from the Los Angeles Times, December 7, 2003, "Stealth Merger: Drug Companies and Government Medical Research." Millions of dollars are paid by drug companies to get their products on the market regardless of what the safety trials reveal.

> "If you rush to take it (a new drug), do so with the full knowledge that you are being a guinea pig. The longer a drug is on the market, the more will be known about the side effects." Robert Mendelsohn, M.D.

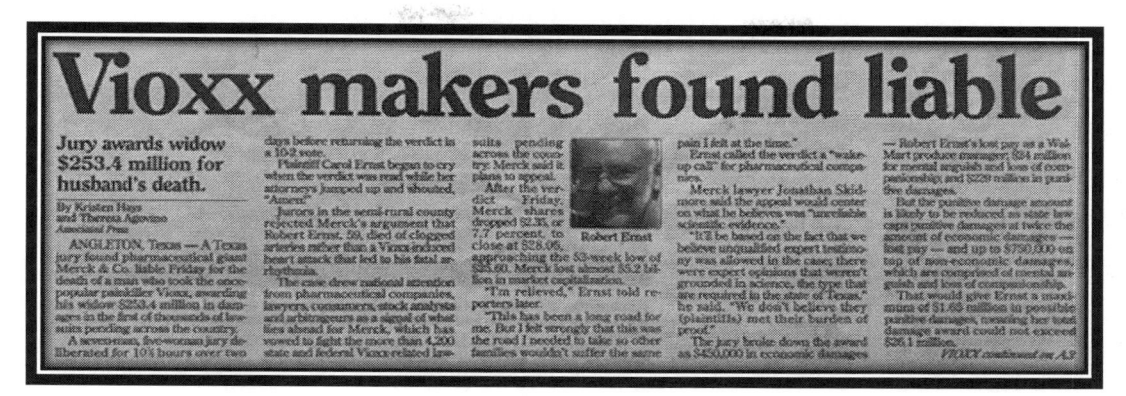

Vioxx – A Killer Drug – Deemed Safe & Effective By FDA

Vioxx makers found liable

Jury awards widow $253.4 million for husband's death.

By Kristen Hays and Theresa Agovino
Associated Press

ANGLETON, Texas — A Texas jury found pharmaceutical giant Merck & Co. liable Friday for the death of a man who took the once-popular painkiller Vioxx, awarding his widow $253.4 million in damages in the first of thousands of lawsuits pending across the country.

A seven-woman, five-woman jury deliberated for 10½ hours over two days before returning the verdict in a 10-2 vote. Plaintiff Carol Ernst began to cry when the verdict was read, while her attorneys jumped up and shouted, "Amen!"

Jurors in the semi-rural county rejected Merck's argument that Robert Ernst, 59, died of clogged arteries rather than a Vioxx-induced heart attack that led to his fatal arrhythmia.

The case drew national attention from pharmaceutical companies, lawyers, consumers, stock analysts and arbitrageurs as a signal of what lies ahead for Merck, which has vowed to fight the more than 4,200 state and federal Vioxx-related lawsuits pending across the country. Merck said it plans to appeal.

After the verdict Friday, Merck shares dropped $2.35, or 7.7 percent, to close at $28.06, approaching the 52-week low of $25.60. Merck lost almost $5.2 billion in market capitalization.

"I'm relieved," Ernst told reporters later.

"This has been a long road for me. But I felt strongly that this was the road I needed to take so other families wouldn't suffer the same pain I felt at the time."

Ernst called the verdict a "wake-up call" for pharmaceutical companies.

Merck lawyer Jonathan Skidmore said the appeal would center on what he believes was "unreliable scientific evidence."

"It'll be based on the fact that we believe unqualified expert testimony was allowed in the case; there were expert opinions that weren't grounded in science, the type that are required in the state of Texas," he said. "We don't believe they (plaintiffs) met their burden of proof."

The jury broke down the award as $450,000 in economic damages — Robert Ernst's lost pay as a Wal-Mart produce manager; $24 million for mental anguish and loss of companionship; and $229 million in punitive damages.

But the punitive damage amount is likely to be reduced as state law caps punitive damages at twice the amount of economic damages — lost pay — and up to $750,000 on top of non-economic damages, which are comprised of mental anguish and loss of companionship.

That would give Ernst a maximum of $1.65 million in possible punitive damages, meaning her total damage award could not exceed $26.1 million.

VIOXX continued on A3

    The FDA showed that people taking **Vioxx** increased their risk of heart attack by nearly 400 percent! Get rid of your arthritis pain and die of a heart attack. Who in their right mind would risk this? The truth of the matter is, when you start researching the possible side effects from different drugs, the wise person is scared into using an alternative, natural and safe approach.

> "The people in charge (FDA officials) don't say, 'Should we approve this drug? They say, 'Hey, how can we get this drug approved?'" Michael Elashoff (Ex-FDA Biostatistician)

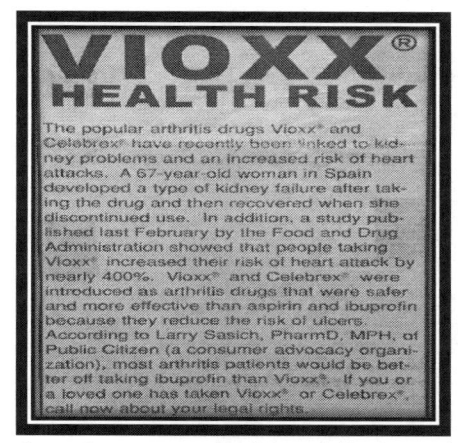

VIOXX® HEALTH RISK

The popular arthritis drugs Vioxx® and Celebrex® have recently been linked to kidney problems and an increased risk of heart attacks. A 67-year-old woman in Spain developed a type of kidney failure after taking the drug and then recovered when she discontinued use. In addition, a study published last February by the Food and Drug Administration showed that people taking Vioxx® increased their risk of heart attack by nearly 400%. Vioxx® and Celebrex® were introduced as arthritis drugs that were safer and more effective than aspirin and ibuprofen because they reduce the risk of ulcers. According to Larry Sasich, PharmD, MPH, of Public Citizen (a consumer advocacy organization), most arthritis patients would be better off taking ibuprofin than Vioxx®. If you or a loved one has taken Vioxx® or Celebrex®, call now about your legal rights.

    The Associated Press launched a whistle-blowing article by FDA scientist Dr. David Graham on January 3, 2005. Dr. Graham revealed the number of Americans who died from heart attacks or whom Vioxx seriously injured was 139,000, not the original, low, 28,000 estimate. In September 2004, the FDA finally pulled this killer from the market. The Los Angeles Times even reported that witnesses had told the Senate Panel that Merck & Co. and the FDA knew about the possible serious adverse effects Vioxx could have on the heart, but they approved it while ignoring the risks. Once again, our tax dollars pay for the fox to guard the henhouse, while innocent Americans suffer and die.

> **"We are prone to thinking of drug abuse in terms of the male population and illicit drugs such as heroin, cocaine, and marijuana. It may surprise you to learn that a greater problem exists with millions of women dependent on legal prescription drugs."** Robert Mendelsohn, M.D.

It is interesting to note that most drugs are not removed from the market until they have reached a high enough financial status to be worth the manufacture's efforts. For example, Merck spent $160.8 million advertising Vioxx! So how much money did Vioxx make before it was pulled from the market in September 2004? During the five years of doctors prescribing Vioxx to their trusting patients, it was a $2.5 billion grand slam! No wonder drug companies can afford to pay out millions to people who file lawsuits when loved ones are harmed or killed from the dangerous poisons that are supposed to help you feel better, but unfortunately cause heart attacks, strokes and death. What happened to our doctors swearing an oath to "First do no harm?" Why is it that doctors who prescribe these deadly drugs are not held accountable?

Hippocratic Or Hypocritical?

> **"The oath of Hippocrates requires that I administer no poisons to my patients even if I am requested to do so. The ancient teacher also advised his students that the first law of healing was, 'Above all, don't make things worse.' In a report from the World Health Organization, we are advised that one of every four people who die in hospitals is killed by the drugs he or she is prescribed. It is believed that this is the result of the physicians being unfamiliar with the dangers of the new drugs, which they freely prescribe. The 'pill for every ill' approach to disease has backfired. We are killing as many people or more with the 'cure' as does the unchecked disease."** Dr. Irving Stone, 1903-1989

Medical doctors take what is known as the Hippocratic Oath and promise to (primum non nocere) *"First do no harm."* Hippocrates, the father of medicine, was an herbalist and nutritionist. He believed in your food being your medicine. He would be turning over in his grave if he knew that medical doctors swear an oath on his name to not administer anything harmful and then turn around and prescribe toxic drugs that kill 250,000 Americans every year!

> **"My People are destroyed for lack of knowledge."** Hosea 4:6 Holy Bible

One of our clients went in for a shoulder operation. The doctors had him on a combination of drugs that were contraindicated with anesthesia but failed to have him stop taking them before his operation. His body could not handle it, and the chemical drugs exploded in him like a science experiment. When he woke up after surgery, it was as if he had suffered a stroke. His speech was slurred, he was dizzy, and his muscles were extremely weak. His doctor assured him the anesthesia would soon wear off and that he would be back to normal. After days, weeks and months of no improvement they began running tests to find out what was wrong. He was later diagnosed with Lou Gehrig's disease. Could this have been prevented?

> **"It's easier to fool people than to convince them that they have been fooled."** Mark Twain

Medical Myths Of The Past

Before 1976, all medical books stated that the "thymus gland atrophies at puberty," implying that the body no longer needs it. When the 1980s came along, our medical scientists said, "Uh, we made a mistake, that thing called the thymus gland, well it turns out that it is actually the boss of your immune system."

Years ago, Acrodynia or Pink disease caused high blood pressure and tachycardia, mostly in children. Doctors administered calomel, a chloride of mercury, to babies to reduce teething pains because it softened the gums. Once they realized mercury was a poison and stopped using calomel, Pink disease disappeared.

> **"Arrogant ignorance has followed science and medicine throughout history."**
> James P. Carter, M.D., Professor of Nutrition, Tulane University

Fifty years ago, medical doctors prescribed PCP, also known as "Angel Dust," and LSD. Then came heroin, the first synthetic version of opium. It was portrayed to be non-addictive cough medicine by Bayer Pharmaceutical Company. It was just a matter of time before it was discovered to be an addictive life-destroyer. The streets are full of these drugs brought to us by medical science. And just to set the record straight, hydrocodone, an opiate prescription used for pain, is synthetic heroin. The brain and the body see this drug the same way they see heroin. When doctors prescribe opioid medications, they are creating heroin addicts.

> "There are many examples in the history of medicine where routine use of pharmaceutical products and other medical interventions is accepted as 'standard of care' for a period of time before they are found to be flat-out wrong and toxic to human health." Dr. Joseph Mercola

Eli Lilly, the founder of Prozac, made over $200 million every month off Prozac sales alone in the 1990s until its patent expired in 2001, allowing generic versions of Prozac to become available. The antidepressant drug is one of the biggest sellers of all time, bringing in more than $20 billion. Despite over 20,000 Prozac related suicides since 1987, according to the FDA's own analysis, the drug remains on the market.

> "A drug without toxic side effects is no drug at all." Eli Lilly

Removing The Nails In The Tire

Disease is really two words, DIS-EASE. Something is not at ease; it's out of balance. If you have a nail in your car tire, who wants to treat the symptoms by continuing to put air in it? Obviously, the smart thing to do is to remove the cause, which is usually a nail, and patch the hole. In health

Two Main Causes Of Disease
1. **Malnutrition** - 16 vitamins, 60 minerals, 12 essential amino acids & 3 essential fatty acids
2. **Toxins** - metals, pesticides, chemicals, Lyme disease, parasites, mold, fungi, yeast, viruses, bacteria, radiation, EMFs, emotions & stress

care, we want to remove the cause and fix the problem. We want to identify what is causing you to be out of balance and correct that cause, thus eliminating the dis-ease. Nutritional deficiencies and toxins are the two major causes for dis-ease. When you take a drug and your body attempts to break it down, you are left with an acidic, toxic, poisonous residue for your liver and kidneys to deal with, and this is one reason we are seeing more and more people needing dialysis.

> "As a young medical student, and even as a young doctor, I naively believed that the army of detail men who were on the road representing drug manufacturers were there to help me save lives. It didn't take me long to realize that this wasn't the primary motive of pharmaceutical manufacturers. They're out to make money and to make everyone think their products will save lives. ... I watched detail men march in my office ... Of course, they knew and I knew that many of these drugs were dangerous,

untested on humans, and possibly ineffective for the purpose for which they were to be prescribed. As I got to know them better, many of them confessed that what they were doing made them sick." Robert Mendelsohn, M.D.

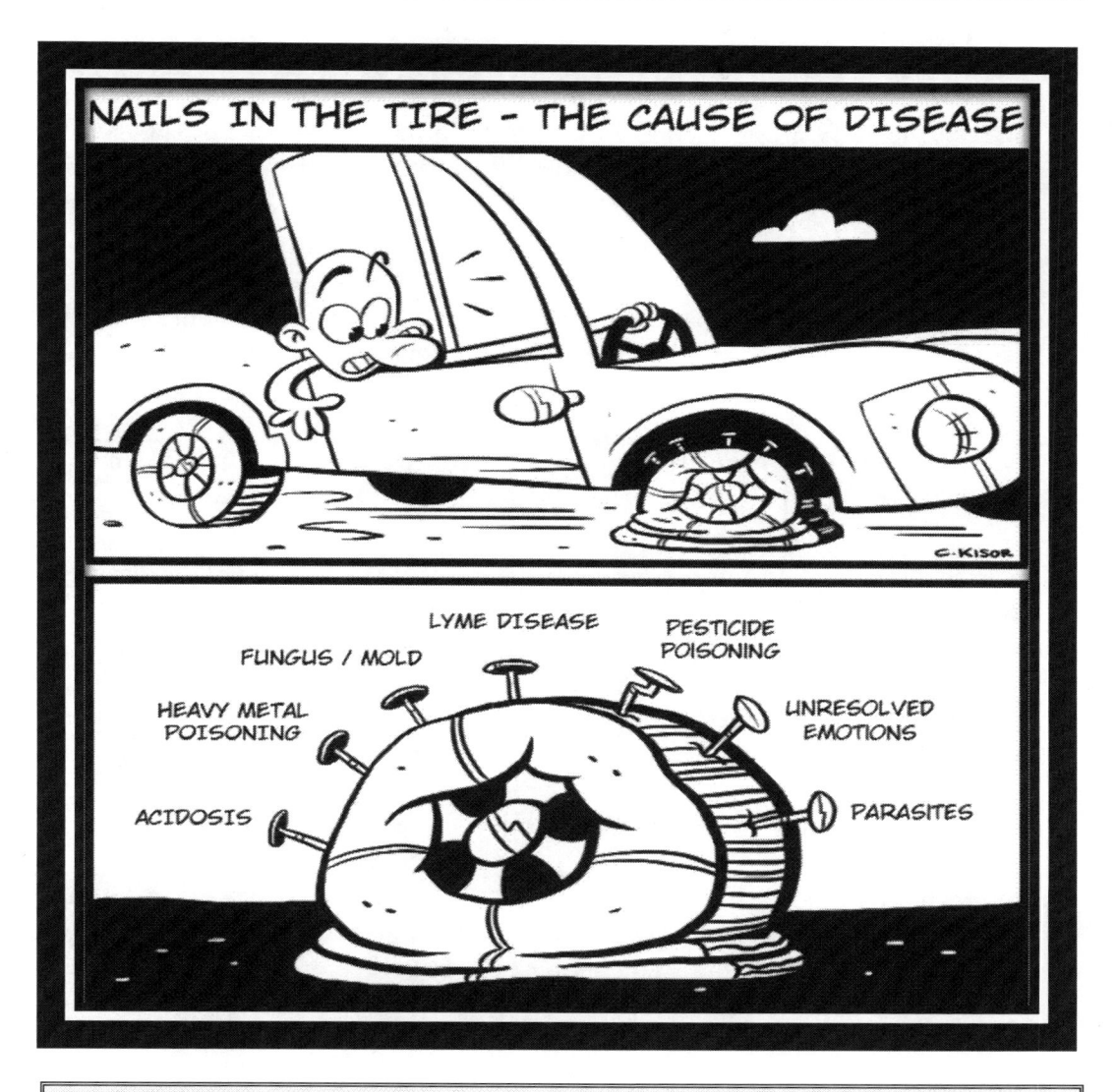

NAILS IN THE TIRE - THE CAUSE OF DISEASE

- FUNGUS / MOLD
- LYME DISEASE
- PESTICIDE POISONING
- HEAVY METAL POISONING
- UNRESOLVED EMOTIONS
- ACIDOSIS
- PARASITES

"You need to be aware that modern medicine is biased, largely unscientific, extremely dangerous, and ignorant of therapies that really can improve your health with virtually no risk." Julian Whitaker, M.D., Whitaker Wellness Institute

According to The Journal of the American Medical Association (JAMA), in 2002, a group of Harvard University professors warned physicians not to prescribe new drugs because their safety had not been proven, despite FDA approval. To support the warning, they pointed out that adverse drug reactions from FDA-approved drugs are the leading cause of death in America.

> "How modern medicine has come to be the No. 1 killer in North America is as incredible as it is horrifying. Doctors certainly don't think of themselves as killers, but as long as they promote toxic drugs and don't learn non-toxic options, they are pulling the trigger on helpless patients." Carolyn Dean, M.D.

The only real differences between what we label a drug versus a poison are dosages and intent. Understand that drugs cannot build new tissue. Only food can do that, and yes, herbs are food. Herbs are loaded with nutrition, including minerals, vitamins, amino acids, fatty acids and enzymes.

> "If all the medicine in the world were thrown into the sea, it would be bad for the fish and good for humanity." Dr. O.W. Holmes, Harvard University

The human body runs on nutrients, not drugs. Like a gallon of gasoline that has the potential to thrust 3,000-pound automobiles 6 miles into the air when extracted in the right form, so do herbs. When combined with organic, whole, living foods and homeopathic remedies, healing miracles become possible. These living plants are packed with antioxidants and contain the vibratory energy frequencies that are the tools for cells to cleanse, nourish and heal the body.

The Paradox Of Modern Medicine

> "If modern medicine really cares about the patients it treats, it shouldn't continue to use questionable drugs and procedures until there is proof that they do kill people; it should be refusing to use them until there is proof that they don't." Robert Mendelsohn, M.D.

JUST SAY NO TO DRUGS. They are too risky. In emergency situations, a drug may be needed to save a life or help you pull through an acute trauma, but to take them long term is playing with fire. When it comes to your health, you deserve something that is (1) SAFE and (2) EFFECTIVE. The facts are, drugs are (1) DANGEROUS and (2) many times INEFFECTIVE with adverse side effects and (3) sometimes FATAL. You are responsible for you; however, some people bow down and worship graven images, even doctors. Wake up to the sad fact that the first thing a smart doctor does is buy malpractice insurance. Why? Because he knows the drugs he or she will be prescribing for you and your loved ones are dangerous, risky, will have adverse side effects and may even kill you.

WARNING: Drugs Deplete Vitamins & Minerals From The Body

DRUG	VITAMIN OR MINERAL DEPLETION
Diabetic medication	B12, B6, CoQ10, zinc, Mag, Pot & Folic acid
Cholesterol (Statins)	CoQ10
Beta Blockers	CoQ10, melatonin
Acid Reflux	B12, Vit D, Calcium
Constipation medication	Vitamins A, D, E & K, calcium, iron, zinc
Antidepressants	Sodium, folic acid, melatonin
Birth Control Pills	B2, B6, B12, C, Zinc, Cal, Mag, Folic Acid
Antibiotics	Inositol, Cal, Mag, Pot, folic acid, all vitamins
Pain medication	Folic acid, Zinc, Vit C, Glutathione
Osteoporosis drugs	Calcium
Thyroid medication	Calcium
Ulcer Drugs	B12, D, calcium, iron, zinc, folic acid

> "Our figures show approximately four and one half million hospital admissions annually due to the adverse reactions to drugs. Further, the average hospital patient has as much as thirty percent chance, depending how long he is in, of doubling his stay due to adverse drug reactions." Milton Silverman, M.D., Professor of Pharmacology, University of California

Prescription Drugs — A Vicious Disease Cycle

Doctor, what caused my diabetes? Most people never connect the dots to their drug-taking puzzle. Young children receive the hepatitis B vaccine at birth, which contains 250 mcg of aluminum, which is 5 times the safety dose level for an adult! The toxic vaccine ingredients cause inflammation and the child begins having ear infections, so an antibiotic is prescribed that causes severe diaper rash due to yeast infection. Then the child is diagnosed with asthma. The doctor prescribes an inhaler and steroid drugs to help them breathe, which causes more yeast infections. After years of drug abuse with an inhaler, the steroid drugs exhaust the adrenal glands, which triggers blood sugar complications. The pancreas cannot keep up with the body's insulin demand nor tolerate the typical American high sugar/grain diet (toaster pastries, pancakes, waffles, toast, cold cereals, etc.), and the poor child is diagnosed with diabetes. Now the doctor displays his dis-ease maintenance plan and instructs the parent how to give diabetic medication or insulin shots. No adrenal, liver and pancreas support is ever mentioned or prescribed. Why? Those are the organs and glands that malfunction when the blood sugar is unstable. The cause is never corrected in mainstream medicine because if it were, the body would no longer need expensive medication to maintain disease.

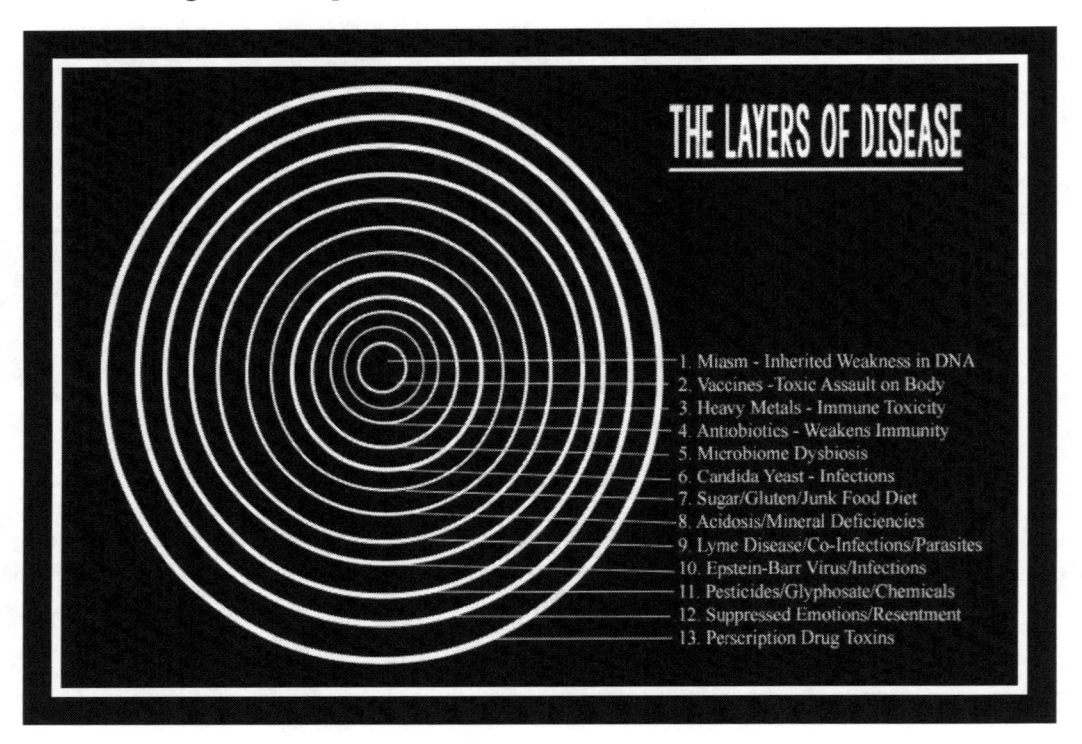

THE LAYERS OF DISEASE

1. Miasm - Inherited Weakness in DNA
2. Vaccines - Toxic Assault on Body
3. Heavy Metals - Immune Toxicity
4. Antiobiotics - Weakens Immunity
5. Microbiome Dysbiosis
6. Candida Yeast - Infections
7. Sugar/Gluten/Junk Food Diet
8. Acidosis/Mineral Deficiencies
9. Lyme Disease/Co-Infections/Parasites
10. Epstein-Barr Virus/Infections
11. Pesticides/Glyphosate/Chemicals
12. Suppressed Emotions/Resentment
13. Perscription Drug Toxins

"Drug companies freely offer this 'education' so they can persuade doctors to 'push' their products. It is evident that the massive quantities of drugs prescribed in this country violate the Hippocratic Oath taken by all doctors to 'First do no harm.' We have been programmed by pharmaceutical corporations to become a nation of prescription drug-popping junkies with tragic results. We need to step back and incorporate the discoveries of quantum physics into biomedicine so that we can create a new, safer system of medicine that is attuned to the laws of Nature." Bruce Lipton, Ph.D.

Heroes In The Emergency Room

Do not be mistaken; there is a time and place for modern medicine. Accidents bring mangled and hurt bodies into emergency rooms on stretchers. Skilled doctors work fast and effectively to give each individual the very best to repair damage. Their knowledge and skills alleviate pain and suffering and save many lives. In some instances, surgery is absolutely necessary, and our emergency room physicians are brilliant geniuses when it comes to patching and mending things back together. I have great respect and appreciation for all those who work in emergency rooms. Thank you for all you do.

If a person undergoes a kidney or heart transplant, the body's T cells will recognize the organ as an illegal alien and begin attacking it because it does not have the proper identification to be in the body. Your cells are highly intelligent and almost every cell has a protein molecule (MHC), like a flag on a ship to indicate which army he represents, so his immune system will know whether he is friend or foe. Doctors administer a drug called cyclosporine, which suppresses the body's immune system from rejecting the life-saving organ so you can live. This type of life-saving emergency medicine is truly awesome and doctors and drug companies that have managed to manufacture drugs like cyclosporine to help save lives deserve to be applauded as well. To them we give credit and say thank you.

> **"A doctor's main focus should always be to get people off drugs and onto dietary supplements."** Carolyn Dean, M.D., N.D.

The problem comes when our non-emergency room physicians begin and continue to hand out toxic, cell-harming drugs for dis-ease maintenance year after year as the poor patient gets sicker and sicker. Doctors who never focus on addressing the cause of dis-ease with nutrition and detoxification routes are doing their patients a great disservice.

> **"What hope is there for medical science to ever become a true science when the entire structure of medical knowledge is built around the idea that there is an entity called disease which can be expelled when the right drug is found?"** John H. Tilden, M.D.

The Cancer Industry

Larry Dossey, M.D., former chief of staff of Medical City, Dallas Hospital sounds the alarm for us to wake up.

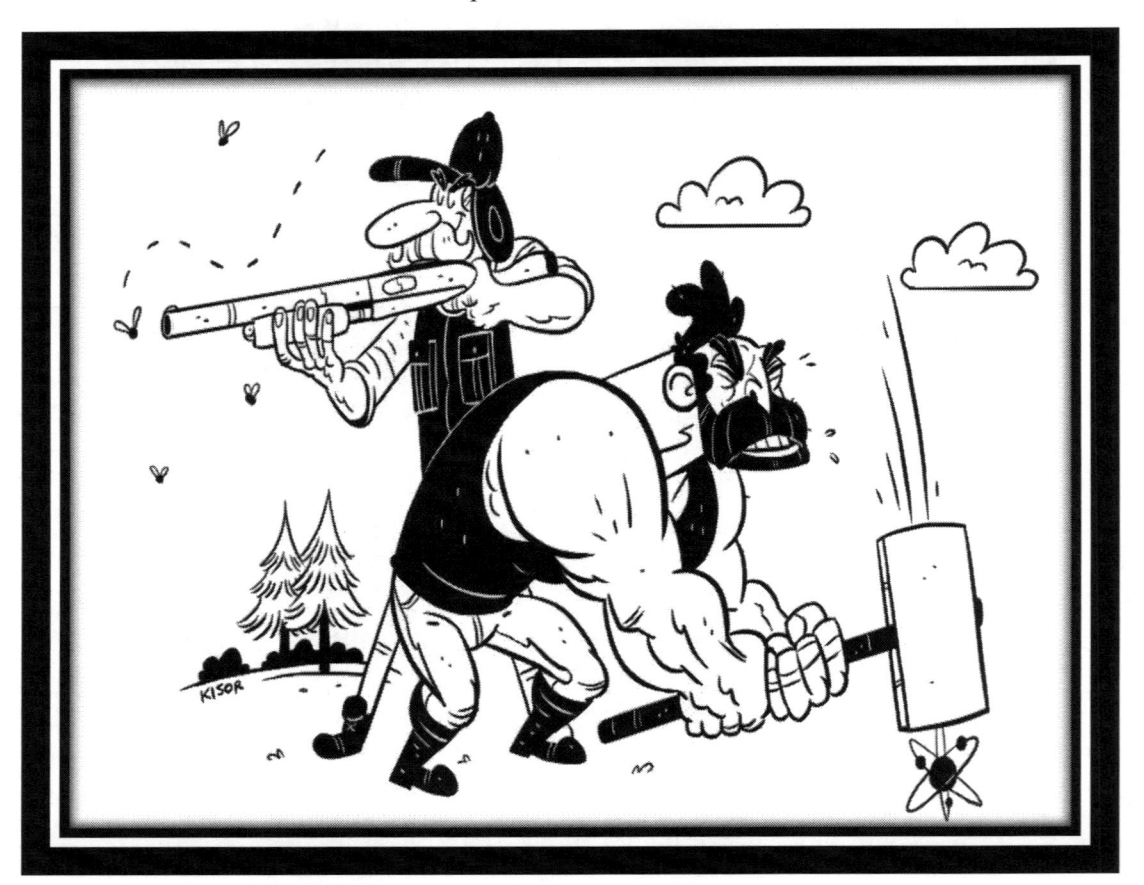

"One does not kill flies with shotguns nor manipulate electrons with hammers; and neither will many human maladies be 'fixable' with our current shotguns and hammers, our drugs and surgical procedures." Larry Dossey, M.D.

Every year, 14 million people worldwide hear the words, "You have cancer." Every day, 1,620 people die of cancer here in the U.S. That's almost 600,000 a year. A hundred years ago, about 1 in 80 Americans were diagnosed with cancer, but now, according to the World Health Organization (WHO), 50 percent of men and 1 in 3 women will be diagnosed with cancer.

> **"My studies have proved conclusively that untreated cancer victims actually live up to four times longer than treated individuals …. Beyond a shadow of a doubt, radical surgery on cancer patients does more harm than good."** Dr. Hardin Jones, University of California

President Richard Nixon declared war on cancer back in 1971 and promised America we would have a cure within five years. He lied. After $200 billion spent on research and $1 trillion spent on therapy, we are losing the war.

> **"To the cancer establishment, a cancer patient is a profit center. The actual clinical and scientific evidence does not support the claims of the cancer industry. Conventional cancer treatments are in place as the laws of the land because they pay, not heal, the best. Decades of the politics-of-cancer-as-usual have kept you from knowing this, and will continue to do so unless you wake up to their reality."** John Diamond, M.D., & Lee Cowden, M.D.

Clifton Leaf, executive editor of Fortune magazine, explains in his March 2004 article, "Losing the War on Cancer," that hundreds of millions of dollars are being wasted by drug companies in pre-clinical models of human cancer. Leaf points out that just because a drug can shrink a tumor doesn't improve a person's chances of survival. What difference does it make if we can shrink tumors but the patient dies? And to make matters worse, the cancer establishment claims chemotherapy was effective if the patient lives at least five years past treatment. It does not matter the quality of life and if he dies one day later after five years, they still claim the cancer treatment was effective.

WHAT DO YOU THINK OF THE WAR ON CANCER?
- "… Largely a fraud." Linus Pauling, Ph.D., twice Nobel laureate
- "… a qualified failure." John Bailar, M.D., Ph.D., former editor of the Journal of the National Cancer Institute
- "A medical Vietnam." Donald Kennedy, former President of Stanford University
- "A bunch of sh_t." James Watson, Ph.D., Nobel laureate, co-discoverer of the DNA code

We are looking for a cure in the wrong place. No man-made chemical drug will ever cure cancer. Believing in such a fairy tale is what the pharmaceutical industry wants you to put your faith and money into. It's their golden calf. You can't cut, burn, kill, drug and radiate your way to good health. It's impossible. Do I sound like a raving lunatic? Good, because so did our founding forefathers when they declared war and won our freedom July 4, 1776. People thought Benjamin Franklin was crazy when he tried to tell everyone about electricity, and they did the same with Thomas Edison when he talked about doing away with candles and using light bulbs. In fact, every great invention or discovery you benefit from was probably laughed and scoffed at before it became popular.

> **"There is only one thing more powerful than all the armies of the world, that is an idea whose time has come."** Victor Hugo

It's time to transform modern cancer treatments from the kill, kill, kill approach with radiation and chemotherapy to strengthening the immune system so it can do what God designed it to do, eradicate abnormal cancerous cells. The foundation for a strong immune system starts with the microbiome in the gut. This is where 80 percent of the immune system originates. Dr. Ryke Geerd Hamer with his "New German Medicine" taught that cancer is not a disease, but a survival mechanism of the body designed to remove toxins that are causing harm.

> **"If everyone is thinking alike, then no one is thinking."** Benjamin Franklin

Cancer Is Not A Genetic Disease, It's A Metabolic Disease

One of the greatest myths about cancer, autism or any other disease is that bad genes predetermine your health. Russian researchers studied adopted children, who did not know they were adopted, and reported that they developed "inherited diseases" from the adopted parents without having any genetic connection. The true cause of disease is our lifestyle, eating habits and how we deal with stress — basically, our learned behavior, not bad genetics.

The more money we raise for cancer research, the more cancer we seem to get, says Boston College professor Dr. Thomas Seyfried, who shatters the gene theory myth in his book, *Cancer as a Metabolic Disease,* while modern medicine still focuses their money and research in the wrong direction, on gene mutations. Dr. Seyfried explains that the gene dogma has indoctrinated physicians and scientists to focus their research on gene mutations, which are the effects and not the cause of cancer. Dr. Seyfried, explains, "If you take the nucleus from the normal cell and put it into the tumor cell's cytoplasm, you get dead cells or tumor cells.

This is the opposite of what you would expect if cancer were a nuclear-driven genetic disease."

> "Preventive oncology is an oxymoron. We have so much information on cancer prevention, which we are not using. I wouldn't give a damn if we didn't do any more research for the next fifty years." Samuel Epstein, M.D., Professor of Occupational Medicine, The School of Public Health, University of Chicago

Mammograms Cause Cancer

The American Cancer Society recommends all women over the age of 45 receive mammograms on an annual basis. Researchers state that mammograms are only 58 percent effective in detecting internal breast abnormalities. The dilemma is, squeezing your breast between two solid plates with 50 pounds of pressure could possibly rupture a tumor and spread cancer cells to other areas, making your situation considerably worse. Every compression during a mammogram procedure leads to microscopic ruptures in the breast tissue and if there is cancer, this is the worst thing you could do! Dr. Russell Blaylock warns, "Doctors are taught that once a lump is found, you don't press it — not even during an examination — because you will cause the cancer cells to spread." Dr. Raymond Hilu, M.D., medical director of the Hilu Institute in Spain, explains that compressing potentially cancerous breast tissue risks unleashing a torrent of cancer cells into other tissue and possibly the blood. Instead of mammograms, Dr. Hilu recommends high-resolution blood analysis (HRB), which amplifies the blood up to 18,000 times to detect immune dysfunction, heavy metal poisoning and free radical damage. It is a safer, nontoxic way of diagnosing what's occurring in the body.

> "I am dying with the help of too many physicians." Alexander the Great 356–323 B.C.

Mammograms emit harmful ionizing radiation. In fact, one single mammogram emits 1,000 times the amount of radiation of a typical chest X-ray. The National Cancer Institute estimates that among women under the age of 35, routine mammograms cause about 75 new cases of breast cancer for every 15 they actually

Cancer Screening Alternatives
1. Thermography
2. High Resolution Blood (HRB)
3. Anti-Malignin Antibody In Serum (AMAS)
4. Human Chorionic Gonadotropin (HCG) Urine Immunoassay
5. Oncoblot Test
6. Thymidine Kinase Test
7. Nagalase Test

identify. Researchers caution that mammograms are 300 to 400 percent more carcinogenic than the high-energy radiation given off by atomic bombs.

The British Medical Journal reports that at least 20 percent of all mammograms issue false positives and the largest study ever done, involving 90,000 women that lasted 25 years, found that death rates from breast cancer were the same in women who got mammograms as those who didn't.

> **"In conclusion, our data show that annual mammography does not result in a reduction in breast cancer-specific mortality. The data suggest that the value of mammography screening should be reassessed."** British Medical Journal

We all have cancer cells. Since the day we were born, our immune system has been eradicating mutated, damaged cancerous cells. Our bodies produce over 100,000 cancer cells every day. Cancer cells do not show up in standard tests until they have multiplied to several billion. It is estimated that cancer occurs six to 10 times in a person's lifetime. The strength of your immune system determines whether you are clinically diagnosed or not. Most women have naturally occurring cancer cells in their breasts, and men have them in their prostates. Many cancers are extremely slow-growing, taking about 10 years to become the size of a pinhead and another 10 to 20 years or more to grow to the size of a pea, then to a grape. Researchers estimate that it takes breast cancer seven to 10 years before it can even be diagnosed. Research published in the International Journal of Cancer after a 25-year study concludes that 80 percent of early stage breast cancers do not progress to invasive breast cancers even after 20 years.

> **"Breast Cancer Awareness Month was actually initiated by the companies that make Tamoxifen. The devices for mammograms are made by General Electric, and General Electric is in a relationship with the people behind Breast Cancer Awareness Month, so there is a huge industry that is invested in breast cancer. Although the goal is noble, to me it is obscene that these companies are using the symbol of the pink ribbon for commercial purposes only. Very few dollars ever make it to really help women."** Dr. Sherrill Sellman, Author of *What Women Must Know to Protect their Daughters from Breast Cancer*

Just as jabbing a needle into a water balloon is a sure way to cause leakage, so is piercing a mass in the breast with a needle biopsy. If there is cancer, now those cells can spread. Do we really want this? The body forms a tumor to encase abnormal cells and keep them from spreading and then we turn around and puncture it so they can flood into other areas.

Men who have PSA tests for prostate cancer and women who undergo mammograms receive many "false positives." Many experts conclude that these tests pose more risks than benefits. Even the National Cancer Institute warns that women under 35 who have mammograms are exposing themselves to unnecessary radiation and trauma to the breast tissue that increases their risks of developing cancer. Statistics show that a third of all patients diagnosed with breast cancer never had it in the first place. They were false positives and treated unnecessarily.

> **"Mammograms increase the risk for developing breast cancer & raise the risk of spreading or metastasizing an existing growth."** Dr. Charles B. Simone

Safer and more accurate testing procedures are infrared thermograms. Unlike mammograms that can only detect a tumor after it has reached a certain size, thermography utilizes the power of infrared heat to detect physiological abnormalities or "hot spots" indicative of possible cancer. This is a safer option for cancer detection with no mechanical pressure or radiation. Dr. Christine Northrup, M.D., informs *"The most promising aspect of thermography is its ability to spot anomalies years before mammography. With thermography as your regular screening tool, it's likely that you would have the opportunity to make adjustments to your diet, beliefs, and lifestyle to transform your cells before they became cancerous. Talk about true prevention."* Thermography can also detect signs of cancer as much as 10 times earlier than either mammography or a physical exam.

> **"Thousands of women are being deceived by the national cancer program. They are led to believe that early detection of cancer will save their breasts. Half of the women with 'early' breast cancer are having mastectomies that might be later proven unnecessary. It is definitely a false promise that if due to some kind of screening the cancer is detected early and the woman's breast can be saved!"** Dr. Michael Baum, University College Hospital in London

Anti-malignin antibody in serum testing (AMAS) is another cancer screening method that can detect any type of cancer with 95 percent accuracy after one test and over 99 percent accuracy after two tests. We all have AMAS antibodies in our blood serum. It becomes elevated when cancer starts to spread, thus making it the earliest cancer detection test available. It is nontoxic and extremely accurate.

> "Cancer is the cure. People don't understand that. Cancer is there to save your life. When your body is so toxic that you are going to die of the poison, the body builds a bag and stuffs all the poison in there and locks it up — the tumor." Dr. Leonard Coldwell

Modern medicine likes to ridicule any theory or treatment plan using natural remedies to build and balance your immune system because if they can't patent a drug and make billions, they are not interested in the treatment, regardless of how successful it may be. And when the check they draw each week depends upon them not understanding something, then that becomes the leash that leads them to research and study only topics that line up with that source of money. The average cancer treatment plan costs over $200,000 a year. Gleevec, a drug to treat leukemia, costs roughly $70,000 to administer.

According to California oncologist Dr. Peter Eisenberg, oncologists receive a financial kickback every time they prescribe chemotherapy drugs. He explains, *"The significant amount of our revenue comes from the profit, if you will, that we make from selling the drugs. ... so the pressure is frankly on to make money by selling medications."* Perhaps if there were no incentive to make a profit on chemotherapy, oncologists wouldn't be so eager to prescribe it for cancer treatment. What would happen if oncologists started receiving a kickback every time they recommended Graviola, Essiac tea, Laetrile, frankincense oil, Vitamin C and turmeric?

> "The medical profession would have abolished slash-burn-and-poison (surgery, radiation and chemotherapy) treatment long ago because the records of success simply aren't there. But the profits are, and these are too alluring for those in the cancer industry to turn down." Burton Goldberg, Author of *An Alternative Medicine Definitive Guide to Cancer*

Is The PSA Test For Prostate Cancer Reliable Or Necessary?

The Prostate Specific Antigen (PSA) test is usually recommended for men over the age of 50 to screen for cancer. The problem is, the PSA test is not always accurate, yielding at least 20 percent false positives. The PSA protein is present in every prostate and a reading above 4 is considered "dangerous." However, a man could have a reading of 0.5 and still have cancer while a reading of 11 may indicate no cancer at all, which makes this test very confusing and misleading. According to several medical journals, the majority of prostate cancer will never progress to a clinically meaningful stage if left undiagnosed and untreated during a man's lifetime. And the discoverer of the PSA test, Richard Ablin, Ph.D., in his book, *The Great Prostate Hoax,* explains how the PSA screening causes serious harm to millions of men as they go through unnecessary and debilitating treatments and has become a public health disaster. Dr. Ablin himself has never had a PSA test and informs that there is no reason for a healthy man to do so because PSA, contrary to what you've been told, doesn't work as a cancer indicator, yet we spend over $3 billion a year in the U.S. on this unnecessary test.

> **"I never dreamed that my discovery four decades ago would lead to such a profit-driven public health disaster. ... The test is hardly more effective than a coin toss."** Richard Ablin, Ph.D. (Discoverer of the PSA Test)

American men have a 16 percent lifetime chance of being diagnosed with prostate cancer but only a 3 percent chance of dying from it. The fact is, the majority of prostate cancers grow very slowly. Many factors such as stress, a simple infection, constipation, a long bike ride, recent sexual activity, low testosterone/high estrogen, consumption of dairy and the use of over-the-counter drugs such as ibuprofen can elevate PSA numbers. When the PSA levels are elevated, most doctors assume the worse and begin procedures that may be unnecessary and have disastrous side effects. Dr. Thomas Stamey published the original study on PSA screening in the New England Journal of Medicine, declaring, *"Our study raises a very serious question of whether a man should even use the PSA test for prostate cancer screening anymore."* He went on to say, *"I removed a couple hundred prostates I wish I hadn't."* Even JAMA has stated, *"A blood test to detect cancer may lead to more problems than it is worth. The PSA test will lead many healthy men to undergo needless surgery for prostate cancer, damaging their quality of life while raising the country's medical bills."* And the U.S. Preventive Services Task Force cautions, *"Prostate-specific antigen-based screening results in small or no reduction in prostate cancer-specific mortality and is associated with harms related to subsequent evaluation and treatments, some of which may be unnecessary."*

> **"PSA-based screening results in small or no reduction in prostate cancer-specific mortality."** New England Journal of Medicine

If you have a PSA test and your number is higher than 4, then you most likely will be referred to a urologist for a biopsy which consists of inserting a hollow needle through the wall of the rectum and into the prostate to remove

> **Causes For Prostate Swelling Or High PSA**
> - Stress – nervous system disorder, emotions, high cortisol
> - Elevated Estrogen (soy products, GMO foods, pesticides, Plastic containers-water bottles, alcohol consumption)
> - Low (DHT) Testosterone
> - Statin Drugs (cholesterol lowering) JAMA 1996
> - Elevated Insulin (sugar, grains, breads, pasta, corn, rice)
> - Liver Problems– sluggish, fatty, toxicity issues
> - Heavy Metal Toxicity (mercury, aluminum, cadmium)
> - Mycotoxins from mold & fungi (corn, wheat & peanuts)
> - Dairy Consumption (milk, cheese – contains growth hormones)
> - Pelvic Trauma – injury to prostate
> - Dehydration – not drinking enough water

samples of prostate tissue to be examined under a microscope. Usually about 12 samples are taken in one session. Researchers report that one month after a biopsy, 40 percent of men have problems with erectile dysfunction, and 6 months later, 15 percent have trouble with their sex life. Once again, before doing a biopsy, if there is cancer, the needle biopsy may allow cancer cells to spread. Professor Paul Frame, M.D., from Rochester School of Medicine and Dentistry, stated that clinical trials have not shown that the PSA test actually saves lives.

As mentioned previously, many men have prostate cancer just as many women have breast cancer. The intelligence of the body encapsulates abnormal cells and incarcerates them in the form of tumors, which keeps them from spreading to the rest of the body. Your body's wisdom keeps cancer in check. When radical surgery is performed and the prostate is removed, you run the risk of suffering from incontinence and having to wear a diaper for the rest of your life, not to mention impotency, sabotaging a man's ability to engage in sexual activity.

What causes an enlarged prostate? Tight-fitting clothes such as a tight belt and tight shorts or anything that restricts lymphatic flow may be a factor. Elevated estrogen levels from soy products, pesticides, genetically modified foods, food and beverages from plastic containers and alcohol consumption might contribute. Statin drugs interfere with cholesterol, the basic building blocks

> **What To Do For A Healthy Prostate**
> 1. Exercise regularly
> 2. Have 2-3 bowel movements daily
> 3. Avoid alcohol & caffeine
> 4. Avoid prolonged sitting
> 5. Enjoy a healthy sex life
> 6. Kegel exercises (stimulates blood flow)
> 7. Soak in warm Epsom salt baths
> 8. Take nutritional supplements
> 9. Get enough sleep (deep REM)
> 10. Eat cruciferous vegetables (broccoli)

for healthy hormone levels in the body, which may be a factor with an inflamed prostate. Eating more cruciferous vegetables such as kale, spinach, broccoli, collard greens and beets can help detoxify excess estrogen, along with nettle root and saw palmetto. Ginger is great to support lymph flow, and ashwagandha helps balance hormones, reduce stress and lower cortisol. Eating walnuts helps protect against prostate cancer. The American Journal of Clinical Nutrition stated that, *"Vitamin K2 may reduce your risk of prostate cancer by 35 percent."*

Prostate Support
- Saw Palmetto
- Nettle Root
- Juniper Berry
- Pygeum
- Graviola
- Ginger
- Ashwagandha
- Flaxseed oil
- Zinc
- Selenium
- Magnesium
- Potassium
- Boron
- Molybdenum
- Vitamin D
- Vitamin K2

Insulin increases growth, so eating a high carbohydrate diet with lots of breads, cereals, pasta, corn, rice, oats and sugar increases inflammation. If you have a fatty liver or it is toxic, this can cause inflammation in the prostate as well. Dairy products contain growth hormones from pregnant cows designed to feed a growing calf. The prostate acts as a sponge for these growth hormones, and it can stimulate and cause prostate inflammation. Vegetable oils from fried foods and salad dressings contain omega 6 oils such as soy oil, corn oil and canola oil, which are genetically modified and inflammatory to the prostate. Olive oil, coconut oil, vinegar and lemon are fine.

Constipation or sluggish bowels will cause pressure to be put on the prostate, so stay hydrated and keep the bowels moving daily. Sex keeps the prostate gland secreting prostate fluid, a component of semen. The prostate muscles help propel seminal fluid into the urethra during ejaculation. What you don't use, you lose. Kegel exercises can be beneficial for toning the muscles in the reproductive region and help eliminate excessive dripping and erectile problems. Kegel exercises are great for women who may experience incontinence and they also help to make multiple orgasms possible. Simply tighten your pelvic floor muscles as if you are trying to stop urination in midstream. Hold for 5 seconds and then relax. Do these 10 times in a row 3 or 4 times a day, to increase blood flow and strengthen your muscles.

> **"To discover and understand the physical causes of cancer, you will first need to let go of the idea that cancer is a powerful disease that must be fought. You never fight a symptom; you heal the carrier of the symptom. You get what you focus on. If you focus on the cancer, then you get more cancer. If you focus on health, that is what you get."** Dr. Leonard Coldwell

Healing Cancer

Nails In The Tire - Causes For Cancer	
Heavy Metals	Mercury
Pesticides	Glyphosate
Chemicals	Miasms
Lyme Disease	Vaccinations
Acidosis	Emotions

Is there a cure for cancer? Yes, there is. Is there a cure for a flat tire? Yes, there is. Remove the nails and patch the holes. Is there a cure for your car that won't start? Yes, there is. You have to troubleshoot it to find out what's causing the problem. Is it out of gas? Does it have a bad battery, a clogged fuel filter or fouled spark plugs? Once you find the cause and fix the problem, the car starts and the tire holds air. Everything has a cause, and so does cancer, and it's not a deficiency of chemotherapy. Like your car, some testing is required to see what's causing it. The most common culprits we see are acidosis, heavy metals, toxic liver and kidneys, poor circulation, miasms, mold, fungi, chemical and pesticide poisoning, radiation exposure, allergies (gluten) and emotional wounds. Miasms are inherited weaknesses in your energetic DNA that leave you susceptible to disease. Once we identify the toxins in your body and remove them, your body can heal. Just as a nail in your tire keeps it going flat, so do toxins in the body keep deflating your immune system. What are the nails deflating your immune system so cancer can thrive? Chemotherapy and radiation do nothing to remove those nails, the cause of disease.

7 Warning Signs Of Cancer By PositiveMed
1. Change in bowel or bladder habits
2. A sore throat that does not heal
3. Unusual bleeding or discharge
4. Thickening or lump in breast or any body part
5. Indigestion or difficult swallowing
6. Obvious change in warts or moles
7. Nagging cough or hoarseness

"Each one of us produces several hundred thousand cancer cells every day of our lives. Whether we develop clinical cancer or not depends upon the ability of our immune systems to destroy these cancer cells. That's because cancer thrives in the presence of a deficient immune system." Douglas Brodie, M.D.

When former chief orthopedic surgeon of San Francisco General Hospital **Lorraine Day**, M.D., was diagnosed with breast cancer with a tumor the size of a grapefruit, she had to make a decision about how to treat herself. Did she choose chemotherapy or radiation? No. Why not? She explains in her own words, *"Cancer doesn't scare me anymore. I had it ... and got well by natural, simple therapies that you seldom hear about. I refused mutilating surgery, radiation and chemotherapy because studies in the medical literature and common sense told me that you* *shouldn't destroy your immune system while you are trying to get well."* To order her videos on how she healed herself of cancer, call 760-343-0965 or go online to www.drday.com. Her videos are simple, easy-to-understand, raw-foods diet instructions. She promotes a strict vegetarian diet.

> **"Everyone should know that the 'war on cancer' is largely a fraud, and that the National Cancer Society and the American Cancer Society are derelict in their duties to the people who support them."** Dr. Linus Pauling (Two-time Nobel Laureate)

30 Cancer Healing Remedies & Modalities

1.	Rife Technology	16.	Wheatgrass Juice
2.	Graviola	17.	Raw Food Organic Diet
3.	Essiac Tea	18.	Fasting
4.	Hoxsey Tonic	19.	Frankincense oil
5.	Gerson Therapy	20.	Myrrh oil
6.	Vitamin B17/Laetrile	21.	Hydrogen peroxide 35%
7.	Capsol T	22.	Oxygen/Ozone therapy
8.	Cannabis (Hemp)	23.	Enzyme Therapy
9.	Vitamin C	24.	Protocel
10.	Turmeric	25.	Issels Immunotherapy
11.	Bloodroot	26.	Burzynski's Antineoplastons
12.	Vitamin D/sunlight	27.	DMSO/Cesium chloride
13.	Trphala (Ayurvedic)	28.	Chinese Happy Tree
14.	714X	29.	Dr. Johanna Budwig protocol
15.	Reishi, Maitake & Shiitake Mushrooms	30.	German New Medicine

The United States Pharmacopoeia listed the herb Bloodroot as a cancer remedy from 1820 to 1926. Can you guess who was in charge of having it removed? In 1997, German scientists began adding bloodroot to animal feed because it was safer and more effective than antibiotics.

Discussing cancer, Robert Atkins, M.D. informed, *"There is not one, but many cures for cancer available. But they are all being systematically suppressed."* The Lancet medical journal reported a study that compared chemotherapy to no treatment at all. The conclusion was that no treatment proved a significantly better policy for patients' survival and for quality of life.

> **"My doctor gave me six months to live, but when I couldn't pay the bill, he gave me six months more."** Walter Matthau

Dr. James Hawver taught that cancer patients always have four main issues:

(1) Poor circulation — Arterial plaque (calcium) restricting blood flow.
(2) Acidosis — The body's pH is too acidic.
(3) Miasms — Inherited genetic weaknesses.
(4) Emotional issues — Something eating them up inside.

1936 — Dr. Otto Warburg Was Awarded The Nobel Prize For Discovering The Cause Of Cancer.   (1) OXYGEN DEPRIVATION & (2) ACIDOSIS

If Dr. Warburg discovered the cause of cancer, then why do the American Cancer Society and oncologists ignore his discovery of acidosis and oxygen deprivation and focus on chemotherapy, radiation and surgical procedures? Why aren't cancer patients put on strict alkaline diets? Could it possibly be that Big Pharma doesn't want you to get well?

> **"Insanity is doing the same thing over and over and expecting a different result."** Rudyard Kipling

Tumors thrive in an oxygen-deprived environment. Oxygen gets to cells via the blood; therefore, if your circulation is compromised in a certain area of the body, then most likely there will be low oxygen levels, and this is the terrain that favors the growth of cancer.

> **"It is my position that the truly healthy body and mind rarely need chemical drugs. Within each of our own bodies exists a far more powerful and efficient weapon with which to combat disease than any drug could possibly provide: the human immune system."** Jau-Fei Chen, Ph.D., Author of *Nutritional Immunology*

As mentioned earlier, an acidic body provides the environment to favor cancer. Everything you eat either feeds cancer or helps to eradicate it by influencing your pH. Sugar and flour (bread/gluten) feed cancer cells and weaken the immune system. Cancer also feeds on mucus, so eliminating milk and most cheese from the diet is beneficial. Substitute cow's milk with almond, coconut or raw goat's milk. Almost all living foods, including vegetables, fruits and berries, are alkaline-forming, which provides an unfriendly terrain for cancer. Dr. Max Gerson proved that he could stop cancer growth in 14 days by putting patients on a fully organic raw-food diet.

Cancer Warning Signs — If Not Corrected
1. Headaches – continually suppressing with pain killers
2. Acid Reflux – continually taking medicine for heartburn
3. Fatigue – can't function without coffee, soda, tea or energy drinks
4. Frequent colds, sore throats, fevers & coughs – using antibiotics
5. Irregular bowel movements – not eliminating every day
6. Feeling stressed out – no time to relax, rest, sleep & have fun
7. Eating junk foods to alleviate anxiety or depression
8. Dissatisfaction – Constantly hating your job, spouse or life
9. Unforgiveness – Holding a grudge or hating someone
10. Drug & Alcohol Abuse – Numbing yourself to avoid your feelings

Cancer cells do not just randomly spread throughout your body. Like every other living entity, they seek the environment that feeds them. They lodge themselves in areas that are congested, acidic and oxygen-deprived. Cancer is no different than any other living form of life. Take, for example, tomatoes. To grow tomatoes, you need good soil that is fertilized as well as oxygen, water and sunlight. Remove any one of those vital elements and tomatoes won't grow. Change the terrain in your body and stop feeding cancer sugar and starches and you'll starve it to death.

Many people have cured themselves of cancer by fasting. When you stop eating, your body will begin to metabolize toxins and abnormal cells for energy. The fibrin coating around cancer cells, made of protein, acts as a shield to protect it from your immune system. Fasting forces your body to go into a cleanse mode and begins to digest and metabolize diseased cells, including cancer.

> "The cancer cell shields itself from anticancer agents by forming a fibrin coating around each individual cell; this fibrous coating is made of protein. Proteolytic enzymes digest this protein coating, which allows the body's white cells to attack the cancer cells and destroy them." Dr. Harold W. Manner

Eating an all-organic, living-foods diet with an emphasis on wheatgrass juice and barley greens has proven effective for beating cancer as well. The Ann Wigmore Foundation or Hippocrates Health Institute is a healing center that has helped thousands of sick people overcome all types of so-called incurable diseases by learning the Living Foods Lifestyle. They use the healing power of wheatgrass juice, which contains chlorophyll, a toxin neutralizer, filled with over 100 healing elements. They offer educational retreats on how to prepare and eat healthy foods to empower your body to heal. They have retreat centers in San Fidel, New Mexico (505-552-0595), West Palm Beach, Florida (561-623-1002), and Puerto Rico (787-868-2430). Look them up at hippocratesinst.org.

> "When the pH is off and our bodies are becoming more acidic, our cells get less oxygen. Cancer thrives under an acid tissue pH/oxygen-deficient environment." Dr. Otto Warburg

Is Cancer A Fungus?

Similarities Between Cancer & Fungus
1. Cancer & Fungi both feed on sugar.
2. Cancer & Fungi both die in the absence of sugar.
3. Cancer & Fungi both thrive in anaerobic environments.
4. Cancer & Fungi can both metabolize nutrients in the absence of oxygen.
5. Cancer & Fungi both produce corrosive lactic acid.
6. Cancer & Fungi both need an acidic environment to survive.
7. Cancer cells & Fungi are both white, with an uneven texture.
8. Cancer & Fungi both respond to antifungal medicines.

In 1951 researchers at Lankenau Hospital in Pennsylvania identified fungi present in every cancerous tumor they examined. Milton White, M.D., taught that cancer is a chronic, infectious, fungal disease. In every sample of cancer studied, he identified fungal spores. And researchers at Johns Hopkins have demonstrated that the drug Sporanax, used to treat toenail fungus, could also block the growth of new blood vessels (angiogenesis) commonly seen in cancers, indicating that antifungal medicine is anti-cancer.

> "The highest form of ignorance is when you reject something you don't know anything about." Dr. Wayne Dyer

Healthy cells use glucose and oxygen to produce ATP, which is the main source of energy for cells. Unlike healthy cells, cancer cells use glucose fermentation for fuel that comes from simple carbohydrate foods like sugar and grains (breads and pasta). As your body becomes more acidic, your cells get less oxygen. When cells become anaerobic (they live without oxygen), in an acidic environment (5.3 pH or lower), feeding on sugar, they become pathogenic organisms much like a yeast, fungus or mold. If you take cancerous tumor cells and culture them, you find the fungus Mucor racemosus fresen. Remember, Dr. Otto Warburg stated that when we become acidic, our cells get less oxygen and this is the terrain that favors fungus and cancer growth.

Fungal Mycotoxins
- Aspergillus
- Fusarium
- Penicillium

An overgrowth of yeast or fungi feeding on sugar produces poisonous byproducts called "mycotoxins." Thousands of mycotoxins have been identified and are linked to human illness. The three major genera of mycotoxin-producing fungi are Aspergillus, Fusarium and Penicillium. Yes, penicillium is the fungus and penicillin (the antibiotic) is the mycotoxin. In 1993, researchers Bernstein and Ross discovered that two months or more of taking a penicillin antibiotic significantly increased the risk of non-Hodgkin's lymphoma. Could using the fungi/mold-derived antibiotics feed cancer?

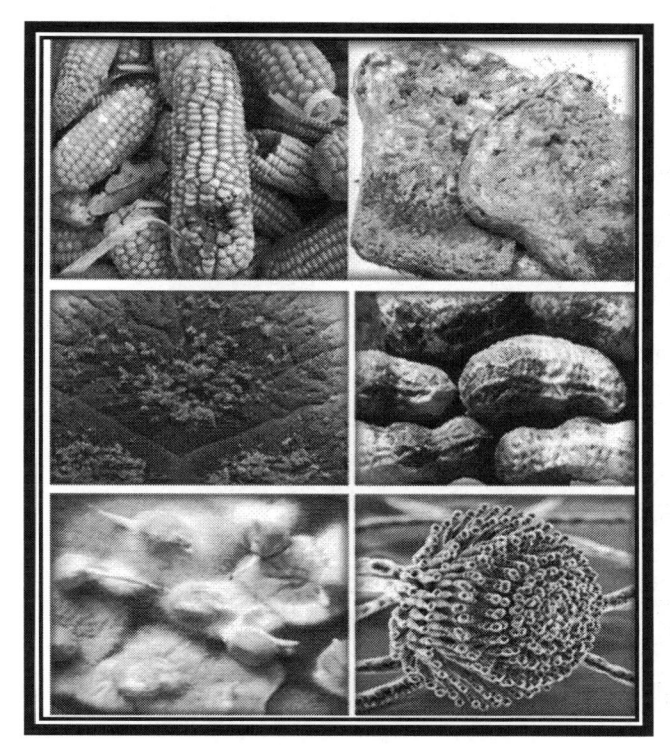

When these harmful mycotoxins from yeast or fungi begin overwhelming your body with their poisonous wastes, symptoms are sure to follow. If not corrected, the mycotoxin acetaldehyde is created by yeast's fermentation of sugar or alcohol. The most common symptoms are sinus problems, allergies, chemical sensitivities, anxiety, paranoia, fatigue, weight gain, feeling spaced-out, mucus discharge, nail fungus, skin rashes, rectal itching, prostatitis, ringworm, PMS and vaginal itching/yeast infections. As your body becomes overburdened with acids and microbial wastes, it stresses your immune system, which can lead to overstimulation of the adrenals and thyroid, causing chronic fatigue along with thyroid disorders. Keep in mind that most corticosteroid prescription drugs such as Cortisone, Prednisone and Advair (asthma drugs) can greatly increase your risks of developing serious fungal infections.

Aflatoxins are poisonous cancer-causing (carcinogens) toxins produced by mold. The International Agency for Research on Cancer classifies naturally occurring aflatoxins from the mold aspergillus as a human carcinogen, with aflatoxin B1 being the most toxic. It can cause liver cancer and has been found in the blood of children with leukemia. Aspergillus can grow in balls in the lungs called "aspergillomas," and they mimic pulmonary malignancy (lung cancer). If you have been diagnosed with lung cancer, it may be aspergillus, since thoracic malignancy and fungus are indistinguishable on X-rays.

As researcher and author Doug Kaufmann points out, when scientists deliberately give laboratory animals cancer to do clinical research, they actually inject them with aflatoxin B1, which is mycotoxicosis. After the animals become sick, they change the name from mycotoxicosis to "cancer."

Aspergillus Mold Produces Carcinogenic Aflatoxin B1

Most of the American grain supply — corn, wheat, barley, peanuts, tobacco (dried) and cotton — is commonly contaminated with these poisonous fungal mycotoxins. Much of the grain used to make alcoholic beverages is usually contaminated with mycotoxins, since the cleanest grains are used for table foods.

Dangerous Fungal Mycotoxins Are...
- Carcinogenic (cancer causing)
- Capable of causing tremors & seizures
- May cause birth defects to developing embryo
- Poisonous to our DNA & nerves
- Immune system suppressant
- Poisonous to the heart & blood vessels
- Poisonous to the liver & kidneys
- Poisonous to the lymphatic system & skin

Antifungal/Mold Remedies

Garlic	Niacin
Oregano	Tea tree oil
Clove oil	Pau d' Arco
Olive leaf	Cat's claw
Zinc	Coconut oil
Psyllium	Citrus oils
Chaga	Echinacea
Dill oil	Baking Soda
Black seed	Colloidal silver

A hangover after a night of drinking is really mycotoxicosis, or mycotoxin poisoning, from the saccharomyces of brewer's yeast used in the fermentation process to make alcohol. Research has shown that 87 percent of cottonseed is impregnated with aspergillus fungi, which produces aflatoxin B1. The American Cancer Society defines mycotoxins as "mutagenic carcinogens." If you go to www.pubmed.com and type in "aflatoxin causes cancer," 2,009 published research papers show up on the fungus/cancer connection.

Test For Candida (Yeast)
1. First thing in the morning, before putting anything in your mouth, spit some of your saliva in a glass of water.
2. Check the water every 15 minutes for 1 hour. If string-like legs from the saliva are traveling down into the water, you have candida. Cloudy saliva that sinks to the bottom or cloudy specks suspended in water also indicates candida.
3. If nothing develops in 45 minutes you probably don't have candida.

One of the reasons fungal infections such as cryptococcus neoformans are difficult to eliminate is because the fungus "escapes phagocytosis (white blood cells attacking infections) because the spores are surrounded by a thick viscous capsule," according to medical textbook, *Mechanisms of Microbial Disease*. Histoplasma capsulatum, a fungus that can cause a deadly disease called histoplasmosis, is sometimes found in macrophages (immune cells). Macrophages gobble up and digest pathogenic debris, like the Pac-Man video game does pellets. In histoplasma capsulatum, the macrophages, oddly enough, do not kill the fungus, but begin assisting them, by hiding them from the rest of the immune system. This strange phenomenon occurs when DNA from fungus marries DNA from your white blood cells, and forms a new hybrid tumor. And since this new tumor is 50 percent human, the immune system no longer attacks it as non-self.

> **"Cancer begins when the DNA from fungus and the DNA from our white blood cells merge to form a new hybrid 'tumor, or sac.' This hybrid attains a life of its own now, bypassing our immune defenses because it is 50% human, and therefore just enough to be recognized as 'self.' Cancer is a fungus that will do what all fungi do – form colonies and spread throughout the host area."** Dr. Tullio Simoncini

We humans have a special cancer tumor suppressor gene (p53) that protects us from cancer. It kills tumor cells; however, in over 50 percent of all cancers, doctors have found that the patient's p53 gene was mutated and unable to kill the cancer. The medical journal, Liver International, in 2011, states, *"aflatoxin genotoxicity is associated with a defective DNA damage response bypassing p53 activation."* And in 1993, the National Academy of Science declared that the mycotoxin, aflatoxin B1, is known to cause p53 mutations.

> **What Causes Our Cancer-Protector p53 Gene To Mutate?**
> ❖ Aspergillus Fungus - Aflatoxin B1 Causes DNA Damage, Bypassing p53 Activation
> (Source: Liver International, 2011 & National Academy of Science, 1993)

Remember, Dr. Thomas Seyfried teaches that cancer is not a genetic disorder, but rather a metabolic disease. In other words, genes don't determine whether you get cancer. The consumption of contaminated grains with mold- and fungus-producing harmful mycotoxins and deadly aflatoxins are what cause metabolic changes to occur that can damage the DNA, thus leaving you susceptible to cancer.

> **"First, you know, a new theory is attacked as absurd; then it is admitted to be true, but obvious and insignificant; finally, it is seen to be so important that its adversaries claim that they themselves discovered it."** Dr. William James 1842-1910

Chemotherapy – Deadly Mustard Gas – Causes Cancer

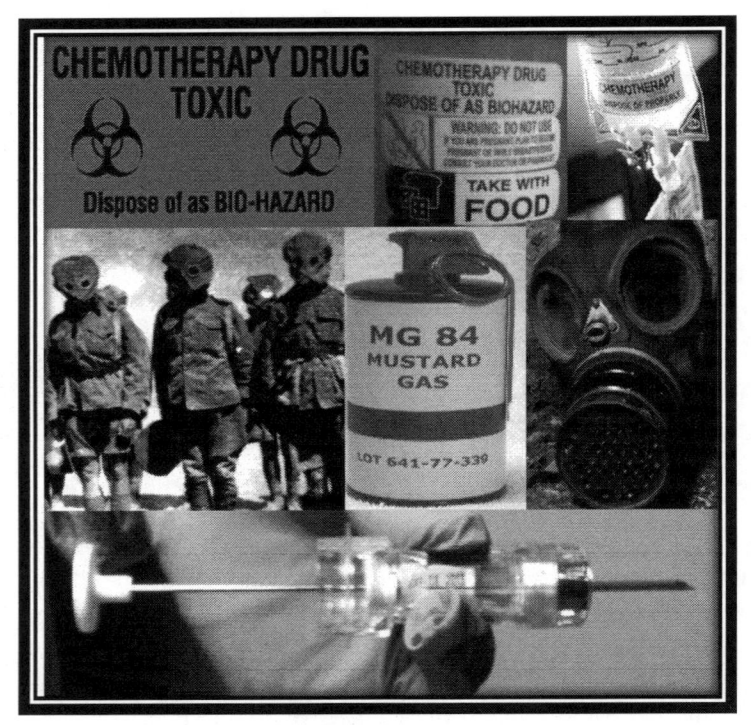

Chemotherapy, a descendent of chemical weapons and biological warfare, is repackaged mustard gas used to kill soldiers during World War II. Chemotherapy causes cancer. How? It strengthens cancer cells by turning them into stem cells so they can reproduce more cancer cells. That is why someone goes through chemo and the oncologist says, "we got all the cancer," and then a few years later it comes back, but this time it comes back with a vengeance. In a 2014 study published in PLOS ONE, 88.3 percent of oncologists confessed that if diagnosed with cancer, they would never receive chemotherapy, high-intensity care.

Cancer cells divide more rapidly than normal cells. Chemotherapy works by damaging the RNA or DNA that tell the cells how to copy themselves in division. The problem is, your immune system possesses rapidly dividing cells too, not just cancer cells, and the chemo doesn't have a brain to distinguish between the two — it annihilates the good, the bad and the ugly. This is why oncologists check your white blood cells often, to see how much damage your immune system is sustaining during the poisoning process. Too much will kill you. When your hair

Chemotherapy Facts
- Chemo kills healthy cells & cancer cells
- Chemo kills rapidly dividing cancer cells, but not all cancer cells are fast growing
- Chemo does not kill cancer stem cells
- Chemo damages the immune system, disabling it from removing cancer cells from the body.
- 90% of chemo patients die 10-15 years after treatment
- Chemo patients are 14 times more likely to develop leukemia

falls out, you feel nauseated and become extremely weak, is this not evidence enough of your cells screaming for you to stop poisoning them?

> **"Please hear this: In the end, there is nothing manmade that can heal cancer. Your immune system has to finish the job. In fact, there's nothing manmade that I know of that can actually heal any disease."** Ben Johnson, MD, N.M.D, DO 1950-2019

Chemotherapy is so poisonous that if you spill a few drops on your hand it can severely burn you, and if spilled in a hospital, it is classified as a major biohazard that requires professionals in biohazard suits to come in and clean up the toxins and dispose of them properly. After having just one chemotherapy treatment, you are no longer eligible to be an organ donor.

> **"When 250 million people believe in a bad idea, it's still a bad idea."** Terry A. Rondberg, D.C.

Chemotherapy has roughly a 2 percent success rate. According to a 14-year study published in the Journal of Clinical Oncology of 154,971 cancer patients from Australia and the U.S. who had 22 different types of cancer, only 2.3 percent and 2.1 percent, respectively, survived longer than five years after chemotherapy treatments. (Morgan, G, 2004 Dec;16(8):549-60)

> **"Chemotherapy and radiotherapy make the ancient method of drilling holes in a patient's head to permit the escape of demons look relatively advanced. Toxic chemotherapy is a hoax. Cancer treatment popular today effectively closes the door on cure."** Dr. Ernst T. Krebs, 1911-1996

Poison For Health?

In naturopathy, we believe there is a cause for the cancer. If a doctor fails to identify the cause and remove it, then the person's chance to heal and live is drastically reduced. Poisoning the body with chemotherapy is as ridiculous as spraying weed-killer all over your lawn to get rid of dandelions. Of course you'll kill the dandelions, but you'll kill the grass too! Just as we don't want to kill the grass to get rid of dandelions, we don't want to poison you with harmful chemicals to kill cancer.

> "To an industry that does not even know how to cure heartburn, we have given $600 billion to come up with a cure for cancer. Gee, I wonder why we aren't any closer to a cure since Richard Nixon declared a war on cancer (44 years ago)." Dr. Peter Glidden

Mustard gas is a poison. Chemotherapy is a poison. We have many poisons to kill. Does it make sense to poison ourselves to kill cancer cells? I don't think our Creator intended for us to poison our bodies in an attempt to be healthy.

> **"Treating cancer with chemotherapy is like treating alcoholism with vodka. It's like treating heart disease with cheese, or like treating diabetes with high-fructose corn syrup. Cancer cannot be cured by the very thing that causes it. Don't let some cancer doctor talk you into chemotherapy using his fear tactics. They're good at that. So next time he insists that you take some chemotherapy, ask him to drink some first. If your oncologist isn't willing to drink chemotherapy in front of you to prove it's safe, why on earth would you agree to have it injected in your body?"** Mike Adams, The Health Ranger

A survey was done on 64 oncologists at The McGill Cancer Center in Montreal to see how they would treat cancer if they or someone in their family were diagnosed. This is one of the largest and most esteemed cancer treatments centers in the world and 91 percent of these doctors said chemotherapy was unacceptable due to the fact that it's ineffective and highly toxic! So why do we continue to use surgery, radiation and chemotherapy for cancer? Because the cancer industry in this country spends over $100 billion a year on cancer treatments alone! Some cancer drugs cost more than $35,000 each month. To fight cancer with chemotherapy generally costs over $100,000 a year. The average cancer patient in the U.S. spends $350,000 on treatment before he or she dies, leaving many completely bankrupt. In 2018, the drug company Pfizer made $53.6 billion on drug sales, with $11 billion being for cancer drugs.

> **"The greatest part of all chronic disease is created by the suppression of acute disease by drug poisoning."** Henry Lindlahr, M.D.

Cats are born with a natural instinct to hunt, kill and eat mice. It's part of their diet just as humans inherit an instinct to eat fruits and vegetables. Get rid of cats and you'll have mice everywhere as long as there is something for them to eat. Imagine that your body is similar to a house and mice are like pathogens (viruses, fungi, bacteria, cancer, etc.) that are looking for a place to live and something to eat. Suppose cats are like killer T-cells, the special forces of your immune system, roaming around hunting those foreign invaders, cancer cells that we don't want.

How do you get rid of mice? You could put poison out to kill them, but if the family pet or young child eats it, it may kill them too. Or you could keep your cats healthy and hungry so they will go out and do what God created them to do naturally — kill and eat mice. Just as cats know how to kill mice, your immune system knows how to kill cancer and other harmful pathogens. The answer is not to poison everything to death. We will never win the war on microbes, trillions of them are everywhere, including in your own body, especially your gut. Optimizing your immune system so that you live in harmony with the microbes is the foundational key to good health. Healthy cats keep mice away just as a strong and balanced immune system keeps harmful pathogens in check.

The kill, kill, kill with antibiotics, chemotherapy and radiation approach to health is a disastrous train wreck. It's time to shift our focus to strengthening what God has already created — your highly intelligent immune system — so that it can function at an optimal level to keep you dis-ease free. It does require some maintenance, proper care and tools to fight foreigners who do not have permission to be in your body.

> "Why would a patient swallow a poison because he is ill, or take that which would make a well man sick." L.F. Kebler, M.D.

After over 30 years of practicing medicine and serving as National Director of Project Head Start's Medical Consultation Service and Chairman of the Medical Licensing Committee for the State of Illinois, Dr. Mendelsohn concludes the following about modern medicine.

Robert S. Mendelsohn, M.D. – Says …

- I believe that the greatest danger to your health is the doctor who practices Modern Medicine.

- I believe that Modern Medicine's treatments for disease are seldom effective and often more dangerous than the ailments they're employed to treat.

- I believe that the dangers are compounded by the widespread use of dangerous procedures to treat non-diseases, procedures that produce real diseases that the doctor will then address with even more dangerous procedures in his efforts to repair the damage he has done.

- I believe that Modern Medicine endangers its victims by attacking minor ailments with hazardous treatments that should only be used when the patient's life is at stake.

- I believe that most doctors are the willing, if unwitting, tools of pharmaceutical manufacturers. Their patients become human guinea pigs for mass testing of drugs with dubious benefits and potentially lethal side effects that are unknown.

- I believe that more than 90 percent of Modern Medicine could disappear from the face of the earth — doctors, hospitals, drugs, and equipment — and the health of the nation would immediately and dramatically improve.

- I do not believe in modern medicine. I am a Medical Heretic … I haven't always been a Medical Heretic; I once believed in Modern Medicine.

"Let's get one thing straight — The American Medical Association is really the American Murder Association." Rick Kunnes, M.D., American Medical News

Chapter 3
HEALING THE CAUSE OF DIS-EASE

The Lymphatic System

The heart starts beating before you are born and continues to beat until you die. But it only pumps blood. It does not pump lymph fluid. You have three times as much lymph fluid in your body as you do blood. Lymph fluid surrounds your cells and when the cells of the body need nutrients, they have to get it from the lymph fluid. When they excrete metabolic waste, it goes into the lymph. The problem is that we have never taken this mystifying system seriously. For example, we can hear the heart, measure the beat, and monitor the pressure of the blood. But, because the lymphatic system just quietly goes about its job, not making waves, we don't study it. In fact, we have done just the opposite by trying to get rid of it. We started 40 years ago by removing tonsils and adenoids from healthy children. These are two of the drainage organs of the lymphatic system and part of our immune system. We have no love for the appendix either, another lymphatic drainage organ. Removal is in order most of the time a surgeon gets close to one. Lymph veins are stripped from the arms during a mastectomy. When your lymph nodes swell, that means they are working, fighting infection. Should we cut your legs and arms off because they are sore and swollen after a hard workout?

> **"Longevity and beauty are not in your genes; they are in your lymph."** Paul Chhabra's great-grandmother, who lived to be 111

Your house has a septic tank to process wastes when you flush the toilet, and so does your body. It's called your lymphatic system. Your lymphatic system includes the spleen, tonsils, appendix, thymus, adenoids, Peyer's patches, lymph nodes, lymph vessels and lymph fluid. Many people take diuretics to help drain extra fluid. If you are swelling or retaining fluids, this is a red flag warning that your septic tank is backed up. What is the clog?

Wise doctors understand that the lymphatic system is part of your highly skilled military defense — the immune system. Our immune system functions similarly to a military operation, with the tonsils in our throat acting as guards at the gate, protecting us from any incoming harmful pathogens that may try to sneak in through foods and beverages. To remove your tonsils is like assassinating the guards, thus welcoming pathogens into the body. The adenoids are used to guard against any toxins that you may breathe in through your nose. The appendix acts as an overflow valve for the large intestine and guards against foreign invaders that may come in through food. It's important to remember to take care of your guards periodically with some herbal cleanses and nutritional support so they can fight off any unwelcomed guests.

> **"The name of a dis-ease depends upon where the poisons settle."** Bernard Jensen, D.C., N.D., Ph.D.

The immune system fights off invading organisms such as bacteria, viruses, fungi and other environmental toxins. Lymphocytes are white blood cells that clean up the garbage. Each person has about one trillion of them working like little "Pac-Man" garbage eaters. From the time you began reading this sentence, over 800,000 of them have been created and destroyed! The thymus gland is the training camp that sends out special forces we call B and T cells to sound the alarm of danger and fight. These soldiers are transported in your body through the lymph vessels. After the war, all the dead cells are taken to be disposed of in the spleen, the graveyard for dead cells. If the spleen becomes sluggish, you will swell and possibly push the toxins out through the skin in the form of a rash. Skin rashes many times are a sign of a backed-up spleen (septic tank).

> **"Disease cannot live in a body spiritually and physically clean and well nourished."** LaDean Griffin, Author of *Is Any Sick Among You?*

Your lymphatic system has 2.25 million miles of lymphatic vessels and 650 lymph nodes. When did your doctor do a lymph check last? They ignore it because they don't have a drug to help it drain. In fact, most prescription drugs inhibit the lymphatic system from being able to filter out waste material. Have you ever wondered why people in hospitals on so many medications swell? Many need heavy diuretics to help remove the excess fluids from a stagnant lymphatic system.

Every solid structure in the body is bathed in lymph. The average human has about 12 quarts of lymph circulating in the body, constantly filtering harmful micro-organisms out in special collection sites (garbage cans) also known as lymph nodes. Lymph nodes also act as the army barracks for the immune cells. As the lymph fluid passes through the nodes, it is filtered and cleansed of bacteria, viruses and other unwanted microbes.

When the garbage is not emptied regularly, we attract infection into the body. Swelling and pain are warning signs that our lymph nodes need to be emptied. When they are full, or fighting infection, they swell. That is why sometimes when you have a cold the lymph nodes under the cheekbones become inflamed. That means they are working, fighting infection, cleansing excess mucus and toxins from the body.

When we ignore our swollen lymph nodes and suppress them with diuretics and painkillers, then we can literally drown from our own metabolic wastes. Remember that Dr. Carrel proved how important it is to keep waste materials cleaned out when he kept a chicken heart alive for 29 years? It died when someone failed to remove the wastes. We too die if our lymphatic system stops circulating and fails to remove the wastes.

> **"When the lymphatic system is stagnant, cells begin to suffocate because nutrients can't get in and waste can't get out. The body has to find other means to cope with the potential infection, and it turns to inflammation. Inflammation is a normal response to an abnormal condition, and it's part of how our bodies cope."** Samuel N. Grief, M.D.

Firemen Put Out Fires & Lymph Nodes Fight Infection

Suppose you live in a city where criminals are burning businesses. So, the city mayor sends out an order for detectives to crack down on crime and find out who's starting the fires. After a few months, five more businesses have burned with no arrests. Out of frustration, the mayor throws up his hands and says, "I don't know what to do. Buildings keep burning, and the only common denominator that our detectives see at the fires are firemen." So, the mayor concludes that firemen must cause fires, and he sends out an order to destroy the fire stations. Complete absurdity, right? Fire stations are where the firefighters come from to put out the fires! Because every time there is a fire (swelling), the mayor (doctor) sees firemen (swollen lymph nodes), he assumes the fires are caused by firemen, not realizing the firemen are there to extinguish the fire. Only a fool would get rid of fire stations in an attempt to stop fires from happening, but doctors who remove swollen tonsils and adenoids without finding out what's causing the infection or inflammation are destroying your immune system's fire stations.

Doctors prescribe antibiotics to crack down on infections (crime). After months of antibiotics failing to get rid of the inflammation and infection, the doctor, like the mayor, throws his hands in the air and says, "We're going to have to do surgery and remove your tonsils and adenoids and destroy the fire stations." Are you going to find out what caused the fire and what's the best extinguisher to put the fires out with, or are you going to cut lymph nodes out and destroy fire stations? Use wisdom when doctors recommend surgery.

> "Some people study all their lives, and at their death they have learned everything except to think." Domergue

Support For Swollen Tonsils
- Echinacea
- Elderberry
- Goldenseal
- Myrrh
- Licorice
- Cats Claw
- Garlic

The solution to reduce swelling and clear up infections is to drink plenty of water. You can't flush a toilet without water and your body can't drain wastes efficiently when dehydrated. Taking herbal and homeopathic remedies to cleanse the blood, expel mucus and support the immune system is important. Some may argue, "My tonsils stay inflamed and infected all the time!" The question is, what are you eating to feed the infection? Does your diet include cow's milk, corn, wheat, cereals, breads (flour/gluten products), sugar and chemicals in packages and processed foods? Stop pouring gas on the fire by consuming inflammatory foods and start eating fresh vegetables, fruits, berries and healthy fats like avocados, nuts, seeds and coconut oil. Fermented vegetables help build up your microbiome in the gut, which is where most of your immune system resides. Eating garlic, onions, ginger and turmeric daily will many times clear up the inflammation fast. Drinking some warm bone broth daily can help. Let your food be your medicine, taught Hippocrates. Drinking a tablespoon of apple cider vinegar with some water twice a day can be beneficial. An EDS scan can identify allergies (food or inhalant) that can be contributing to inflammation along with identifying which herbs are best to put out the fires and clear out infections in your body.

"If Indian ink is rubbed into the gums, it is promptly absorbed and it reappears in the tonsils which eliminates it. If the bacilli of tuberculosis are inserted into the tonsils of healthy calves, they are not infected because the tonsils destroy the bacilli. It therefore follows that the tonsils are not portals of entry for tubercular infection, as had previously been assumed. On the other hand, if the bacilli are allowed to enter the lungs of calves, the calves become tuberculous and the bacilli are found in the previously healthy tonsils. This indicates that the tonsils take part in eliminating and destroying the germs of disease." Dr. Alfred Tienes, 1934

A fish aquarium circulates water through filters to remove toxins. If the water stops circulating, it turns a dark, murky color

Drink Half of Your Body Weight in Ounces of Water Each Day.

and fish die because of the disease-producing environment of stagnant water. The fish are alive, and living creatures excrete waste material. Just as circulation is essential in having a clean aquarium, so is circulation essential for good health.

The Lymphatic System

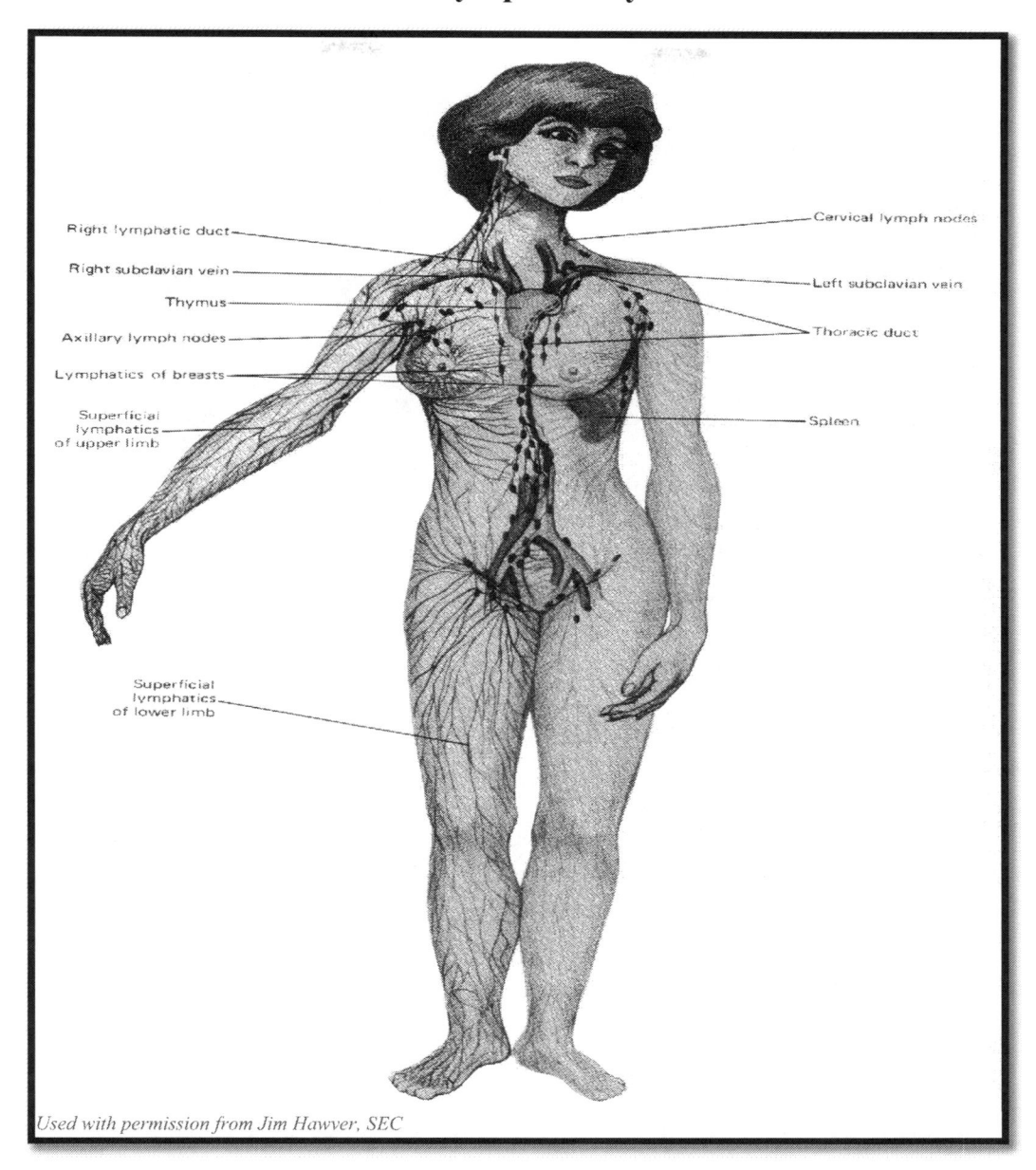

Used with permission from Jim Hawver, SEC

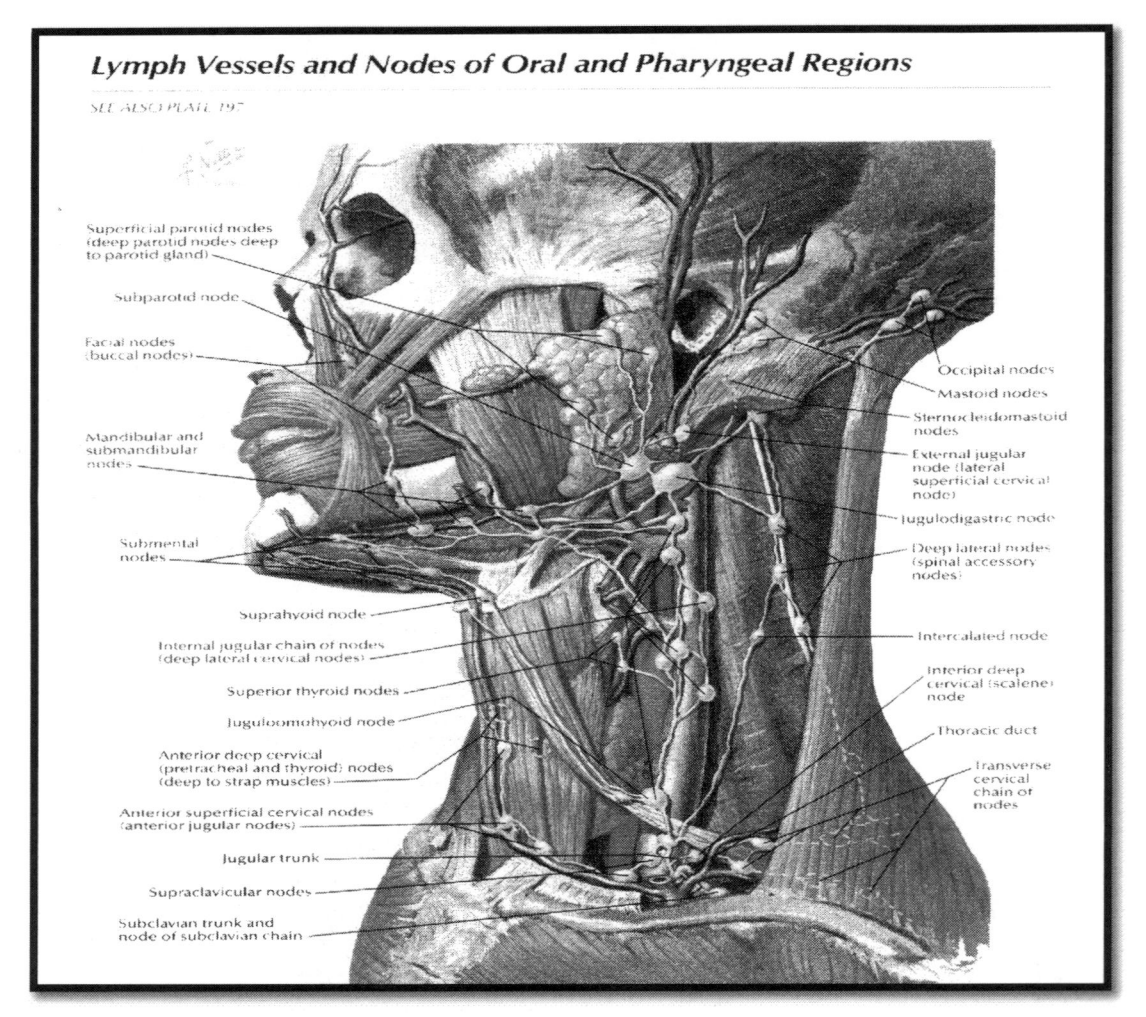

Lymph Vessels and Nodes of Oral and Pharyngeal Regions

Used with permission from Jim Hawver, SEC

Notice how many lymph nodes are in the neck and under the cheek bone. It is common for the nodes to swell when you have a cold or are fighting infection.

Can you wash the dishes or clean a dirty table with a diet soda, milk, orange juice, sweet tea or coffee? Of course not, because they contain sugars or nutrients that must be broken down in the digestive system. Water is a cleanser necessary for disposing of wastes. If your water gets turned off so you can't clean, you have a problem. Just as your toilet needs to be flushed, so do your cells in the body to expel toxins. Insufficient drainage due to dehydration is common. Many people drink coffee, tea, orange juice, sports drinks and colas, but very little water is consumed because they are full from their favorite beverages. You need water to cleanse your body. Constipation and headaches are the two biggest symptoms of dehydration.

> **"If the lymphatic system stops circulating for just 24 hours, death will occur."**
> Arthur C. Guyton, M.D., Text Book of Medical Physiology

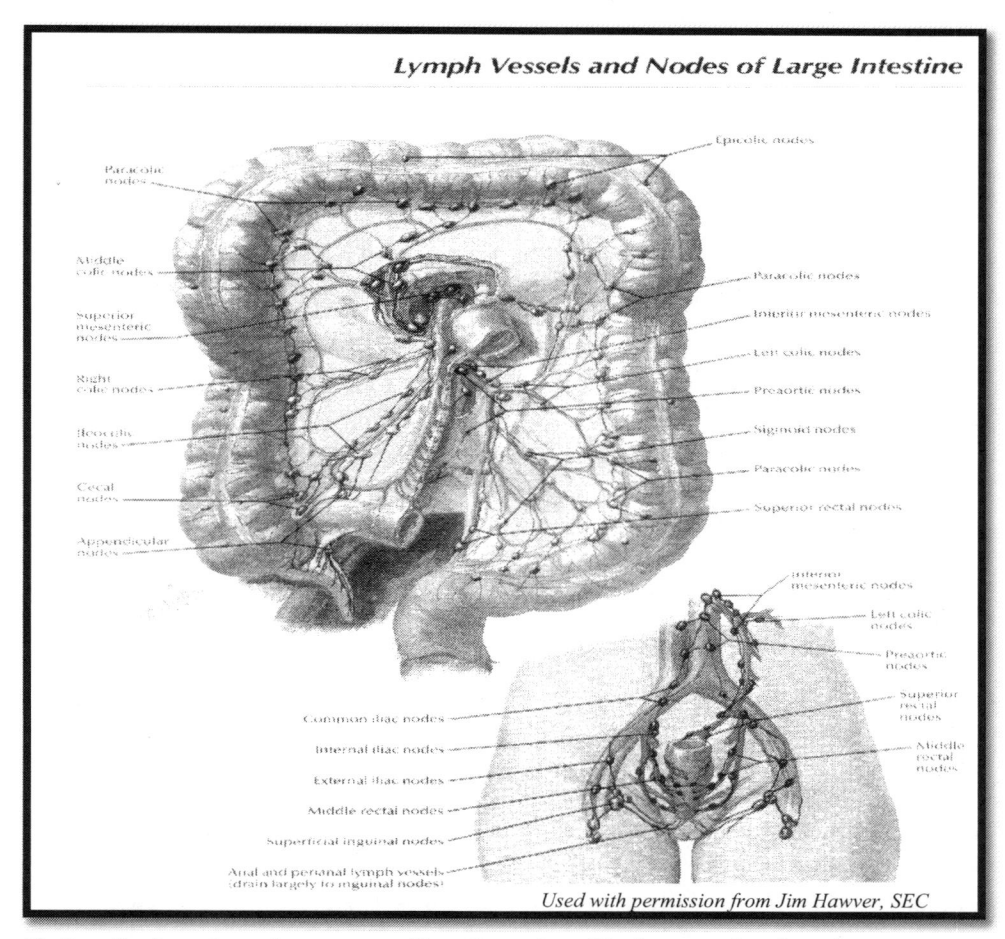

Notice the lymph nodes surrounding the colon. Having regular bowel movements daily is crucial for optimal health.

Rebounding (Lymphasizing)

Exercise is vital to pump the lymph fluid through the body. We are born with a natural instinct to bounce. Children demonstrate this well as they naturally love to jump on the couch, bed, pogo sticks, trampolines and anything else that is bouncy. When small babies cry, what do we do? Bounce them, of course, because the bouncing motion pumps the lymphatic system, which soothes inflammation and makes us feel better. As we grow older, some of us stop bouncing with life. We would be healthier if we all had a label on our foreheads like salad dressing that said, "SHAKE WELL BEFORE USING."

> **"Every cell generates an electrical field. It is an actual electrical generator."** C. Samuel West, D.N., N.D.

A rebounder is a small mini-trampoline that enables you to use it almost anywhere. By bouncing, you activate the lymph flow as much as 10- to 30-fold. The up and down motion while rebounding activates the one-way lymph valves to their maximum. A good quality rebounder can be purchased online at ReboundAIR. Look them up or call 1-888-464-5867.

> **"Rebounding is by far the most efficient, the most effective form of exercise yet devised by man."** Albert Carter, The National Institute of Reboundology and Health

Rebounding a few minutes every morning to pump the lymphatic system and strengthen every cell in the body is energizing and invigorating. The human body functions through electricity produced by the sodium-potassium pump of each cell. Rebounding is an effective way to generate a tremendous amount of electrical energy within, so you are empowered to reach your goals.

Do Drugs Heal Disease?

> **"We doctors are taught in our medical training that virtually 80 percent of diseases have no known cause. We are not taught to treat the underlying cause of the disease, we are only taught to treat the symptoms. This does not get a person well."** Lorraine Day, M.D., Former Chief Orthopedic Surgeon, San Francisco Hospital

How many people do you know who have been cured of arthritis, diabetes or multiple sclerosis by taking prescription drugs? If you don't look for the cause, how are you going to heal it? Prescription drugs do not heal, they only mask symptoms. That creates major imbalances in the body and pushes the toxins deeper into the tissue only to manifest later on in a different form or fashion.

You and your doctor never connect the dots, but many cancerous tumors are caused from years of prescription drug abuse by suppressing your symptoms, and now the piper must be paid. You reap what you sow. Just because a drug magically makes your symptoms disappear like the great magician David Copperfield does animals in cages and girls in sparkling clothes, it does not mean that you have fixed the problem. As a matter of fact, you are creating the terrain that will favor major disease in the future. This is not health; it is disease maintenance. It is nothing more than an illusion created by a clever scientist's drug to make your current symptoms disappear so you think the problem has been solved.

> **"Well, Ralph, what did you learn in school today? Did you learn how to think or did you learn how to believe?"** (Ralph Nader's father)

If the body has the power to inflame a joint or grow a tumor, then it has the power to remove it. If it has been created, then it can be uncreated. You have that power. Take responsibility and be the cause, not the effect. You are far more powerful than what you know, your body is divine, and it can and will perform miracles when given a chance. YOU are the source!

Mother Nature's Food Chain

Mother Nature has a food chain in place working perfectly. When a rabbit is killed on the road, vultures gather around for dinner. Flies come and lay eggs and maggots emerge. We have been and always will be exposed to millions of germs that science can identify under a microscope. Bacteria, viruses, molds, fungi, parasites and any other type of microbe or pathogen we can think of will always be in our midst, despite how much hand sanitizer you use. They are everywhere; there is no way to escape the microbes. As long as you live on planet earth you will encounter millions of these "germs."

If you want to get rid of flies in your house, what do you do? Oh sure, you can buy poisonous fly spray and poison them to death or you can spend all day swatting them against the wall with a fly swatter, but more flies will eventually come back in time. They'll come back because the cause is still there. What's the cause? Probably a dirty trashcan, food left out or maybe a dirty bathroom with something for flies to eat. The environment either attracts or repels different life forms to it, especially within your own body.

Clean your house and get rid of the fly-attracting food and you cure it. If there's nothing there for the scavenger flies to eat or lay eggs in, they leave. They cannot survive in a clean environment. It's Mother Nature's way of cleaning house.

It keeps the world turning. If something needs cleaning up, she sends ants, maggots, flies, mice, vultures, etc., to clean up the mess, and they do an excellent job. Just leave a piece of candy out and watch the ants devour it within a few hours. Watch the vultures feast on a dead carcass next to the road. What is trash to one is a meal to another. Mother Nature has things figured out. We would be wise to work with her, instead of attempting to manipulate her. Be calm, relaxed and harmonized with the universe. Stop resisting what God has created. Cleanse yourself from within and give up the need to worry about the evils outside.

You reap what you sow. Every living thing eats something. Everything has a purpose. If you plant carrots in the garden, you won't harvest tomatoes. Put a low-octane fuel in your car and never change the oil, air filter or spark plugs, and it will run sluggishly. Eat a lot of processed, dead food packed with sugar, flour, nitrates, chemical dyes and artificial colors and you'll catch colds and every virus that comes your way.

Every time you eat sugar, it has a paralyzing effect on your immune system. A candy bar and cola suppress the immune system for up to six hours. How many kids get sick right after Halloween from eating lots of candy? Cold and flu season always accompanies the holidays because we fire an assault on our immune system with all the Thanksgiving and Christmas goodies. The consumption of large amounts of sugar and flour leaves us wide open to illness. Of course, a lack of Vitamin D from less sun exposure in the winter months plays a role as well.

> **"If you want to watch your flowers grow, treat the roots, not the leaves. If you want to heal disease, treat the cause, not the symptoms."** Anonymous

The Germ Is Nothing — The Terrain Is Everything

What's the solution to good health? Ingest antibiotics every week to kill bacteria? Of course not, because new ones will come your way as fast as you kill the first. If we want to heal dis-ease and get rid of infections, then we have to change our body's terrain so that it no longer is susceptible to infection and illness.

We all have streptococcus bacteria; in fact, the average human has about 500 types of bacteria in their mouth. It is estimated that your body houses roughly 100 trillion bacteria and one quadrillion viruses! We only get sick with strep

How Much Bacteria Is In The Average House?
• Door handle – 121 bacteria/square inch
• Light Switch – 217 bacteria/square inch
• Phone – 133 bacteria/square inch
• Bathroom Faucet Handle – 6,267 bacteria/square inch
• Bathtub Drain Area – 119,468 bacteria/square inch

throat when the mouth becomes acidic and the microbe changes to our new environment, then the microbe's secretions, not the germ itself, causes us to become ill with a sore throat, cough, congestion etc. This is why, if someone has the flu or a cold, not everyone around them is going to get it, only those with a weakened immune system.

> **"Antibiotic resistance comes mainly because of inappropriate or improper use of antibiotics by physicians. Some 150 million prescriptions are written annually in this country. And 60% of them — that translates to 90 million prescriptions — are for antibiotics. Of those, 50 million are absolutely unnecessary or inappropriate."** Dr. Philip Tierno, Director of Clinical Microbiology and Diagnostic Immunology, New York University Medical Center

When you take your child into the doctor for an ear infection and he or she prescribes an antibiotic that doesn't work, it is probably because the infection wasn't caused by bacteria. Many ear infections are caused by a virus or fungus, and antibiotics only work against bacterial infections.

Nature's Detoxifying Foods	
Garlic	Cacao
Onions	Hemp
Turmeric	Beets
Bee pollen	Kelp
Goji berries	Lemon
Coconut oil	Alfalfa
Chlorella	Spirulina

Do you know people who start on one antibiotic and it seems that every four months they are sick again? That's because they did nothing to change the terrain that has allowed the bacteria to exist in the first place. The solution is to break the food chain cycle. Stop poisoning your body so the critters have something to eat. Clean up the dead rabbit on the road and the vultures and flies won't come around. Cleanse the body of undigested proteins, mucus, built-up fecal matter, etc., and these microbes will have nothing to consume. Microbes only proliferate in an unclean body where there is much garbage to feed on, like vultures do flattened opossums on the side of the road.

The survival of every human, animal, insect, fish, plant, bird, virus, bacteria, fungus, mold, germ, microbe or whatever you can identify big or small that is alive only continues living if its environment allows it. You will never see polar bears living naturally in the Sahara Desert nor alligators at the North Pole, because these animals cannot survive in those environments. Everything either lives or dies depending upon its environment. We become diseased when our internal terrain favors disease, not by coming in contact with a "germ" when someone coughs or sneezes next to you.

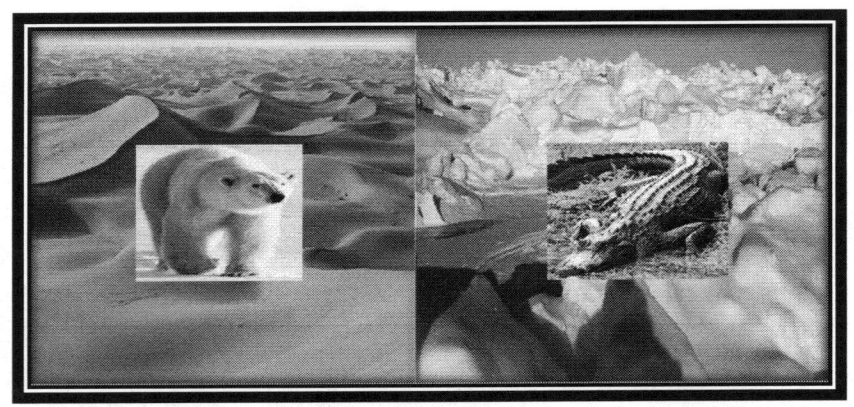

Germs are very seldom the cause of disease; in most cases, they are the result of disease. When your body's pH (fluid in and around your cells) is acidic, then your immune system is weakened. Undigested proteins and excess mucus backed up in the lymphatic system sets the stage for infection and illness.

> **"DNA does not control biology and the nucleus itself is not the brain of the cell. Just like you and me, cells are shaped by where they live. In other words, it's the environment, stupid."** Bruce Lipton, Ph.D.

Drugs are very acid-forming and contribute to a terrain that favors dis-ease. On the other hand, herbs are alkaline-producing foods that help balance pH. Doctors who understand how the body truly heals will recommend remedies that reverse cellular acidosis, not drugs that cause it. Healthy people have a pH (saliva) of about 6.8.

People around the world who eat and drink only wholesome organic foods and beverages rarely get sick. Some can honestly say they haven't had a cold, the flu or a headache in 10 years. How can this happen when they are around sick, coughing, sneezing people all the time? The secret is, healthy people don't get sick. If your immune system is balanced, you have nothing to fear because the minute a pathogen like a flu virus enters your body, it is destroyed and eliminated by the guards at the gate in your lymphatic and immune system.

> **"Disease symptoms are an effort of the body to eliminate waste, mucus, and toxemia. This system assists Nature in the most perfect and natural way. Not the disease but the body is to be healed; it must be cleansed, freed from waste and foreign matter, from mucus and toxemia accumulated since childhood."**
> Professor Arnold Ehret – German Naturopath, 1866-1922

Fever (Leukocytosis) — How Your Body Destroys Pathogens

Leukocytosis is when the body heats up to increase immune function and fight infection. Just as we clean our ovens with high temperature heat for about 4 hours (clean mode) to rid it of junk, so does the body produce a fever to rid itself of pathogenic toxins. Viruses and bacteria cannot live beyond certain high temperatures, so the body heats up to speed up the immune response to destroy them. Cancer cells don't like heat either; in fact, 108 degrees for one hour will kill cancer cells while leaving healthy cells alone.

Fevers & Flu in Children
Children's Composition Plus
- Yarrow
- Peppermint
- Elder Flowers
- Lemon Balm
- Chamomile
- Essential Oils

> **"Artificially induced fever has the greatest potential in the treatment of many diseases, including cancer."** Dr. Josef Issels, German Physician, 1907-1998

What do most mothers do as soon as a child gets a fever? They run and grab a fever-reducing drug to lower the body temperature. Taking acetaminophen to reduce a fever is interfering with the body's intelligence, what the doctor within is attempting to do, which is to get you well. When your military-like immune system identifies foreign invaders such as bacteria or viruses, it automatically heats up to march in the marines, your white blood cells, and destroy the infection-causing pathogens. And then you come along and turn the thermostat back down with a fever-reducing drug, which stops the marines from rushing in to kill the enemy and terminate the infection. Why would you do this? When the body is not given a chance to raise the temperature high enough to increase white blood cells to go after pathogens, then we are forcing it to burrow deeper into the tissue to surface at a later date and in a different fashion. This is dangerous and may cause many future health problems. Wisdom beckons us to stop interfering with the way that God engineered the human body to clear out infections. Anything done to reduce the temperature such as drugs or sponging is counterproductive.

> **"Every doctor learns during the preclinical years of medical school that for every degree of rise in temperature the rate of travel of the disease-fighting leukocytes in the bloodstream is doubled. This process is known as leucotaxis. I can't comprehend why a doctor would want to put the brakes on a mechanism that is striving to make his patient well."** Robert Mendelsohn, M.D.

Research has shown that regular use of fever-reducing/pain-killing acetaminophen (Tylenol) medications is linked to higher rates of asthma and chronic obstructive pulmonary disease (COPD).

A fever is nature's way of bringing toxins and impurities to the surface to be eliminated. When channels of elimination are not removing waste materials fast enough, the body sometimes will spike a fever. Viruses and bacteria die when body temperatures rise. For example, if you have a 104-degree fever, the ability of your white blood cells to move through the body and fight infection is increased 64 times compared to normal body temperature of 98 degrees. It is your innate intelligence's way of saving your life. It isn't something to fear but to be thankful for because the body is heating up to speed up the healing process. If your fever lingers on, an enema, especially a coffee enema, helps detoxify the liver and can speed up the recovery process tremendously. Garlic enemas have been proven to be beneficial as well.

> **"Give me the chance to create fever and I will cure any disease."** Parmenides (2,000 years ago)

How high can a fever get before it becomes dangerous? Every parent would be wise to read Dr. Mendelsohn's book, *How To Raise A Healthy Child In Spite Of Your Doctor*. He states that fevers below 105 degrees do not pose any lasting threat to one's health. Very seldom will fevers go over 105. Brain damage from a fever generally will not occur unless the fever is over 107.6.

> **"Natural forces within us are the true healers."** Hippocrates, Father of Modern Medicine, 460-370 B.C.

Many doctors have shown that the body produces a fever to prevent infection from spreading to other areas. Experiments performed by G.W. Duff and S.K. Durum have demonstrated that at 2 degrees Centigrade of fever, T-cells and antibodies rapidly increased by 2,000 percent above their normal number at regular body temperature. If fever increases our ability to fight pathogens, is it possible that a low body temperature, people with hypothyroidism, are more susceptible to infections?

> **"The Intelligence within you is the same Intelligence that created this entire planet."** Louise L. Hay, Author of *You Can Heal Your Life*

Colds

> **Master Tonic Immune Formula**
> ¼ cup chopped garlic
> ¼ cup chopped white onions
> ¼ cup grated ginger
> 2 Tbsp. grated horseradish root
> 2 Tbsp. turmeric powder
> 1 habanero pepper or
> 1 tsp. cayenne (optional)
> 24 oz. Apple Cider Vinegar
> (Organic Bragg)
> Fill a 1-quart Mason jar with dry ingredients and mix well. Pour in vinegar and shake daily for 2 weeks. Strain, squeeze well and drink. Take 1 Tbsp. up to 6 times a day.

A wise person has locks on their doors and a weapon to defend their home against intruders. Your immune system will be primed and ready when you supply it with nature's colds and flu busters. I suggest arming yourself with the Master Tonic Immune Formula listed on the left. It is simple, inexpensive and easy to make, and stays good for years. It can be taken daily as a general tonic preventive, or used in time of infections and sickness. It stops sore throats and colds dead in their tracks. Every house should be armed with it. I never leave home without it when I travel.

The common cold is your body's way of cleaning house and expelling toxic garbage, which produces symptoms we call a cold. A stuffy or runny nose, sneezing, cough, diarrhea or rash are typical house-cleaning symptoms known as catabolism. Typically, this inner-cleansing process lasts three to 10 days. Of course, most people run and get an antibiotic, and when they start to feel better, they give the antibiotic the credit, when in reality, their body's intelligence was doing some house-cleaning and had everything under control all along.

Remember, only sick people get sick. If you are healthy, your body would never need a cold to cleanse mucus and other toxic sludge that impairs your immune system. The doctor within knows when to automatically clean, and when he snaps his fingers, all 100 trillion cells crack their heels and salute. Your body is a house of order. When told to clean, the cells begin cleaning, and as a result, you begin draining mucus and expelling toxins

> **Sore Throat Spray**
> - Colloidal Silver
> - Oregano Oil
> - Lemon Oil
> - Peppermint Oil
> Mix all ingredients in a spray bottle and spray in throat every hour.

through the sinuses. Coughing and sneezing are the body's ways of expelling metabolic trash. Anything done to suppress it usually causes the illness to last longer.

When the sinuses are compacted with mucus and there's no blood flow to bring in the marines (white blood cells) to fight infection, this allows congestion to linger for lengthy periods. The head basically becomes a human petri dish full of mucus breeding bacteria. People with congestion are usually heavy dairy and gluten (grains) consumers.

> **Sinus Congestion Neti Pot Cleanse**
> 1. 8 oz. purified water (if using tap water, boil for 5 minutes)
> 2. 3 tsp. raw salt (do not use iodized salt)
> 3. 1 tsp. baking soda (optional)
> 4. 1 tsp. hydrogen peroxide (optional)
> 5. Mix all ingredients in 8 oz. of warm (not too hot) water. Pour in neti pot or irrigation device.
> 6. Tilt your head sideways over sink. Press the spout of your device into upper nostril and slowly begin to irrigate while breathing through your mouth and let water run out bottom nostril.
> 7. Rotate your head and repeat on the other nostril.

> **"Disease is nothing else but an attempt on the part of the body to rid itself of morbific matter."** Dr. Thomas Sydenham, Famous 17th-century English Physician

> **Hydrogen Peroxide Miracle for Colds**
> Lay down on your side and pour one capful of hydrogen peroxide (standard 3% grade) in ear and let bubble and fizz for 3 minutes. Turn over and do the same for the other ear.
> This clears out infection in the ears, throat and sinuses and helps eliminate allergies and candida yeast. It is very beneficial to do once a week for general maintenance.

A cold develops after we have abused the body with the typical American junk-food diet. Too much wheat (gluten), pasteurized dairy and processed foods laden with sugar and trans-fats acidify the body and lead to constipation, which produces toxicity in the body. Periodically, the body has to punch the red panic button to clean house so the cells are able to function. When cold symptoms hit and you feel terrible with sinus drainage, your body is in a mucus-eliminating cleanse. Bacteria, viruses and germs of all types thrive only in a toxic body that provides a hospitable environment for them to exist. Your diet, your response to stress and emotions are usually the difference between staying healthy or coming down with a cold.

> **"Echinacea and garlic are the 'one, two punch' for the common cold!"** Dr. Richard Schulze

THE IMMUNE SYSTEM - FIGHTING TO KEEP YOU HEALTHY

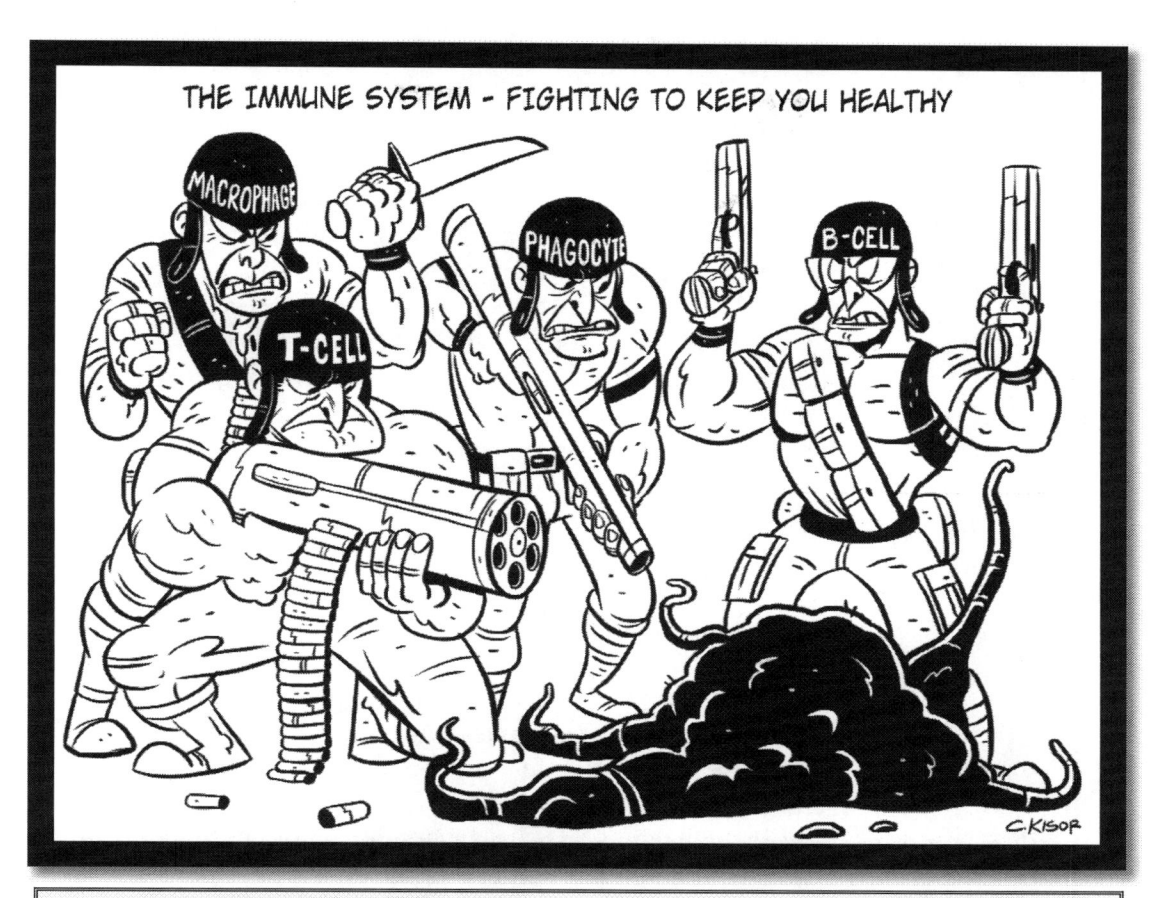

"Whenever the immune system successfully deals with an infection, it emerges from the experience stronger and better able to confront similar threats in the future. Our immune system develops in combat. If at the first sign of infection, you always jump in with antibiotics, you do not give the immune system a chance to grow stronger." Andrew Weil, M.D.

Cold & Flu Busters	
Echinacea	Olive leaf
Elderberry	Cat's claw
Goldenseal	Cinnamon oil
Ginger	Oregano oil
Garlic	Beta Glucan
Colloidal Silver	Zinc
Vitamin C	Vitamin D
Astragalus	Cayenne

At the first sign of a cold, you would be wise to start on echinacea and elderberry immediately three times a day. Eating raw garlic chopped up and taken with bites of food will help knock out viruses and bacteria. Supplementing with Vitamin C (1,000 mg five times a day) along with Vitamin D (20,000 IU per day)

117

and zinc (100 mg per day) will supercharge your immune system. Spending one hour in direct sunlight will give you about 50,000 mg of Vitamin D, so get out in the sunlight. Putting three drops of oregano oil in a large glass of water and drinking it several times a day can finish off most cold and flu viruses fast. Putting a teaspoon of colloidal silver in a glass of water and drinking it three times a day can help clear out infections as well.

Sinus Support
- Myrrh Plus
- Adrena Plus
- Hista Plus

Attempting to stop a cold with drugs is interfering with the natural cleansing process your intelligence automatically ordered. A cold should be allowed to run its course and you would be wise to support it in its effort to save your life by eliminating congestion. Consuming warm bone broth (chicken or beef), fermented vegetables, homemade kefir or yogurt with fresh fruits, berries and vegetables along with herbal teas gives the body optimal nutritional support. A massage and bouncing on a rebounder (mini-trampoline) can help get the lymphatic system draining. Sleep as much as you can for two days. The body heals while sleeping. Drink plenty of water. Soaking in a hot Epsom salt (2 cups) bath for 20 minutes with some essential oils (20 drops of lavender) may be very beneficial, especially if you are stressed out and congested. Running a diffuser to breathe in essential oils (clove, lemon, cinnamon, eucalyptus, rosemary) is good.

Lung Support
- Mullein Plus
- Pneumo Plus
- Adrena Plus
- Mold X

If the bowels are not eliminating properly, then toxins will be reabsorbed from your colon into your body and you'll feel terrible and the cold may linger on for days. Doing an enema, especially a coffee enema, can help eliminate toxins and expedite the healing response. Allowing a cold to run its course results in you having more vibrant energy in the long run. Stopping a cold with drugs results in future health challenges and less energy.

Years ago, poor people in India and Russia, who couldn't afford to go to the doctor, ate garlic to stay healthy. Garlic is considered "Russian penicillin." Research has proven that garlic stimulates natural killer cells, which are our main defense against cancer. Garlic with purplish skin is the best. Eating a little garlic with your meals raw or cooked with food is a great way to keep the immune system in tip-top shape. And if you want the best for your immune system, eat garlic, onions, ginger and turmeric every day. Those four gems are Mother Nature's pathogen destroyers.

> **"Stop judging. Celebrate everything. Yes, even your disease. It is your blessing."** Dr. Richard Schulze

Own Your Dis-ease & Be Healed

Negative thoughts and fear-based emotions weaken your immune system. Have you ever had an argument or been really angry with someone and the next day woken up sick? Do you have someone at work or in your family that's a real pain in the neck or just gets under your skin? These stressors are nails in your tire continuing to weaken your immune system.

> **"No man is free who is not master of himself."** Epictetus

Poor people are usually blamers and complainers. They always have an excuse, and it's always someone else's fault. As long as you blame someone or something else, you are giving away your power and will continue to be powerless. One of the first steps to healing is to take full responsibility for your illness and own it. Empowerment comes from taking ownership of your situation and realizing that we create our experiences. God gives us our free agency to experience whatever we choose by the thoughts we choose to think, the feelings we dwell upon and the choices we make.

> **"I can do all things through Christ which strengtheneth me."** Philippians 4:13

If I have the power to create something, then I also have the power to uncreate it. Give up the need to be a victim of your circumstances. Stop giving away all your power to cancer or whatever you have been diagnosed with. You have given something else more power than yourself when you do this. Healing occurs when you take ownership of the illness. Be the source of it. Be the creator of it. By owning it, you can do what you want with it. Instead of it controlling you, you control it. This belief in your mind is crucial in order to heal. This is empowerment. If you are the source of it, meaning you created it, then you also have the power to destroy it and create something different. When you do this, you begin to live powerfully. This is being rich. This is being one with the source. This transformation aligns you with Divinity. Live the life you love and love the life you live.

> "Everything you see has its roots in the unseen world. The forms may change, yet the essence remains the same. Every wonderful sight will vanish; every sweet word will fade, but do not be disheartened. The source they come from is eternal, growing, branching out, giving new life and new joy. Why do you weep? The source is within you. And this whole world is springing up from it."
> Jelauddin Rumi 1207-1273

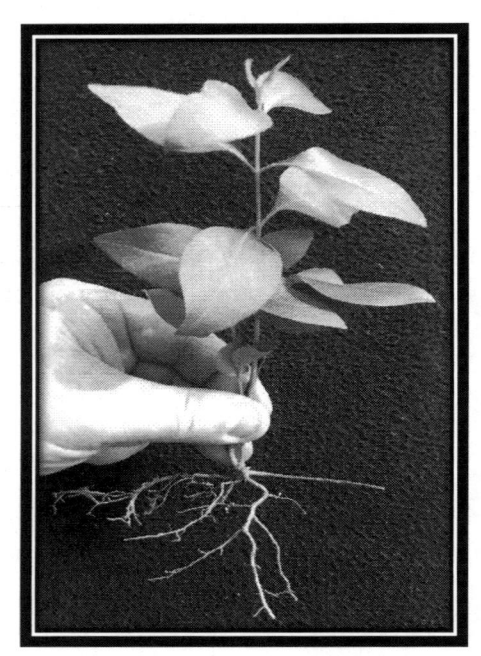

If you have a disease like cancer and you believe and feel you are a poor innocent victim, then you will have a difficult time healing. Oh sure, surgery, chemotherapy and radiation might get rid of it for the time being, but nothing has been done to pull the roots out that nourished it to grow in the first place; therefore, you are not truly healed. Many times, those roots are negative mental/emotional patterns that cause you to self-destruct (subconscious way of committing suicide). Without changing your destructive thought patterns, or healing the unresolved emotional hurts from the past, that same illness will be recreated perhaps in a different form or part of the body. In the meantime, your doctor has performed another magic trick to make the cancer look like it is gone, but if he is honest, he will admit it is impossible to get 100 percent of the cancer cells. They'll be back again, it's just a matter of time, and when it does, it will come back with a vengeance.

Sick people have lots of faith. They have a tremendous amount of faith in the wrong thing. What do you worry about? What is your biggest fear? Whatever you allow your mind to dwell upon is where your faith is. In the Bible, there is a story about Job. By focusing on what he didn't want, is what he got. He was plagued with boils.

> "What lies behind us and what lies before us are small matters to what lies within us." Ralph Waldo Emerson

What you dwell upon creates your reality. Focus on what you want, not what you don't want. What you dwell upon is what you give your power to. Like

Job, if what you don't want is what you give your attention to, then it will eventually manifest itself in your life. What you feed grows. Your life is a reflection of your innermost thoughts and beliefs. Take ownership of your situation. If it is cancer, then own it. If it's a troubled relationship, then own it so that you have the power to create something different, because what you previously created isn't working. Like an artist painting a masterpiece, your life is whatever you choose to create. What you choose to create is who you are BE-ING. If you don't like that, then create something different.

> **"Reality is that which, when you stop believing in it, doesn't go away."** Philip K. Dick

De-Nile is not just a river in Egypt. Accept full responsibility for your condition. See and feel yourself completely healed. Give your attention to health, not disease. If you want to lose weight, stop focusing on losing weight. Start focusing on being healthy and see yourself fit and in shape. Put those thoughts and energetic vibrations of health in your mind so they can physically manifest in your life.

> **"Who looks outside, dreams; who looks inside, awakes."** Carl Gustav Jung

Exercise For Weight Loss & Healthy Blood Sugar

BURST TRAINING

1. Warm up for about 3 – 5 minutes.
2. Pick an exercise that you can't do longer than 30 seconds, such as bicycling (recumbent bike), elliptical machine, running sprints, box jumps or swimming. These are excellent to get the heart rate up very high so you are gasping for air with a good burn in the muscles. This is crucial to kick start your metabolism and stabilize blood sugar! I like to run or hop football stadium stairs. By the time I hit the top, my legs are on fire and I'm breathing as hard as I can. I also love to run sprints or bicycle as fast as I can up a steep hill. I change up my routine so I never get bored.
3. Exercise as hard and fast as you can for 30 seconds. (Beginners will have to work up to this but try to do 8 to 30 seconds). You should be completely exhausted so that you can't go any longer. If you can keep going after 30 seconds, the exercise is too easy.
4. Recover for about 90 seconds, still moving but at a much slower pace.
5. Repeat this cycle 5 to 7 times.
6. Cool down by slowing down your pace until you are breathing normally again.
7. Total workout time should be 20 minutes or less. It may take several months to work up to being able to go as hard as you can for 30 seconds for a total of 7 cycles. Work at your own pace. Obviously a 220-pound NFL running back will have more stamina than an office worker who is 60 pounds overweight. Be smart, go at your own pace and don't compare yourself to others. It doesn't matter where we start, only that we reach our health goals.

High Intensity Interval Training or BURST TRAINING for 20 minutes three times a week is the most effective way to lose weight and stabilize blood sugar levels. Some people spend an hour at the gym every day working out inefficiently. Exercising too much may be counterproductive. Remember, more is not always better.

> **"Vigorous exercise is a better antidepressant than Prozac."** Mark Hyman, M.D.

When you work out hard, you create tiny tears in your muscles and they rebuild bigger and stronger during rest, which is the healing process. Therefore, it is wise to only train each muscle group with weights two or three times a week. It gives the muscles time to recuperate. When I competed in powerlifting years ago, I suffered injuries from over-training and ignoring my body. Be smart and be consistent with your workouts.

Exercising increases blood flow, bringing a fresh supply of oxygen, vitamins and minerals to every cell in the body, rejuvenating you. This is why you feel good after exercising. Your cells, especially those far away from your heart, finally get some nourishment and new oxygen after a long famine. This is the reason we tell people who are tired all the time to start working out, because exercise creates more energy, not less.

Exercise is one of the best remedies for depression, better sleep and more energy. When you exercise, many neurotransmitters are triggered in the brain that release endorphins that help you feel energized, happy and in control. These antidepressant endorphins are serotonin, dopamine, GABA and glutamate. Have you ever noticed that happy people exercise and depressed people just don't feel like it, because they're too tired? It sounds like an oxymoron, but exercising will give you more energy and definitely help you sleep better.

Exercising reduces the stress hormone cortisol, which triggers insulin resistance and sugar cravings, and excess cortisol causes you to put on belly fat. Exercise dramatically increases hormonal levels that govern every process and function in the body as well as improving sexual function. It also helps reduce your risk of heart disease and strokes.

Research has proven that exercising for lengthy periods, like jogging or doing cardio machines at the gym, is inefficient compared to burst training. In fact, by doing burst training, you can exercise less and still burn 9 percent more body fat. Burst training can improve your insulin sensitivity by almost 25 percent with a fraction of the time invested, compared to cardio training. And exercising in the morning before breakfast while fasting is very beneficial to help break down stored fat. Don't worry, the muscles being exercised will not break down, but it is wise to eat within 30 minutes after exercising in the morning and break-your-fast to help muscles recuperate.

Burst training also helps stimulate Human Growth Hormone (HGH), which helps slow down the aging process and keeps you strong, vibrant and robust. Usually by age 30 and beyond, the body slows down the production of HGH considerably. This is another reason why burst training is so needed as we age.

One of the worst things you can do before a workout is carb-loading. Many people are misled into thinking you need carbs for energy to work out. Eating granola (energy bars), breads, pasta or rice, or using sports drinks with sugar and caffeine, will all sabotage weight loss and blood-sugar-stabilizing goals.

The Facts About Fats

> "Your health and life span are determined by the proportion of fat versus glucose you burn throughout your lifetime. And that is determined by what you choose to eat." Ron Rosedale, M.D.

We've been lied to. Fats don't make you fat, carbohydrates (sugar and starches) do. Your body burns either fats or sugar (carbs) for fuel. Fats are the best fuel for your body, especially your brain. In fact, we really don't even need carbs. We were meant to burn fats as our primary source of fuel. Just as souped-up racecars require a high-octane fuel for top-notch performance, we humans function our best when fueled by fats instead of carbs.

Eat Healthy Fats/Oils	Avoid Unhealthy Fats/Oils
▪ Coconut oil	○ Canola oil
▪ Olive oil	○ Soybean oil
▪ Avocados	○ Sunflower oil
▪ Olives	○ Corn oil
▪ Eggs	○ Safflower oil
▪ Raw Nuts & Seeds	○ Grapeseed oil
▪ Butter	○ Peanut oil
▪ Ghee	○ Cottonseed oil
▪ MCT oil	○ Vegetable oil
▪ Avocado oil	○ Margarine
▪ Hemp seeds	○ Crisco
▪ Chia seeds	

Ketones are made by mitochondria in your liver from stored fats and are used as an alternative source of fuel to glucose. Because ketones are water soluble, they can pass through cell membranes and right into the brain for immediate fuel. Many doctors still hold on to the outdated and false belief that the brain only uses sugar for fuel. This is false, as Dr. George Cahill has proven. When you fast and the body gets low in carbohydrates, your body converts fats into ketones and will burn ketones from stored fat for energy. This is how some people can fast for prolonged periods of time and stay mentally sharp.

Not all fats are the same. Avoid trans-fats from vegetable oils such as shortening, corn oil, French fries, vegetable oil shortenings, salad dressings and margarine. Margarine is one of the worst foods you can eat because it coats your cells, changing the permeability so they can't breathe. If you put a plastic bag over your head, you suffocate and die. When you eat margarine, you are basically consuming liquid plastic that is equivalent to putting a bag over the lipid bi-layer of cells so they can't breathe. One of the biggest frauds to ever sucker-punch Americans in the gut is the false belief that eating margarine instead of butter is a healthier choice. Nothing could be further from the truth.

Margarine is one molecule away from plastic, and shares 27 ingredients with paint.

Trans-fatty acids are made by taking oils under high pressure and exposing them to high temperatures in the presence of a metal catalyst such as nickel and aluminum. Hydrogen atoms are shifted to unnatural positions. The end product of partially hydrogenated oil contains small amounts of aluminum and nickel, both of which are linked to serious health problems. These trans fats interfere with your insulin receptors and lead to diabetes and cardiovascular diseases.

The key to reversing diabetes and permanent weight loss is to reprogram the body to burn fats instead of carbs for energy. The truth is, we thrive on a high-fat, or very low-carbohydrate diet. Coconut butter is excellent to give you energy and make you feel full. Fat is like rocket fuel for the brain. It is simply the best fuel. Research has proven that low-fat diets and statin drugs put you at a higher risk for neurological and brain problems such as dementia, Alzheimer's and Parkinson's.

"Fat — not carbohydrate — is the preferred fuel of human metabolism and has been for all of human evolution." David Perlmutter, M.D., Author of *Grain Brain*

Fats help you lose weight and give you energy. Healthy fats are coconut oil, avocados, olive oil, olives, butter, eggs, raw nuts and seeds. So, how do we reprogram the body to burn fats? Simply get off carbs and replace them with healthy fats as mentioned above. Obviously, we want to continue eating lots of vegetables. Berries and some fruit in moderation are good. Organic meats such as salmon, trout, chicken, turkey and steak provide us with good protein if used in moderation.

Coconut Oil – Fuel For Life

Coconut oil is loaded with health promoting goodies such as Vitamin E, caprylic acid and lauric acid, an anti-inflammatory which when

> **Which Coconut Oil IS Best?**
> - Use virgin, organic, cold-pressed & unrefined
> - Avoid deodorized or bleached
> - For cooking, expeller-pressed, unrefined is OK

consumed is converted to monolaurin by your body and will destroy lipid-coated viruses such as HIV, herpes, influenza, giardia, measles and gram-negative bacteria. Its antimicrobial properties have also been shown to eradicate bacteria, fungi and parasites (protozoa) along with supplying you with healthy antioxidants. Monolaurin is found in breast milk to boost a baby's immune system as well as colostrum. These are the true flu- and cold-busters, not a needle loaded with foreign toxins like the flu shot provides. Researchers compared the antifungal effects of coconut oil to the anti-fungal drug Diflucan, and the coconut oil proved to be more effective. (J Med Food. 2007 Jun 10(2):384-87) Not only is coconut oil highly beneficial for the immune system, but it's also super fuel for your cells, metabolism, blood sugar, bones, brain, energy and stamina. It works great for dry skin and skin infections as well.

Oil pulling has become popular because of its ability to clear up infections and bind to toxins. Swishing a spoonful of coconut oil in your mouth every morning for about 5 minutes helps eliminate toxins. Make sure and spit it out and do not swallow it, since it absorbs toxins from the mouth.

Dr. George Cahill from Harvard Medical School teaches that beta-hydroxybutyrate (beta-HBA), a ketone body produced from fasting, is superior fuel for the brain, especially for Alzheimer's and Parkinson's. It is also easily obtained by adding coconut oil to your diet. It improves antioxidant function, increases mitochondria and supports the growth of new brain cells. Coconut oil also helps boost the absorption of fat-soluble vitamins. And researchers at the University of Adelaide report that lauric acid, a main ingredient in coconut oil, destroyed 93 percent of colon cancer cells in a 48-hour period in vitro.

Intermittent Fasting

> **"A little starvation can really do more for the average sick man than can the best medicines and the best doctors."** Mark Twain

Fasting turns on your survival genes so that your body begins using stored fat for fuel. When we eat 3 meals a day, the body's glycogen stores are never fully emptied.

Benefits Of Fasting	
Stabilizes blood sugar	Metabolic rate increases
Lowers insulin	Hunger decreases
Improves insulin resistance	Damaged cells removed
Digestion gets a rest	Cancer hormones eliminated
Ketones are produced	Brain health improved
Fat is burned for fuel	Body fat is shed
HGH is released	Immune system regeneration
Free radicals decrease	Antiaging support increases

Most of us have plenty of glycogen stored up in the body in the form of fat from our typical high sugar and grain diets. This unused energy has been stored there from eating too many carbs. When we stop eating during a fast, after about three days, the liver begins to break down stored body fat to burn as fuel, also known as ketosis. Ketones are produced by the liver and used as an energy source when glucose is not available.

When we practice intermittent fasting and allow the glycogen stores to empty then we reprogram the body to burn fat for fuel again. Waiting until 11 a.m. to eat and not eating past 7 p.m. can really help with weight loss and stabilizing blood sugar levels. Fasting also allows your body to go through a repair and rejuvenation period and will break down old and diseased cells.

It is interesting to note that most religions around the world practice fasting for spiritual purposes but also to cleanse the temple physically. Fasting helps us have self-discipline, and after constantly resisting the hunger signals to eat, when you do break your fast, you appreciate your food so much more. Fasting increases our gratitude.

The heart and the brain function more efficiently on ketones rather than blood sugar. Cancer cells can only burn sugar for fuel. Dr. Giulio Zuccoli of the University of Pittsburgh School of Medicine published a case of treating glioblastoma (the most aggressive brain cancer) with a ketogenic diet with promising results.

"The best of all medicines is resting and fasting." Benjamin Franklin

Breast Milk

If you were breastfed as an infant, congratulations, thank your mother, because she started you out on the right foot. Breastfed babies start life out in ketosis. As mentioned earlier, we were created to run on ketones, not glucose. Mother's breast milk, the most perfect food on earth, contains 54 percent saturated fat. If fats were bad for us, like we have been brainwashed to believe, why would our Creator put such a high amount in mother's milk? All of your cells in the body with those delicate membranes are 50 percent saturated fats. Fats are healthy! The richest source of Docosahexaenoic acid (DHA), which is brain food, is human breast milk.

The British nonprofit organization Save the Children estimates that 830,000 newborn deaths could be prevented every year if all infants were given breast milk in the first hour of life. And babies who are fed breast milk exclusively for the first 6 months of life are protected against many major childhood diseases. By contrast, a child who is not breastfed is 15 times more likely to die from pneumonia and 11 times more likely to die from diarrhea. The organization states that breast-feeding is the most effective of all ways to prevent disease and malnutrition that cause death.

Blood Sugar

Which Of The Following Foods Spikes Your Blood Sugar Most?
A. Snickers Candy Bar   B. Slice of Whole Wheat Bread
C. Banana   D. 1 Tbsp. White Sugar

The test on the left is one Dr. David Perlmutter, a neurologist, gives to see how many people understand which foods cause the greatest surge in blood sugar levels. He is the author of an informative book, *Grain Brain*. He explains how the consumption of grains leads to diabetes and neurological disorders such as Alzheimer's disease and dementia after years of spiking the blood sugar and damaging the delicate nerve endings. So, it's probably obvious by now that the answer to the test above is a slice of whole wheat bread spikes your blood sugar more than straight sugar, a Snickers candy bar or banana!

Eating a low- or no-grain diet with high-quality fats helps reverse high blood sugar (diabetes). Saturated fats help keep your bones healthy and enhance your immune system. They actually protect your liver from harmful toxins and help promote cardiovascular health. The sick-care industry wants you to believe that saturated fats cause cardiovascular disease, and this is false.

Cereal Killers & Gluten – Food Or Poison?

Gluten means "glue" in Latin. Gluten is a type of protein found in wheat, barley, rye, spelt and kamut. No human can completely digest these proteins. They cause inflammation in the body. Grains and cereals contain phytic acid that interferes with calcium and zinc absorption. Breads in particular are high in phytic acids that bind with zinc molecules, making it difficult for the body to absorb zinc.

Gluten Sensitivity Signs
- Fatigue After Eating
- Brain Fog
- Dizziness
- PMS
- Migraine Headaches
- Mood Swings
- Joint Pain
- Gas/Bloating
- Constipation/Diarrhea

Gluten-Free Grains & Starches

Amaranth	Quinoa
Arrowroot	Coconut Flour
Rice	Almond Flour
Buckwheat	Sorghum
Corn	Soy
Millet	Tapioca
Oats	Teff

Every 15 years, the number of recorded cases of celiac disease doubles. You may or may not have symptoms when you eat gluten. Don't make the mistake of thinking that just because you don't feel bad or have symptoms immediately after eating something, that you don't have an allergy to it. Many things happening at the cellular level don't always manifest symptoms to make you feel bad. How many colon cancer patients felt perfectly fine until they were diagnosed?

Dr. Mark Hyman cautions, *"If you eat two slices of whole wheat bread, you're going to raise your blood sugar more than if you ate a candy bar."* Avoid eating grains. Grains spike the blood sugar and then send your energy levels crashing. This blood sugar roller coaster leaves you feeling hungry, craving carbs and overeating, which causes you to put on belly fat. Consuming grains will eventually damage your brain due to surges in blood sugar. That is why Alzheimer's disease is now considered type 3 diabetes. Avoid all grain breads (even 100 percent whole wheat and Ezekiel breads), pasta, oatmeal, rice, corn, cereals, cornbread, crackers & chips. A good gluten- and grain-free substitute for white flour is coconut flour or almond flour so you can bake grain-free breads.

Gluten Containing Grains

Barley	Rye
Bulgur	Semolina
Couscous	Spelt
Farina	Triticale
Graham flour	Wheat
Kamut	Wheat germ
Matzo	

"Modern grains are silently destroying your brain." David Perlmutter, M.D.

If a farmer wants to fatten his animals before taking them to the butcher, he puts them on a high-carb diet with corn and grain. The grains spike their blood sugar and cause them to gain weight. Just as farmers know which foods to feed animals to fatten them up, weightlifting bodybuilders who want to lose as much fat as possible before a show, while bulking up and retaining as much muscle mass as possible, understand this concept and have been using it for years. It's simple. Eat lots of vegetables, fats and proteins in the form of meats, vegetables, nuts, seeds, eggs, healthy oils and cheese and leave the carbs (breads, pasta and sweets) alone. Starving the body of carbs puts you in ketosis, and the body is forced to burn fat for energy. While working out, your muscles get bigger and your body fat decreases as the body burns your fat for fuel. This is how a bodybuilder sheds extra stored fat while sculpting a massive physique of muscle.

> **"Gluten is the most commonly recognized environmental trigger that sets off any autoimmune reaction."** Dr. Tom O'Bryan

At the root of most chronic degenerative conditions is inflammation. So, if we can get rid of inflammation, we fix many problems. This is why supplements such as Vitamin C, turmeric

Inflammatory Foods
1. Gluten (wheat, barley & rye)
2. Sugar

and essential fatty acids, omega 3s (fish oil, flaxseed oil, krill oil) are so healing. They are naturally anti-inflammatory. But the question remains, what's causing the inflammatory condition in our body? Gluten in wheat and sugar are the two major culprits for inflammation. Alessio Fasano, M.D., the chair of pediatric gastroenterology at Massachusetts General Hospital, has researched gluten extensively at Harvard University. His research reveals that gluten in wheat causes intestinal permeability in every human. If we want to put the fires out that are causing inflammation, we have to stop throwing gas on the fire by eating gluten and sugar.

> **"No human has the enzymes to fully digest the proteins of wheat, rye and barley. These grains will cause inflammation and intestinal permeability every time they are eaten."** Dr. Tom O'Bryan

Molecular Mimicry

The proteins gliadin and gluten are found in wheat. As your body attempts to digest these proteins, they absorb into the bloodstream through microscopic holes in your digestive tract. This is referred to as "leaky gut." If you are sensitive to these proteins, your immune system will recognize these proteins as harmful invaders and begin attacking them. The problem is, whatever cells these proteins attach themselves to, the body will attack. So, if

Causes Of Molecular Mimicry
- Gluten
- Heavy Metals
- Lyme Disease
- Vaccinations
- Epstein-Barr Virus
- Infections

the proteins end up in the thyroid, then the immune system begins attacking your thyroid. If they are in the pancreas, then your body attacks the pancreas. This is referred to as molecular mimicry. This is another reason why wheat (gluten) can be so notorious in causing inflammatory response, which leads to autoimmune disorders. So, if you have an autoimmune disorder such as rheumatoid arthritis, lupus, multiple sclerosis, Type 1 diabetes or Hashimoto's disease, I highly suggest a gluten/grain-free diet. Just a note, about 75 percent of Americans have undiagnosed food sensitivities (allergies). You may not have the dreaded celiac disease, but at the cellular level in some part of your body there may be a silent battle occurring right now. By eating gluten, you are giving your enemy guns and ammo that cause inflammation. Once your body can no longer keep patching the holes in your intestinal tract to keep you healthy, then you have a high probability of being diagnosed with irritable bowel syndrome, colitis or Crohn's disease.

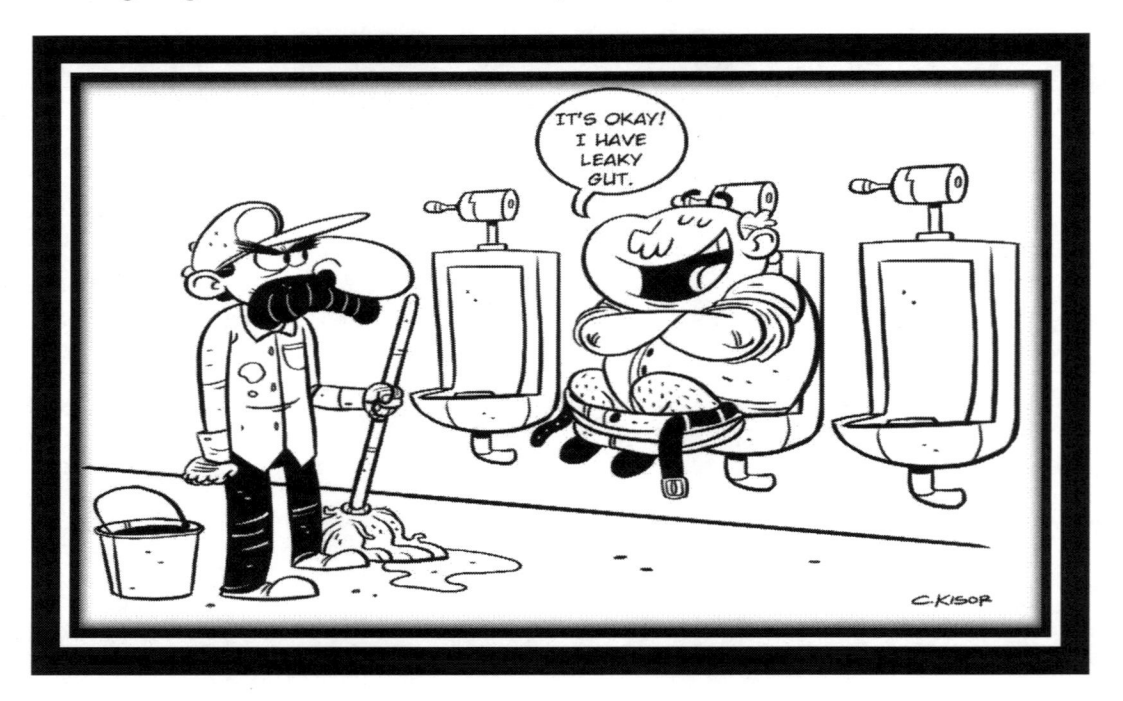

You Crave What You Are Allergic To

Dr. Christine Zioudrou and her colleagues teach how gluten can produce a high. *"If you've ever felt a rush of euphoric pleasure following the consumption of a bagel, scone, doughnut or croissant, you're not imagining it and you're not alone. We've known since the late 1970s that gluten breaks down in the stomach to become a mix of polypeptides that can cross the blood-brain barrier. Once they gain entry, they can then bind to the brain's morphine receptor to produce a sensorial high. This is the same receptor to which opiate drugs bind, creating their pleasurable, albeit addicting, effect."* This helps us understand why people crave what they are allergic to.

Do You Have Allergies Or A Digestion Imbalance?

All chemical changes within the cells of humans are performed by the action of enzymes. A deficiency of enzymes can cause malfunctioning of your digestion and metabolism. A newborn baby has 100 times more enzymes in their bloodstream than that of an elderly person.

Digestive Enzymes
1. Protease - proteins
2. Lipase - fats
3. Amylase - carbs

> **"Minerals are the basic spark plugs in the chemistry of life, on which the exchanges of energy in the combustion of foods and the building of living tissue depends."** Dr. Henry Schroeder

A mother brought her 10-year-old son, Evan, into our office because he had terrible sinus congestion. The pediatrician had him take five rounds of antibiotics in the last 6 months, and it failed to help improve his breathing. We ran an EDS scan and found that he didn't have an infection. He had a gluten allergy that was off the charts. We put him on some digestive enzymes and probiotics to repair the damage the antibiotics caused to his gut and put him on a gluten-free diet. Within a week he was breathing 90 percent better. He and his mother were amazed. The gluten was throwing gas on the fire, inflaming his sinuses. Then one day he went to a cousin's birthday party and ate pizza and cake, and the sinuses became totally inflamed again. This 10-year-old boy saw firsthand that the gluten was poison in his body and was motivated to stop eating it from that day on, because it made him feel so bad. His mother says that now he walks down the aisles in the grocery store checking labels for gluten. He's determined not to eat it because he can't breathe when he does.

Many of our foods are not properly digested, and Dr. Edward Howell states that many bacteria, yeast cells, large protein molecules and fats (especially if you don't have a gallbladder) can slip through the walls of the intestines and into the bloodstream. Most of us have some degree of leaky gut. When this happens and your body is lacking the necessary enzymes to digest those molecules, then allergies develop. Allergies are the body's way of removing foreign protein molecules. If allergic reactions are suppressed with drugs, then the body is forced to store the allergen in the body. After years of toxic allergen accumulation, degenerative disease is the result.

Many allergies, sinus congestion and headaches are caused from poor digestion. If you aren't breaking down your fats, carbs and proteins, these undigested food particles, especially fats and proteins, absorb into the blood. The undigested foods cause inflammation in the sinuses and head. As the body recognizes them as foreigners and releases histamines in an attempt to expel them, you experience swelling and discomfort. Two ways to eliminate this problem are first to stop eating foods that cause inflammation, then to supplement your meals with digestive enzymes so you can digest your foods properly, thus eliminating inflammation.

> **"It takes an average of 17 years for research findings to work their way down to your local doctors. The problem is that you don't have 17 years to waste."**
> Dr. Tom O'Bryan

Stomach Acid – Your Friend For Life

In 2014, $5.9 billion was spent on Nexium to treat acid reflux and heartburn symptoms. Acid-blocking drugs like Nexium and Prilosec deplete magnesium from the body and interfere with the absorption of Vitamin B12, which leads to osteoporosis. What is causing all the indigestion? First of all, if you eat three times a day, you should have two to three bowel movements per day. Let's analyze this for one moment. You eat lunch. You chew your food and mix it with saliva, which contains the enzyme ptyalin. This is the first step in digestion. It's important for you to chew your food and completely break it down to a smooth liquid before swallowing. The longer you chew your food, the more digestible it becomes.

> **"Most doctors don't know anything about nutrition, because medical schools are so oriented toward intervention that they virtually ignore nutrition as an element in the prevention or cure of disease."** Robert Mendelsohn, M.D.

After you swallow food, hydrochloric acid (0.8 pH) and pepsinogen enzymes are secreted by parietal cells to mix and break it down in the stomach, which usually takes about 4 hours. The stomach is one area of the body that needs to be acidic (pH of 1.5 - 2.0) for proper digestion. These stomach acids are powerful enough to dissolve a thin metal bar. A mucus lining, coating the stomach, provides protection from these powerful acids that are necessary to properly break down food. Hydrochloric acid also acts as a natural disinfectant that kills any bacteria that we may eat or drink. Acid blockers stop the secretion of hydrochloric acid in the stomach, which invites any bacteria from food or drinks to come in and proliferate.

If the mucus lining in the stomach isn't able to keep the acid away from the stomach wall, then it can become irritated and ulcers can form. People who are under lots of stress have a tendency to get ulcers because their body uses up its magnesium and potassium reserves to balance the nervous system. Once depleted, the stomach is unable to manufacture its needed digestive juices, including the mucus, to protect against the strong stomach acids. This leaves you susceptible to ulcerative conditions and infections such as Helicobacter pylori bacteria.

Low Stomach Acid Symptoms
- Asthma
- Celiac disease
- Autoimmune disorders
- Chronic hives
- Dermatitis
- Diabetes
- Eczema
- Thyroid (hyper or hypo)
- Lupus
- Osteoporosis
- Pernicious anemia
- Rheumatoid arthritis
- Rosacea

If the stomach isn't acid enough, then it cannot absorb calcium and iron. This can cause anemia. Calcium and iron have a positive charge, as does the lining of the intestinal tract. Minerals will go right through the intestinal tract without being absorbed because like repels like. However, when the stomach has enough acid, then the minerals pick up an extra positive charge from the acid, which allows them to bind with a protein so that they can be properly assimilated. This is why taking acid-blockers is so dangerous. They prevent assimilation of nutrients. If you are anemic, you may have plenty of iron, but are unable to absorb it due to low stomach acid and digestive enzymes. Once the food in the stomach has been mixed and churned properly with gastric juices and broken down into what is known as chyme, then the pyloric valve opens to release the food into the duodenum, the first part of the small intestine. This acidic liquid activates the pancreas to release enzymes to break down proteins (protease), carbohydrates (amylase) and fats (lipase). Alkaline digestive juices (sodium bicarbonate) and enzymes are secreted to further break down the food. Bile is secreted from the gallbladder to help break down fats and lubricate the intestines. If your gallbladder has been removed, then you will have difficulty metabolizing your fats.

Digestive Support
- Alpha Gest – for acid reflux
- Alpha Gest II – for burning & reflux
- Alpha Gest III – for reflux, gas & bloating
- Alpha Zyme III – for gas & bloating
- Diadren Forte – for digestion/blood sugar
- Beta Plus – for those with no gallbladder
- Dia Zyme – for diabetics
- BR-SP – for stomach irritation/ulcers
- Kava Kalm – for H. pylori bacteria
- Intestinal Formula – for constipation
- Cape Aloe – bowel lubricant/constipation
- Fiber Life – Colon Cleanser

The surface of the small intestine, if stretched out, would cover an area the size of a tennis court. The small intestines are covered with millions of fingerlike villi that constantly sway back and forth like palm trees in the wind, sucking up digested food. The villi have lymph vessels that suck up the fat. They also have veins that pick up food and take it to the main transport vessel called the portal vein, which carries the food up to the liver for the processing of nutrients. If you are constipated, old fecal matter putrefying in the intestines will seep back into the bloodstream from the portal vein, causing headaches, skin rashes, sinus congestion and joint pains. This stresses the body, weakens the immune system and leaves you highly susceptible to illness. Layers of mucoid plaque, which is another way of saying undigested food, accumulates in your intestinal tract and can cause the beer belly bulge. That bulge could be an accumulation of perhaps 10 to even 70 pounds of undigested food. Fasting, and taking psyllium husk and bentonite clay, is highly effective for cleansing the intestinal area. My favorite intestinal cleanse program comes in a complete kit with guide. It's Dr. Richard Anderson's Arise & Shine program. Look it up at ariseandshine.com or call 800-688-2444. Other good bowel lubricants and cleansers are aloe vera concentrates, cascara sagrada and senna leaves.

> **"In the 50 years I've spent helping people to overcome illness, disability and disease, it has become crystal clear that poor bowel management lies at the root of most people's health problems."** Bernard Jensen, D.C., N.D., Ph.D.

Waves of muscular contractions in the intestinal tract, also known as peristalsis, push food through the intestines and eventually into the colon. By the time your food reaches the colon, it is largely made up of unwanted materials and water, commonly known as stool. Water is needed to mix with waste to form stool. Without enough water, your bowels do not move. Many constipated people simply need to increase their water consumption to hydrate the bowels so they can move.

If an individual is highly stressed, or eating a highly acidic diet, which is typical of many Americans, then it is common for the magnesium and potassium levels to become depleted as mentioned above. These minerals along with zinc are needed to produce hydrochloric acid to properly break down food. As we age, the production of hydrochloric acid is reduced. Indigestion symptoms such as heartburn, gas and bloating can all be caused from this imbalance. Some people do well to take digestive enzymes with each meal to ensure proper digestion.

Heartburn is most often caused by the flow of gastric juices up the esophagus. This causes a burning discomfort that is usually made worse by lying down. When someone begins having heartburn or acid reflux, they usually take a chalky antacid like Rolaids or Tums, which neutralizes the acids and stops the burning but creates a major disturbance in the digestive process. The stomach, which needs to be highly acidic, has now just been flooded with a medicine to neutralize the acids. Think about it. The body wants the food in the stomach acidic in order to digest it and we swallow chalky calcium to neutralize it. This disrupts digestion and consequently you do not properly break down your food. This chalky calcium is equivalent to pouring cement on the villi in the small intestine, which inhibits proper absorption of nutrients. When autopsies are performed on deceased individuals, it's easy for the pathologist to identify Tums and Rolaids consumers because the intestinal tract will be heavily lined with white chalk.

Some of the doctor-prescribed proton-pump inhibitors (acid blockers), like Prilosec or Prevacid, work like a charm at stopping heartburn, and the individual sings praises to their doctor for giving them something that relieves their discomfort. However, what the patient isn't taught is that now they have just shut down the secretion of digestive juices. How will your body get calcium and magnesium into the bones? Now your foods will not be properly broken down and digested. The body will become malnourished. This will lead to arthritis as bones become malnourished and brittle. Organs and glands will be deprived of nutrients. The patient is basically trading in his or her heartburn for arthritis and other diseases if the medication is continued long enough.

The solution for healing heartburn or acid reflux is to get the pH of the body in the 6.8 to 7.0 range. As mentioned earlier, magnesium, potassium and zinc are crucial for proper digestion. Taking betaine hydrochloric acid (HCL) and Pepsogin supplements with meals will ensure that your stomach has what it needs to mix your foods. Once the stomach acid is sufficient, then a signal is sent out to close the esophageal sphincter so acid won't go up the esophagus and burn. Burning sensations, acid reflux and heartburn are usually symptoms of your digestive system not having enough hydrochloric acid, as opposed to the common myth that you have too much. When the stomach has enough acid, the valve closes. When it doesn't have enough acid, it stays open, thus triggering acid reflux.

Taking a tablespoon of apple cider vinegar 15 minutes before a meal helps the stomach prepare to digest food and can eliminate acid reflux. Some need more and others need less. It's a very simple, healthy and inexpensive way to solve heartburn or acid reflux issues.

> "There is no natural death. All deaths that come from so-called natural causes are merely the end point of progressive acid saturation. Many people go so far as to consider that sickness and disease are just a 'cross' or an element which God gave them to bear here on this earth. However, if they would take care of their body and cleanse their colon and intestines, their problems would be pretty much eliminated and they could eliminate their 'cross' by proper diet, proper exercise, and in general, proper living." George C. Crile, M.D., Head of the Crile Clinic in Cleveland (One of the world's greatest surgeons)

Healthy bowels move two to three times every day and should produce a stool that looks like a brown banana. If you see blood, mucus, undigested foods or loose stools, you have an imbalance in the digestive system. We have some people come in who only have one or two bowel movements a week. If a person has eaten three meals a day for seven days, equaling 21 meals without a bowel movement, where do you suppose all of that material is accumulating? If each meal weighs a pound, that is 21 pounds of food going in, with nothing coming out. Fecal matter backed up in the intestinal tract causes toxicity throughout the whole body, lowering your immune system and zapping your energy. Sure, you can treat the symptoms with painkillers, caffeine and cortisone, but does that make any sense? Expelling old fecal matter from the body gives your cells room to work and takes pressure off capillaries and organs, which reduces inflammation, and many symptoms clear up on their own. Why? Because we are eliminating the cause of inflammation. Back pain sometimes can be the result of backed-up fecal matter, putting pressure on nerves and vertebrae as well. A tablespoon of psyllium husk before bed ensures that you have good bowel movement the next morning.

> **"Every tissue is fed by the blood, which is supplied by the bowel. When the bowel is dirty, the blood is dirty, and so on to the organs and tissues …. It is the bowel that invariably has to be cared for first before any effective healing can take place."** Bernard Jensen, D.C., N.D., Ph.D.

The colon is like a balloon. When it gets full, it keeps expanding and stretching. As mentioned earlier, any toxic substance left in the colon has the capability of being absorbed right back into your blood stream through the portal vein. A clean colon, liver, kidneys and spleen result in clean blood. Clean blood equals a healthy immune system. A healthy immune system allows you to be around sick people and remain healthy. This is foundational for good health. Keep the colon clean and you'll eliminate 90 percent of your health problems.

> Toxins in the bowels = toxins in the blood = toxins in organs = toxins in the cells = DIS-EASE.
> Where the toxins settle, and how they manifest, is the disease you are diagnosed as having.

> **"Of the 22,000 operations that I have personally performed, I have never found a single normal colon, and of the 100,000 that were performed under my jurisdiction, not over 6 percent were normal."** Harvey Kellogg, M.D.

According to many health experts like Dr. Bernard Jenson, digestion is the great secret of life. Many people we see with arthritis are suffering from poor digestion. If you aren't absorbing nutrients from your food, then how are you going to build strong bones, tendons and ligaments? Discs deteriorate because they are literally starving for nutrition. Meat takes 24 to 72 hours to move through your colon. Have you ever noticed how tired and sluggish you feel after stuffing yourself at Thanksgiving dinner with lots of meat and all the goodies? That's because you have just overloaded your system with way too much protein. All your energy goes to break down the meal you've just consumed, leaving you exhausted.

If someone gets food poisoning, what does the body do? It will create diarrhea or vomiting, two ways to get poisons out of the body. Diarrhea is often constipation in disguise. When the bowels are so toxic that they can't function in a normal fashion, then the cells call a special cleansing party and the diarrhea helps expel the toxins.

Your Gut Flora (Microbiome)

"All diseases begin in the gut." Hippocrates

Optimizing Gut Flora
- Eat organic fruits & vegetables
- Eat healthy fats
- Eat fermented vegetables
- Eat organic grass-fed meats
- Eat wild-caught Alaskan salmon
- Increase Omega 3's (fish oil)
- Avoid grains (gluten)
- Take probiotics

About 80 percent of your immune system resides in your gut. The average person has 100 trillion bacteria living in the gut, weighing 3 to 5 pounds, with over 500 different species. These bacteria make up your gut flora, or your microbiome, and they outnumber cells in the body 10 to 1. These bacteria are extremely important to your health, because they keep harmful bacteria and yeast in check. Gut flora aids in the digestion and absorption of carbohydrates, (B vitamins), minerals and the elimination of toxins. They are foundational to a strong immune system and aid in the ability to fight infections by helping to produce antibodies to combat harmful pathogens. Like drill sergeants in the army, they teach your immune system to distinguish between the good guys and bad guys and when to attack. So, if you have an autoimmune disorder, most likely the problem is with the microbiome in your gut.

As mentioned previously, allergies many times are triggered when your immune system becomes too hyper from eating inflammatory foods like gluten and dairy. Once we give your microbiome a tune-up, many allergies disappear by eliminating the cause. It's also important to know that your microbiome plays a large role in the functioning of the thymus gland, which is responsible for releasing

T cells to fight infections and cancer. When you support your gut health, and avoid inflammatory foods, your immune system is primed and ready for anything that could threaten your health.

The microbiome in the gut is your second brain. It originates from the same type of tissue as your brain. Have you ever had a gut feeling something wasn't right? Before a competition or game, many competitors get "butterflies" in their stomach. Why? Because the gut is your second brain, and it actually produces more neurotransmitters than the brain. In fact, researchers have discovered that the largest concentration of neurotransmitters such as serotonin, which helps us feel happy, is actually found in your intestines.

Yeast / Fungi Eliminators	
Garlic	Oregano oil
Pau D'Arco	Tea tree oil
Olive leaf	Clove oil
Cats claw	Dill oil
Chaga	Citrus oils
Echinacea	Coconut oil
Zinc	Niacin

> "We digest not only food, but thoughts, emotions, and spiritual and sexual experiences." Dr. Keesha Ewers

Infants who suffer from eczema are usually dealing with an allergy caused by an imbalance in the microbiome. Providing the child with a probiotic (friendly bacteria) is important. Nursing mothers can even put probiotic powder on their pinkie finger or nipple to give the infant.

Antibiotics are extremely damaging to the microbiome. They kill off everything, leaving the gut like a devastated city after being bombed in a war. We use about 24 million pounds of antibiotics every year in America, and 19 million of those are used in animal feed. This leads to antibiotic-resistant superbugs that antibiotics can no longer kill. Antibiotics are useless against viral and yeast infections. They only kill bacteria, that is why so many children who go to the doctor with ear infections never get better from the antibiotic. It's because the ear infection is caused from a virus or yeast infection.

Antibiotic means "Against Life"
Probiotic means "For Life"

Prescription Drugs That Disrupt Your Microbiome	
Antibiotics	Steroids
Antacids	NSAIDS
Birth control pills	Antidepressants
Statins	Chemotherapy

Antibiotics upset the delicate balance in your intestinal tract, allowing naturally occurring yeast to multiply out of control. This imbalance in the microbiome is referred to as dysbiosis. The yeast (fungi) use their hyphae (tendrils) to poke holes through the lining of your intestinal wall and make their way into the blood. This is called leaky gut.

This leads to candida overgrowth, which causes itchy vaginal yeast infections and may produce a cottage cheese-like discharge. This is why women usually come down with yeast infections after taking antibiotics. Skin rashes, toenail fungus and jock itch are usually caused from systemic yeast as well.

> **"Optimizing your gut flora is far superior to getting a flu shot."** Dr. Joseph Mercola

GUT-HEALING SMOOTHIE
1-2 cups coconut milk or unsweetened almond milk
½ avocado
2 frozen bananas
1 cup frozen blueberries
2 tablespoons ground flaxseeds
1 tablespoon unflavored gelatin powder
1 teaspoon cinnamon
1 tablespoon hemp hearts

Place all ingredients in a blender and blend on high until smooth. Add extra water if too thick.

Our gut flora is populated during childbirth. If you were born by a natural, vaginal birth then you inherited your microbiome from your mother. This is one of the most important things a mother can do to provide her child with a strong and healthy immune system. At the end of pregnancy, high concentrations of the Prevotella bacteria begin to colonize in the vaginal tract. When the baby comes through the birth canal, these beneficial bacteria cover him or her, signaling for the infant's gut to start creating digestive enzymes to break down breast milk. This is why C-section babies tend to have a higher risk of asthma, ADD, allergies, eczema and colitis. Their little immune systems have been short-changed from the very beginning of life.

The microbiome plays a vital role in digesting amino acids and converting them to neurotransmitters in the brain, which controls how we feel. If the gut is inflamed with toxic foods like dairy, gluten, corn and sugar, and we aren't breaking down our fats, carbs and proteins, then neurotransmitters in the brain will be subpar. The neurotransmitters help us feel good, energized and in control. They give that spark to life. Depression, anxiety, ADD, ADHD, mood swings, brain fog, sluggish metabolism, obesity and memory loss can all be triggered by an unhealthy microbiome that prevents proper metabolism of nutrients, amino acids and neurotransmitters.

> **"Show me a patient who is chronically ill with virtually any condition and I'll show you a person who is toxic with a major imbalance in their GI tract."** Dr. Rashid Buttar

I grew up on a wheat farm in Moses Lake, Washington, and my mom used to make whole wheat bread. After eating a bowl of Cream of Wheat with homemade toast for breakfast, is it any wonder why I felt lethargic and sleepy at school in the mornings? I was spiking my blood sugar with wheat and then crashing. How many of our kids eat processed grain cereals for breakfast with toast, and then we wonder why they can't sit still, pay attention and focus at school. Hello, you spike their blood sugar with carbs and then want them to sit still, be quiet, and focus on their schoolwork? Good luck! No wonder so many teachers think kids need to be on ADD/ADHD medication. Stop poisoning them in the morning with high-grain foods such as cold cereals, toaster pastries, doughnuts, toast, waffles, pancakes, bagels, muffins, granola bars and oatmeal. Yes, oatmeal spikes the blood sugar. It's a grain! This is why one in four teenagers is diabetic or prediabetic. If you want to prevent diabetes, you have to stop throwing gas on the fire and eating SAD – the Standard American Diet.

Healthier breakfast options are an egg omelet with vegetables or a smoothie with unsweetened almond milk, blueberries, avocado, egg, almond butter, coconut oil, nuts and seeds so they have some brain food to help them think and learn. Half a banana will sweeten a smoothie, but it can elevate blood-sugar levels. Avoid toast, cold cereals and orange juice.

> **"Tell me what you eat, I'll tell you who you are."** Anthelme Brillat-Savarin 1755-1826

Healthy living involves eating the majority of your diet from the vegetable category. We would be wise to consume most of our diet from the garden. If you don't like green vegetables, then I suggest making a green smoothie in the blender with kale, berries, lemon and water. If you want to be healthy, you have to get green vegetables in your body every day. Legumes, nuts, seeds, eggs, fermented foods and baked meats in moderation are good. Berries are great, and eat fruits in moderation. We have way too many young kids giving themselves insulin shots. Many times, type 2 diabetes is completely avoidable and reversible by simply giving up grains and sodas.

For those who are wheatgrass juice consumers, keep in mind that at about day 17 of the wheat sprout's life, the plant will start producing gluten, so it is best to harvest your wheatgrass between days 11 to 14 to avoid getting any gluten.

Diabetes – Insulin Resistance

In 1994, the American Diabetes Association recommended that Americans should consume 60 to 70 percent of their calories from carbohydrates. Can you guess what happened? Diabetes skyrocketed. From 1997 to 2007, the number of cases of diabetes actually doubled. In the 1980s, children with diabetes was very rare, but by the year 2000, nearly one in 10 kids was pre-diabetic or was diagnosed as diabetic. By 2008, one out of every four teenagers was pre-diabetic or had type 2 diabetes.

> **ATTENTION DIABETICS:**
> The FDA warns if you have taken Invokana, Invokamet, Farxiga, or other SGLT2 inhibitors for diabetes you could be at risk of serious injury or death
> Side effects may include:
> Kidney failure, Heart attack, Stroke or hospitalization for Diabetic Ketoacidosis

> **MEDICAL ALERT**
> **ZYPREXA® LINKED TO DIABETES AND PANCREATITIS**
> If you or a loved one have taken Zyprexa and susequently suffered from Diabetes, Pancreatitis, Ketoacidosis (Coma) or Death, you/they may have a valuable claim. Call our office now for a free consultation.

We consume 152 pounds of sugar and 146 pounds of flour per person, per year, and 70 percent of American adults and 40 percent of children are overweight. Sadly, the majority of kids, 70 percent, are too fat and unfit to serve in the military now. It's time to make some changes in our diet, and it starts with education. Flour from grains like wheat spikes your blood sugar more than straight sugar. Low-fat yogurt contains more sugar than a can of soda. We have been misled on what is healthy and what is diabetic fuel.

> **"When we eat foods that have a high glycemic index, the grains and sugars in corn, wheat, rice, then we're creating an environment that promotes fungal overgrowth, and that's going to cause inflammation and that's going to, again, incent cells to turn to cancer cells!"** Dr. Roby Mitchell

When we eat carbohydrates like cold cereal, toast, bagels, muffins, toaster pastries, breads — yes, even 100 percent organic whole wheat — white rice, potatoes and orange juice, the pancreas secretes insulin. The more insulin you have in your blood, the more signals your body receives to store fat. This spiking of insulin causes diabetes and weight gain. Eating high-carb foods will cause you to feel hungry and crave even more carbs. To the contrary, eating high-fat foods will stabilize blood sugar, give you energy and satisfy your hunger.

Nearly one in three people have some form of diabetes or pre-diabetes in the U.S. Improper insulin and leptin signaling is the cause for diabetes. The SAD

(Standard American Diet), which is high in carbs and grains, begins to desensitize our cells to insulin, which causes insulin resistance. The cells then begin to ignore insulin and struggle with getting glucose out of the blood. The pancreas begins to pump out more insulin in order to get sugar into the cells. Diabetes, or high blood sugar, occurs when leptin signaling malfunctions and more insulin is needed to unlock the doors to get sugar (glucose) into the cells. As insulin levels increase, cells become less responsive to open the door to let sugar in, so it builds up in the blood and then the pancreas pumps out more insulin. The blood sugar may be normal, but the insulin may be sky high. Excess insulin causes you to feel hungry and store belly fat.

    Leptin is a hormone produced in your fat and other cells that helps regulate appetite and body weight. It signals your brain to eat when you are hungry and to stop when you're full. Consuming a diet high in fructose, carbs, sugars and grains causes the leptin signaling to become sluggish. Have you ever sat at the dinner table and kept eating because you didn't feel full and then an hour later wished you wouldn't have had that last portion? That's your leptin levels being lazy.

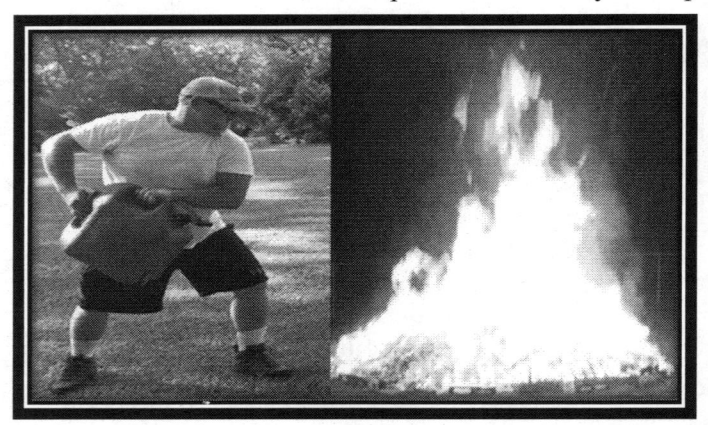

Type 2 diabetics do not need more insulin. What they need is help getting the blood sugar into the cells. Taking insulin to lower blood sugar actually makes their insulin resistance worse. Many doctors are starting to see that taking insulin is like throwing gas on the fire for diabetes. Research published in JAMA Internal Medicine (174 no. 8) June 30, 2014, suggests that insulin therapy in type 2 diabetes may be doing more harm than good.

> **"Many physicians are seriously confused about (insulin resistance) and give insulin to type 2 diabetics to lower their blood sugar, which actually makes their insulin resistance worse and contributes to their premature death."** Dr. Joseph Mercola

Blood Sugar Levels
▪ 70-80 mg/dl – Fasting Blood Sugar (morning) = Good
▪ 120 or lower – 2 Hours After Eating = Good
▪ 140 or higher – 2 Hours After Eating = Pre-Diabetic
▪ 200 or Higher = Diabetes

A1C Blood Glucose Test
▪ 3 or lower = Excellent
▪ 4.8 – 5.4 = Good
▪ 6 or higher = Diabetes

The best time to take your fasting blood sugar is first thing in the morning, before eating. Your fasting blood sugar should be 70-80 mg/dl. It's good to check your blood sugar two hours after a meal as well. If the reading is under 120 mg/dl, you are doing well. If it's over 140, you are pre-diabetic. If it's over 200, you have type 2 diabetes.

The hemoglobin A1C test measures your average blood sugar over the past six weeks. A healthy A1C is in the 4.8 to 5.4 range and preferably below 5. If you are below 3, you are doing excellent. Anything over 6.0 is considered diabetes.

> **"Type 2 diabetes is brought on by constantly having too much insulin and leptin circulating secondary to the same diet that has been recommended to treat diabetes and heart disease, a high-carbohydrate, low-fat diet. Then giving these diabetics more insulin is adding gasoline to the fire. Doctors couldn't be doing more harm if they tried."** Ron Rosedale, M.D.

Insulin is the hormone that takes excess carbs and stores them in the form of fat, for future energy shortages. Unfortunately, most Americans never dip into their fat storage because as soon as we get hungry, we run to eat. If we eat grains three times a day, we are sending those carbs to the food storage house, usually referred to as your "love handles" or "beer belly." So, it's not a bad idea to practice some intermittent fasting occasionally, to burnup our fat storage supplies.

The glycemic index refers to how carbohydrates or sugars in foods affect blood glucose levels after being eaten. Generally, foods that have a value of 55 or less are more slowly digested and are a healthier choice for stabilizing blood sugar. Notice how many grains and cereals are high on the list.

> **"Sugar is eight times more addictive than cocaine. And what's interesting is while cocaine and heroin activate only one spot for pleasure in the brain, sugar lights up the brain like a pinball machine."** Dr. Mark Hyman

Sugar is more addictive than alcohol, cocaine and heroin! No wonder so many people love it, crave it and eat it. Dr. Serge H. Ahmed performed a study and concluded that sugar was eight times more addictive than cocaine. And artificial sweeteners are even more addictive than sugar! This is why so many Americans walk around with their diet colas, because they are addicted to the artificial sweeteners.

Glycemic Index Chart

103 Dates	71 Grape-Nuts	42 Yogurt
95 French Baguette	70 Bread, white	41 Snickers Bar
93 Corn Flakes	69 Special K	40 Apple Juice
93 Potato, red, baked	68 Bread, wheat	40 Strawberries
91 Rice Crackers	68 Cornmeal	39 Milk, skim
89 Rice Chex	68 Taco Shell	39 Plums
87 Rice	68 Sugar, white	39 Pinto Beans
84 Pretzels	67 Croissant	38 Navy Beans
84 Special K	67 Wheat Thins	36 Apples
83 Corn Chex	66 Oatmeal	35 Carrots, raw
83 Rice Krispies	66 Potato Chips	34 Lentils
82 Rice Cakes	66 Pineapple	33 Butter Beans
80 Pancakes	65 Spaghetti	32 Lima Beans
78 Jelly Beans	65 Cantaloupe	29 Kidney Beans
78 Gatorade	65 Sugar, brown	27 Milk, whole
76 Doughnuts	64 Macaroni & Cheese	25 Grapefruit
76 Waffles	64 Raisins	22 Cashews
76 Maple Syrup	63 Colas	22 Cherries
75 Shredded Wheat	61 Honey	15 Tomato
75 French Fries	60 Pizza, cheese	15 Spinach
74 Cream of Wheat	60 Ice Cream, vanilla	15 Cucumber
74 Cheerios	58 Pears	15 Celery
74 Graham Crackers	54 Sourdough Bread	15 Prunes
74 Saltine Crackers	53 Bananas	15 Walnuts
74 Bread Stuffing	51 Mangos	15 Almonds
74 Bran Flakes	47 peaches	15 Peanuts
73 Raisin Bran	46 Orange Juice	15 Olives
72 Corn Chips	46 Grapes	14 Yogurt, plain
72 Watermelon	44 Sweet Potato	10 Broccoli
72 Rice, brown	44 Baked Beans	10 Eggs, boiled
72 Bagel	43 Oranges	10 Avocado
72 Popcorn	42 Peaches	5 Beef

High fructose corn syrup in most sodas is much worse than regular sugar because it blocks the appetite-control hormones (leptin) that tells your brain when you are full. In other words, your brake never gets pulled to tell you when to stop eating. The other major problem with high-fructose corn syrup is that it contains mercury and leads to leaky gut, according to Dr. Bruce Ames.

FOODS TO EAT	FOODS TO AVOID
Foods to Help Lose Weight & Stabilize Blood Sugar	*Foods That Cause Weight Gain & Diabetes*
Most Vegetables - (all green vegetables) Jerusalem artichokes, asparagus, bell peppers, carrots, celery, cucumbers, kale, mushrooms, okra, peas, radishes, green beans, avocados, broccoli, garlic, onions, brussels sprouts, cabbage, cauliflower, chard, Collard greens, lettuce, turnip greens, spinach, squash, tomatoes, zucchini, parsley **Meats** - salmon, trout, tuna, tilapia, chicken, turkey, beef, venison **Nuts & Seeds** - almond butter, almonds, flaxseeds, chia seeds, hemp seeds, pumpkin seeds, sunflower seeds, walnuts, hazelnuts, Brazil nuts, macadamia, pecans **Oils** - cook with coconut oil. olive oil & butter are good, sesame oil, ghee **Legumes** - black-eyed peas, chickpeas, kidney beans, lentils, lima beans, pinto beans, split peas **Eggs** **Cheese** **Tart Fruits & Berries** - apples, grapefruits, apricots, kiwi, pears, plums, lemons, limes, raspberries, cranberries, blackberries, blueberries, strawberries, cherries **Fermented Foods** - kefir, sauerkraut, unsweetened yogurt, miso, natto, tamari, tempeh, cottage cheese **Flour Alternatives** - buckwheat (is a seed, not a grain), coconut flour, almond flour, arrowroot **Stevia**	**All Refined Carbohydrates** **Sugar**/high fructose corn syrup soft drinks/diet drinks **Fruit Juice** **All Grains** **White Flour/Whole Wheat Products** breads, pasta, noodles, crackers, chips, cold cereals, Cheerios, Corn Flakes, Rice Krispies, pastries, cakes, muffins, pretzels, cookies, rice, corn, microwave popcorn, granola, oatmeal, cornbread **Fruits** – avoid sweet fruits like watermelon & raisins **Vegetables** - beets, parsnips, potatoes, pumpkin, yams, sweet potatoes, butternut squash **Milk**, ice cream **Smoked or Cured Meats** - breaded meats, bacon, hot dogs, luncheon meats, sausage, ham, spam, bologna **Margarine**, shortening, hydrogenated oils **Coffee** **Alcohol** **Artificial Sweeteners** - Aspartame, Splenda

Foods that spike your blood sugar are addictive. And just because a food or drink has a fruit in front of it, doesn't necessarily make it healthy. For example, orange juice contains more sugar than soft drinks. Fruit juices are way too high in sugar and should be avoided.

> "Normalizing your insulin level is the most important factor in optimizing your overall health and helping to prevent disease of all kinds, from diabetes to heart disease to cancer and everything in between." Dr. Joseph Mercola

Healthy Meals & Snacks

Breakfast – Egg omelet with onions, tomatoes, spinach leaves and mushrooms.
Snack – 1 Tbsp. coconut oil mixed with 1 Tbsp. raw almond butter on a celery stick. (Great for sugar cravings & low energy)
Lunch – Grilled chicken garden salad with spinach leaves, purple onion, cucumbers, tomatoes, feta cheese with olive oil salad dressing.
Snack – Almonds & fresh blackberries or chicken salad on celery sticks
Dinner – Baked salmon, steamed broccoli, carrots & asparagus or homemade vegetable beef stew. Slow-cooker chicken or bone-broth beef soup with added vegetables.
Snack – Two hard-boiled eggs or unsweetened yogurt with strawberries
Dessert – Half an apple with almond butter or unsweetened yogurt with fresh raspberries & blueberries

Here are some healthy low-glycemic breakfast shake recipes that give you energy, help you feel full, stabilize blood sugar levels and help you lose weight. Remember, healthy people eat fats. Grains and sugary (high-carb) foods lead to diabetes, weight gain and dis-ease.

Breakfast Shake #1	Breakfast Shake # 2	Breakfast shake #3
½ cup blueberries	1-2 scoops whey protein	¾ cup of spinach
½ cup cranberries	1 Tbsp. chia seeds	3 slices of cucumbers
1 Tbsp. raw almond butter	1 Tbsp. hemp seeds	½ stalk celery
1 Tbsp. pumpkin seeds	½ avocado	1 tsp. organic cinnamon
1 Tbsp. chia seeds	10 oz. unsweetened coconut milk or almond milk	2 frozen strawberries
1 Tbsp. hemp seeds	Mix in blender	1 Tbsp. flaxseeds
2 raw walnuts		½ cup blueberries
2 raw Brazil nuts		8 oz. unsweetened almond milk
¼ avocado		Mix in blender
½ Tbsp. coconut butter	**Breakfast shake #4**	
1 cup unsweetened Almond milk	2 raw eggs	**Kale Shake #5**
(1 scoop SEC Greens optional)	1-2 scoops whey protein	Handful kale
Mix in blender	10 oz. unsweetened almond milk	Frozen berries
	1 Tbsp. sunflower seeds	1 scoop SEC Greens
	1 Tbsp. flaxseeds	Mix in blender with water
	Mix in blender	

These shakes may be altered according to your taste. Coconut milk or almond milk (unsweetened) is fine for most recipes. If you like your shakes cold, add ice cubes. If you like it thick, don't add water or decrease the amount of almond or coconut milk used. Most berries are good to add in your shakes. Adding half a banana will sweeten the drink considerably but is high in carbs (sometimes needed for kids to like it). If you like lemon, add in a half a lemon. Adding a pinch of cinnamon will help sweeten a shake, and raw cacao (real chocolate) provides added flavor. A small piece of ginger root adds a zing to a shake. Some stevia may be added to sweeten the shake. Find what you like best and start your day off with a healthy shake that tastes good.

Once you have your blood sugar levels balanced, adding in some occasional brown rice, quinoa, millet, oats, tiff and amaranth is usually OK if used in moderation.

> **"Diets very high in fat and low in carbs can reverse type 2 diabetes."** Mark Hyman, M.D.

Coconut milk or almond milk can be used as a substitute in any recipe that calls for milk or dairy. When buying oils, look for cold-pressed or extra-virgin. Avoid sauerkraut from the store since they add sodium benzoate to stop the fermentation process. Beans do contain carbs and may trigger blood sugar spikes in some people, so use with caution.

> **"To say diabetes is genetic is an evasion of the truth. The incredible rise in the incidence of diabetes does not indicate a sudden change in genes but points to an environmental cause."** Carolyn Dean, M.D., N.D.

Type 2 diabetes was unheard of before we started processing foods and injecting our children with massive doses of vaccines at a young age. Hydrogenated fats and oils are found in so many of our processed foods, like crackers, chips, desserts and the fake butter substitute, margarine. Almost everything that comes in a box or package contains these highly toxic health-destroyers. This man-made junk is like putting silicon sealer on the cells of your body. It seals cellular glucose receptor sites, keeping glucose out and insulin up. The result of consuming this plastic-like substance is diabetes, not to mention the clogging of arteries. Only a fool would eat silicone sealer; however, when we ingest these hydrogenated oils, we are sealing glucose receptor sites and arteries. This is why diabetics always have poor circulation in their feet and run the risk of infections that lead to amputations.

> **"I have found the ingredients that have been scientifically and historically proven to reverse (cure) diabetes."** James Chappell, D.C., N.D., Ph.D., M.H.

> **The Seven Remedies Dr. Chappell Has Identified To Reverse Diabetes**
> 1. Cinnamon 2. Bitter Melon 3. Gymnema Sylvestre 4. Nopal Cactus
> 5. Fenugreek 6. American Ginseng 7. Chromium Picolinate

Chromium

In 1955, Dr. Walter Mertz discovered that he could cause mice to develop type 2 diabetes by removing chromium from their diets.

Chromium is the mineral that supports proper blood sugar levels.

Cinnamon

Dr. John Anderson of the United States Department of Agriculture (USDA) discovered a polyphenol compound called MHCP in cinnamon that mimics insulin.

Laboratory experiments show that cinnamon lowers glucose, blood fat and cholesterol levels along with neutralizing free radicals.

Research indicates that the positive effects of cinnamon last for at least 20 days after people stop taking it. *"I don't know of any drug or product whose effects persist for 20 days, cinnamon must be an exception,"* reports Harvard professor Dr. Frank Sacks.

Bitter Melon

"Pharmacological and clinical evaluations indicate that bitter melon had a significant blood glucose-lowering effect and that the long-term use may be advantageous over chemical drugs in alleviating some of the chronic diseases and complications caused by diabetes. The use of natural agents in conjunction with conventional drug treatments, such as insulin, permits the use of lower doses of the drug and/or decreased frequency of administration, which decreases the side effects most commonly observed."

Journal of Phytotherapy, Dr. W Jia, W Gao and L Tang

Gymnema Sylvestre

Gymnema sylvestre in Hindi means "sugar destroyer" because it actually blocks the sugar receptor sites. This plant has been used to treat diabetes in India for over 2,000 years. It has proven to be effective in enabling cells to take in glucose while preventing adrenaline from stimulating the liver to produce glucose, thus reducing blood sugar levels.

Harvard Medical School along with Natural Standard states, *"There is evidence to suggest that gymnema can lower blood sugar levels in people with Type 1 and Type 2 diabetes."*

Nopal Cactus

The ancient Aztecs in Mexico used this "prickly pear" to treat and cure diabetes and it is still being used in Latin America today. Nopal cactus blocks absorption of sugar in the intestinal tract, which results in lowered blood sugar levels. It is also good for lowering blood pressure, cholesterol and triglycerides. It helps curb the appetite and break down fat.

In The Archives of Medicine as reported by the Department of Internal Medicine in Mexico, Drs. AC Frati, N Diaz Xiloti state, *"Diabetic patients had a significant decrease of serum glucose reaching from 41 percent to 46 percent when taking nopal cactus."*

American Ginseng

Ginseng is considered "the king of all herbs" in Asia. It is very effective for chronic

fatigue, stress, mercury poisoning, circulation, memory, nervous system disorders and diabetes. It is also antibacterial and anti-viral. Ginseng lowers blood glucose levels.

Dr. Jing-tian Xie from Pritzker School of Medicine, University of Chicago, stated, *"American ginseng possesses significant anti-hyperglycemia and thermogenic activity and may prove to be beneficial in improving the management of Type 2 diabetes. American ginseng berry possesses significant anti-hyperglycemic and anti-obese effects."*

Fenugreek

"Fenugreek significantly reduced blood sugar and improved the glucose tolerance test with a 54 percent reduction in 24-hour urinary excretion," states Drs. R.D. Sharma, T.C. Raghuram and N.S. Rao from the National Institute of Nutrition, Council of Medical Research, Hyderabad, India.

Blood Sugar Support
- Chromium
- Vanadium
- Vitamin D3
- Cinnamon
- Gymnema Sylvester
- Juniper Berries
- Bitter Melon
- Fenugreek
- Nopal Cactus
- Licorice root
- Alpha Lipoic acid
- Ginger

One reason reversing type 2 diabetes on the ketogenic or paleo (no-grain) diet is fairly simple is because you stop consuming the grains (corn and wheat) that harbor poisonous mycotoxins produced from mold and fungi. Avoiding peanuts and peanut butter is also wise, since they, along with corn and wheat, produce mycotoxins. It has been noted that many diabetics develop gout, caused from too much uric acid. Uric acid is a byproduct of yeast. Aspergillus and penicillium fungi produce several poisonous mycotoxins, which include aflatoxin, ochratoxin and patulin. Aflatoxins interfere with glucose metabolism in the liver, causing elevated blood sugar levels. Ochratoxins create insulin resistance and are very damaging to the kidneys. Patulin interferes with our cells' ability to use oxygen, which provides a favorable environment for fungus, since it can live anaerobically. Once you remove the grains and peanuts containing toxic poisons from your diet, you stop throwing gas on the fire and blood sugar levels stabilize. So, why don't we focus on ridding the body of fungus? Because treating diabetes is huge money. The average Type 2 diabetic patient generates about $400,000 of income for doctors, drugs and hospitals over the course of 20 years. Do you think they really want you to reverse your diabetes? A patient cured is a customer lost for the pharmaceutical industry.

> **"A junkie is a junkie, whether he or she is using legal or illegal drugs. … Other than the fact that your drug supply was doctor-prescribed, your situation hardly differs from that of the ordinary street addict."** Robert Mendelsohn, M.D.

Why Can't I Lose Weight?

As we continue to manufacture more chemicals (cosmetics) and plastics, we have an increase in xenoestrogens, chemicals that mimic the effect of estrogen in the body and are fat soluble, meaning they are stored in your body. These chemicals are endocrine gland disruptors and can affect hormones, cause weight gain and put you at a higher risk for cancer. These toxins have flooded our environment and are causing young children to start puberty earlier. We are now seeing girls start to develop breasts and start their periods at age 7 or 8. Xenoestrogens are feminizing agents that cause some boys to no longer want to be boys.

> **"The availability of specific types of bacteria is one of the primary criteria to examine when people are unable to lose weight, even on calorie-restricted diets."** Dr. Tom O'Bryan

Stop counting calories. All calories are not created equal. Calories from a bagel or orange juice are completely different than calories from eggs or spinach leaves. Some foods are healing and some are inflammatory; however, they may contain the same number of calories. Food does more than just give us energy; it is information for the body.

Researchers took 154 countries and studied their diets and calorie consumption. They found that when 150 calories a day were added into the diet, it had little or no significant rise in the risk for diabetes, but when they added those 150 calories from soda, then the risk of diabetes skyrocketed to 700 percent.

> **"One can of soda a day increases a child's risk of becoming obese by 60 percent. One can of soda a day increases a woman's risk of type 2 diabetes by 80 percent."** Mark Hyman, M.D.

Have you tried cutting out sweets and other junk foods and exercised every day and still can't lose weight? Do you feel like no matter how hard you try, the scale just won't budge? No doubt you are frustrated. You are not alone. Every day we have people telling us how strict their diet is and how intensely they exercise, and they still can't seem to lose weight. Chances are, you have a problem in your gut.

Microbiome Imbalance Symptoms
- Indigestion
- Yeast infections
- Rectal itching
- Acne
- Iron deficiency
- Fatigue
- Amenorrhea
- Bruising

If for most of your life you have consumed the typical American diet and have taken just one antibiotic, then your microbiome is in desperate need of a tune up. Years of eating processed packaged foods and taking prescription medications along with an occasional antibiotic allows harmful bacteria and fungi to grow out of control, creating an imbalance, thus leaving you susceptible to all kinds of diseases and the inability to lose weight. Why? Because beneficial bacteria in your microbiome plays an important role in the digestion of certain nutrients like amino acids and converting them into neurotransmitters that help us feel good, have energy, sleep well and lose weight by regulating metabolism. That's why so many people who can't lose weight also suffer with low energy, insomnia, depression and anxiety. Their microbiome needs a tune up to regulate neurotransmitters and bring them back into balance. In simple terms, the bad bacteria and fungi in your gut are sabotaging your ability to lose weight and feel good.

Microbiome Damaging Drugs
- ✓ Antibiotics
- ✓ Antacids
- ✓ Birth Control Pills
- ✓ Steroids
- ✓ NSAIDS
- ✓ Antidepressants
- ✓ Statin (cholesterol) Drugs

"Taking an antibiotic is like dropping a bomb on your microbiome: The drug damages or destroys everything in its path, including both good and bad bacteria." Dr. Tom O'Bryan

Microbiome Healers
- Probiotics
- Vit D3
- Glutamine
- Fish Oil
- Colostrum
- Licorice Root
- Frankincense
- Zinc Carnosine

It is interesting to note that autoimmune diseases began showing up in the same time frame that we started using antibiotics. Do you know someone who takes an antibiotic for a sinus or urinary tract infection and then within the same year they are back at the doctor's office with another reoccurring infection? In these situations, the bacteria has become resistant to the antibiotic. Numerous studies have been done on this. Every time you take an antibiotic, your immune system becomes weaker. Every time you allow your immune system to eradicate an infection naturally, it becomes stronger. This is why antibiotics should be used with extreme caution and only in very severe situations.

> **"An abnormal microbiome will create inflammation and can cause intestinal permeability all by itself, even with a squeaky-clean diet."** Dr. Tom O'Bryan

Some people eat very healthy diets and they still struggle with health issues. Why? The missing puzzle piece is usually caused from an issue with the microbiome. If you have tried everything out there and have done 16 liver and colon cleanses and still have health challenges, it's time to give your microbiome a tune-up.

Fermented Vegetables — Balance Your Microbiome

> **"Literally, one serving of fermented foods is equal to an entire bottle of a high-potency probiotic."** Dr. Tom O'Bryan

Fermented Vegetables Ingredients
- 1 large cabbage
- 3 large carrots
- 1 beet
- 4 radishes
- 1 peeled garlic
- Habanero or jalapeno peppers, optional
- 2 cups of freshly made celery juice
- Starter culture or probiotic mix
- 1 or 2 quart-size canning jars

Shred all your vegetables in a food processor or slice with knife. Add probiotic or starter culture to celery juice. Pour liquid over vegetables in large mixing bowl. Pack vegetables into jars. Put lids on loosely and let sit in cooler to ferment at room temperature for 3 to 4 days. Tighten lids and store in fridge.

Making your own fermented vegetables is easy and possibly one of the healthiest things you can add in to your diet for a tune-up. Eating a forkful a day is equivalent to taking a whole bottle of probiotics to promote beneficial bacteria growth, which supports a healthy immune system. I like to make 12 quarts at a time and share with friends. Obviously, the recipe below is for a smaller batch. Keep in mind, you can alter the recipe however you want. If you're a good old German and prefer sauerkraut because that's what grandma always had, then use just cabbage and make sauerkraut. There is no right or wrong. The goal is to provide your gut with healthy bacteria from fermented foods.

Mix your chopped veggies in a large bowl. Mix starter culture with freshly made celery juice or filtered water (if you don't have a juicer). Tightly pack veggies in jars. Pour in celery juice with starter culture. Make sure all veggies are covered in juice. Top with cabbage leaf. Put the lids on loosely so when the fermentation process begins and gases are produced, your mixture can expand.

Healthy Fermented Foods
- Fermented Vegetables
- Sauerkraut
- Pickles
- Kombucha
- Miso
- Kimchi

Put the jars in a large cooler so if they leak it doesn't make a mess on your floor. Let jars sit for anywhere from a few days, to a couple of weeks. The longer they sit, the stronger the fermentation. They will ferment faster in the summer than winter months. Keep at room temperature or 72 degrees while in cooler. After a few days or a week, sample your veggies. The longer they ferment, the stronger and softer they will be. When you have the mixture where you want it, put jars in the fridge. They will keep for about 6 months. Eat a forkful a day with a meal. Always use a clean fork so you don't contaminate your batch with bacteria from your mouth.

Consuming just a spoonful of fermented vegetables a day provides about 10 trillion CFUs of bacteria. Fermented foods grow beneficial bacteria on them. They help boost your immune system, reduce allergies and inflammation and remove toxins from the body. Sauerkraut and fermented foods from the store like pickles are not the same, because all the bacteria has been deactivated. It is crucial to ferment your own vegetables to ensure you are getting all the "good" bacteria.

BONE BROTH RECIPE (Beef or Chicken)

4 pounds beef bones with marrow (short ribs & knuckle bones are good) **or**
4 pounds chicken carcass (neck, feet, skin, wings)
***Use organic beef or chicken
½ cup raw apple cider vinegar
4 quarts filtered water
4 celery stalks, chopped
4 carrots, chopped
3 onions, quartered
4 garlic cloves, smashed
Handful of fresh parsley
1 teaspoon oregano
3 sprigs fresh thyme
2 bay leaves
1 teaspoon sea salt

Bone Broth

BONE BROTH INSTRUCTIONS

1. Place bones in a slow cooker, add apple cider vinegar and water, and let the mixture sit for 1 hour. (The vinegar leaches the minerals out of the bones)
2. Add more water if needed to cover the bones.
3. Add the vegetables (use parsley later) and bring to a boil. Reduce heat to simmer for 6 hours. Skim the scum from the top and discard.
4. Cover and cook on slow, low heat (chicken, 24 hours, or beef, 48 hours).
5. During the last 10 minutes of cooking, throw in a handful of fresh parsley for added flavor and minerals.
6. Make sure all marrow is knocked out of the bones and into the broth.
7. Let the broth cool and strain it, discarding the layer of fat that hardens on the top. Add sea salt to taste and drink the broth as a beverage or store in fridge up to 7 days or freezer up to 6 months for use in soups or stews.
8. Drink 8 ounces 1 to 2 times daily plain or in a soup.

Bone broth helps heal the gut and reduces joint pain and inflammation, courtesy of chondroitin sulfates, glucosamine and other compounds extracted from the boiled-down cartilage. It is also loaded with healing amino acids and minerals to build healthy bones and strengthen the immune system. Bone broth is very beneficial for healing the gut and gastro-intestinal disorders such as IBS, leaky gut, autoimmune disorders, allergies, skin issues, autism and arthritis.

Diet Drinks Sabotage Weight Loss

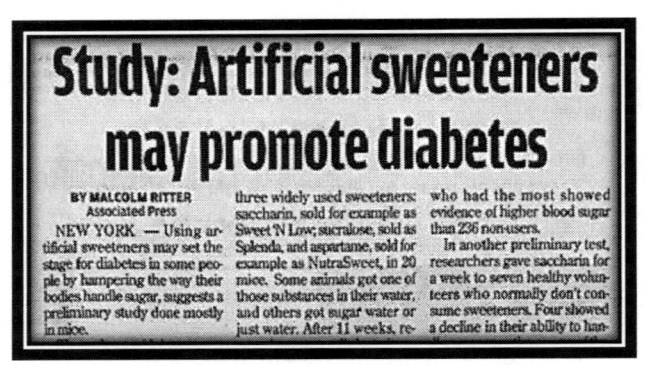

The U.S. has jumped on the bandwagon against sugar. Popular artificial wonders such as NutraSweet, Equal and Splenda taste like sugar minus the calories. These artificial sweeteners have been incorporated into some 9,000 food products. It may surprise you to know that Splenda (sucralose) originated as an insecticide with a deadly "organochlorine" or very toxic form of chlorine. The by-products of these sweeteners put in our foods and diet drinks are known poisons that slowly kill you: methanol, phenylalanine, and aspartic acid.

Diet drinks make people fat. If you are drinking diet drinks and using artificial sweeteners to reduce your calories, you are shooting yourself in the foot. Research has shown that specific bacteria in your gut that is used to digest saccharin actually triggers your body to store energy in the form of fat while altering the microbiome. So, you drink a diet drink thinking you will lose weight because you're not consuming calories, but in actuality it causes you to pack on even more weight.

Recent research reveals that diet drinks actually raise the risk of diabetes more than regular sweetened sodas. How could this be? Artificial sweeteners are hundreds to thousands of times sweeter than regular sugar, which stimulates our desire for sweets more than any other food. Complicating things even more, artificial sweeteners send out a deceiving message to the body, that sugar is on the way and as a result the pancreas begins pumping out insulin. With all the extra insulin secreted from the pancreas from the diet drink, with no actual sugar to drive into the cells, the body is forced to store it in the form of belly fat, the very thing you're trying to prevent and get rid of! Irony at its finest. If that's not bad enough, artificial sweeteners switch your metabolism into slow gear, so you burn fewer calories, and with the extra insulin release, you feel hungrier and crave high-carb foods. Another paradox for those wanting to lose weight.

Aspartame: An Addictive Excitoneurotoxic Carcinogenic Drug

> **"Artificial sweeteners make you fat and diabetic."** Mark Hyman, M.D.

The FDA claims that aspartame is safe. When you look at all the studies that claim how safe aspartame is, you will find that roughly 90 percent of them were funded by the food and beverage companies themselves. If you look at independent studies, that have no financial ties to any manufacturers, 90 percent of them report serious health problems associated with aspartame. The point is, always look at who is funding the research. It just might influence the conclusion of the research. Money has a tendency to influence research results just a tad.

> **"Aspartame (NutraSweet) is a neurotoxin and should be avoided like the plague. Aspartame has been shown to cause birth defects, brain tumors and seizures, and to contribute to diabetes and emotional disorders."** Carolyn Dean, M.D., N.D.

Aspartame contains three components: aspartic acid, phenylalanine and methyl-ester. When aspartame-containing products such as NutraSweet and Equal are used as sweeteners and the product reaches a temperature higher than 86 degrees Fahrenheit (when ingested), then methyl-ester converts to methyl alcohol, a deadly wood alcohol also known as methanol. An ounce of this poison can blind or kill an adult. As it breaks down further, it converts into formaldehyde, which is grouped in the same class of drugs as cyanide and arsenic, which are deadly poisons. Next it converts into formic acid, which is used as fire-ant venom. After aspartame goes through these series of chemical breakdowns, it produces diketopiperazine, a known brain tumor agent. Aspartame has been proven to be a class A carcinogen that affects the respiratory, gastrointestinal and central nervous systems.

Romania Banned Aspartame Why? Because It Causes Cancer

Many scientific studies indicate that systemic lupus is triggered by aspartame poisoning. Multiple sclerosis in many cases is methanol poisoning. The neurological problems associated with aspartame can trigger seizures. It also interferes with dopamine levels, which only worsens the condition for Parkinson's disease.

In 1969, the Searle Company approached Dr. Harry Waisman to study the effects of aspartame on primates. Seven infant monkeys were fed the artificial sweetener in milk. One died after 300 days and five others had grand mal seizures. Searle deleted these findings when they submitted this study to the FDA. Some researchers define NutraSweet as nerve gas that eradicates brain and nerve functions. Even the FDA's own toxicologist, Dr. Adrian Gross, reported to

Congress that at least one of Searle's studies, *"has established beyond any reasonable doubt that aspartame is capable of inducing brain tumors in experimental animals."*

Dr. H.J. Roberts, a specialist in diabetes and world expert on aspartame, has warned us of the dangers of it in his book, *Defense Against Alzheimer's Disease*. He explains how aspartame poisoning is escalating Alzheimer's disease. It damages the cellular powerhouses, the mitochondria, and debilitates cell function. Dr. Roberts reports that when he got his patients off aspartame, they lost an average of 19.5 pounds. He says, "I now advise all patients with diabetes and hypoglycemia to avoid aspartame products."

A study performed at Purdue University by Dr. Susan Swithers and Dr. Terry Davidson tested two groups of rats given yogurt to eat. The first group consumed yogurt with sugar and the second group consumed yogurt with saccharin. After 14 days, the group consuming yogurt with saccharin began to eat significantly larger amounts of food as their appetites became overstimulated. This study revealed that rats who consumed the artificial sweetener in their yogurt gained a significant amount of weight, compared to the group that consumed no saccharin, and their core body temperature decreased, which results in a more sluggish metabolism.

Dr. Luis Elsas, Pediatrics Professor of Genetics at Emory University, has testified before Congress stating that in his lab tests, animals given aspartame developed brain tumors. It is also interesting to note that when brain tumors in humans are removed and examined, many contain high levels of aspartame residue.

Aspartame should be avoided by diabetics because it causes unstable blood sugar levels, may lead to serious vision problems and can cause death. Dr. Betty Martini exposes 92 side effects from aspartame poisoning that have been reported to the FDA.

Aspartame is a neurotoxin, capable of going past the blood brain barrier and damaging vital neurons in the brain, leaving you susceptible to Alzheimer's and Parkinson's. It can also trigger diabetes, explains neurosurgeon Dr. Russell Blaylock, author of *Excitotoxins: The Taste That Kills*.

> **"The ingredients of aspartame stimulate the neurons of the brain to death, causing brain damage of varying degrees."** Dr. Russell Blaylock (Neurosurgeon)

NutraSweet and Equal are amongst some of the deadliest toxins in our society because they are hidden in so many of our foods, including children's vitamins, medicines, powdered drink mixes, chewing gum and gelatin as well as being found on tables in restaurants.

Next time you reach for a "sugar-free" product or "diet drink" you might want to reconsider. If Americans are ever going to win the war on cancer, diabetes or any disease, we have to start by not throwing gas on the fire.

Fetal tissue cannot tolerate methanol. Dr. James Bowen calls NutraSweet instant birth control. The fetal placenta can concentrate phenylalanine and cause mental retardation. He also points out that, "aspartame is a known destroyer of DNA. The mitochondrial DNA (MtDNA) is especially damaged, causing consuming mothers to pass this on to future generations. Aspartame tests on animals showed that it causes brain and mammary tumors." Attorney James Turner states, *"It is impossible to say that aspartame is not a carcinogen."* Is it any mystery that after drinking diet drinks for 20 years, we wonder why so many women have breast cancer and men have prostate cancer?

Common Symptoms Associated With Aspartame Poisoning

Headaches	Depression	Slurred Speech	Fibromyalgia
Vertigo	Rashes	Chronic Fatigue	Brain Tumors
Cancer	Epilepsy	Graves' Disease	Birth Defects
Joint Pain	Numbness	Tinnitus	Anxiety Attacks
Loss of Taste	Vision Loss	Seizures	Retinal Problems

Why is this deadly poison still in our foods and on the market if it has been proven so lethal? Once again, if we examine it like forensic detectives do a murder mystery, the clues line up. Monsanto, the big manufacturer of aspartame, funds the American Diabetes Association, the American Dietetic Association and the Conference of the American College of Physicians. When millions of dollars are donated in their behalf, usually the recipients don't turn around and bite the hand that feeds them.

Soft Drinks

Brominated vegetable oil (BVO) is derived from corn or soy and bonded with bromine. It is added to roughly 15 percent of all sodas in the U.S. to prevent citrus flavoring from separating and floating to the surface. Bromines are endocrine gland disruptors. Women who drink soft drinks run the risk of having hormonal issues. BVO has been banned in more than 100 countries, including most of Europe and Japan, but not here in the USA.

If you want to be healthy and prevent dreaded diseases, then you must become a label reader. If there are ingredients in your food and drinks that you can't pronounce, then it might be a wise idea not to put them in your mouth. Some diet drinks contain polyethylene glycol, which is used in anti-freeze and as an oil solvent. These harmful chemicals were never meant to be consumed, yet we wonder why we have abnormal liver tests and our kidneys are on the verge of needing dialysis.

Phosphoric acid is found in most soft drinks. The phosphorus in the acid upsets the body's calcium-phosphorus ratio and dissolves calcium from the bones. How many people do you know with arthritis who drink soft drinks on a daily basis? The phosphoric acid also interferes with hydrochloric acid in the stomach, causing digestive problems, and then we wonder why we have acid reflux.

The large amounts of corn syrup found in these drinks can induce hypoglycemia or hyperglycemia, both of which lead to diabetes. Consuming these sugary drinks overtaxes the adrenal glands. Once the sugar high burns off, you are left feeling tired and drained.

Aluminum cans are common containers for soft drinks. The acid in the drink eats away at the aluminum so that every time you drink a soft drink, you ingest trace amounts of aluminum. Aluminum is very toxic and builds up in the body. It interferes with proper brain function and has been linked to Alzheimer's disease and dementia.

Most soft drinks are very acidic with a pH of about 2. Remember that our ideal pH should be 6.8 to 7.0. So, if we are continually drinking acidic, carbonated beverages throughout the day, how do we expect our pH to be in a healthy range? It won't, and that is one reason we have so many diseases in this country.

> **"Soda (soft drinks) is the No. 1 acid-producing substance ingested into the body. Thus the country's No. 1 killer is really soda!"** Johnnie Strickland, M.D.

Caffeine

Caffeine, when ingested, triggers the release of dopamine (the reward, feel-good neurotransmitter); however, when it wears off, it causes you to crave more sugar. The reason why we have coffee cake is because after drinking a cup of stimulating coffee, the caffeine accelerates your desire for sweets.

Hot Epsom Salt Detox Bath
- Fill tub with hot water
- Add 2 cups Epsom salt
- Add ½ cup baking soda
- Add 15 drops lavender oil
- Soak for 20 - 30 minutes

Coffee contains 208 different acids. These acids interfere with your insulin and glucose levels. Decaffeinated is not much better because the acids are still there.

As you stop consuming diet drinks and caffeine, some people experience a caffeine withdrawal headache. To minimize the ill effects, start by consuming half of your normal dosage for a couple of days and then cut your dosage in half again. Slowly weaning off can prevent nagging headaches. If you are feeling bad, drink extra water, take some Vitamin C (2,000 to 4,000 mg a day) and take a hot Epsom salt bath (2 cups) with 15 drops of lavender in the water and soak for 20 to 30 minutes.

All Calories Are Not Created Equal

Stop counting calories. All calories are not created equal. A calorie from a piece of toast and a bowl of Corn Flakes is completely different than a calorie from an egg or avocado. If the majority of your calories come from sugar and grains such as crackers or chips and granola bars, you are conditioning your body to burn sugar as the primary fuel. When you eat sugar and grains, the body releases insulin and leptin, hormones that regulate energy intake and expenditure. If you don't need the energy, the body stores the sugar as glycogen in the liver and muscles. Once your glycogen store is filled, any additional sugar you consume is converted to fat (stored energy). After being on a typical American diet, your body may develop a resistance to insulin and leptin and you will require more and more insulin to get glucose into the cells. This causes you to stay hungry and crave sweets as the body continues to store the excess energy (fat) around the belly. This leads to you gaining weight and the development of diabetes.

A great snack when craving sweets and experiencing low energy is to eat 1 tablespoon of coconut oil with 1 tablespoon of raw almond butter on celery. Adding the coconut oil and almond butter with a glass of kefir can really help too, especially with hypoglycemic symptoms like headaches, irritability, weakness and tremors. Macadamia nuts and pecans are great snack foods because they are lower in protein as compared to some of the other nuts.

Weight Loss Without Trying

> "I know what Victoria's Secret is. The secret is that nobody over 30 can fit into their stuff!" Gary R. Oberg, M.D.

Twenty-five-year-old Rhonda came into our clinic after her chiropractic physician sent her to the emergency room because he suspected she was having a heart attack. In the emergency room, all the tests came back normal, so they sent Rhonda home with painkillers, despite her pounding heart that felt like it was going to explode. She was also experiencing tightness in her throat, fatigue, nausea, high blood pressure and severe panic attacks. She came in our clinic and complained that she felt like she was having a nervous breakdown and was so jittery that she couldn't even drive, her mother had to bring her.

We did an EDS scan. Within 15 minutes of testing, we found a major imbalance in her gallbladder, spleen and thyroid. Further testing revealed her nervous system was causing these organs and glands to be compromised. Checking her body for nutritional deficiencies, we detected her magnesium and potassium levels to be extremely depleted. We immediately opened a bottle of magnesium and potassium and had her take three capsules. Within 10 minutes the nervous, panicky, jittery feeling decreased dramatically and she reported that she felt 90 percent better. "Wow! That is powerful stuff. Can it really work that fast?" she asked. Why didn't the emergency room doctors check her magnesium levels? Magnesium is the mineral to help us calm down and relax. It's great for anxiety, insomnia, muscle cramps, twitches, angina, fast/irregular heart beat and high blood pressure.

She left our clinic with some nutritional supplements and some herbal formulas to detoxify her gallbladder and spleen. We also gave her some circulation support, kelp and thyroid support. Six weeks later, Rhonda came back a new person. Her nervous system was stable, her energy levels were up and she had lost 20 pounds without even changing her diet.

Balancing the endocrine system and hormones is a key to losing weight. Stress increases cortisol levels, which affect the adrenals and thyroid. When we support the nervous system and thyroid, which controls body temperature and metabolism, then the body lets go of excess weight. Unfortunately, most medical doctors do blood work to check the thyroid, which is many times inaccurate. Emotions, diet, stress, exercise and menstrual cycles can all influence the blood chemistries, which may or may not give us accurate thyroid readings. Dr. Broda Barnes taught that thyroid hormone exerts its influence on every cell in the body

---

Barnes Basal Temperature Thyroid Test

- Immediately upon awakening place thermometer in armpit and leave for 10 minutes while laying perfectly still. Do this for 5 consecutive days.
- If the average temperature is less than 97.8 then you may have hypothyroidism.
- If the average temperature is above 98.2 you may have hyperthyroidism.
- Women who are menstruating, record your temperature starting on the second day of menstruation. This is the best time.

---

inside the cells, while the blood tests only measure the circulating thyroid hormone levels outside the cells. The bottom line is, thyroid blood tests are not an accurate way to check for thyroid imbalances. We have many people who come in with their blood work to show us that their thyroid checked well; however, when we run an EDS scan, we usually see an imbalance with the thyroid, adrenals and sometimes the pituitary and hypothalamus.

"I am more convinced than ever that solely relying on the patient's (thyroid) blood tests without taking into account the physical exam as well as the patient's history will result in a misdiagnosis for many patients." David Brownstein, M.D.

We recommend the Barnes Basal Temperature Test, a mercury thermometer check of your temperature. Keep the thermometer on your nightstand next to the bed so you don't have to get up. Obviously, if you get up and move around, your body temperature elevates. We want an accurate reading, so first thing in the morning, put the thermometer in your armpit, and go back to bed for 10 minutes and then check your temperature. Record your readings for several weeks. Normal temperature should be 97.8 to 98.2 degrees Fahrenheit. If your morning temperature consistently registers less than 97.8 degrees, then you most likely have a sluggish thyroid. If the readings are higher than 98.2, you probably have a hyperthyroid.

After about 50 years of research, Dr. Broda Barnes, M.D., Ph.D., claims that no less than 40 percent of the adults in the U.S. suffer from hypothyroidism (low thyroid).

> **"When medication is needed to treat hypothyroidism, I believe that using a desiccated glandular thyroid product (e.g., Armour Thyroid, Nature-Thyroid or Westhroid) are much more effective treatment options as compared to using T4 derivatives. My clinical experience with using desiccated thyroid has shown that it is a superior product as compared to the synthetic versions of thyroid hormone presently available (such as Synthroid or Levothroid)."** David Brownstein, M.D.

Hypothyroidism Symptoms

Weakness	Dry flaky skin	Lethargic	Slow Speech
Swelling	Cold hands/feet	Diminished Sweat	Thick Tongue
Coarse Hair	Pale Skin	Constipation	Weight Gain
Hair falls out	Breathing (labored)	Swollen Feet	Hoarseness
Loss of Appetite	Irregular Menses	Nervousness	Heart Palpitations
Brittle Nails	Slow Movement	Poor Memory	Emotional Instability
Depression	Headaches	Sleepiness	Goiter (enlarged neck)
Ringing in Ears	Acne	Irritable	Mental Dullness
Numbness	Low Energy	Low Sex Drive	High Cholesterol
Cold Intolerance	Morning Fatigue	Mood Swings	Unsuccessful Dieting
Infertility	Miscarriage	PMS	Muscle/Joint Aches

> **"I believe that 40 percent of the population is suffering from hypothyroidism."** David Brownstein, M.D.

When you have an underactive thyroid (hypothyroidism), typical symptoms are feeling sluggish and tired (especially in the mornings), gaining weight easily, feeling cold all the time, feeling achy, having your hair fall out and losing the outside of your eyebrows. An underactive thyroid will cause you to walk with the back of your hands rotated forward. Birth control pills contain estrogens that interfere with thyroid hormones.

When the thyroid is overactive (hyperthyroidism), your body kicks into high gear. Your heart rate speeds up, and you feel nervous, jittery and shaky. A balanced thyroid is essential to feeling healthy and vibrant.

Goiters

> "Without thyroid, there can be no complexity of thought, no learning, no education, no habit formation, no responsive energy for situations as well as no physical unfolding of faculty and function. No reproduction of kind with no sign of puberty at expected age and no exhibition of sex tendencies thereafter."
> Louis Berman, M.D., World Renowned Endocrinologist

Thyroid Support
- Kelp Complex – 50 drops twice daily
- Thyro Plus – 2 capsules twice daily

An enlarged thyroid gland, where the individual's neck swells, is called a goiter. Why does it swell? All your blood (about 5 quarts) circulates through the thyroid every hour to take hormones to your cells. Every cell in the body requires thyroid hormones to catalyze metabolism, similar to your car's engine needing spark plugs to ignite the fuel. When the thyroid is not getting enough iodine, it swells in an attempt to capture more iodine from the blood. We don't need a drug or radiation to shrink the thyroid. What we need is to give the thyroid the nutritional support it is screaming to get. Sea kelp is the best source of iodine. Magnesium, Vitamin A, B2 (riboflavin) and amino acids may also be needed to balance the thyroid.

> "There are doubtless a great many people who are mildly deficient in thyroid hormone and would be benefited by taking it orally but are not ill enough to see a physician." Dr. Roger J. Williams, Discoverer of Pantothenic Acid

Healthy Glandular Thyroid Medications
- **Armour Thyroid** – contains desiccated porcine & cornstarch
- **Westhroid** – contains desiccated porcine – **corn-free**
- **Nature-Throid** – contains desiccated porcine – **corn-free**

If you must take a thyroid medication, using a more natural one is usually best. Synthroid provides T4 and Cytomel T3. Natural desiccated thyroid hormones taken from animal thyroid glands such as Armour, Westhroid and Nature-Throid contain all forms of thyroid hormones, which includes T1, d2, t2, T, T3, and T4, providing a more complete set of nutrients for the thyroid to regulate itself. Dr. David Brownstein explains how much better most of his patients do when they make the switch to a natural glandular support like Armour. If you have an allergy to corn, avoid Armour and switch to Nature-Throid or Westhroid, since they do not have cornstarch as a binder. If you have an autoimmune thyroid disease, such as Hashimoto's, you may do better with a corn-free version such as Nature-Throid or Westhroid as well.

Thyroid Gland Disruptors	
Birth Control Pills	Surgery
Estrogen	Fluoride
Beta Blockers	Lead
Steroids	Mercury
Lithium	Pesticides
Phenytoin	Soy
Theophylline	Radiation
Alcohol	Chlorine
Bromine	Stress
Soft drinks	Plastic bottles

It has been shown that after removing the thyroid from test animals, arteriosclerosis develops. Dr. Kocher of Switzerland found that after performing surgery to remove thyroids (thyroidectomy) from individuals with goiters, they developed arteriosclerosis just like the test animals (Journal of Clinical Endocrinology & Metabolism June 2003, 88(6): 2438-2444). Austrian pathologists have also concluded that thyroidectomy contributes to hardening of the arteries.

We are bombarded in our environment with thyroid receptor site toxins that prevent thyroid hormones from getting into our cells. Some of the notorious ones are chlorine, fluoride and bromine. When you take a hot shower, you breathe in massive amounts of chlorine and fluoride through the steam that goes right in to the lungs and into the bloodstream. You essentially create a toxic gas chamber! If you feel dizzy or light-headed after a hot shower, you are getting a heavy dose of chlorine toxicity. I highly suggest getting a shower filter to remove chlorine and fluoride. You can order one from **www.berkeywaterfilter.com** or find one on amazon.com. Bromines are found in pesticides, plastics, soda, bakery goods, swimming pools, hot tubs and medications. This is one reason I'm not a fan of drinking out of plastic water bottles or swimming in chlorinated pools. Drink out of glass or stainless steel and swim in saltwater pools instead of toxic chlorine pools.

> **"A hypothyroid is just one more symptom of Epstein-Barr Virus."** Anthony William

By addressing the cause of dis-ease and not just suppressing symptoms with drugs, we can bring the body back into balance with natural remedies. When we do this, symptoms disappear. This is called health and it is earned by giving your body the nutrition it cries out for by sending warning signals most Americans view as annoying symptoms. Listen to your body. It is trying to get your attention so you will make a change. You don't ignore the red warning light on your dash in your car when it comes on. How much more important is your health than your car? Stop ignoring the warning signals and suppressing them with drugs and fix the problem before you end up in the emergency room. Your body is talking for a reason. Give it what it needs to heal.

> **"Those who fail to take time to be healthy will ultimately have to take the time to be sick."** James Chappell, D.C., N.D., Ph.D.

It is important to know that many drugs (sulfa and antidiabetic) interfere with the formation of thyroid hormones by blocking iodine uptake. Prednisone and estrogen (for women on birth control or hormone replacement therapy), according to Stephen Langer, M.D., should be used very cautiously because these drugs indirectly worsen already subnormal thyroid function. He also warns that cough medicines, lithium and aspirin can also contribute to hypothyroidism. If you look at all the medicines Americans take, it is easy to understand why so many have sluggish thyroids that lead to obesity, depression, fatigue and cold hands and feet. We trade in one bag of symptoms for another.

Birth control pills and Premarin increase certain protein levels, which decrease the thyroid hormone thyroxin. This leads to chronic fatigue syndrome. Dr. John Lowe claims that 63 percent of individuals diagnosed with fibromyalgia have laboratory signs of hypothyroidism.

> **"Cellular health depends upon three factors, a steady supply of nutrients, oxygen and thyroid hormones."** Broda O. Barnes, M.D., Ph.D.

Some individuals are cold all the time. No matter what they do, they can't get their basal temperature up. If your thyroid medication doesn't seem to help, chances are, there is an issue with heavy metal poisoning, usually mercury. This is the first layer of the onion. The second is usually an overgrowth of candida yeast. Reoccurring vaginal yeast infections, skin rashes and a white coating on the tongue are sure signs of yeast.

> **"Hidden in the throats of unsuspecting millions is the reason for many — if not most — heart attacks: a subnormal thyroid gland."** Stephen E. Langer, M.D.

Losing Weight & Keeping It Off

One of the keys to weight loss is having a balanced endocrine system, which is where your hormones are manufactured. Even if you only eat one small meal a day, you will not lose weight if your endocrine system is out of balance. The biggest culprit with obesity is stress. Stress revs the adrenal glands into high gear, which pulls the thyroid out of balance. The thyroid regulates metabolism and body temperature.

Heavy metals and pesticides can accumulate in the body and interfere with glandular functions. Mercury tends to accumulate in the thyroid. If heavy metals are interfering with glandular functions, then you probably won't have much success balancing hormones until the metals are detoxified from your body. An EDS scan will test for heavy metals toxicity.

> **"A friend of mine confused her Valium with her birth control pills. She had 14 kids, but she doesn't really care."** Gary R. Oberg, M.D.

It may surprise you to know that the average glass of store-bought milk contains over 100 different antibiotics. A large dairy farmer I know told me his best milk cows produce 16 gallons of milk a day. Back in the 1940s, my grandfather hand-milked 20 cows in St. Ignatius, Montana. His best cow would produce 4 gallons of milk a day. How can we go from 4 gallons to 16 gallons a day? Steroids. We eat the meat, eggs, cheese, yogurt and drink the milk from these animals and receive a plethora of concentrated forms of these steroid growth hormones and antibiotics and then wonder why we can't lose weight. Just as massive bodybuilders have 22-inch arms and Holstein milk cows are pumping out 16 gallons of milk a day, you eat the animal products fed these growth hormones and bulk up too and then wonder why you can't lose weight. Buy organic foods and stop poisoning your body with these weight-gaining chemicals.

You eat what's in your house. Foods like boiled eggs, raw almonds, pecans, walnuts, almond butter/coconut butter, celery sticks, frozen berries and canned Alaskan salmon are good snacks. If you have a food pantry filled with breakfast toaster pastries, chips, snack cakes, cookies and crackers, plus ice cream in the freezer, you are setting yourself up for failure. Get rid of the junk food! If it's Friday night and you have done well on your diet all week, then maybe it's time to reward yourself with a good dinner and dessert. Remember, all things in moderation.

What's The Healthiest Water To Drink?

Some people believe that if they drink water, they will feel bloated and gain weight. This is false. Dehydration is one of the biggest inhibitors of weight loss. When people are dehydrated, they retain fluids. The body's cells are intelligent, like camels crossing a desert that know how to conserve water when they haven't received enough in the past. If you wait until you are thirsty to drink, you are way too late. First thing in the morning upon arising, drink 16 ounces of purified room-temperature water. Squeezing fresh lemon or lime in it is good. This will tell your cells from the start of the day that you won't be crossing the desert and that they can use an abundance of water to clean, bathe and flush out toxins. This hydrates the colon so you can have a healthy bowel movement.

As mentioned previously, drink at least half of your body weight in ounces of water a day. Of course, if you are roofing a house in August and it is 100 degrees, you will need more water than the secretary sitting at her desk in an air-conditioned office. Be smart and use good judgment. If you drink water and then need to urinate immediately after, because "water runs right through me," as some say, then most likely you are deficient in trace minerals.

What type of water to drink is probably one of the most controversial topics in the health-care field. Everyone has an opinion. Clean, purified water that is not contaminated with chlorine, fluoride, heavy metals, pesticides, hormones and microbes is best for drinking. Natural spring water from a clean source is good, if you have access to one. A whole house water purification system is great, so you drink clean water and bathe with non-fluoridated/chlorinated water.

After nearly losing his son to fluoride poisoning from their drinking water that contained a carbon block filter, Fred Van Liew, also known as "The Water Doctor," developed an excellent reverse osmosis water purification system to remove chlorine and fluoride along with a structured water unit. He also has shower filters. Look him up at eWater.com.

Distilled water is clean and pure, but dead, water. If using distilled water, I would add a pinch of pink Himalayan salt to each gallon. A Berkey water filter with fluoride removing filters is good. They also make a shower filter. www.berkeyfilters.com.

After purifying your water, it is a wise idea to energize and harmonically structure it to ensure the water can penetrate your cells for better hydration and enhance cellular communication. Dr. Gerald Pollack, bioengineering professor at the University of Washington, explains how hexagonally structured or vortexed water hydrates the cells more effectively and enhances biochemical processes in the body.

The best way to alkalize the body is by eating fruits and vegetables. The pH of the stomach is very acidic. Drinking alkaline water neutralizes the acid in the stomach, inhibiting proper digestion.

> **"Great spirits have always encountered violent opposition from mediocre minds."** Albert Einstein

More than 50 percent of the human body is water. Dr. Masaru Emoto of Japan, author of *The Hidden Messages in Water*, demonstrates that distilled water has no structure, but when a word such as love or peace is written on the container holding the water and then it is analyzed under an electron microscope, the water forms a beautiful, symmetrical, crystal structure. When a word such as hate or evil is written on it, the crystal structure becomes jagged and chaotic with no symmetry. Similar patterns occur when water is exposed to different types of music as well. When heavy metal rock music is played, the crystal structure becomes a chaotic, jagged blob, but when classical music such as Bach or Beethoven is played, the water takes on a beautiful, symmetrical, harmonious structure. So, when you walk around all day in your body that's more than 50 percent water, is it balanced with harmonious, healthy thoughts, or are the water structures in your cells chaotic and angry, living in fear, producing a dis-eased state? Your innermost thoughts, words you speak and emotions are constantly resonating with health and life or fear and disease. What you think and feel has a profound impact on your health.

Stevia – Mother Nature's Sugar Substitute

> **"Stevia has virtually no calories. It dissolves easily in water and mixes well with all other sweeteners. I use it myself in a delicious homemade ice cream that is extremely low in carbohydrates."** Robert C. Atkins, M.D. (1930-2003)

Most Americans consume too much sugar, which causes weight gain and blood sugar disorders. Stevia is an herb from Paraguay that is 200 to 300 times sweeter than sugar with no calories. This makes it an excellent 100 percent, all-natural sugar/artificial sweetener substitute. A couple of drops will sweeten anything you desire. Research has shown that Stevia helps regulate the pancreas and stabilize blood sugar levels.

> **"Stevia is not only non-toxic, but has several traditional medicinal uses. A digestive aid and also has been topically applied to help wound healing. Recent clinical studies have shown it can increase glucose tolerance and decrease blood sugar levels. Of the two sweeteners (Aspartame and Stevia), Stevia wins hands down."** Julian Whitaker, M.D.

Healing Skin Issues

Pus and blood oozed out of huge open lesions on Fran's legs. The open sores smelled and looked terrible. She came to us because all of her previous six medical doctors had failed to help her. They all tried prescribing every type of cream and salve available. They put her on antibiotics, round after round, but to no avail. She had been suffering for 13 years and no doctor had been able to help her. She came in to our clinic to see if a "naturopathic doctor" using natural remedies could help.

> **"The necessity of teaching mankind not to take drugs and medicines is a duty incumbent upon all who know their uncertainty and injurious effects; and the time is not far distant when the drug system will be abandoned."** Charles Armbruster, M.D.

We began our full investigation with an EDS scan to identify the cause of her skin lesions. We found that her skin lesions were not caused from a deficiency of antibiotics, cortisone creams or any other man-made drug. It's a good thing doctors can't cut your skin off and throw it in the trash like they can a gallbladder, tonsils or uterus, because if they could, I'm sure it would have already been done.

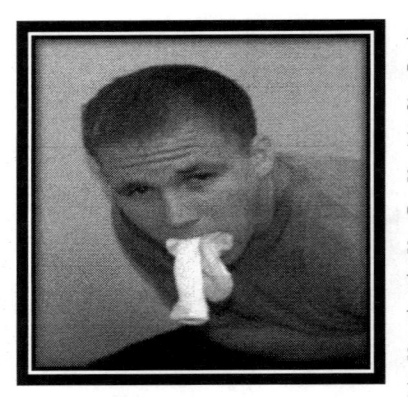

As we tested her for toxicity issues, we found chemicals and heavy metal poisoning. I asked Fran about her history and found out that she used to work in a chemical manufacturing facility. Her liver and spleen were resonating at a very low frequency. The cause had nothing to do with the skin. Due to her liver, spleen and lymphatic system being unable to drain toxins efficiently, her body was excreting the toxins through her skin. When the internal filters (liver, spleen and kidneys) of the body become clogged, instead of shutting down and dying, our body will save its life by pushing the toxins out through the skin. This is how awesome we are made! Your intelligence always does what is best for you, every time, whether you or your doctor understand it or not. Your body's intelligence always works for your greatest good. Trying to stop toxins from coming out through the skin is equivalent to stuffing a sock in your mouth when vomiting. We want the toxins out of the body, and once we support the filters, which are the liver, kidneys and spleen, then we eliminate the root cause and the skin clears up.

> **"Medical practice has neither philosophy nor common sense to recommend it. In sickness, the body is already loaded with impurities. By taking drug-medicines, more impurities are added; thereby, the case is further embarrassed and harder to cure."** Elmer Lee, M.D., Vice President, Academy of Medicine

Our skin is capable of eliminating 3 pints of poison a day. Anything we do to suppress the body from detoxifying is counterproductive. It is believed that if we were to inject those 3 pints of poison back into the blood, we would die in three days of blood poisoning.

As Dr. Bernard Jensen taught, always remember, if you step on a cat's tail, it's the other end that yells. Just because the problem manifests on the skin doesn't necessarily mean that's what needs the attention. Always look for the cause and work with the body to eliminate it and then the symptoms usually clear up on their own.

> **"The problem is not where the pain is."** Dr. Burt Espy

We put Fran on a homeopathic lymphatic drainer as well as a heavy metal/chemical detox formula and an herbal liver and spleen cleanse. Within three weeks, the sores on her legs were completely healed!

> "It's supposed to be a secret, but I'll tell you anyway. We doctors do nothing. We only help and encourage the doctor within." Albert Schweitzer, M.D., Nobel Laureate, 1940

Don't Ignore Your Body's Warning Signs

Choosing to ignore the warning signals in your body is no different than you putting duct tape over an annoying red, low-oil light in your car. The wise automobile manufacturers put the oil warning light there to prevent disaster when the oil level gets dangerously low. Like the warning lights on the dash of your car, The Creator engineered your body with warning signals as well. Headaches, swelling, pain, heartburn, diarrhea, hunger, thirst, lightheadedness, fatigue, etc., are some of those signs you come equipped with. Most of us address the hunger and fatigue signals by eating and sleeping, but suppress the other signals with drugs, which is equivalent to putting a strip of duct tape over the light thinking we solved the problem.

> "All symptoms are manifestations of the body's attempt to rebalance itself." Humbart "Smokey" Santillo, N.D.

A fever allows us to sweat out toxins. Diarrhea, vomiting, sneezing and coughing are ways the body expels toxins from the inside. Anything done to suppress what the body does naturally is inviting disease to stay and thrive and eventually become cancer. Edema (swelling) and pain are warning signs from your body crying out for help. Mainstream medicine teaches us to ignore those vital warning signals by suppressing them with painkillers, diuretics and anti-inflammatories. The surgeon for the King of England understood this healing secret long ago when he stated,

> "There is but one disease and that is deficient drainage." Sir Arbuthnot Lane, M.D., Surgeon for the King of England

In his book, *The Biology of Belief*, cell biologist Bruce Lipton, Ph.D., from Stanford University's School of Medicine, relates a story to illustrate how absurd it is to continue to suppress symptoms with drugs without ever addressing the cause.

"Our drug mania reminds me of a job at an auto dealership I held while in graduate school. At 4:30 on a Friday afternoon, an irate woman came into the shop. Her car's 'service engine light' was flashing, even though her car had already been repaired for that same problem several times. At 4:30 on a Friday afternoon, who wants to work on a balky problem and deal with a furious customer? Everyone was quiet, except for one mechanic who said: 'I'll take care of it.' He drove the car back into the bay, got in behind the dashboard, removed the bulb

from the signal light and threw it away. Then he opened a can of soda and lit a cigarette. After suitable time, during which the customer thought he was actually fixing the car, the mechanic returned and told the woman her car was ready. Thrilled to see that the warning light had stopped flashing, she happily drove off into the sunset. Though the cause of the problem was still present, the symptom was gone. Similarly, pharmaceutical drugs suppress the body's symptoms, but, most never address the cause of the problem."

> **"Most diseases are the result of medication which has been prescribed to relieve and take away a beneficial and warning symptom on the part of Nature."** Elbert Hubbard, Philosopher

Americans have foolishly been taught by a money-oriented medical system to "cut the wires" so we can go on our merry way with life and not be annoyed with warning lights and symptoms. Like a businessman once told me as he swallowed his painkillers, "I don't have time for this nagging headache and this little pill does the trick." There's no doubt that drugs do a wonderful job at keeping the signals suppressed; however, we run the risk of burning up the engine. When he's lying in a hospital bed because he just had a heart attack, kidney failure or liver cancer, then he'll suddenly have time. When your health fails, you have all the time in the world to lie in bed and mope around sick because you can't work or play. Don't wait until you are flat on your back in the hospital to start focusing on health. An ounce of prevention is worth a pound of cure, and your health is your wealth.

> **"Drugs never cure disease. They merely hush the voice of nature's protest, and pull down the danger signals she erects along the pathway of transgression. Any poison taken into the system has to be reckoned with later on even though it palliates present symptoms. Pain may disappear, but the patient is left in a worse condition, though unconscious of it at the time."** Daniel H. Kress, M.D.

Chapter 4
HEALERS OR DRUG DEALERS?

Epilepsy Healed

A businessman brought his son in and said, "I don't believe in what you do, but I'm here because I have no other options. The best doctors around tell me there is no cure for my son's epileptic seizures. Do you think you could help him?" Mike had been suffering with epilepsy, narcolepsy, sleep apnea and restless leg syndrome. After spending over $300,000 on the best medicine in the country and not getting any relief, they came to see if a naturopathic approach could provide any solutions.

We ran an EDS scan, and after two months of being on a detox and nutritional program, Mike's seizures were completely healed, after having three a week, for the last 20 years of his life. Was it a miracle? No, that's what the body does when you give it the nutritional support it needs and open up the channels of detoxification.

> "Half of what we have taught you is wrong. Unfortunately, we do not know which half." Dean Burwell, M.D. (Addressing medical students at Harvard University)

People always ask, "Can you cure epilepsy, cancer or multiple sclerosis?" The answer is no, we can't cure anything and neither can any other doctor; however, your body can heal itself of disease once it receives correct nutrition and the nails in the tire, or toxins, are removed.

Mike's father was left baffled. How can you spend over $300,000 on the best medicine in America with all the tests being inconclusive and drugs that don't help, and then go to a naturopath and for about $600 worth of products and testing fees, the boy is completely healed of epileptic seizures? How could insurance cover all the expensive medical testing that failed to help and then refuse to cover a naturopathic approach that allowed his son to be healed? The father asked why insurance does not cover what we do. When you understand the monopoly that has been formed in this country involving oil, drugs and insurance, then you understand why they do not cover natural medicine.

What were the nails in the tire causing Mike's seizures? An EDS exam identified energetic disturbances in his nervous system, pituitary gland and circulatory system. Mercury poisoning was the first major nail in the tire, interfering with his nerves and glands. Uncovering his symptoms, layer by layer like an onion, we also found Toxocara Cati (cat roundworms) causing chaos in the nervous system. And the last nail was a major nervous system toxin, called the

> **CALIFORNIA**
> **Doctors find tapeworm larva in man's brain**
>
> NAPA — A California man says he went to an emergency room with a terrible headache and nausea, slipped into a coma, and was told a tapeworm larva had been living in his brain when he woke up.
>
> College student Luis Ortiz, 26, of Napa, said doctors told him he needed immediate surgery to remove it.
>
> "I was shocked," Ortiz said. "I just couldn't believe something like that would happen to me. I didn't know there was a parasite in my head trying to ruin my life."
>
> The surgery and the aftermath have greatly impacted his life, Ortiz said. He had to drop out of school, move back home and find a temporary place for his dog. He can't drive or work.
>
> "My memory is like a work in progress," he said. "It gets better from therapy," but he has to remind himself to do his memory exercises and other daily tasks.

syphilinum miasm. These were the toxins causing him to manifest epileptic seizures. Drugs do not pull nails out, they have no power to detoxify cells, but herbs and homeopathic remedies were created for that purpose and they do it safely, effectively and powerfully.

In naturopathy, we focus on health, not disease. We balance the body with nutritional and detoxification supplements so that healing occurs. So next time you go to another doctor's visit, remember, your doctor will only find what he is looking for, not what's necessarily causing your problem and then prescribe a drug to maintain the symptoms. This is not health care, it's disease maintenance.

> **"The best of our popular physicians are the ones who do the least harm. But unfortunately some poison their patients with mercury, and others purge or bleed them to death. There are some who have learned so much that their learning has driven out all common sense; and there are others who care a great deal more for their own profit than for the health of their patient — a physician should be the servant of Nature, not his enemy; he should be able to guide and direct her in her struggle for life, and not throw by his unreasonable influences fresh obstacles in the way of recovery."** Paracelsus, Swiss doctor, 1493-1541

When we scanned Mike to check his nutritional levels, which includes all minerals, amino acids, vitamins, fatty acids and enzymes, we found him to have a raging magnesium/potassium deficiency. He was also low in calcium, zinc, taurine, iodine, choline, inositol and pantothenic acid. His serotonin levels were also out of balance. We put him on detoxification support with homeopathic remedies and herbal drainage formulas, as well as nutritional support supplements. Diseases don't have to be these mysterious incurable illnesses; we just need to find out what's causing them and support the body in detoxifying. The doctor within has access to the DNA library that contains all the healing wisdom of the ages. It knows how and can heal any dis-ease when given the correct nutritional and detoxification tools to do what God engineered you to do — HEAL!

Pathological blood work is usually a poor diagnosis to check for mineral deficiencies because the body will do everything in its power to maintain homeostasis. In other words, when the blood begins to change and deficiencies are detected, then we know the organs and glands have been deprived for a dangerously long time. The blood is the last to change. For example, the body will rob magnesium from the heart to keep the blood levels balanced. So, you may have a raging magnesium deficiency, but your lab work shows normal, while your heart is beating irregularly with severe chest pains, insomnia, muscle cramps, restless legs and anxiety – all classic magnesium deficiency symptoms, as your doctor smiles and says, "Everything looks good according to the blood work." We see this often. Do not wait for deficiencies to manifest themselves in bloodwork to take action. Most of us need to supplement with minerals daily because our foods are grown in soils that are depleted.

> **"Out of four thousand cases recently examined in a New York hospital, only two were not suffering from a lack of calcium."** Journal of the American Medical Association

Toxic Chemicals In The Environment

We live in a toxic world bombarded with pollutants and chemicals in our foods, water and air we breathe. Chemicals surround us in our environment. The United States Office of Technology Assessment informs that the EPA lists more than 65,000 chemicals in its inventory of toxic chemicals. What's even more alarming is that every year they receive more than 1,500 notices of intent to manufacture new chemicals. We eat, drink and breathe in 75,000 micro clustered chemicals every day that cause health problems. It doesn't matter how natural and organic you are, these chemicals are everywhere.

The majority of all cereal in the USA contains BHT (a preservative) which has been banned in England, because it has been shown to cause chemical changes in the brain. And we wonder why so many people are depressed, have anxiety, bipolar disorders and ADD. How many Americans start the day off with a bowl of BHT-laced, blood-sugar-spiking, gluten-packed cereal with pasteurized milk containing antibiotics and steroids?

Dioxins from PVC products (plastic piping) are found in fish and shellfish. Polychlorinated biphenyls (PCBs) that were used to make paint, ink, hydraulic fluids and electrical transformers were banned in the late 1970s, but concentrations are still found in most farm-raised salmon.

Furans, similar to dioxins, and PCBs are associated with endocrine and hormonal disorders. Propylene Glycol is

Avoid These Toxins For Optimal Health	
Sugar	Artificial flavors
Hydrogenated oil	High fructose corn syrup
Enriched flour	Monosodium glutamate
Vegetable oil	Palm oil
Wesson oil	Margarine
Splenda	Aspartame
Artificial colors	Soy

used in antifreeze and hydraulic fluids. It is also used in vaccinations, cosmetics, deodorants, lotions, shampoos, toothpaste and processed foods. It has been shown to absorb through the skin, causing kidney/liver damage, immune-system disruption, respiratory damage and nervous system complications. Parabens are found in shaving gels, moisturizers, spray tans, makeup, toothpaste and deodorant. Parabens mimic estrogen and have been found in breast tumor samples.

Asbestos is found in buildings constructed in the 1950s and 1960s that were insulated with cancer-causing materials. The microscopically small fibers get into the air we breathe and irritate cells and cause cancer. Organochlorine insecticides (DDT and chlordane) were used to kill insects, mainly mosquitos, after World War II. DDT has been banned in the USA; however, India, China and North Korea still continue to use the deadly poison. Phthalates are chemicals found in soft plastics and used to lengthen the shelf life of cosmetics, hair spray, mousses and fragrances. They are notorious for harming the liver, kidneys, lungs and testicles in teenage boys. Volatile organic compounds (VOCs) are petroleum-based chemicals found in toiletries such as aftershave lotions, shampoos, perfumes, air fresheners, household cleaners, furniture polish, plastics, foams and adhesives. If you live on planet earth, you are exposed to harmful toxins every day.

Bisphenol A (BPA) used in the manufacturing of plastic water bottles is an estrogen-mimicking hormone that causes man boobs in males. Avoid plastic water bottles, use glass or stainless steel containers. Another reason we are seeing such an issue with cancer of the reproductive organs (ovaries, uterus, breast, prostate), obesity and hormonal issues is because most pesticides produce an estrogenic effect, which means they mimic estrogens in our bodies. Add this with all the growth hormones in our dairy products and meats along with birth control pills and we increase our risk for cancer exponentially. Science news published a study that showed a link to household pesticide use and childhood leukemia. Families who use professional exterminators in their homes increase the risk of childhood leukemia three times as much, compared to those who did not use exterminators. Young children, 2 years old or younger, are at highest risk. Also, pregnant women who are exposed to pesticides double the risk of their baby developing leukemia. Use a natural insecticide! Essential oils are great.

Natural Insect Killer	
1 cup witch hazel	
1 cup apple cider vinegar	
Lemongrass oil	75 drops
Citronella oil	75 drops
Tea Tree oil	75 drops
Eucalyptus oil	75 drops
Peppermint oil	75 drops
Mix in spray bottle	

The weed killer 2,4-D, when mixed with other chemicals, becomes highly toxic. It is used in lawn-care products for killing dandelions and other weeds and is heavily used on crops, especially wheat, golf courses, parks and school playgrounds. Farmers who spray the weed killer have been shown to have an increase in cancer, especially non-Hodgkin's lymphoma. In fact, non-Hodgkin's lymphoma has increased in farm workers (especially in wheat-growing areas) by 75 percent over the previous 20 years. Attorneys are advertising heavily to call if you were exposed to Roundup weed killer and have been diagnosed with the dreaded cancer.

> **"Drugs put a tremendous strain on the liver, the organ responsible for providing enzymes to metabolize the drugs and dispose of their toxic waste products."** Candace B. Pert, Ph.D.

According to Stephen B. Edelson, M.D., *"The liver accumulates rather than eliminates toxins ...."* He points out that one of the most serious yet overlooked toxins in our society is mercury. Not only is it found in dental fillings but also in seafood, water, pesticides, fertilizers, paints, solvents, bleached flour, processed foods and even fabric softeners.

Chemical Detoxifiers
• Milk Thistle
• Chlorella
• Spirulina
• Garlic
• Selenium

We recommend having an EDS evaluation at least once a year to check for possible toxins that could be affecting your health. We change oil and filters in our automobiles on a regular basis to keep the engine running strong so it will last as long as possible, so shouldn't we give our bodies the same or better? Your liver and kidneys are bombarded with harmful chemicals on a daily basis. A wise person does a cleanse periodically to keep dis-ease at bay. Natural health care puts responsibility upon the patient. We teach **"Response-Ability**," which is your ability to respond to life in a health-promoting way. Doctors prescribe poisonous drugs that sometimes cause worse symptoms than what you are taking the drug for in the first place. How many so-smart doctors gave their patients Vioxx and other health-destroying drugs that have harmed and killed good Americans so many times that the FDA finally pulled the killer from the market? You trusted him with Vioxx. Which drugs are you trusting him with now that will be recalled next year?

Dangerous Dis-ease Causing Toxins

Bisphenol A (BPA)	Aspartame	Soy lecithin (E322)	2,4-D
Hexane	Monosodium glutamate (MSG)	Polysorbate 80 (E433)	Asbestos
Glyphosate	Artificial dyes	Carbon monoxide	Fiberglass
Triazines	Sodium benzoate (E211)	Potassium bromate (E924)	Nuclear radiation
Organochlorines	Potassium benzoate (E212)	Brominated vegetable oil (BVO)	Birth control pills
Organophosates	Calcium benzoate (e213	Sodium nitrite (E250)	X-rays, radiation
Pyrethroids	Parabens (E214, E215, E218, E219	Hydrogenated oils	Vaccines
Carbamates	Propyl gallate (E310)	Sulfites (E223)	Triclosan
Arsenal pesticides	Neonicotinoids	Carrageenan (E407)	Chronic stress

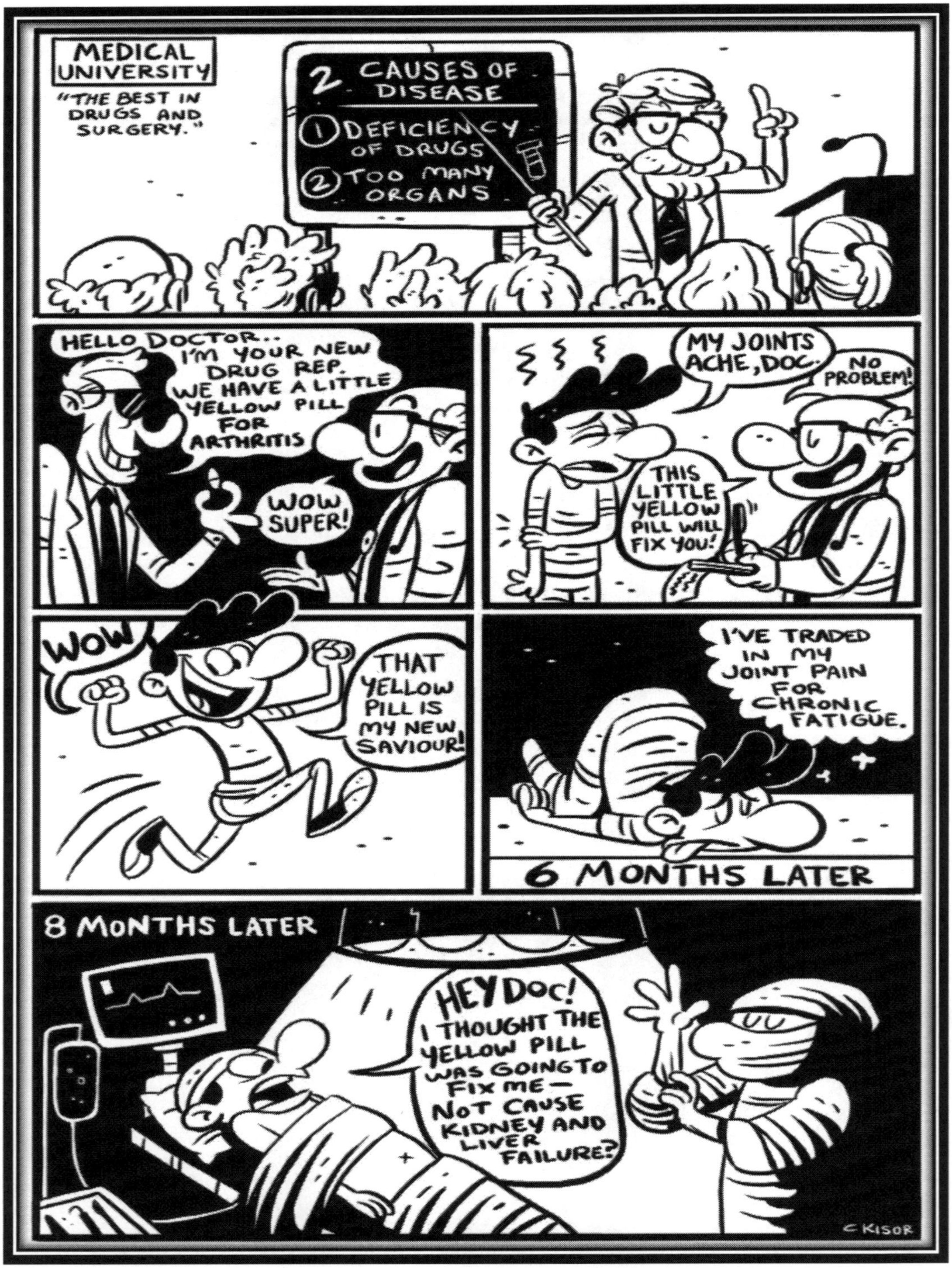
MEDICAL UNIVERSITY
"THE BEST IN DRUGS AND SURGERY."
2 CAUSES OF DISEASE
1 DEFICIENCY OF DRUGS
2 TOO MANY ORGANS
HELLO DOCTOR.. I'M YOUR NEW DRUG REP. WE HAVE A LITTLE YELLOW PILL FOR ARTHRITIS
WOW SUPER!
MY JOINTS ACHE, DOC.
NO PROBLEM!
THIS LITTLE YELLOW PILL WILL FIX YOU!
WOW
THAT YELLOW PILL IS MY NEW SAVIOUR!
I'VE TRADED IN MY JOINT PAIN FOR CHRONIC FATIGUE.
6 MONTHS LATER
8 MONTHS LATER
HEY DOC! I THOUGHT THE YELLOW PILL WAS GOING TO FIX ME— NOT CAUSE KIDNEY AND LIVER FAILURE?
C KISOR

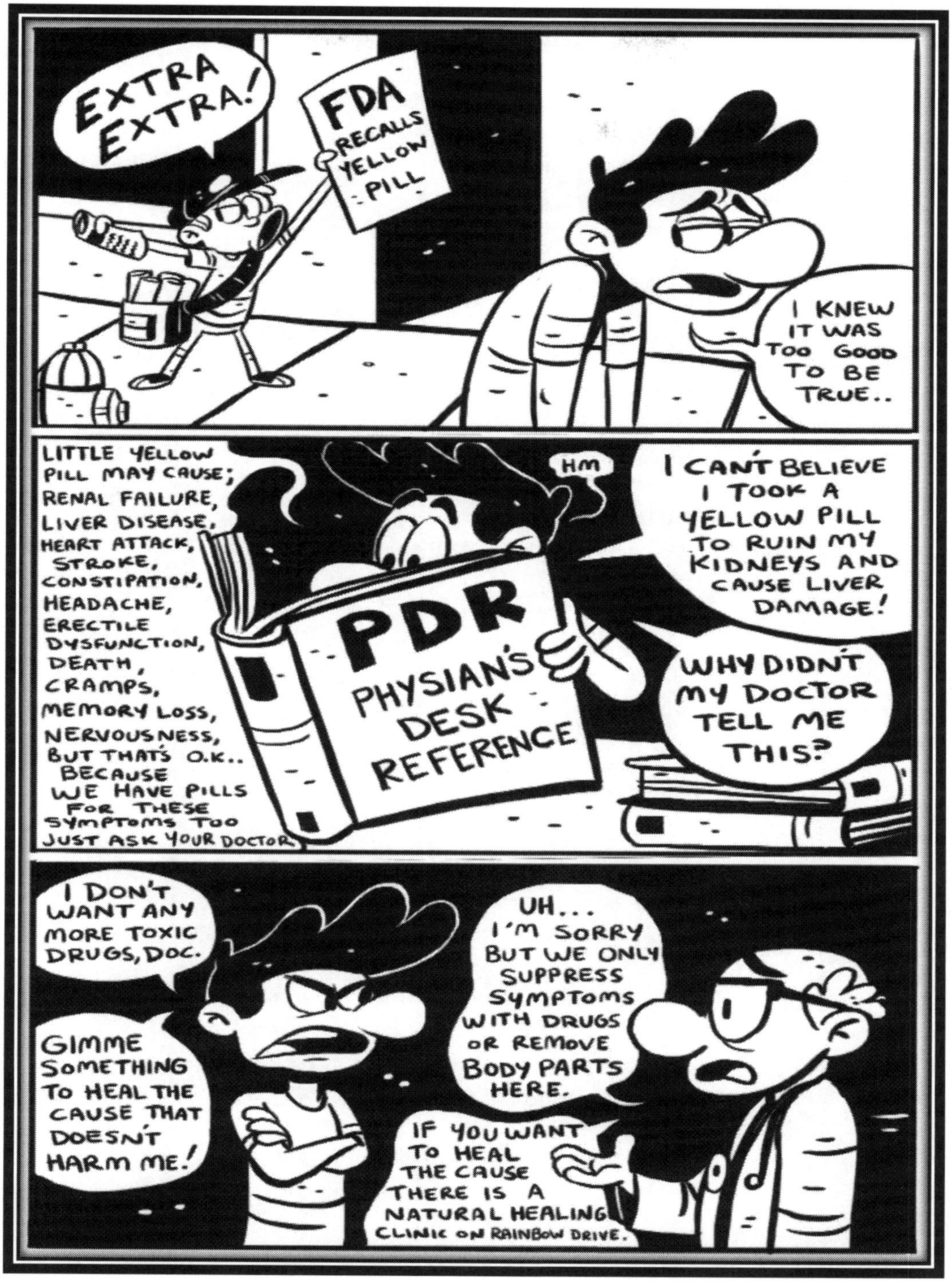
EXTRA EXTRA!
FDA RECALLS YELLOW PILL
I KNEW IT WAS TOO GOOD TO BE TRUE..
LITTLE YELLOW PILL MAY CAUSE; RENAL FAILURE, LIVER DISEASE, HEART ATTACK, STROKE, CONSTIPATION, HEADACHE, ERECTILE DYSFUNCTION, DEATH, CRAMPS, MEMORY LOSS, NERVOUSNESS, BUT THAT'S O.K.. BECAUSE WE HAVE PILLS FOR THESE SYMPTOMS TOO JUST ASK YOUR DOCTOR
HM
PDR PHYSIAN'S DESK REFERENCE
I CAN'T BELIEVE I TOOK A YELLOW PILL TO RUIN MY KIDNEYS AND CAUSE LIVER DAMAGE!
WHY DIDN'T MY DOCTOR TELL ME THIS?
I DON'T WANT ANY MORE TOXIC DRUGS, DOC.
GIMME SOMETHING TO HEAL THE CAUSE THAT DOESN'T HARM ME!
UH... I'M SORRY BUT WE ONLY SUPPRESS SYMPTOMS WITH DRUGS OR REMOVE BODY PARTS HERE.
IF YOU WANT TO HEAL THE CAUSE THERE IS A NATURAL HEALING CLINIC ON RAINBOW DRIVE.

Case Study

Most of my adult life I have had numerous health problems. About 14 years ago I was stricken with a strange flu-like virus that would not go away. After seeing two or three medical doctors and 6 months later, I was finally diagnosed with Chronic Epstein-Barr. I was told there was no known treatment. For many years I had experienced chronic fatigue, especially after overexertion or periods of stress.

I was diagnosed with Hypothyroidism in the early 1960s. In this last decade, I have been diagnosed with Chronic Fatigue Syndrome, mini-stroke, osteoporosis, food and inhalant allergies, gastrointestinal problems, high triglycerides, anxiety attacks, depression, TMJ, and fibromyalgia. The fibromyalgia contributed to many of my problems. The debilitating fatigue was probably the hardest to deal with. Household activities were very limited, while church and social events were practically nonexistent.

The medical doctors only knew to keep adding prescription drugs for treatment of all my medical problems. The cost of treatment for my medical problems, along with menopause and hypothyroidism, was a $600 to $700 pharmacy bill a month. As I was taking all the medication prescribed by the medical doctors, I realized that the drugs were slowly killing me. I was in constant pain and discomfort. I couldn't sleep, and riding in a car was almost unbearable. My digestive system was extremely messed up, and I got very little relief with any medication prescribed for the stomach.

For all my medical problems, I was sent from doctor to doctor and had scans, X-rays, MRIs, echo-cardiograms, colonoscopies, endoscopies, neurological testing, and blood work of every type. With all the testing, evaluations and medication, nothing corrected my problems. I have been under the care of several different chiropractors during the last decade. I am not a "doctor hopper" as it may sound, but several of the doctors who treated me threw up their hands and gave up on me.

*My latest doctor of internal medicine, who I have been seeing for the last four to five years, knew **I was developing an interest in alternative medicine since the medical field gave me no hope or lasting help.** In April 2004, my medical doctor admitted medical science had no cure for me and she suggested I seek other means of help if I chose to do so. She said if I found a naturopathic doctor whom I felt comfortable with, to go with her blessings. This was a big change of direction for me, because I was indoctrinated to follow only mainstream medical practice.*

I checked several places of alternative medicine within driving distances, but was not satisfied that they were right for me. My present chiropractor, Dr. Jon Alan Smith, recommended I see a naturopathic doctor in Gadsden. After talking with Dr. Sainsbury on the phone, I knew that I was being led in the right direction. On June 3, 2004, I had my first visit Dr. Sainsbury. I went with some hesitation, but I knew if I were to have a better life, or life at all, I had to try a different approach. I carried a bag full of medication (nine prescription drugs plus over-the-counter stuff). Dr. Sainsbury cued in on my multitude of problems and began addressing the most pressing problems by addressing the cause with natural supplements.

Since Dr. Sainsbury has been working with me, replacing drugs with natural supplements, I have shown remarkable improvement physically, emotionally and mentally. At the present, I am taking two to three very small doses of prescription drugs, and before long, I hope to be off all the chemicals. The last two months, my pharmacy bill has been $35 instead of $600 to $700. My internist is elated with my state of health. My weight has dropped 20-plus pounds, and all my blood work and physical exams are good. Although medical insurance does not cover Dr. Sainsbury's programs, as I told my medical doctor, I would rather be where I am health-wise today than have the amount of money used for the programs. To quote her, "There is no price you can place on good health."

I am far from where I was health-wise in June 2004, and on January 18, 2005, I am not where I want to be. By God's grace and using Dr. Sainsbury as His instrument, I will be where I want to be health-wise soon.

I now have a "HOPE" for some quality years ahead. Jeremiah 29:11

Thank God for Dr. Reed Sainsbury.

B.R.
Albertville, Alabama

"Doctors are men who prescribe medicines of which they know little, to cure diseases of which they know less, in human beings of whom they know nothing." Voltaire

---

Healing Cancer With Whole, Living Foods

When I was a young teenager, my dad took my brother and me to meet Scott and Gladys Forsyth in Moses Lake, Washington. They were health enthusiasts who grew wheatgrass and juiced it along with other healthy practices, such as composting their own soil for gardening. Many years ago, Gladys was diagnosed with cancer and Scott had previously suffered from a heart attack. Like most Americans, they sought the best help available and began chemotherapy treatments for Gladys. Her body did the natural thing: rejected the poison chemotherapy. In an effort to get rid of the toxins, she began vomiting frequently and her hair fell out. Deep down, she knew there was a better way.

One night as her husband sat by her side, she told him that she couldn't stand feeling sick like this anymore and if this is how her life was going to be, then she would rather go home and die in her own house. She didn't want to suffer in this awful state any longer.

Being very religious people, they decided to get on their knees and pour out their hearts to God for help. They prayed for deliverance from the hell they were experiencing and asked that if there be a way to heal this cancer to please make it known. Shortly after, they learned from a friend about The Ann Wigmore Living Foods Lifestyle in Boston, Massachusetts. This natural healing center is built upon the principal and belief:

> *THE NAME OF THE DISEASE IS NOT IMPORTANT. IF YOU PUT NOTHING BUT WHOLE LIVING FOOD INTO YOUR BODY IT WILL HEAL ITSELF.*

"My doctor became extremely upset and said, 'you'll die' if you don't take this chemotherapy," explained Gladys. Since her doctor admitted to her that he couldn't promise the chemotherapy would work and allow her to live, she chose something different. Going against her doctor's orders, she stopped the chemo treatments and left with her husband and flew to Boston to The Ann Wigmore Living Foods Foundation. They stayed for two weeks, eating organic whole foods along with lots of wheatgrass juice and "rejuvelac," which is a probiotic-rich, fermented drink made from sprouted wheat berries. They felt strongly that God had heard and answered their prayers.

> **"The food you eat can either be the safest and most powerful form of medicine, or the slowest form of poison."** Ann Wigmore

The days went by and Scott and Gladys continued making and drinking "rejuvelac," along with eating raw living foods. These raw living foods are high in enzymes, chlorophyll and easy to digest. They are cell foods, meaning they feed, nourish and cleanse the cells of the body. This is what your body has been engineered to burn for fuel, to receive energy and health, despite not being practiced by mainstream medicine due to obvious financial reasons.

The Forsyths began to feel better and their quality of life drastically improved. Three months later, still being on their whole foods diet and drinking freshly squeezed wheatgrass juice daily, they went back to their doctor to check the status of the cancer. The doctors ran tests and rechecked their previous reports to see if perhaps they had made a mistake in diagnosing Gladys with uterine cancer. They couldn't believe it, but the cancer was completely gone! Not a single trace of it showed up! It had been healed completely.

> **"Let thy food be your medicine and your medicine be your food."** Hippocrates

Was Gladys getting a clean bill of health a miracle? Absolutely not! That is just how God created your immune system to work when you get sick. Stop poisoning it and start feeding it living foods that cleanse and rebuild and dis-ease cannot exist. But yes, the fact that God created your immune system so intelligently, that as soon as you give it cell foods, it knows how to heal, is a testament of Divine Intelligence unfolding before our very eyes.

> **"No physician can ever say that any disease is incurable. To say so blasphemes God, blasphemes Nature, and depreciates the great architect of Creation. The disease does not exist, regardless of how terrible it may be, for which God has not provided the corresponding cure."** Paracelsus

You are a living person. If you want to live and be healthy, you must eat living foods. One fruit or vegetable can contain over 10,000 phytochemicals. Those plant chemicals are in there for a reason. Eat living foods to live.

The Healing Energy Of Plants

Medical schools do not teach herbology or homeopathy courses to medical doctors in this country, so they have not been taught about the healing power of plants. Herbs are ingeniously created in a perfect balance far beyond any scientist's comprehension. These healing entities are balanced with minerals, vitamins, amino acids, essential fatty acids and enzymes. The best-kept secret and most important ingredient in herbs is the living intelligent life force. This healing vibrational energy is the spark that your cells use to cleanse, nourish and regenerate your body back to health.

About 70 percent of pharmaceutical drugs originate, in some form, from herbs. For thousands of years in India, snakeroot herb has been used to help calm people down. The pharmaceutical industry makes a tranquilizer drug from this, called Reserpine. Quinine has been used as a fever reducer in cases of malaria and it is extracted from the Cinchona tree, also known as Peruvian bark. Vinblastine is used for treating leukemia. It is derived from periwinkle plants. The list goes on and on.

> "Keep in mind that twenty-five percent of our conventional prescription drugs are derived directly or indirectly from plants and these twenty-five percent of drugs furnish the template for ninety percent of modern synthetic drugs." Varro Tyler, Ph.D., Professor, Purdue University

Drugs Derived From Herbs

DRUG	HERB	USED FOR
Digitalis	Foxglove	Heart medicine
Aspirin	Willow Bark	Blood thinner/pain
Taxol	Pacific Yew	Ovarian cancer
Coumarol	Sweet Clover	Blood clots
Reserpine	Snakeroot	High blood pressure
Quinine	Cinchona Tree	Malaria
Vinblastine	Periwinkle	Leukemia
Hydrocortisone	Yam tubers	Inflammation/allergies
Morphine	Opium Poppy	Pain Reliever
Sudafed, Meth	Ephedra	Decongestant
Atropine	Belladonna	Pupil dilator/eye test
Menthol	Eucalyptus	Cough Medicine
Tubocurarine	Curare tree	Muscle relaxant

Scientists rearrange molecular structures of plants and isolate certain ingredients to manufacture a drug. Once they finalize their concoction, they can put a patent on it, so others can't copy it and sell it for a fortune. Why do they tear the plant apart? Because you can't put a patent on echinacea, ginseng or garlic growing wild in the woods. Isolate an ingredient and mix it with some other substances and *voilà*, we have a magic drug formula to be sold by a pharmacist for $609 a bottle, like Eliquis.

The ingredients in herbs are synergistically balanced to give the cells in your body nourishment. Man comes along and messes everything up by tearing the plant apart and isolating certain ingredients to make a drug. God put all those ingredients together in the plant for a reason. Just because millions of dollars haven't been spent to figure out why does not make a pharmaceutical employed chemist smarter than Mother Nature working under the direction of The Almighty. If they would leave the ingredients alone, just how nature created them in the first place, there wouldn't be adverse side effects. But then again, without the opportunity to make billions of dollars off patented drugs, there's no incentive to find what really works.

> "And God said, Behold, I have given you every herb bearing seed, which is upon the face of all the earth, and every tree, in which is the fruit of a tree yielding seed; to you it shall be for meat ... wherein there is life, I have given every green herb for meat." Genesis 1:29-30

It is estimated that less than 10 percent of some 300,000 plants have actually been researched. An herb is defined as a medicinal plant. Weeds are simply plants that we haven't found medicinal purposes for yet. Through a process called photosynthesis, plants (herbs) combine sunlight, carbon dioxide and water to release oxygen that we humans breathe. So, the next time you hear someone say, "I don't believe in herbs," tell them to stop breathing because they are using the oxygen produced by herbs.

The only difference between chlorophyll (the green lifeblood of the plant) and human blood (hemoglobin, the protein of red blood cells) is one molecule. The metallic atom in a molecule of human blood is iron, while that of chlorophyll is magnesium. We humans have more in common with herbs and plants than most realize.

Mother Nature's Intelligence

> **"Man does not weave this web of life. He is merely a strand of it. Whatever he does to the web, he does to himself."** Chief Seattle

Nature baffles the mind of man with sacred geometry, also referred to as the blueprint for all creation. If you look, you can see it everywhere. Bees create perfectly hexagonal cells to store their honey. A spider's web is a highly organized geometry that optimizes their function. Plants follow the Fibonacci sequence by placing each leaf along the stem in a geometrical pattern, maximizing the access to sunlight and rain. Trillions of snowflakes are all perfectly symmetrical, following hexagonal geometry. The Greek philosopher Pythagoras taught that sacred geometry was the basis of all forms of matter. The Greeks believed that sacred geometry was embodied in the energy patterns that create and unify all things in the universe.

The miracle of life surrounds us everywhere, yet we are indoctrinated to believe that somehow man's products are better than nature's for healing. Take an acorn the size of a thimble and in 50 years it grows into a massive 80-foot-tall oak tree. What is in that little seed that has the potential to evolve into something that massive? Can a scientist duplicate that? That seed possesses the secret to life. It also contains the secret to healing. It is the secret "unseen" universe that man has only yet to begin to scratch the surface.

Inside every seed is life-force intelligence. It knows what to do when it comes in contact with dirt and water. Intelligence directs it which way to send its roots and which way to push to get sunlight. Plants know how to lay dormant in the long, cold winter months and magically come back to life in springtime. How do they do all that? They just know. God created them with intelligence. If the intelligence contained in seeds and plants have enough knowledge to do all this, then does it not make sense that when we eat these living foods and herbs, we are providing our bodies with a tremendous amount of powerful intelligent wisdom? Even more miraculously, these herbs know how to heal when they go into your body. They know how to attack cancer cells while leaving healthy cells alone. Only a fool would argue against the fact that one little apple seed, if planted in dirt, will grow into a massive tree that will produce thousands of delicious apples every year.

The apple tree is intelligent. No programming is necessary. It just produces naturally. That intelligence is what provides your body with the tools necessary to heal disease.

When scientists take their limited knowledge and put that into man-made synthetic drugs, and then put those drugs into the human body and hope they don't react adversely with the billions of other cellular activities occurring, that is risky. Why would you choose man's synthetic drug concoctions with toxic side effects when you could have living intelligence in the form of herbs go into your body and do what they know how to do? The intelligence they were created with from the beginning of time was created for healing purposes. Are we evolving or regressing? Mother Nature's pharmacy is packed with intelligence from on high. Man's chemical drugs have no life force or intelligence, but plenty of adverse side effects, enough to kill 250,000 Americans each year. You choose.

A SHORT HISTORY OF MEDICINE
2000 BC   Here, eat this root.
AD 1000   That root is heathen. Here, say this prayer.
AD 1850   That prayer is superstition. Here, drink this potion.
AD 1940   That potion is snake oil. Here, swallow this pill.
AD 1985   That pill is ineffective. Here, take this antibiotic.
AD 2019   That antibiotic is artificial. Here, eat this root!
                                                                Anonymous

---

"Perhaps in time the so-called Dark Ages will be thought of as including our own." George C. Lichtenberg

Is It God's Will Or Are You Justifying Eating Junk Foods?

Some people, who have the best of intentions, walk around giving God all of the responsibility for their lives. They proclaim, "If it's God's will, then I will die of cancer." Is it God's will that you ate three doughnuts packed with inflammatory gluten and sugar, fried in grease for breakfast, two cancer-causing sodium nitrate-packed hot dogs made of leftover scraps in a slaughterhouse for lunch and a preservative-packed TV dinner radiated in your microwave for supper with a neurotoxic-aspartame-containing diet cola? You reap what you sow. God has given you free agency. You are free to do what you choose. If you drink a bottle of fingernail polish remover and die, I sure hope your family isn't naive enough to stand around mourning your death in the cemetery saying, "It was God's will that she died." Whatever you eat and drink has consequences. Everything you put in your mouth either feeds cancer or helps eradicate it. Be responsible for what goes in your mouth. We reap what we sow.

> **"When diet is wrong, medicine is of no use. When diet is correct, medicine is of no need."** Ayurvedic Proverb

Case Study

Since the time I was about 13, I have been plagued with migraines. As I got older, not only did the migraines worsen in severity but also frequency. I would sometimes get them three to six times a month, and they would last anywhere from one day to four days, not including the 24-hour recovery time needed to get all the drugs out of my system.

I tried every migraine drug I could get my hands on and when all else failed I was prescribed strong painkillers. About three times a year I was taken to the ER or my doctor's office for a shot because nothing would take the pain away. I was terrified of becoming addicted to painkillers, but even more terrified of the horrendous pain of the migraines that disabled me. I remember so many times that the pain was so excruciating that I would crawl to the bathroom, lay my head on the toilet to throw up and just lay on the floor with my hands clutching my head sobbing in pain.

I felt as though every time I got a migraine, I lost a part of my life that I could not get back. It seemed as though I revolved around my pain. Most days, I woke up in pain from a "normal" headache, afraid that this would turn into a migraine. After a change in my typical pattern of migraines I was sent once again for a MRI/MRA. This time an abnormality showed up which sent me once again to a neurologist. The abnormality turned out to be scarring in the brain matter, similar to people who have MS or who have had a stroke. I was put on several different types of medicine, the last being a nerve medicine used to treat shingles.

I finally had enough of all the doctor's appointments, the therapy, and especially all the medicine. At this point, I was on nine various types of medications and began to wonder if I had a serious medical problem. All the treatments had failed.

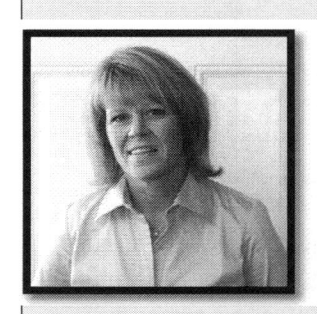

In July 2007, I got serious and started flying from Michigan to Alabama to see Dr. Sainsbury every eight to 10 weeks. He did an EDS exam and found many imbalances in my body causing the migraines. He found allergies and I was given remedies to desensitize them. Chemical poisoning showed up causing an imbalance in my liver. My pituitary gland was way out of balance as well. He put me on nutritional support and detoxification formulas and I began to improve.

> *I have now been three months without a headache or migraine. I am invigorated when I wake up every morning, without even a trace of pain. I am now down to only two prescriptions on a regular basis instead of nine. It is wonderful that I no longer need painkillers, migraine medicine or anti-depressants. This experience has been a life-altering event for me!*
>
> *Annette Morgan*
> *Clinton Township, Michigan*

"There is no such thing as an incurable disease, only incurable people." Dr. John R. Christopher

A Headache Healed

A throbbing, nonstop headache has suddenly come upon 22-year-old Lauren, a first-year teacher who, until now, has had nearly perfect health her whole life. But for six days, she has been bogged down with a nagging, relentless headache. The pain in her head is unbearable. She goes in to see her medical doctor and explains the pain that she is having. In less than 2 minutes, he sends her out the door with three prescriptions, two painkillers and one for sinus congestion, despite her not having any congestion. When she questions him, he says it's just in case there is some congestion triggering the headache. No testing of any kind is performed to determine the cause of the headache. And he does not ask about her bowel movements. He merely guesses which drug to give her.

"When doctors learn to do more educating, they will be able to do less medicating." Bernard Jensen D.C., Ph.D., N.D.

Skeptical about taking these drugs, she calls our clinic and makes an appointment to get a second opinion. We perform an EDS test that is noninvasive and painless. Within 15 minutes of testing, the root cause of the headache is found. No, it's not a deficiency of acetaminophen, antibiotics or any other man-made substance. Her gallbladder, uterus and adenoids do not need to be taken out and thrown in the trash, nor does she need some other radical surgical procedure as if to say, "Sorry God, but the human body really doesn't need all those things you put in there so I'm going to fix what you didn't get right." The culprit for Lauren's headache is a simple magnesium deficiency along with some low amino acid levels. For a $20 bottle of magnesium and potassium, the nagging headache is completely gone by the next morning. The prescriptions were never taken, and Lauren is back to feeling good again, headache-free. Problem solved, through simple, cost-effective, natural medicine. No drugs or painkillers were ever needed, and no adverse side effects were experienced. And best of all, no vicious cycle of drugs was ever started to leach vital nutrients out of her already deficient body. This is basic naturopathy 101.

> **"There is a true glory, the glory of duty done."** General Robert E. Lee

If Americans started demanding that their doctors look for the cause of the symptoms and stop administering poisonous drugs, then we might start making some progress with cancer and other supposedly incurable diseases. How are you going to cure a disease if you don't find the cause? It's time for change. It's time to heal our poisoned-medicine, disease-maintenance system. It's time to start finding the cause of dis-ease and then give the body what it needs to heal, with non-toxic remedies. This is called health care.

> **"Remember, it is pure food, simply and appetizingly prepared, and not drugs that bring back the glow of health to the cheek, and maintains maximum health in those who are well."** Hans Anderson, Author of *The New Food Therapy*

Remodeling Your House

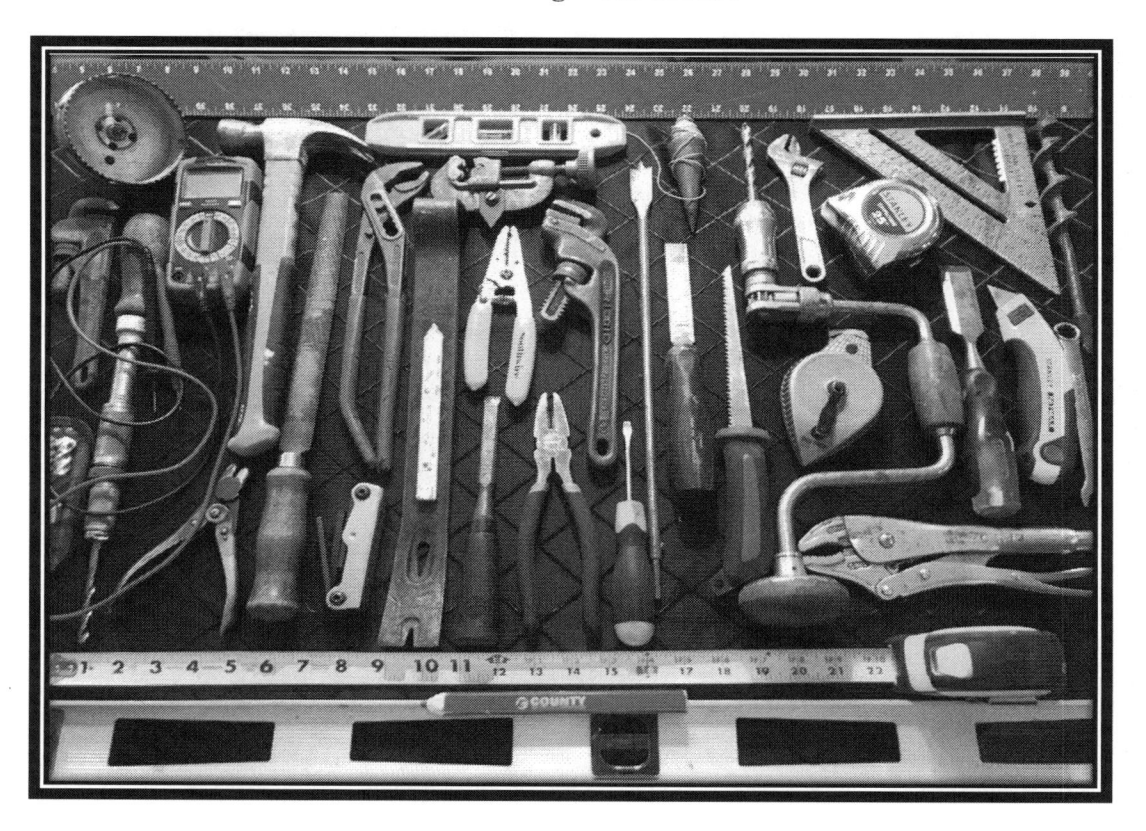

> **Cellular Health Tools**
> - 60 Minerals
> - 16 Vitamins
> - 12 Essential Amino Acids
> - 3 Essential Fatty Acids

Remodeling a house requires the correct tools. Just as a carpenter needs a good hammer, level, saw, chalk line and tape measure to build or remodel a house, so do the cells of your body. What are the tools your cells need? Good wholesome nutrition is foundational. Most organic, raw living foods grown in healthy soils contain all 60 minerals, 16 vitamins, 12 essential amino acids and three essential fatty acids. Of course, our foods today don't always contain these nutrients, because the soils are depleted of minerals from our farming methods. This is why it is wise to supplement our diet with a vitamin/mineral formula, preferably plant-derived. Liquid seems to be more easily absorbed in the body.

DNA & Your Divine Intelligence

> **"Intelligence makes the difference between a house designed by an architect and a pile of bricks."** Deepak Chopra, M.D.

One drop of blood, so small you can't see it with the naked eye, contains the entire genetic code of a human being. The most revolutionary discovery about the human body during the latter half of this century is DNA (deoxyribonucleic acid). Half of the DNA comes from the sperm of the father and half from the egg of the mother. Once the egg and sperm share their inheritance, the DNA chemical ladder splits down the center of every gene such as the teeth of a zipper pulled apart. DNA re-forms itself each time the cell divides: 2, 4, 8, 16, 32 cells, each with the identical DNA. Along the way cells specialize, but each carries the entire instruction book of 100,000 genes. A nerve cell may operate according to instructions from volume 4 and a kidney cell from volume 372, but both carry the whole compendium. It provides each cell's sealed credential of membership in the body. Every cell possesses a genetic code so complete that the entire body could be reassembled from information in any one of the 100 trillion cells of the body. Scientists have identified at least six billion steps of DNA in a single cell. The DNA is so narrow and compacted that all the genes in an entire body's cells would fit into an ice cube, yet if the DNA were unwound and joined together end-to-end, the strand would stretch from the earth to the sun and back more than 400 times. That's 74 billion, 320 million miles! Trying to understand the complexity and intricate precision of a single cell is humbling to the intellect, to say the least.

According to Dr. Carl Sagan, if all the information contained in the DNA of one cell could be written down in book form, it would take a huge library to hold the complete set. There would be about 4,000 books the size of the Bible to hold this information. The DNA in each cell is so complex and precise that it can be compared to the entire universe. And even more amazing is that every year, almost every cell in your body dies and is replaced with a new one. So, in a year, you basically have a brand-new body. The reality is, no doctor or scientist can even begin to understand how intelligent the human body is and the capabilities it possesses to heal from disease, when given correct nutrition and detoxification support. Your body is divine. It continues to baffle the greatest minds in the world. You are, whether you believe it or understand it, intelligent design. The dilemma is, most people don't believe it. They can't even fathom it.

> **"I have said, Ye are gods; and all of you are children of the most High."** Psalms 82:6

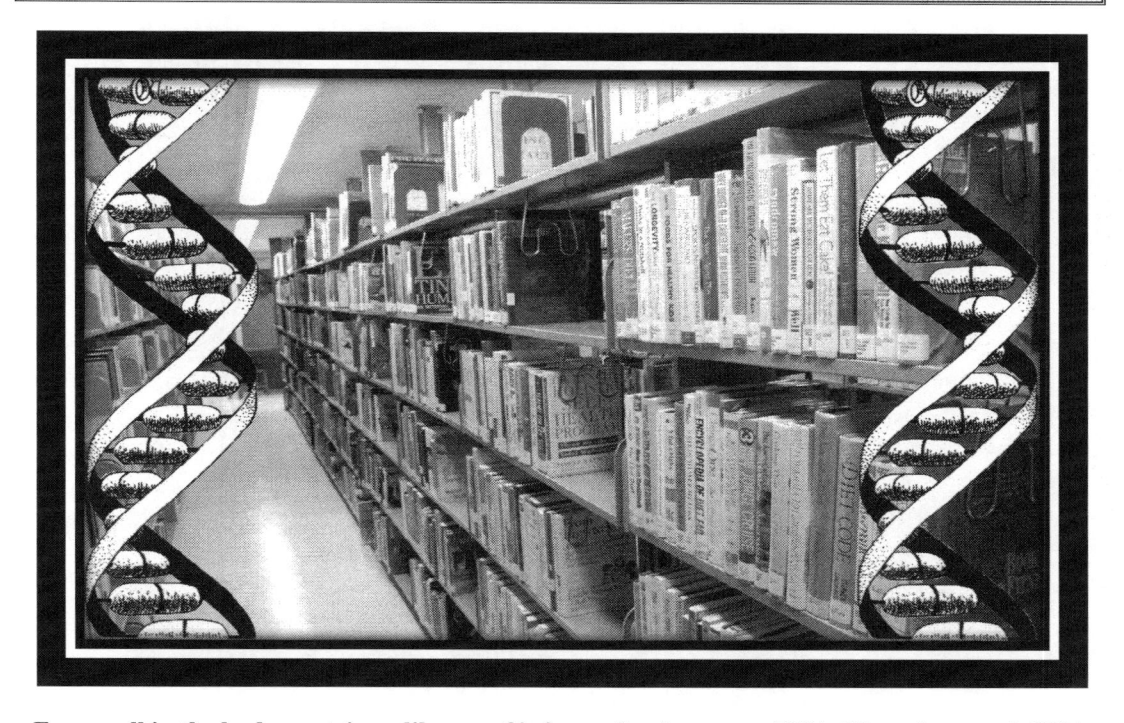

Every cell in the body contains a library of information known as DNA. There is enough DNA in each cell to produce a whole new you.

> **"Each patient carries his own doctor inside him. We are at our best when we give the doctor who resides within a chance to go to work."** Albert Schweitzer, M.D., Nobel Laureate, 1940

Chapter 5
MEDICAL MYTHS EXPOSED

Your Gallbladder — Crucial For Healthy Digestion

Most Americans go to their medical doctor for routine checkups. Doctors check their blood pressure, cholesterol, blood sugar, etc., and then send you home with a prescription if any of those numbers don't fit into their "normal" box. Then one day you have some indigestion, nausea and pain. It gets worse, so you go back to your doctor. They begin running tests and sure enough, it's a sluggish gallbladder filled with stones and possibly infection. "We need to do surgery and remove it as soon as possible," the doctor informs. Why didn't the doctor check the gallbladder last time you were in for your checkup? The answer is obvious. Doctors don't check the gallbladder or appendix when you are feeling well. They wait until something breaks or malfunctions and then the only thing left for them to do is antibiotics and surgery. True health care involves practicing what Thomas Edison taught, *"An ounce of prevention is worth a pound of cure."*

When a person comes into our clinic with a headache, chronic fatigue, overweight or arthritis … it doesn't matter what symptoms they have, we are going to check the gallbladder and every other organ, gland and system to see what needs support. By correcting imbalances in the body before they turn into full-blown problems that require surgery, we can eliminate problems BEFORE they happen.

Case Study

For many years I have had problems with heartburn and indigestion. I had to take antacids after every meal or I would be completely miserable. I thought this was just the way it was for some people.

One day at work I really started having problems with heartburn. It got so bad that I couldn't stand up straight for an extended period of time. I had sharp pains between my shoulder blades and in my chest. I went into the medical clinic at work and they thought that I was having a heart attack. The doctor wanted me to go to the emergency room immediately. I didn't feel like that was what I needed to do. Instead, I called and made an appointment with Dr. Sainsbury.

Dr. Sainsbury did an EDS scan on me to determine the cause of my symptoms. No energetic disturbances were detected with my heart and circulation. But when he checked my gallbladder it was very high and my stomach and small intestine points checked very sluggish on the computer. Dr. Sainsbury found the supplements that checked the best to flush out my liver and gallbladder. He also recommended digestive enzymes and hydrochloric acid to support my digestive system.

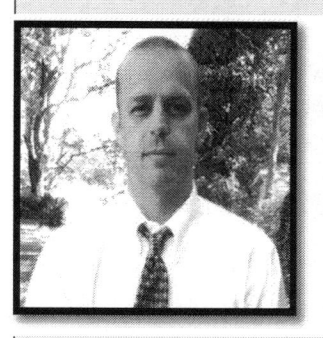

I started taking the products and by the next day I was feeling much better. As the days went by, I kept improving. It wasn't long before my heartburn and indigestion stopped altogether. I am now healthy and no longer experience heartburn and indigestion. The products gave my body the tools it needed to heal. Now I don't even have to take antacids after meals and I feel great. I know that if I would have gone to the hospital, they would have removed my gallbladder and that would have led to future health problems.

I have total confidence in Dr. Sainsbury and the way that he addresses the cause of symptoms by giving the body what it needs to heal. I take my wife and children to him whenever any of them have problems. I highly recommend Dr. Sainsbury and his natural healing programs for anyone who has health problems. I am the type of person who has to see or experience something in order to believe it. He made a believer out of me. I am convinced that natural healing works!

Joey Nelson
Rainbow City, Alabama

"The most serious potential danger associated with experimental orthodox medicine is that a patient may avoid or delay receipt of safe, natural healing care in a timely fashion leading to irreversible damage caused by toxic drugs, mutilating surgeries and medieval carcinogenic radiation." James Chappell, D.C., N.D., Ph.D.

Gallstones, most of the time, are caused by a deficiency of organic sodium in the body. Our high-protein diets, with lots of meats, heavy flour/gluten, fried foods, hydrogenated oils, sugar and processed foods cause us to be acidic. When the body becomes too acidic it uses its mineral reserves to buffer the acids, thus leaving us depleted of calcium, magnesium, sodium, potassium and iron. The key to preventing gallstones is to eat more alkaline foods such as fruits and vegetables containing organic sodium.

Table Salt Vs. Organic Sodium

Inorganic, commercially produced sodium chloride (table salt) comes from rock and is not completely soluble in water or the blood stream. Table salt is made

> **Pink Himalayan Salt Contains 80 Trace Elements & Is Water Soluble**

by taking sodium chloride and heating it to around 1200 degrees and then adding aluminum hydroxide and other anti-caking additives with it. When humans ingest it, it will adhere to the walls of the arteries, thus causing high blood pressure. Therefore, doctors tell you to restrict your salt intake. Yes, table salt may cause hypertension and edema. However, organic sodium found in celery, carrots and spinach is what your cells need to lower blood pressure, reduce water retention and promote overall general health. These vegetables have been balanced with sodium and potassium perfectly in nature to nourish your body. Other great sources of sodium include spirulina, watercress, Irish moss and dulse. The next best source of sodium after fruits, vegetables and herbs is Pink Himalayan Salt or Celtic Sea Salt in its natural, unaltered state, which contains over 80 trace elements and minerals and is soluble in water and OK for human consumption. However, keep in mind the best source of sodium comes from plants.

Sodium is responsible for making blood minerals soluble. This is why drinking carrot and celery juice can heal so many diseases. It balances the sodium levels, so the body can absorb calcium, magnesium and other bone-strengthening minerals. When these health-restoring minerals are supplied to the cells, diseases like arthritis and gout vanish, because the nutritional deficiencies that caused them have been removed.

Sodium helps neutralize acids in the body, thus alkalizing the cells. When we don't have enough sodium, joints will crack. Cracking joints tell us we have too much calcium and not enough sodium, which will eventually lead to calcium deposits in the joints, arthritis and possibly gout. Pregnant women with morning sickness usually need extra sodium.

Sodium Rich Foods	
Kelp	Okra
Irish moss	Carrots
Olives	Apples
Dulse	Beets
Figs	Plums
Swiss chard	Dates
Beet greens	Parsley
Celery	Asparagus
Kale	Cucumbers
Spinach	Radishes
Strawberries	Turnips
Bone Broth	Collard greens
Asparagus	Egg yolks
Cucumbers	Fish
Radishes	Lentils
Veal joint broth	Peppers
Raw goat milk	Spirulina
Watercress	Parsley
Powdered whey	Prunes
Sesame seeds	Raisins
Sunflower seeds	Apricots

Diuretics, or water pills, for edema (swelling) are dangerous because they pull fluid out of the body along with vital minerals. They are notorious for depleting the body of sodium and potassium, which triggers many health problems. This is why so many people who are on diuretics have muscle cramps, twitches, heart palpitations and joint problems. The diuretic drugs are depleting them of their vital minerals needed for health! It is interesting to note that in Japan, they consume a diet high in sodium with lots of miso soup, salted vegetables and fish, yet they have one of the longest life expectancy rates in the world.

> **"Organic sodium keeps calcium in solution in the human body. The type of salt the body needs is bio-organic sodium salts, which are formed in plants by the internal process of living cells**." Dr. Bernard Jensen

Gallbladders need to be cleaned and serviced periodically, or they can become sluggish, stop working, form stones and possibly get infected, especially if you are eating SAD (Standard American Diet). Many digestive disturbances, joint pains, headaches, sinus congestion and allergies are caused by liver and gallbladder issues. Microscopic parasites that are undetected on most doctors' diagnostic exams will often make the gallbladder their home, causing inflammation and possibly infection. Doing a simple gallbladder cleanse periodically can clear up annoying symptoms such as fatigue, hives and shoulder, upper arm, back and joint pain. If you experience burning pain between your shoulder blades, especially after eating fried or greasy foods, that is usually caused from a sluggish liver/gallbladder.

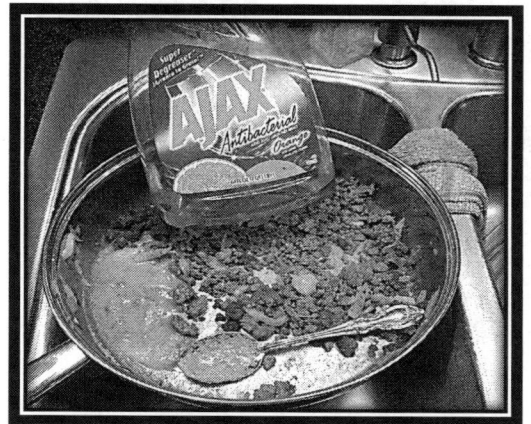

What good is a gallbladder anyway? Did God make a mistake when He created you with a gallbladder? Just because your doctor seems to think it's no big deal to cut it out and throw it in the trash does not necessarily mean that's what is best for you. Every day, your liver manufactures 1 to 1 ½ quarts of bile and then stores it in the gallbladder. When we eat, especially fatty foods, the gallbladder squeezes itself empty and the bile is used to help break down our fats and also lubricate the intestines for proper elimination. If you cook fatty hamburger meat tonight and let the pan sit on the stove and cool off, a thick, white layer of grease coats the pan. Dish detergent in hot water is required to cut the grease. Your gallbladder secretes bile, which is the dish detergent in your body to digest fats. By surgically removing the gallbladder, you throw away your dish detergent bottle. Now when you eat fats, the liver, which in most Americans is already overloaded with toxins, has an extra burden placed on it to secrete more bile, to emulsify fats. Without a gallbladder, and the ability to digest fats, you become much more susceptible to diabetes and heart attacks.

When the body fails to secrete enough bile (soap) to break down fats, then these undigested fats absorb into the bloodstream, causing inflammation. Inflammation in the head causes pressure on the capillaries, triggering migraines and headaches. A toxic liver/gallbladder is the No. 1 culprit we find that causes headaches. If these undigested fats accumulate in the sinuses, you will have congestion, and if they settle in the joints, you will have achy, arthritic pain. When they settle in the muscles, you will feel burning and discomfort. What is fibromyalgia? Your doctor will tell you inflammation, but what causes it? Undigested fats and proteins cause a lot of it. Proper digestive support can eliminate headaches, congestion, allergies and muscle and joint pains.

Liver/Gallbladder Support	
Lecithin	Choline
Dandelion	Inositol
Milk thistle	Betaine HCL
Artichoke	Lipase

Once you cleanse your liver/gallbladder and give it support, 90 percent of migraines and headaches no longer exist, because we have removed the nail from the tire that was causing the inflammation. People who drink a lot of pasteurized milk or eat a lot of cheese (dairy) many times will be stuffy all night long and wake up unable to breathe through their nose. There's your clue that you are not digesting your fats, and if you have dairy allergies, then it's a double whammy for mega-inflammation.

Gallstone/Kidney Stone Dissolver	
• Hydrangea	50 drops 3 times daily
• Stonebreaker Plus	50 drops 3 times daily
• E Plus	50 drops 3 times daily

We are seeing an overwhelming number of people having their gallbladders removed, then being diagnosed with diabetes because they are not breaking down their fats. Your doctor probably failed to inform you that by removing your gallbladder, you significantly increase your risk of diabetes. When undigested fats build up and begin coating your cells, and this interferes with insulin's ability to get sugar into the cells, you are diagnosed with diabetes. If not corrected, the fat build-up will accumulate in the arteries and may cause blockages and then — bingo, you have a heart attack. Once again, no one ever connects –the dots.

One of the best ways to avoid diabetes and heart disease is to keep your liver and gallbladder working properly. This requires a cleanse periodically so that it stays functioning in tip-top shape to break down fats in your body. Avoid eating artificial trans-fats and hydrogenated oils such as margarine, shortening, vegetable oil or corn oil that cause major damage and blockages in the body, leaving you susceptible to diabetes and heart disease.

Supporting your body's ability to break down fats includes digestive enzymes and possibly betaine and pepsin if needed. Certain herbs and essential fatty acids like flaxseeds, krill oil, fish oil and evening

Liver/Gallbladder Fat Digestion Support	
• Alpha Gest III	2 capsules with meals
• Beta Plus	2 capsules with meals

primrose oil are beneficial for fat metabolism and removing plaque from the arterial walls.

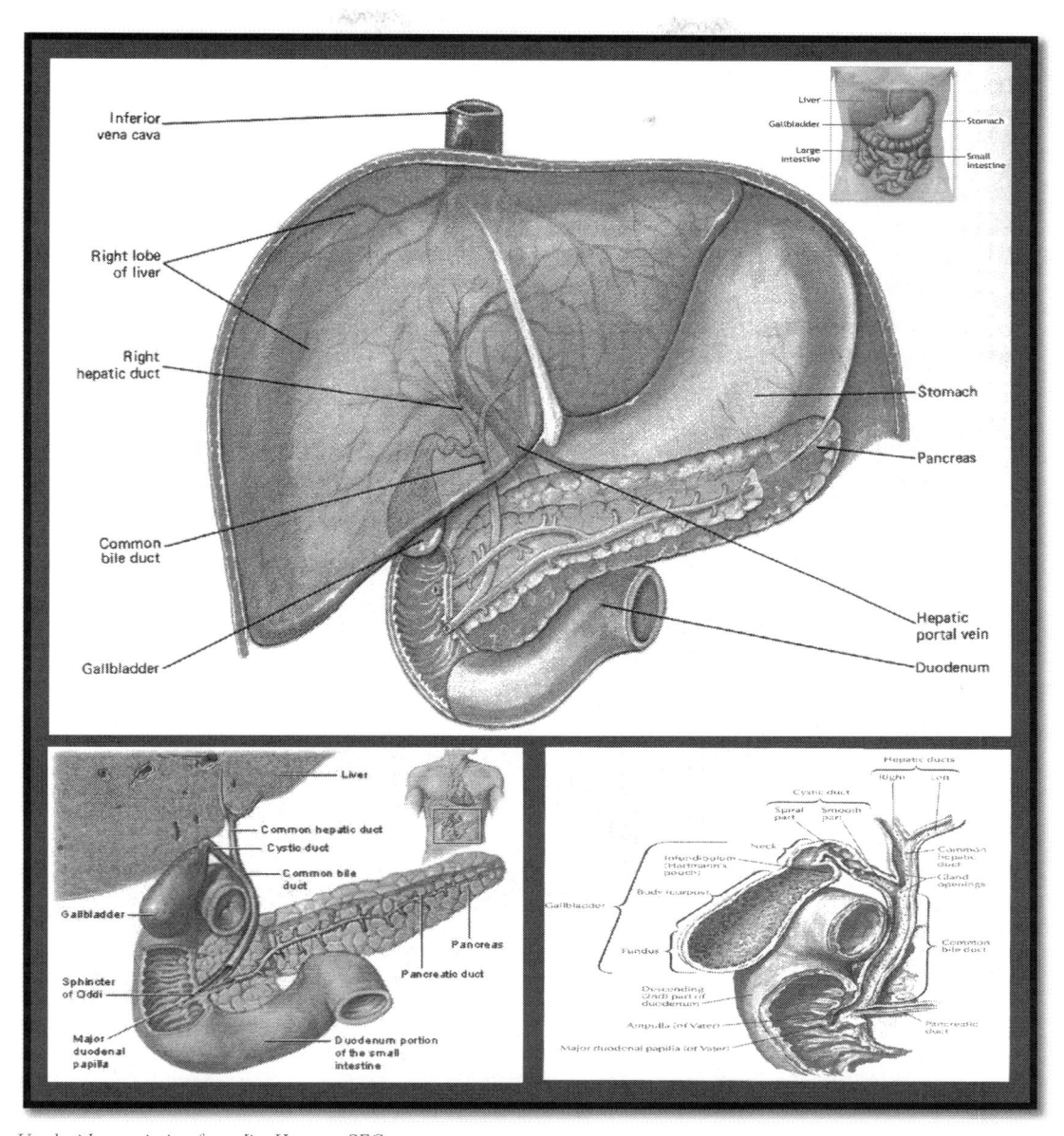

Used with permission from Jim Hawver, SEC

*The liver and the gallbladder play a crucial role in your health. Notice how the bile duct from the gallbladder goes directly to the small intestine. Bile is stored in the gallbladder and then secreted to break down fats.

"The yellow pigment in bile that causes the characteristic yellowing of jaundice sufferers may not be simply a body waste after all, scientists say. Bilirubin,

195

long thought to have no value, may be beneficial in thwarting cancer, aging, inflammation and other health problems, researchers from the Berkeley and San Francisco campuses of the University of California have found. The researchers say bilirubin appears to be a powerful antagonist of oxygen compounds that play a role in numerous diseases and conditions. Roland Stocker, the lead investigator in the study, said the results indicate scientists should examine other wastes from chemical processes in the body to see if they also have other functions. Reporting in the most recent issue of Science, Stocker and his associates said in test-tube studies, bilirubin acted much like anti-oxidants Vitamin C and E, neutralizing so-called oxygen radical compounds that destroy beneficial Vitamin A and linoleic acid, a common fatty acid that is a major component of cell membranes. 'Instead of spending 95 percent of our time developing means to get rid of bilirubin, we should spend time on possible beneficial roles of bilirubin,' Stocker said."
(Vancouver Sun, March 7, 1987)

> **"In my years of medical practice, I've seen a lot of surgery performed because surgeons believe that God blundered mightily when He created the human physique. You're supposed to regard it as providential that they're around to repair God's mistakes."** Robert Mendelsohn, M.D.

Liver/Gallbladder Flush For Stones
From Hulda Clark, Ph.D., N.D. "The Cure For All Diseases"

Ingredients:
4 tablespoons **Epsom salts**
Half cup **Olive oil** (light olive oil is easier to get down)
½ cup fresh (you squeeze yourself) pink **grapefruit juice**
4 to 8 **Ornithine capsules** (amino acids) for sleep. (Don't skip this or you may have the worst night of your life!)
Pint jar with lid
Black Walnut Hull tincture, (10 to 20 drops, to kill parasites coming from the liver.)

Choose a day like Saturday for the cleanse, since you will be able to rest the next day. Take no medicines, vitamins or pills that you can do without. They could prevent success. Eat a no-fat breakfast and lunch such as cooked cereal, fruit, fruit juice, bread and preserves or honey (no butter or milk), baked potato or other vegetables with salt only. This allows the bile to build up and develop pressure in the liver. Higher pressure pushes out more stones. Limit the amount you eat to the minimum you can get by on. You will get more stones. The earlier you stop eating the better your results will be, too. In fact, stopping fat and protein the night before gets even better results. Finish eating by noon with only sips later.

2 p.m. <u>Do not eat or drink after 2 o'clock</u>. If you break this rule you could feel quite ill later.

Get your Epsom salts ready. Mix 4 Tbsp. in 3 cups water and pour this into a safe jar. This makes four servings, ¾ cup each. Set the jar in the refrigerator to get ice cold (this is for convenience and taste only).

6 p.m. Drink one serving (¾ cup) of ice-cold Epsom salts. If you did not prepare this ahead of time, mix 1 Tbsp. in ¾ cup water now. You may add ⅛ tsp. You may rinse your mouth, but spit out the water.

Get the olive oil and grapefruit out to warm up.

8 p.m. Repeat by drinking another ¾ cup of Epsom salts. You haven't eaten since 2 o'clock, but you won't feel hungry. Get your bedtime chores done. The timing is critical for success.

9:45 p.m. Pour ½ cup (measured) olive oil into the pint jar. Squeeze the grapefruit by hand into the measuring cup. Remove pulp with fork. You should have at least ½ cup, more (up to ¾ cup) is best. You may top it off with lemonade. Add this to the olive oil. Also, add Black Walnut Hull tincture. If you haven't gotten stones out in the last few cleanses, add citric acid to bring success. Also, using ⅔ cup water for Epsom salts instead of ¾ can bring success. Close the jar tightly with the lid and shake hard until watery. (only fresh citrus juice does this).

Now visit the bathroom one or more times, even if it makes you late for your 10 o'clock drink. Don't be more than 15 minutes late. You will get fewer stones.

10 p.m. Drink the potion you have mixed. Take 4 Ornithine capsules with the first sips to make sure you will sleep through the night. Take eight if you already suffer from insomnia. Drinking through a large plastic straw helps it go down easier. You may use salad dressing, syrup, or straight sweetener to chase it down between sips. Take it to your bedside if you wish. Get it down within 5 minutes (15 minutes for very elderly or weak persons). If you had difficulty getting stones out in the past, add ½ tsp. citric acid to the potion. You may put it in capsules.

Lie down immediately. You might fail to get stones out if you don't. The sooner you lie down, the more stones you will get out. Be ready for bed ahead of time. Don't clean up the kitchen. As soon as the drink is down, walk to your bed and lie down flat on your back with your head up high on the pillow. Try to think about what is happening in the liver. Try to keep perfectly still for at least 20 minutes. You may feel a train of stones traveling along the bile ducts like marbles. There is no pain because the bile duct valves are open. (thank you Epsom salts!) **Go to sleep**. You may fail to get stones out if you don't.

Next Morning. Upon awakening, take your third dose of Epsom salts. If you have indigestion or nausea, wait until it is gone before drinking the Epsom salts. You may go back to bed. Don't take this potion before 6 a.m.

2 hours later. Take your fourth (the last) dose of Epsom salts. You may go back to bed again.

After 2 more hours you may eat. Start with fruit juice. You may add another ½ tsp. citric acid to it (or capsules) and get even more stones. Half an hour later, eat fruit. One hour later, you may eat regular food but keep it light. During the day, take the parasite-killing herbs. By supper you should feel recovered.

Alternative Schedule 1: Omit the first Epsom salts dose at 6 p.m. Take only one dose, waiting till 8 p.m. Change nothing else. Many people still get stones with one less dose. If you do not, do the full course next time.

Alternative Schedule 2: Add ½ tsp. citric acid to the oil-grapefruit mixture. Stir till dissolved. Next morning, add ½ tsp. citric acid again to the first fruit juice you drink when done with Epsom salts.

Alternative Schedule 3: For brain and spinal cord cancers, caffeic acid is the antigen to be avoided. This includes grapefruit. Blend whole apples instead, Red or Golden Delicious. Strain to get ½ cup juice. Add ½ tsp. citric acid to oil-juice mixture.

If you don't get stones …

*   Use slightly less than ¾ cup water for each Epsom salts dose.

CONGRATULATIONS! You have taken out your gallstones without surgery!

How well did you do? Expect diarrhea in the morning. This is desirable. Use a flashlight to look for the gallstones in the toilet with the bowel movement. Look for the green kind since this is proof that they are genuine gallstones, not food residue. Only bile from the liver is pea green. The bowel movement sinks but gallstones float because of the cholesterol inside. Count them all roughly, whether tan or green. You will need to total 2,000 stones before the liver is clean enough to rid you of allergies or bursitis or upper back pains permanently. The first cleanse may rid you of them for a few days, but as stones from the rear travel forward, they give you the same symptoms again. You may repeat cleanses at two-week intervals. Never cleanse when you are ill.

Sometimes the bile ducts are full of cholesterol crystals that did not form into round stones. They appear as "chaff" floating on top of the toilet bowl water. It may be tan colored, harboring millions of tiny white crystals. Cleansing this chaff is just as important as purging stones.

With gallstones, much less cholesterol leaves the body, and cholesterol levels may rise. Gallstones being porous can pick up all the bacteria, cysts, viruses and parasites that are passing through the liver. In this way "nests" of infection are formed, forever supplying the body with fresh bacteria. No stomach infection such as ulcers or intestinal bloating can be cured permanently without removing these gallstones from the liver.

Epsom salt is not the healthiest thing to put in the body but it sure does help in cleansing gallstones. For those who do not want to use the Epsom salts, there is another cleanse that takes a little longer, but is still effective.

> **"The laws of God and Nature are immutable: They cannot long be broken without retribution. Life in its fullness is Mother Nature obeyed."** Weston Price, D.D.S.

#2 Liver Flush Without Epsom Salts for Gallstones

For this flush, you will need 144 ounces of organic apple juice and 1 bottle of Alpha-Ortho-Phos. This flush is done during two days of fasting, so be prepared not to eat (this is best done over a weekend). For the first two days, drink six 12-ounce glasses of the apple juice each containing 50 drops of the Alpha-Ortho-Phos (this is to soften the stones). Make sure to spread the apple juice throughout the day so as to lessen the hunger and blood sugar drop.

On the third day upon arising, take 8 ounces of Extra Virgin olive oil and the juice of one lemon and mix together well. Drink the mixture and go back to bed, lying on the right side with the right knee pulled up to the chest. The olive oil forces the gallbladder to push the stones out. In two or three hours, you should pass the stones in a bowel movement. They will be greenish-blue in color. There could be very many pieces or one greenish-blue bowel movement. Once the movement has passed, you may resume your normal pattern of eating.

The Cholesterol Myth – Busted For Fraud

> **The diet hypothesis that suggests that a high intake of fat or cholesterol causes heart disease has been repeatedly shown to be wrong, and yet, for complicated reasons of pride, profit and prejudice, the hypothesis continues to be exploited by scientists, fundraising enterprise, food companies, and even governmental agencies. The public is being deceived by the greatest health scam of the century."** Dr. George Mann, Framingham Heart Study

Mediterranean cultures, Greece and Italy consume 40 percent of their calories from fat. Pacific Islanders, like Tokelau from New Zealand, along with Maasai warriors from Kenya eat a very high saturated fat diet, roughly 66 percent fat, and have some of the lowest rates of heart disease in the world. And Eskimos of Greenland consume a diet consisting of mostly seals, whales and cold-water fish that contain high levels of omega 3 fatty acids. Their diets are about 75 percent fat, yet they have a very low incidence of heart disease, diabetes, dementia and cancer. How can that be? We've been told to stay away from fats because they cause cardiovascular disease, right? Wrong! A high-fat diet does not cause high cholesterol and heart disease. It actually helps prevent it.

Mother's milk is the most perfect food on the planet for infants, and it is over 50 percent fat, and most of it is saturated fat! If cholesterol wasn't healthy for us, why would God make human breast milk with so much fat and cholesterol? Mother Nature puts all that fat in breast milk because cholesterol is healthy! Every cell in your body needs cholesterol. Commercial baby formulas are low in fat and cholesterol, thus failing to provide the proper nourishment to the developing brain, nervous system and hormones of the child. Mothers who choose not to breastfeed deprive their babies of the best nutrition in the world. Research shows that breastfed babies have a lower risk for obesity, type 2 diabetes and heart disease later on in life, despite having higher cholesterol levels.

Cholesterol has been blamed for heart disease, and it's time to expose the fraudulent scam perpetrated by the pharmaceutical giants for their greedy, billion-dollar profits. Why have we been lied to? So, 1 out of 4 Americans will take a statin drug, making the pharmaceutical companies about $29 billion a year. End of story. It has nothing to do with health and everything to do with money. Lipitor is the best-selling drug of all time. We have seen people with cholesterol counts over 600 who have no arteriosclerosis, no blockages, no high blood pressure and no heart disease. On the other hand, we see people with very low cholesterol counts of 100, after being on statin drugs, who have had heart attacks and required triple bypass surgery. Research published in 1996 found that 50 percent of heart attacks and 80 percent of patients with coronary artery disease have normal cholesterol levels.

> "There hasn't been a published study in the last 30 years that has unequivocally demonstrated that lowering serum cholesterol by eating a 'low-fat, low-cholesterol diet' prevents or reduces heart attack or death rate." Dr. Donald W. Miller, Cardiac Surgeon, Professor of Surgery, University of Washington

Your Body Needs Cholesterol For...

- Building & maintaining healthy cell membranes
- Healthy brain function – memory & serotonin (feel good) receptors
- Manufacturing sex hormones (testosterone, estrogen, progesterone & DHEA)
- Balancing hormones = emotional balance & neurotransmitters
- Libido (sex drive)
- Precursor for making steroid hormones (cortisol & aldosterone)
- Healthy neurons & nerve function, myelin sheath – insulation for conduction of nerve impulses
- Acts as an antioxidant & free radical scavenger
- It's the building block for all bodily tissue & protects against free radicals
- Healthy immune system – production of lymphocytes, T-cells, helper T-cells
- Improves cell signaling of T-cells & B-cells
- LDL inactivates many strains of bacteria (**It's a natural antibiotic**)
- Helps the liver produce bile acids for intestinal absorption of fats as well as fat-soluble Vitamins A, D, E, & K.
- Helps intestinal function, prevention of leaky gut & repairs damaged cells
- Helps mineral absorption, such as calcium
- Cholesterol is a precursor molecule for making Vitamin D
- Higher cholesterol contributes to longevity & overall good health

Why would you take a dictator drug to deprive your body of these benefits?

With so many people being diagnosed with cancer, we could all benefit from extra immune support, and professor David Jacobs and Dr. Carlos Iribarren have informed us that higher cholesterol levels have been shown to reduce vulnerability to infection, intestinal disease and respiratory disease. Dr. Meyer Texon, a pathologist at New York University Medical Center, explains that accusing saturated fat and cholesterol for hardening of the arteries is as foolish as accusing white blood cells of causing infection.

> "**Cholesterol is the most important molecule in the body, next to water. ...Lowering cholesterol causes your body to fall apart.**" Shane Ellison, M.S. – The People's Chemist

Cholesterol 150 Or Lower May Cause:	
Emotional Instability	Aggression
Hormonal Imbalance	Anxiety
Poor Memory	Suicide
Erectile Dysfunction	Depression

The moneymaking myth that high cholesterol is a major cause of heart disease and stroke has been strategically orchestrated by the pharmaceutical industry to sell their cholesterol-lowering drugs. A large study named PREDIMED published in the New England Journal of Medicine in 2013 showed that eating fat actually reduced the risk of heart attacks and deaths by 30 percent. (2013 Apr 4;368(14):1279-90) Back in the 1960s, cholesterol levels around 360 were considered normal. In order to sell statin drugs, "the normal" keeps getting lowered. Who do you think is responsible for that? Cholesterol levels lower than 160 are very dangerous. Oxford professor, Dr. David Horrobin teaches that cholesterol levels below 200 can cause emotional instability, aggression, violence and suicide. We have people come in the office complaining of brain fog, poor memory, low libido and muscle weakness. When I ask them if they are taking a statin drug, they surprisingly look at me as if I'm psychic and wonder how I knew. It's quite obvious when they have all the classic symptoms of cholesterol deficiency. Healthy and normal cholesterol levels hover in the 250 range.

> "Eating high-cholesterol foods has no impact on our actual cholesterol levels, and the alleged correlation between high cholesterol and high cardiac risk is an absolute fallacy." David Perlmutter, M.D.

Our bodies need cholesterol for health. Cholesterol is not the bad guy it is made out to be. The fact is, your cell membranes are 50 percent cholesterol. Cholesterol builds and maintains a healthy nervous system and brain. A strong immune system and your white blood cells require cholesterol to recognize and destroy invading germs and to go after cancer. Your sex hormones need cholesterol in order to be balanced. The reality is, without cholesterol we would die. It's a vital nutrient for health! Cholesterol is our friend and very much needed for optimum health.

> "Your brain is 60 percent fat, and much of it is made of omega-3 fats and cholesterol. When you eat a low-fat diet, you are starving your brain." Mark Hyman, M.D.

Cholesterol is used in our bodies to make hormones such as blood sugar-regulating hormones, stress hormones and sex hormones. Do you know people who get on cholesterol medication and lose their sex drive, gain weight, become depressed, experience hot flashes and have low energy? Hmm, could it be that the statin drugs are throwing vital hormones out of balance, causing serious health problems? Without enough cholesterol, our testosterone, estrogen and cortisone levels are in trouble. Cholesterol is necessary to make testosterone. Without testosterone, your sex life will peter out. How many men take statin drugs and then stand in their doctor's office asking for some Viagra? A study published in the Journal of Clinical Pharmacology and Therapeutics (21:89-94, 1996) reported that men taking statin drugs increased the frequency of sexual dysfunction by 50 percent. Oh, but don't worry, that same drug company will turn around and be glad to sell you a bottle of Viagra to perk things up since they caused it to fizzle out in the first place. How convenient: sell a drug to zap your sexual function and then another one to spring it back into action.

Low-Fat Diets May Cause...
▪ Depression
▪ Suicide
▪ ADD
▪ Autism
▪ Aggressive behavior
▪ Dementia
▪ Alzheimer's Disease
▪ ALS
▪ Stroke
▪ Neurodegenerative Diseases

> **"If you are taking a statin drug, there is no way you can have normal hormone balance."** Dr. Patrick Flynn

Cholesterol is a waxy fat that is attached to a protein for transport in the blood. Cholesterol is so important that your body manufactures it in the liver, if you're not getting enough from your diet. In fact, most cholesterol is manufactured in the liver and does not come from your diet. Researchers have shown that 80 percent of all cholesterol in the blood serum is produced by the body from foods that do not contain cholesterol. The difference between what is considered "good" cholesterol and "bad" cholesterol is the protein to which the cholesterol is attached.

Low Density Lipoproteins (LDL) is considered "bad cholesterol" (a term invented by the pharmaceutical companies to sell their drugs) because it is found as plaque in the arteries. If what we are told about high cholesterol causing heart attacks is true, then when people die from heart attacks, we would see elevated blood cholesterol levels, right? What story do autopsies tell? Half of all heart attacks and strokes occur in people without elevated cholesterol levels. (Ridker PM. Clinical Cardiology. 2003 April; 26(4 Suppl 3): III39-44)

LDL (Low Density Lipid) proteins manufactured in the liver transports cholesterol to a problem area in the body where there is a need for more cholesterol. It's used to heal a cut, make extra hormones or patch leaky blood vessels. LDL is the delivery truck driver to drop off supplies (cholesterol) to make repairs. After LDL has carried cholesterol to specific areas and made repairs, then HDL (High

Density Lipid), which is considered "good cholesterol" proteins, are the second delivery truck that picks up the remaining (supplies) cholesterol and takes it back to the factory we call the liver.

> **"First and foremost, cholesterol is a vital component of every cell membrane on earth. In other words, there is no life on earth that can live without cholesterol. That will automatically tell you that, in and of itself, it cannot be evil. In fact, it is one of our best friends. We would not be here without it. No wonder lowering cholesterol too much increases one's risk of dying. Cholesterol is also a precursor to all the steroid hormones. You cannot make estrogen, testosterone, cortisone, and a host of other vital hormones without cholesterol."** Ron Rosedale, M.D.

Let's suppose you were a crime scene investigator or the fire chief, and every time there was a fire, you were called to investigate what caused it. As you investigate, the only consistent item you saw, at every fire, were a bunch of firemen, so you conclude that fireman must be the cause for house fires. That would be absurd, wouldn't it? Just as fireman are there to put the fires out, cholesterol is utilized in your body to strengthen cell membranes and repair cracks in your arteries. Blaming heart disease and strokes on cholesterol is as ridiculous as blaming house fires on firefighters. The clever pharmaceutical companies have bamboozled most doctors into believing this hoax and in the meantime innocent people continue to "lose their minds" literally, and sexual function, from taking statin drugs, robbing them of the basic building blocks for healthy cell membranes, blood vessels, hormones, nerves and brain cells. It's one of the biggest scams ever perpetrated on the American people.

A statin drug works by disrupting the liver (the processing factory for nutrients). If you were to get rid of all your LDL, you would die. The idea that low cholesterol is good for health is as ridiculous as saying low engine oil improves motor function. Just as a motor will burn up with insufficient oil, so will your brain, nerves and hormones malfunction without adequate cholesterol.

> **"Cholesterol is one of the most important players in maintaining brain health and function."** David Perlmutter, M.D.

Your brain weighs 3 pounds and has 100,000 miles of blood vessels, and is the fattest organ in your body, at 60 percent fat. Your brain and nervous system require cholesterol to function optimally. Statin drugs deprive your neurons and cell membranes of healthy cholesterol. It's been shown that in order to grow new synapses in the brain, cholesterol is vital. It helps latch cell membranes together so that signals can jump across the synapse. The myelin coating around neurons requires cholesterol to transmit messages. Without cholesterol, your brain and nervous system is like a house with all the fuses removed from the breaker box, preventing the electricity from flowing to lights, switches and outlets. Research has proven that when cholesterol levels are low, brain health suffers, and we are at a higher risk for developing dementia and other neurological disorders such as Alzheimer's and Parkinson's disease.

Could statin drugs be the reason we are seeing Alzheimer's disease escalating? The sixth-leading cause of death in this country is now Alzheimer's disease, killing 150,000 Americans each year. There has been an 89 percent increase in deaths due to Alzheimer's between 2000 and 2014. It is interesting that this terrible memory-destroying disease started skyrocketing about the same time doctors started prescribing statin drugs. Coincidence?

"If you deprive cholesterol from the brain, then you directly affect the machinery that triggers the release of neurotransmitters. Neurotransmitters affect the data-processing and memory functions. In other words, how smart you are and how well you remember things. If you try to lower the cholesterol by taking medication that is attacking the machinery of cholesterol synthesis in the liver, that medicine goes to the brain too. And then it reduces the synthesis of cholesterol, which is necessary in the brain. Our study shows there is a direct link between cholesterol and the neurotransmitter release, and we know exactly the molecular mechanics of what happens in the cells. Cholesterol changes the shape of the proteins to stimulate thinking and memory." Dr. Yeon-Kyun Shin, Professor of Biophysics, Iowa State

Dr. Stephanie Seneff, a senior research scientist at MIT, explains that low-fat diets and statins may be a major cause of Alzheimer's disease. She informs us that the brain suffers when taking statins because they handicap the liver's ability to make cholesterol, which inhibits the brain's ability to communicate between neurons and produce new brain cells. She also informs that they paralyze the cells' ability to make coenzyme Q10 (antioxidant and energy producer in the cells).

Vitamin D is directly formed from cholesterol. It acts more like a steroid in the body, decreasing inflammation and ridding the body of infections. So, with millions of people on statin drugs, naturally their vitamin D levels will be lowered, thus causing a lowered immune system and making them more susceptible to infections, including cancer. It's interesting to note that more than 200 studies link Vitamin D deficiency to cancer. Optimizing Vitamin D levels can reduce your risk of 16 different cancers, including breast cancer, by half. However, your doctor turns around and prescribes a statin drug that annihilates your Vitamin D levels. If we truly wanted to eliminate cancer, we would stop cutting our own throats by taking liver-damaging statin drugs that lower our cancer-fighting Vitamin D levels.

Is it possible that Big Pharma knows that by lowering millions of American's cholesterol levels with statin drugs, will inevitably lower Vitamin D levels and weaken the immune system, causing more cancer? More cancer patients allow them to maximize their profits off your ill health, caused from the drug that was supposed to make you healthy? Irony at its finest.

> "Why was $150 million spent on cholesterol research involving a drug whose negative effects outweigh the positive? And how did medical science ever get side-tracked with recommending avoidance of dietary cholesterol and saturated fat, a practice which fails to address the basic problem?" Stephen E. Langer, M.D.

CRESTOR (Rosuvastatin Calcium) According to data published by the Food and Drug Administration (FDA), Crestor® may be linked to kidney damage and a **painful muscle condition called rhabdomyolysis**, even in **doses as low as 10 mg. and in people under 50.**

Rhabdomyolysis is a painful condition where muscle tissue is released in the bloodstream and **in severe cases, can lead to kidney failure and death**. Patients with **rhabdomyolysis** typically experience pain in the calf muscles and lower back.

Dr. Eckhard Alt, director of cardiovascular research at Tulane Heart and Vascular Institute, reports that their research has shown that statin drugs prematurely age stem cells, which explains the notorious side effects such as memory loss, muscle problems and increased risk of diabetes. They also discovered that statins prevent stem cells from becoming macrophages, which is necessary to help fight inflammation, generate new bone and cartilage, and prevent osteoarthritis. Dr. Reza Izadpanah, a stem cell biologist, informs, "Our studies show statins may speed up the aging process ... people who use statins as preventative medicine for health should think again, as our research shows they may have general unwanted effects on the body which could include muscle pain, nerve problems and joint problems."

Every burn unit in hospitals throughout the world knows that the fastest way to help patients heal is to feed them lots of eggs (up to 20 hard-boiled a day) because it is the fastest way to speed up the healing process and help rebuild damaged cells. Cholesterol is a healer! We would be wise to embrace it, rather than shunning it like an evil plague.

> "Eating saturated fat does not cause heart disease. There is no consistent evidence that saturated fat in our diet from meat raises our blood cholesterol. In fact, there is plenty of evidence that eating meat actually improves our cholesterol profile when consumed in the absence of sugar and refined carbs." Mark Hyman, M.D.

Dr. Edward Athrens of Rockefeller University has conducted cholesterol research for over 40 years. He does not believe that lowering cholesterol levels reduces heart disease and informs that the low-cholesterol hype is unscientific and foolishness.

Cholesterol is necessary for sperm to join with an egg and to create a new life. When this intelligent life process occurs, they bring along their own supply of cholesterol. When a woman becomes pregnant, her blood serum level of cholesterol rises by about 50 percent in order to nourish the fetus's trillions of new developing cells. Dr. Barnes points out how ridiculous the high cholesterol myth is.

> **"If cholesterol were harmful to arteries, as so many have stated, the fetus would have a heart attack before the baby saw the light of day."** Broda Barnes, M.D.

Cell membranes, myelin sheath and the brain all need cholesterol in order to be healthy. Without cholesterol, your nerve cells cannot transmit signals. NASA astronaut and flight surgeon Dr. Duane Graveline reports that he lost his memory after six weeks of being on Lipitor. He is the author of *Lipitor – Thief of Memory* and explains how after taking Lipitor he could not recognize his wife and house for six hours at a time. After experiencing his own disaster from a statin drug, he did some research, uncovered a rat's nest and wrote a book warning of this giant fraud. If every medical doctor in this country would read his book and stop listening to the pharmaceutical reps, statin drugs would no longer be prescribed, but unfortunately, the golf course is more interesting than scientific research.

> **"And now we have evidence in the scientific literature to prove that when cholesterol levels are low, the brain simply doesn't work well; individuals with low cholesterol are at much greater risk for dementia and other neurological problems. We need to change our attitudes about cholesterol and even LDL; they are our friends, not foes."** David Perlmutter, M.D.

Statin Drug Side Effects

Memory loss	Neuropathy (nerve damage in hands/feet)
Dizziness	Suppressed immune function
Weakness	Muscle aches & pains
Anemia	Dysfunction of the pancreas
Acidosis	Hormonal imbalances
Cataracts	Elevated liver enzymes
Cancer	Emotional instability (depression, suicide)
Depression	Rhabdomyolysis (muscle degeneration)
Lowers CoQ10	Decreased ketone production in liver
Diabetes	Sexual (erectile) dysfunction

Dr. Beatrice Golomb from the University of California reiterates how notorious the statin drugs are for causing memory loss. She reports, *"We have people who have lost thinking ability so rapidly that within the course of a couple of months, they went from being head of major divisions of companies to not being able to balance a checkbook and being fired from their company."* Get your cholesterol where your doctor wants it and lose your job in the process, because your brain is lacking vital cholesterol needed to function. It's time to wake up. Your doctor's drugs are backfiring on you! Learn the facts before you swallow poison, because your doctor told you it's medicine. It's time to heal the poisoned medical system. Just say no to drugs.

Statin drugs disrupt the process in the liver by which the body makes cholesterol, which may cause inflammation in the liver and the breakdown of muscle tissue. Do you know why? Because they are poisonous! Why else would your liver swell and muscles deteriorate? This is why doctors check for elevated liver enzymes. It's a side effect. Stop taking medication that damages your liver, because once your liver fails, you die.

Our immune system needs cholesterol in order to have healthy lymphocytes and T-cells to fight infection. Cholesterol also helps the liver produce bile acids, which help break down fats so toxins can be eliminated. Most likely, your doctor never mentioned any of this to you, did he? Of course not, because Pfizer has promised him a candy bar if he's a really good boy. Doctors are wined and dined and treated like royalty by pharmaceutical reps to prescribe their drugs. They may not get a kickback anymore, with the exception of cancer drugs; however, an all-expense weeks' vacation to a 5-star resort in Mexico is a persuasive incentive.

Paved roadways break down and deteriorate with heavy traffic over time, and so do the blood vessels in the body. Many factors such as free radicals, trans fats, heavy metals, chemicals and viruses cause irritation and inflammation, which weakens the vessels and can cause leakage. Just as road crews repair and seal cracks in the roads with hot tar, so does the body repair cracks and damaged blood vessels with cholesterol in your 70,000 miles of blood vessels.

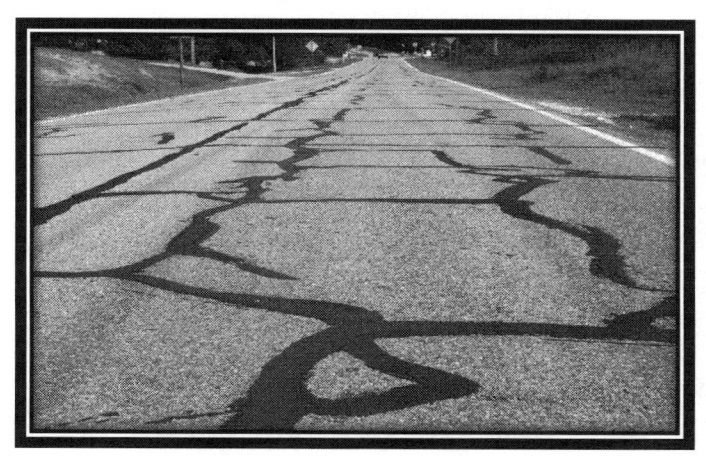

Cholesterol repairs damaged cells, and as we age, the body requires more repairs, so cholesterol production increases. Dr. Harlan Krumholz from the cardiovascular department at Yale University reported in 1994 that older people with higher cholesterol levels died half as often from heart attacks as did those with lower cholesterol levels. And The Framingham Heart Study states that having a total cholesterol lower than 180 actually triples your chances of suffering from a stroke.

Researchers Walsh and Grady from the University of California proclaim that there is NO EVIDENCE from primary prevention trials to prove that lowering cholesterol levels with the use of statin drugs decreases mortality rates from heart disease. (JAMA 1995 Oct 274:1152-1158)

Cholesterol will only attach itself to the artery when the artery is damaged, just like putting a patch on a tire that has a nail hole in it. It's your body's innate way of healing, without you ever being aware of it. If your arteries are healthy, then cholesterol goes right through you without any problems, but when there is a crack, cholesterol is used to patch it.

> **"The American public can no longer blindly trust that its vaunted medical journals and world-class medical experts put the interests of patients first."** John Abramson, M.D.

Another myth-shattering study was published in JAMA in 1987, "Cholesterol and Mortality: 30 Years of Follow-up from the Framingham Study." This study is not well liked by the drug companies because it shows that after the age of 50, there is no increased death rate with elevated cholesterol levels. Even more shocking is the fact that when cholesterol levels did begin dropping lower, then the death rates increased by 14 percent for every 1 mg/dL drop in total cholesterol every year! Basically, this study reveals that when we lower our cholesterol with statin drugs, we die sooner. (JAMA 1987 Apr 24; 257(16):2176-80) Why aren't doctors reading the research published in their own journals?

The European Heart Journal reports a study done with 11,500 patients. Behar and associates discovered that people with cholesterol lower than 160 mg/dL increased their risk of death by 2.27 times higher than those with higher cholesterol. The risk of heart attack was the same in both groups. The report also revealed that people with lower cholesterol increased their risk of cancer.

Would anyone in his right mind trade high cholesterol that isn't even proven to decrease heart disease for cancer? JAMA published a shocking report by Thomas B. Newman, M.D., MPH, that revealed how cholesterol drugs increase your risk for cancer. Rodents that were given cholesterol-lowering drugs (fibrates and statins) developed cancer. (Carcinogenicity of Lipid-Lowering Drugs." JAMA Jan 3, 1996- Vol 275, No. 1.) We have enough problems with all the toxic chemicals in our environment that cause cancer. We certainly don't need to be taking a drug that causes it.

> **"Good brain function depends on saturated fats. In fact, most of your brain is made up of saturated fats and omega-3 fats."** Mark Hyman, M.D.

The Journal of Cardiac Failure published a study for those who have suffered with heart failure. The conclusion after analyzing 1,134 patients is, **"Low** serum total cholesterol is associated with marked increase in mortality in advanced heart failure." In other words, by lowering your cholesterol, you are at higher risk for having a heart attack and dying. This is exactly the opposite of what doctors are telling their patients!

Scientists in Israel examined close to 300 people diagnosed with heart failure for an average of 3.7 years. Those who were on statin drugs with the lowest levels of LDL were found to have the highest death rate. Interestingly enough, those with higher levels of cholesterol had a lower risk of death. Are we still on the golf course?

> **"Conventional medicine is limited to treating the symptoms of secondary risk factors. Drugs blocking the synthesis of cholesterol and other lipid-lowering agents are now being prescribed to millions of people. These drugs are known to cause cancer and have other severe side effects. You should avoid them whenever you can."** Matthias Rath, M.D.

What happens when a medical doctor begins researching "the research?" He begins to untangle a web of lies that have been deliberately told in order for the pharmaceutical industry to sell more drugs. John Abramson, M.D., instructor at Harvard Medical School, exposes enough corruption in what is called "medical science" to make you think twice before you trust your doctor's next prescription. The financial links between FDA officials and drug companies explains how and why dangerous killer drugs are allowed on the market and are prescribed in the USA when they haven't been proven safe or more effective than placebos. For those who want to see how corrupt our medical system has become, read his book, *Overdosed America The Broken Promise Of American Medicine* – HOW THE PHARMACEUTICAL COMPANIES ARE CORRUPTING SCIENCE, MISLEADING DOCTORS, AND THREATENING YOUR HEALTH.

> **"There are multiple layers of people engaged in a conspiracy of not telling the truth."** Dr. Mary G. Enig, Biochemist, University of Maryland

Healthy Cholesterol Support
- Chola Plus   2 capsules with meals
- Omega Complete 2 capsules with meals
- Beta Plus   2 capsules with meals

After seeing how corrupt pharmaceutical companies are with their outright lies in order to sell more drugs, Roni Rabin from Newsday.com writes, "We've been bamboozled about cholesterol risks." How many drugs have you taken or are you taking right now that have been lied about? As we look back at how foolish we were for taking the killer drug Vioxx that caused thousands to die of heart attacks, the time will come, in the near future, when our children and grandchildren will look back at this generation of foolishness knowing that people actually took statin drugs to lower cholesterol. Any serious researcher knows that the true culprit of heart disease is inflammation, caused mainly by sugar consumption and oxidative stress, not cholesterol.

How To Balance Cholesterol Levels
• Avoid trans-fats (hydrogenated oils)
• Avoid deep-fried foods
• Avoid milk (homogenized & pasteurized)
• Avoid eating grains and sugary foods
• Cook with ghee, coconut oil or butter
• Eat avocados, eggs, olives, nuts & seeds
• Eat coconut oil, butter & olive oil
• Eat organic vegetables, fruits & berries
• Eat organic grass-fed meats in moderation
• Take fish oil or krill oil daily
• Exercise daily (30-minute walk is good)

For those who are obsessed with lowering cholesterol, research has proven that eating an organic, non-GMO red apple, carrots and beets every day can significantly help lower cholesterol. Taking CoQ10, garlic and omega 3 fatty acids like fish or krill oil are beneficial as well. If your cholesterol stays elevated even after supporting your liver, you may have parasites blocking the flow of bile in the ducts of the liver. A parasite cleanse can sometimes normalize cholesterol levels.

> "It is sugar, not fat, that is the big driver of heart disease (as well as stroke, obesity, type 2 diabetes, and dementia)." Mark Hyman, M.D.

Sugar, Grains & Carbs Cause Heart Attacks — Not Fat

Saturated fats and palmitic and stearic acid are manufactured in your liver and are found in your blood after consuming sugar and carbohydrates. These are the major contributors to heart disease. It is interesting to note that stearic and palmitic fats do not come from eating meats, only carbohydrates.

> "Animals don't get heart attacks, because — as opposed to humans — they produce their own Vitamin C in their own bodies. Heart attacks and strokes are not diseases but the consequences of chronic vitamin deficiency, and they are therefore preventable." Matthias Rath, M.D.

Eggs

Many researchers believe that eggs may quite possibly be the world's most perfect and complete food because they are packed with all the nutrients required to create new life. Stop throwing out the yolk, as it's the most nutritious part, containing choline, which supports a healthy brain and helps prevents Alzheimer's. Choline is also needed for women to get pregnant. Eggs are a great food to support healthy blood sugar levels as well. Studies have shown that people on a low-carb diet, while including lots of eggs in their diet, improved insulin sensitivity. When you eat an egg, you are getting all of the essential amino acids, vitamins, minerals, and a broad spectrum of antioxidants that give you anti-aging support and help protect you from free radical damage, especially in the eyes and brain.

As previously mentioned, there is no scientific research to prove that dietary fats of animal origin (saturated fats) elevate cholesterol in your blood or increase the risk for coronary heart disease. In fact, it's just the opposite. The cholesterol we eat actually reduces the body's production of serum cholesterol. Dr. Juliet Gray blew the whistle on the cholesterol myth when he published his research, "Eggs and Dietary Cholesterol — Dispelling the Myth." Remember, more than 80 percent of cholesterol in your blood (that shows up on your doctors' test) is produced in the liver regardless of what you eat.

Pasture-raised eggs with dark orange-yellow yolks are the healthiest. Avoid commercial raised eggs with pale yellow yolks. Also, don't cook them in hot oils which oxidize and become carcinogenic. Cooking eggs at low temperature and leaving the yolk runny is beneficial for retaining nutrients, and eating them raw in a smoothie is even better. Poached or soft-boiled is next best.

Deadly Hydrogenated Oils – The True Villains Of Heart Disease

So, what are the culprits that cause arteriosclerosis? Hydrogenated oils stand guilty. In 1911, Proctor & Gamble, with the help of German chemist Edwin Kayser, took liquid fats and made them solid with a prolonged shelf life. Their patented hydrogenated cottonseed oil, also known as Crisco, became the new fat for cooking and to be put in processed foods. This is what is known as trans-fat. Most of our processed foods contain this man-made, indigestible, artery-damaging trash. Start reading labels and you'll find them in baked and pre-packaged foods like breakfast pastries, salty snacks, desserts, fried foods, pastas and breads.

Unhealthy Foods Containing Trans Fats	
Microwave Popcorn	Beef Jerky
Breakfast Pastries	TV Dinners
Fried Foods	Frozen Pizza
Chicken Nuggets	Crisco
French Fries	Non-stick Spray
Peanut Butter (most)	Margarine
Cookies	Cake Frosting
Cakes	Coffee Creamer
Pies	Cold Cereals
Doughnuts	Crackers

Any food you have that lists hydrogenated oil, partially hydrogenated oil or the butter substitute margarine should be shunned like the plague. Most Americans consume liberal amounts of trans fats, and are slowly killing themselves by eating this health-destroying, fake food. Put a container of shortening outside and even flies won't go near it, because it's not food.

In 2013, the FDA finally ruled trans fats "not safe to eat." The dilemma is that foods can be labeled "free of trans fats" and still contain up to 0.5 grams of trans fat content. For example, Cool Whip claims on the label that it contains zero trans fats, but it is mostly made up of trans fats. Confusing? Yes, but since it's mostly air and has less than 0.5 grams per serving, it can claim "free of trans fats." Be careful when reading food labels. The food industry is very deceiving.

Another big artery-damaging terrorist we willingly invite into our bodies is homogenized and pasteurized dairy products. When dairy products are homogenized, they are sent through cylinders that beat the molecules up so badly that the cream will no longer float to the top of the milk. It's very convenient for people who don't want to mess around with cream, but now your body has to attempt to break down another man-made product instead of how nature produced it.

Causes Of Heart Disease
- Hydrogenated oils/Trans fats
- Sugar/High fructose corn syrup
- Grains – gluten in excess
- Cooking at high temperatures
- Smoking
- Heavy metal toxicity
- Calcium plaquing
- Alcohol in excess
- Lack of exercise
- Emotional stress

Pasteurization is the process of boiling milk and dairy products to kill bacteria. Put a few drops of formaldehyde in it and the grocery store can keep it on the shelf for many weeks longer before it spoils. By pasteurizing milk, we destroy all the enzymes and most of the vitamins, amino acids and calcium bioavailability. After man destroys what nature creates, we then force our bodies to deal with the nutrient-depleted, inflammation-causing substance. What's the result? Kidney stones, bone spurs, congestion, ear infections, mucus, colds and arthritis.

> **"INDISPUTABLE FACT: YOU DO NOT NEED DAIRY TO HAVE STRONG BONES AND TEETH."** Karen Urbanek, H.H.P.

It is interesting to note that osteoporosis is most common in the United States, England, Israel, Sweden, and Finland, where large quantities of dairy products and calcium supplements are consumed. On the other hand, osteoporosis is rare in Africa and Asia, where milk consumption is very low.

Humans are the only animals on the planet that continue drinking milk past childhood. All other animals are weaned off mother's milk shortly after birth, and they do not drink milk from other animals, but we humans do.

Store-bought milk does not do a body good. It causes a lot of illness. If you feel you must drink milk, then get it straight from the farmer in its whole, raw, natural form with the enzymes intact to help your body digest it. Goat's milk is superior to cow's milk, as it's easier for humans to digest. Blood type Bs usually do better than other blood types with more dairy in their diet. Almond or coconut milk is a good alternative to store-bought milk. Homemade kefir, fermented milk, is excellent because it provides beneficial bacteria (probiotics) and helps boost immunity.

Deadly Genetically Modified Organisms (GMOs)

Monsanto, the developer of Agent Orange, DDT, saccharin and aspartame, has expanded its enterprise of deadly chemicals to altering the seeds that grow the foods we eat. Genetically modified organisms are foods, plants or meats that have had their DNA artificially altered in a laboratory by genes from other plants, animals, viruses or bacteria to produce foreign compounds in that food. These gene-altered foods have been shown to cause cancer, damage sperm, cause infertility, cause abortions, trigger allergies and alter DNA. With Monsanto's global soybean monopoly, Americans consume 18 billion pounds of soybean oil each year. Most vegetable oils are made from genetically modified organisms (GMOs), including the popular Wesson vegetable oil that comes from GMO soybeans.

Roundup (Glyphosate) Causes:
- Cancer
- Birth Defects
- Spontaneous Abortions
- Skin Diseases
- Neurological Diseases
- Respiratory Disorders

Genetically engineered crops such as wheat, corn and soybeans are Roundup Ready, because they have been created so farmers can spray them and kill the weeds without harming their crops. That's great for farmers but not so great for the consumers of these foods because studies have shown that GMOs cause adverse health effects. Scientists have reported that now GMO Roundup Ready Soybeans produce formaldehyde, which depletes glutathione (a powerful antioxidant needed for detoxification in the body). These man-made genes found in these foods can be transferred to the bacteria in the gut after eating them. Do we really know what wheat GMO proteins are capable of doing inside the human body? I personally don't like to be a guinea pig in a science experiment.

Many countries, 64 of them, require GMO labeling, and all of Europe has banned GMOs. The Austrian government published a study in 2008 showing that the more GMO corn fed to mice, the fewer babies they had and the smaller the babies were. Baylor College of Medicine discovered that rats raised on GMO corncob bedding neither breed nor exhibit reproductive behavior.

According to research published in 2015 in Lancet Oncology along with 17 independent researchers around the world, Monsanto's herbicide Roundup has been linked to cancer. The World Health Organization has even declared that glyphosate (Roundup) is a "probable carcinogen" in humans; however, we still ingest it heavily in this country.

Glyphosate & Aluminum Detoxifiers
- Glycine
- Silica
- Chlorella
- Zeolite

The Appendix

The appendix, according to Dr. Mendelsohn, is regarded by most surgeons as another one of God's mistakes. He explains, *"I can't tell you the number of times I have heard a surgeon tell a woman that the appendix is 'a useless, vestigial organ – some of God's leftover physiological junk.'"*

It is worth noting that in 1975, 784,000 appendectomies were performed in the USA and about 3,000 of those patients died. These surgeries were considered emergency situations, but when the appendixes reached the pathology lab, one out of four were found to be perfectly healthy. Oops! Oh well, a man has to do something for a living, right?

Every organ and gland has a function in your body; unfortunately, most surgeons are trained to remove body parts. The appendix is part of your immune system and helps fight infection. Studies have proven that people who have had their appendixes removed were twice as likely to develop cancer of the bowel. Furthermore, you are left at high risk for other infections as well. The appendix acts as an overflow valve to keep impacted fecal matter from pushing back into the small intestines and being reabsorbed into the blood.

> **"Surgeons are trained to do surgery, not avoid it."** Robert Mendelsohn, M.D.

Don't be mistaken. In some instances, when people have neglected their health and they are in the emergency room because the appendix is on the verge of rupturing, then of course surgery is required. The point is, routine maintenance, a colon cleanse once a year, keeps your digestive system tuned-up and your bowels moving regularly to prevent illness. An EDS exam will indicate what areas of your body need cleansing and toning. A parasite cleanse once a year is good prevention, especially if you have cats or dogs in your house. The appendix and gallbladder are favorite hang-out places for parasites. Don't wait until you have symptoms to do a cleanse. Again, an ounce of prevention is worth a pound of cure.

There Are No Incurable Diseases

> **"We are the physical manifestation of the essence of our collective consciousness. We are the I AM. To see us is to see that which sent us."** James Chappell, D.C., N.D., Ph.D.

The Tarahumara Indians in northwestern Mexico are some of the world's greatest long-distance runners. They die peacefully when they reach old age and choose a time to depart from this mortal life. When they feel they have accomplished what they came to do on earth, they say goodbye and walk out in the woods. Do you know what they do to die? Nothing. They simply sit down and stop moving, and mentally surrender. Once the spirit and mind give the body permission to die, there is no struggle. The lymphatic system shuts down and within 24 hours the physical body dies and the spirit departs.

> **"What a caterpillar calls the end of the world we call a butterfly."** Eckhart Tolle

Some Americans do nothing all day. They sit in front of the TV, lifeless, and the Prozac they are on has them in a zombie-like foggy haze. One of the worse things a person can do in my opinion is to retire. We humans are meant to be productive. If we do not have a project, a cause, a purpose, something exciting that motivates us to get out of bed in the mornings, then we are sick. With all of the millions of awesome opportunities there are in this world, how could anyone possibly be bored? For those who are retired, stay on a schedule with projects, or volunteer to help an organization for a good cause. There are opportunities available, so choose one that resonates well with you and help make the world a better place for someone else. When we become selfish and lazy, only focusing on ourselves, we're going to have health problems. A river in the mountains, in order to stay healthy and clean, has to keep moving and giving of itself abundantly. Once it stops moving and hoards its water, it becomes a swamp or like the Dead Sea, stagnant and filled with disease-causing toxins.

Everyone has talents. We all have the ability to make a difference. Are you part of the problem or part of the solution? Do you sit around complaining and blaming or do you do something to be part of the change? What are you doing to make the world a better place?

> **"If you think you are too small to make a difference, try sleeping with a mosquito."** Dalai Lama

Circulation is a key to life. Get up and move your joints and muscles the way they were meant to move so you can stay limber. Yoga is excellent to get the body moving. If Americans would do 10 minutes of simple exercising every day, then most could avoid wheelchairs and walkers. This is why yoga and other fitness classes are good. They get us moving. How many Americans can't do a full squat with just their body weight? If we were to train our youth to do 25 full squats every day, then by the time they were 75, most would still be able to do them perfectly and pain free. When we stop moving, joints become calcified, like rust on a bicycle chain that is never ridden.

> **"Most of the things worth doing in the world had been declared impossible before they were done."** Louis D. Brandeis, American Judge, 1856-1941

> **Case Study**
>
> *Dear Dr. Sainsbury,*
>
> *First, I want to thank you for all that you have done for me. You have helped me to help myself both physically and emotionally.*
>
> *Initially, when I contacted you, I was unable to get through the day without constant tears, unbelievable fatigue, and severe anxiety. I had been diagnosed with lupus, osteoarthritis, disc bulges, had injections of epidurals (to no avail) and was considered a candidate for back surgery as well as severe bone loss. My fatigue was such that I could not get through the day without at least two naps. Almost immediately after seeing you, the tears stopped, my anxiety decreased to almost non-existence and my energy has returned to a point such as I experienced many years ago. More importantly, through your affirmation CD, I have discovered my much-needed spiritual rebirth. I am now healthy, energized, happy, joyful, and certainly in harmony with the flow of life.*
>
> *Again, I want to thank you for helping me return to a joyful, balanced, harmonized and healthy life style. In my opinion, your efforts have contributed more to my health than any other professional that I have contacted.*
>
> *Please keep up the good work. I pray this will help enlighten anyone who may have any doubts as to the benefits that can be obtained through your natural remedies and counseling.*
> *Sincerely,*
>
> *Doris O'Neil*
> *Collinsville, Alabama*

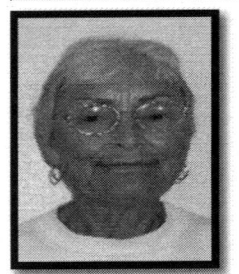

Dis-ease: Your Body's Way Of Filing Bankruptcy

Some have the ignorant belief that arthritis is just part of getting old. In the book *Chemistry of Man* by Dr. Bernard Jensen, he relates the following story, *"There is a myth going around that arthritis is a disease of old age. An elderly lady, so the story goes, went to see her doctor about arthritis pains in her left knee. "How old are you?" the doctor asked. "I'm 65," she said. "I'm 65, and I have arthritis, too," the doctor told her. "There's no cure for it. Just go home and chalk it up to old age." And this little old lady looked at the doctor and said, "I want to tell you *something. My right knee is the same age as my left knee, and it doesn't have arthritis!"*

Your health is like a bank account. If you take, take, take and never put back, then your bank account will be overdrawn and your health will deteriorate. When you take Advil for headaches, Claritin for allergies, Cortisone shots for back pain, Nexium for heartburn, Prozac for depression, Synthroid for a sluggish thyroid, Lipitor for high cholesterol, Losartan for high blood pressure and Ambien to help you sleep, then wonder why you are the poor victim of cancer 10 years later is it really a mystery? The sad reality is, after years of taking harmful prescriptions, making one withdrawal after the other, your bank account and body are completely bankrupt. There's nothing left to give. Your body has been depleted of nutrients. Like weeds growing in a neglected garden, cancer cells thrive in a neglected body, especially after many faithful years of you swallowing your lymphatic-blocking, liver-clogging, kidney-damaging, acidifying, toxic drugs religiously for many years. As soon as you felt that first twinge of discomfort, you ran to the kitchen cabinet to grab your magic pill to make you all better. And magic it has been for all these years. However, now the piper must be paid.

> **"Be not deceived; God is not mocked: for whatsoever a man soweth, that shall he also reap."** Galatians 6:7

The good news about dis-ease is if you created it, then you have the power to uncreate it. God gave us that healing ability within. You have to start by making some deposits in the bank. By deposits, I mean healthy organic foods, liver and kidney cleanses with alkaline herbs and healthy nutritional cell foods such as wheatgrass, alfalfa, barley greens, spirulina, chlorella, blue green algae, bee pollen and fresh fruits, berries and vegetables.

> **"Disease is never acquired. It is always earned. Disease is a natural result obtained from an unnatural lifestyle. ... Disease occurs only when one's internal environment is favorable for disease growth. We create our internal environments. ... As you never see flies in a clean garbage can, you also never see disease in a completely pure being."** Richard Anderson, N.M.D.

CHRONIC FATIGUE CULPRITS

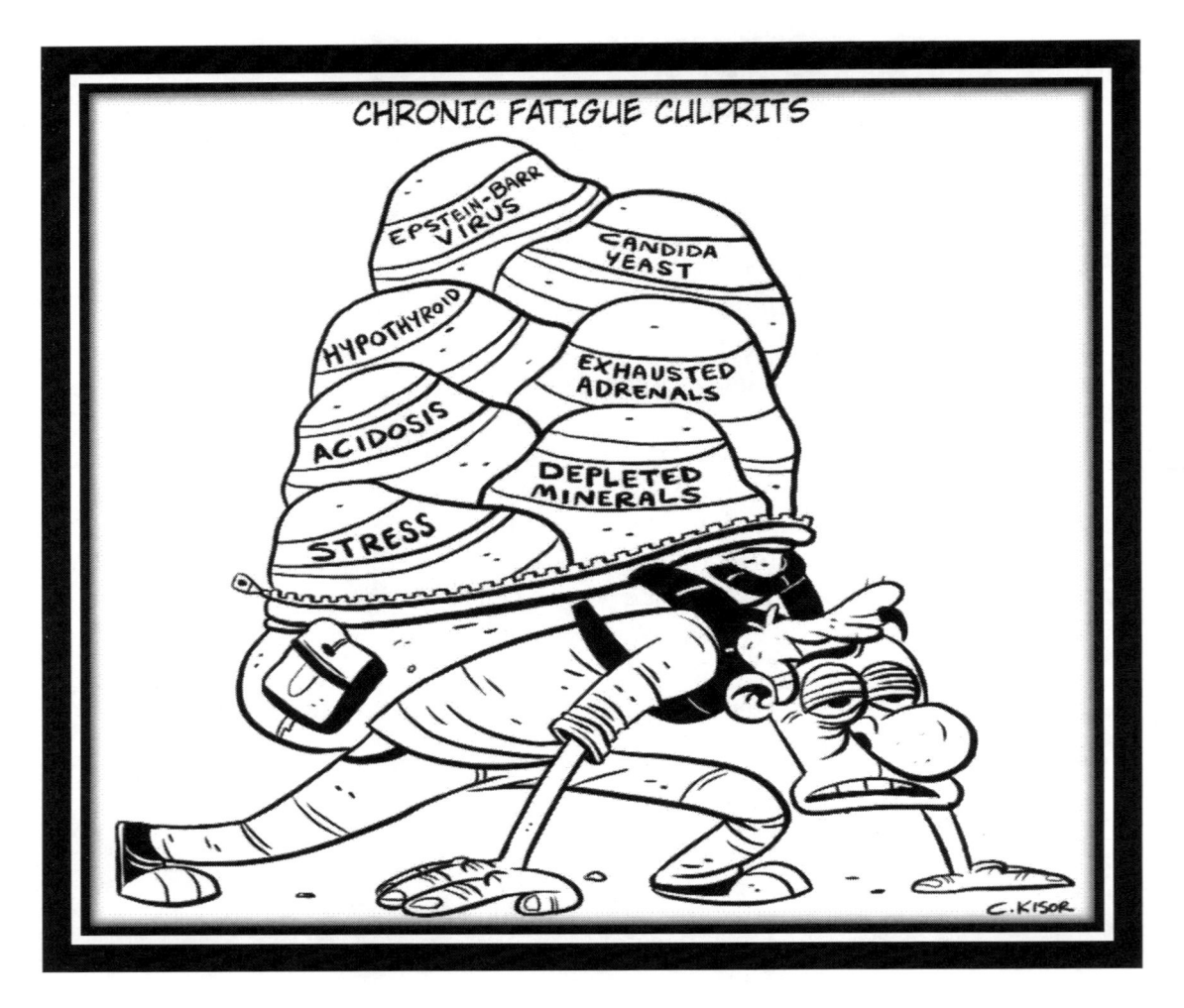

Epstein-Barr Virus, Candida Yeast, Hypothyroid, Exhausted Adrenals, Acidosis, Depleted Minerals, Stress

Antibiotics Weaken Your Immune System & Increase The Risk Of Diabetes

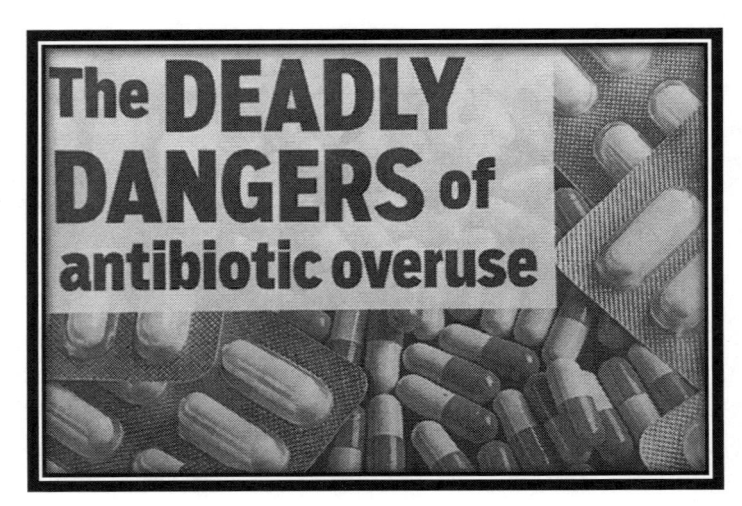

The DEADLY DANGERS of antibiotic overuse

According to the CDC, in 2015, about 269 million antibiotics were prescribed and 47 million, or one in three, of those were completely unnecessary. In fact, they state most antibiotics are unnecessary for respiratory conditions such as colds, sore throats and bronchitis that are caused by viruses. The CDC states that many sinus and ear infections that are bacterial do not always need an antibiotic, and that at least 50 percent of doctors' antibiotic prescriptions are unnecessary.

Antibiotics produce an acidic effect on the body when they kill bacteria. When an antibiotic destroys the bacterial wall of a cell, it releases protein matter that alters the pH and enables surviving endobionts to recreate an infectious cycle of sickness. This is why so many infections are re-occurring.

> **"No antibiotic can be said to have proven successful in truly eradicating any infectious disease in modern times."** Marc Lappe, Ph.D., Professor, University of Illinois

Women get on antibiotics and then are plagued with vaginal yeast infections caused from the antibiotics killing off the good bacteria and disrupting the microbiome in the the gut. Once the naturally occurring yeast in our gut gets in the blood stream, it puts a tremendous strain on the immune system, causing inflammation throughout the body. When candida yeast settles in the muscles and joints, they become inflamed and achy. You run back to the doctor who prescribed the antibiotics that caused the yeast to become systemic (in the blood) and now he diagnoses you as having fibromyalgia, not realizing that his drugs caused it. It zaps your energy and triggers horrible skin rashes, headaches, sinus infections and reoccurring urinary tract infections. Welcome to the antibiotic vicious drug cycle.

> **"Candidiasis is basically a 20-century disease, a disease resulting from medical developments like antibiotics, birth control pills and estrogen replacement therapy."** Leyardia Black, M.D.

Antibiotics are worthless for colds, influenza and upper respiratory tract infections caused by a virus. They only target bacteria. When you allow your immune system to naturally battle infections without antibiotic interference, it develops a memory to specific antibodies of the current infection and many more similar to it. It leaves you stronger, so the next time an infection comes along, your immune system will say like cops do when they see a repeat criminal, "Hey, this guy has a criminal file and he's got a warrant out for his arrest!" In very serious, life-or-death cases, antibiotics can help clear up bacterial infections and may be needed, but most of the time our immune system becomes stronger by letting nature run its course. Antibiotics should be a last resort, not first.

> **"Not only are antibiotics powerless against the viruses that cause colds and flu, but misuse of antibiotics can actually do more harm than good."** Fred Rubin, M.D., Associate Clinical Professor of Medicine, University of Pittsburgh; Contributor, Merck Manual

Children learn to walk by falling. With each clumsy step, a child develops muscle strength and coordination. Through adversity, the child masters the ability to walk, run and jump. To prevent a child from ever falling would deprive them of learning to keep their balance. Similarly, our immune systems are growing and being strengthened as they are challenged by the unseen universe of microbes. We need the adversity of microbes to keep us strong. Like muscles that grow stronger from working out, our immune systems grow stronger from pathogen exposure. Put your leg in a cast and don't walk for three months, and the muscles begin to atrophy. What we don't use, we lose. Any time we ingest antibiotics, we are allowing our immune system to skip a workout that may cost us in the championship match when we meet a nasty virus or gang of cancer cells. Do you know people who lost their championship fight to cancer or some other disease because their immune system was weak from skipping workouts and cheating with antibiotics too many times?

> **"There may be a time down the road when 80 percent to 90 percent of infections will be resistant to all known antibiotics."** Alexander Fleming, Discoverer of Penicillin

Alexander Fleming, the discoverer of penicillin, warned us that what appears to be great may also prove our fate. Experts are concerned about our future because of the massive amounts of antibiotics that are beginning to backfire. In other words, the microbes are beginning to become stronger and resistant to our current antibiotics. We are creating "super microbes" that antibiotics can't touch. Darwin's theory "survival of the fittest" is proving true in the world of microbes.

If you do choose to take an antibiotic as a last resort or in an emergency, make sure and take some probiotics (acidophilus) to replace the good bacteria that the antibiotic will kill off. This will help prevent naturally occurring candida yeast from getting into the blood and becoming systemic.

> **"Antibiotics are indiscriminate killers; they kill bacteria that are required for our survival as efficiently as they kill harmful bacteria."** Bruce Lipton, Ph.D.

A study published in The Journal of Clinical Endocrinology & Metabolism in 2012 reports that Danish researchers found that those who have used two to four antibiotics in the last 13 years had a 23 percent higher risk for developing diabetes, and those who took five or more antibiotics had a 53 percent higher risk for developing Type 2 diabetes as opposed to those who took none.

> **"If you have taken five or more ANTIBIOTICS in the last 13 years, you have a 53 percent higher risk for diabetes."** (Journal of Clinical Endocrinology & Metabolism)

Acidosis – The Terrain That Favors Dis-ease

pH SCALE		
0 ACIDIC	Battery Acid	
1	Stomach Acid	
2	Vinegar	lemon juice
3	Soft Drinks	orange juice, shellfish, pasta, pastries, tobacco smoke, aspartame, wine, cheese, tea, microwaved foods, pork, pickles, Equal, NutraSweet, Sweet'N Low
4	Acid Rain	beer, wheat, popcorn, distilled/reverse osmosis water, bottled water, white bread, beef, peanuts, tomato sauce
5	Coffee	cooked beans, sugar, potatoes, butter, wheat bran, chicken, turkey, canned fruit, pinto beans, lentils, white rice, black beans
6	Urine	milk, yogurt, eggs, brown rice, oysters, soy milk, goats' milk, fish, lima beans, cocoa, oats, coconut, salmon, tuna
7 NEUTRAL	Pure Water	human blood, raw fresh milk, butter
8	Sea Water	apples, tomatoes, pineapple, cantaloupe, oranges, almonds, olives, radishes, cherries, strawberries, grapefruit, avocados, mushrooms, apricots, peaches, bananas
9	Baking Soda	olive oil, zucchini, raw green beans, mangoes, tangerines, grapes, lettuce, sweet potato, blueberries, papaya, melons, alfalfa sprouts, pears, figs, dates, kiwi, borage oil
10	Detergent	raw spinach, kale, cauliflower, broccoli, red cabbage, carrots, cucumbers, asparagus, artichokes, celery, onions, collard greens, lemons, limes
11	Ammonia	
12	Soapy Water	
13	Bleach	
14 ALKALINE	Drain Cleaner	

When it comes to health, we look at the pH (potential of Hydrogen) of the body. A pH scale runs from 0 to 14. On the low end of the scale, 0 means complete acidity. On the high end, 14 indicates complete alkalinity. Obviously, a 7 on the scale is right in the middle, neutral. Healthy individuals have a pH (saliva) that hovers in the 6.8-7.0 range. Healthy urine pH runs somewhere between 5.5-5.8. Most health problems are caused by the body's pH being too acidic. Yeast (Candida), viruses, bacteria, arthritis, cancer and fibromyalgia thrive in an acidic atmosphere. Analyze what you typically eat for breakfast, lunch and dinner and that will give you a good clue as to where your pH hovers. If you are emotionally upset or stressed out, that will cause your pH to become acidic. If we want to be healthy, we must change the terrain of the body by eating more alkaline-forming foods. Most living foods are alkaline, and vegetables are on the top of the list. Fruits and berries in moderation are good.

It's important to understand that some foods, like lemons and grapefruits, are acidic in nature, but once metabolized in your body, they leave an alkaline ash. That is why we call most fruits and vegetables alkaline ash-forming foods, while high-protein foods such as meats, poultry, fish, and grains are acid ash-producing foods.

> "Germs, bacteria, viruses and alike are scavengers and can live only on wasting-away cells, mucous and toxic conditions. They can never exist in a healthy and clean cell structure or body." John Christopher, N.D.

The Terrain, Not The Germ, Causes Dis-ease

The theory that germs cause disease is a myth. Louis Pasteur was famous for discovering that bacteria can cause illness. He subsequently developed the pasteurization process for milk, in which milk is boiled to kill any possible bacteria, thus preventing disease. Pasteur spent his life studying how germs cause illness, but on his deathbed, he confessed the following:

> "I have been wrong. The germ is nothing. The 'terrain' is everything." Louis Pasteur

If you have a tree in your backyard with moss growing on it and you want to get rid of the moss, because let's suppose it is cancer, then what are your options? You could have a doctor poison it with chemicals, like chemotherapy or Roundup weed killer, but then you will probably kill the whole tree in the process. You could have him perform surgery and cut if off with a scalpel. He could freeze it off with

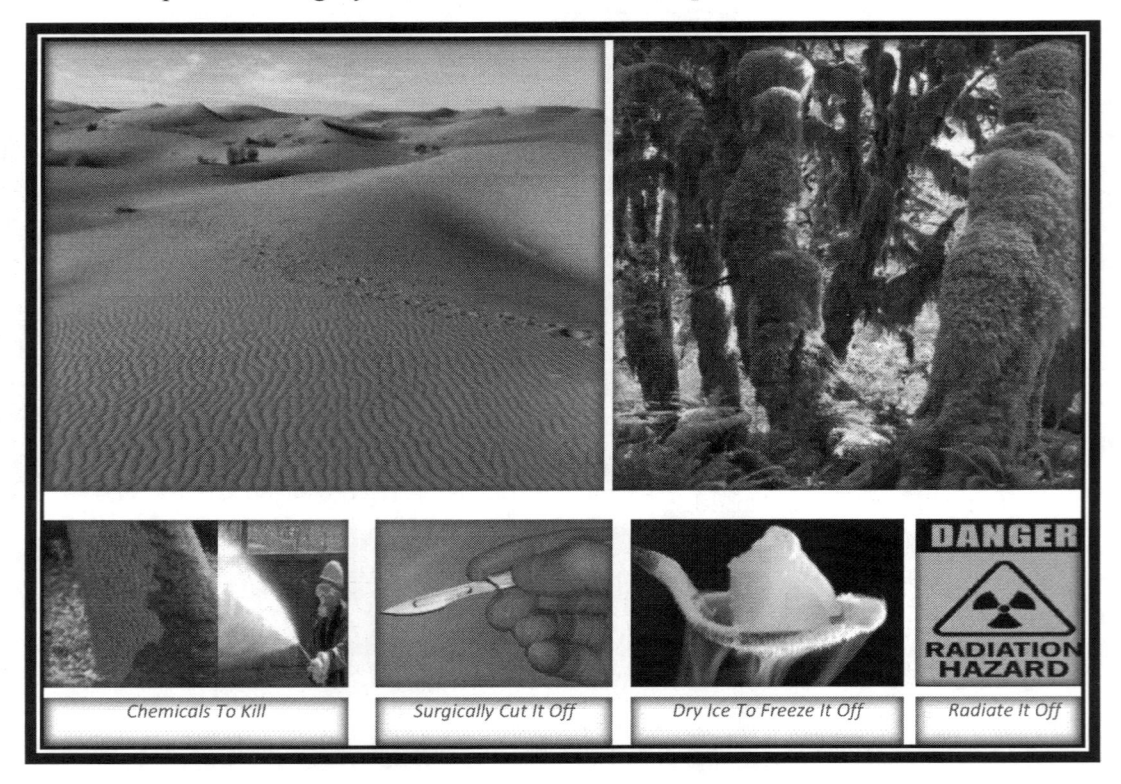

| Chemicals To Kill | Surgically Cut It Off | Dry Ice To Freeze It Off | Radiate It Off |

dry ice, or he could radiate it or destroy it with a laser. All of these are possibilities to treating moss (cancer) on the tree; however, what's going to happen in a year or two? Of course, the moss will grow right back, because we have failed to remove the cause that created it to grow in the first place.

> **"The idea of a microbe as a primary cause of disease is the greatest scientific silliness of the age."** Pierre Antoine Bechamp, France 1816-1908

The Terrain That Causes Moss
1. Moisture
2. Shade
3. Temperature 69-75 degrees

The Terrain That Causes Cancer	
1. Acidosis	4. Malnutrition
2. Toxins	5. Poor Circulation/Low Oxygen
3. Miasms	6. Emotional Issues/Stress

Without moisture, shade and temperatures hovering around 69 to 75 degrees, moss will not grow. This is the terrain or environment required for moss to survive. That is why it usually grows on the north side of trees and buildings. If we were to take a moss-laden tree and transplant it in the Arizona desert, what would happen? Of course, the hot, dry, sunny climate would kill the moss. This is why killing things in the body with antibiotics and chemotherapy is a foolish attempt to achieve optimum health. If we don't want yeast infections, fibromyalgia, arthritis and cancerous tumors, then we have to change the terrain that has caused it to grow in the first place.

> **"If I could live my life over again, I would devote it to proving that germs seek their natural habitat — diseased tissue — rather than being the cause of diseased tissue …."** Dr. Rudolph Virchow, The Father of Cellular Pathology, 1821-1902

If a tumor grows in the body, what caused it? What fed and nourished it? Was it mercury poisoning with an overgrowth of candida yeast, caused from vaccinations and routine antibiotic use? Was it caused from too much estrogen from years of taking birth control pills, or is the liver swamped with chemicals and pesticides along with gluten allergies that keep the immune system suppressed? We have to start looking at the cause if we want to heal. Jumping in with chemo without addressing toxicity issues is about as absurd as an auto mechanic who just starts replacing random parts without doing any testing to identify the cause of the problem.

> **"If the 'germ theory of disease' were correct, there'd be no one living to believe it."** B.J. Palmer, 1882-1961, Developer of Chiropractic

Chemotherapy and radiation do nothing to change the terrain that has favored cancer to exist. Sure, this poison and radiation can very well get rid of cancer, but it also poisons the rest of our cells. Without changing our diet, thoughts and healing emotional trauma from the past, it is just a matter of time before the cancer comes right back to the environment that nourished it to grow in the first place. As most oncologists will tell you, when it does come back, it returns with a vengeance to a body whose immune system is even weaker than before, after undergoing the cell-damaging procedures of radiation and chemotherapy.

> **"Our way of life is related to our way of death."** The Framingham Study, Harvard University

ACID FORMING FOODS

Alcohol	Cornstarch	Lentils, dried	Sardines
Anger	Corn syrup	Lobster	Sausage
Aspirin	Corn oil	Macaroni	Scallops
Aspartame	Corned beef	Mayonnaise	Seeds
Bacon	Crackers	Milk (cow)	Soft drinks
Beer	Currants	Niacin	Soybeans
Blueberries	Dairy products	Nuts	Soymilk
Bran, wheat	Drugs (medicinal)	Oatmeal	Spaghetti
Bran, oat	Eggs	Olives	Squash
Bread, wheat	Flour, whole wheat	Pasta	Sugar -
Butter	Fish (all)	Peanuts	(refined)
Cake	French fries	Peanut butter	Tea, black
Carob	Fruits, canned	Pepper, black	Turkey
Cereals (all)	Fruits, glazed	Peas, dried	Vinegar -
Cheese	Fruits, sulfured	Popcorn	distilled)
Chicken	Hamburgers	Pork	Walnuts
Chickpeas	Honey	Rice, brown	Wheat
Chips	Hot dogs	Rice, white	Wheat germ
Chocolate	Ketchup	Rice milk	Wine
Coffee	Legumes	Salmon	Yogurt
Corn (canned)	Unforgiveness	Worry	Vitamin C

In order to change the terrain of the body, we need to pay attention to the acidic and alkaline foods and drinks that we consume. Yellow vegetables have a calming, laxative effect. Green vegetables help build the blood and are excellent for the anemic (low in iron), sluggish individual. The green chlorophyll in vegetables is also anti- inflammatory and helps the body heal faster. Red fruits and vegetables stimulate the body and are good for circulation.

Most proteins and starches are acidic. Intuition will tell you which foods your body needs. Eat the fruits and vegetables that sound good to you on that particular day. Most people do very well to consume 75 percent of their diet from the alkaline food list, while limiting their consumption of acidic foods to only 25 percent.

ALKALINE FORMING FOODS

Almonds	Apple cider vinegar	Love	Quinoa
Apples	Chlorella	Mangoes	Radishes
Apricots	Cucumbers	Maple syrup	Raisins
Bananas	Dates, dried	Melons, all	Raspberries
Barley juice	Dulse	Milk, goat raw	Rhubarb
Beans, dried	Figs, dried	Millet	Rutabagas
Bee pollen	Alfalfa sprouts	Limes	Yams
Prunes	Garlic	Molasses	Sauerkraut
Beet greens	Ginger	Mushrooms	Olive oil
Beets	Goat whey	Mustard greens	Spirulina
Berries (most)	Grapefruit	Okra	Spinach, raw
Blackberries	Grapes	Onions	Sprouts
Broccoli	Green beans	Oranges	Squash
Brussels sprouts	Green peas	Parsley	Strawberries
Cabbage	Herbs (all)	Parsnips	Stevia
Cantaloupe	Kale	Peaches	Tangerines
Carrots	Kelp	Pears	Tomatoes
Cauliflower	Leech nuts	Peppers	Turnip greens
Celery	Lemons	Pineapple	Watercress
Chard leaves	Lettuce	Plums	Watermelon
Cherries, soups	Lima beans, dried	Potatoes sweet	Wheatgrass juice
Cinnamon	Lima beans, green	Potatoes, white	Collard greens

> "Consider that Americans consume more calcium-rich dairy foods than almost every other nation, and we have one of the highest rates of osteoporosis. There's a disconnect here. Dairy may be rich in calcium, but most dairy foods also produce acid yield." Loren Cordain, Ph.D.

I know many vegetarians who are healthy and vibrant and thrive on a meatless diet. On the other hand, some people, especially blood type Os, seem to do better with some meat in their diet. We have had health nuts come in who are very sick with raging candida yeast infections. The dilemma is, if you don't eat meat, what else do you eat besides fruits and vegetables? Most consume a lot of grains, including wheat, rice, oats and corn — all very acid-forming as well as blood-sugar-spiking foods. And worst of all, grains and fruits feed yeast (fungi) and mold. If you consume a lot of whole wheat bread and sweet fruits, you are providing the terrain to feed yeast and develop diabetes. I believe we are each unique individuals and you have to find the diet plan that makes you feel best. For some, it's vegetarian all the way, and for others, they do better with meats. And most do better to leave grains off completely or eat them sparingly or in moderation. There is no one-shoe-fits-all perfect diet.

> **"Acid wastes build up in the body in the form of cholesterol, gallstones, kidney stones, arterial plaque, urates, phosphates and sulfates. These acidic waste products are the direct cause of premature aging and the onset of chronic disease."** Dr. Stefan Kuprowsky

It is important for us to understand that the way foods are prepared before we put them in our mouths makes a world of difference. For example, raw milk, straight from the cow or goat, is alkaline-forming; however, once it has been pasteurized (boiled), it becomes acid-forming. What the dairy industry fails to mention is the fact that once milk has been pasteurized, it takes more calcium to digest it than it gives back to your bones. It leaves your body acidic, and in order to buffer the acids, the body will use up more minerals to buffer the acids than what the milk provided.

Almonds are alkaline from Mother Nature, but when they have been roasted, they become acidic and are harder to digest. Most grains are acidic until they are sprouted. When the enzymes in them are activated and spring to life, they become alkaline and full of living nutrition.

Some people get all gung-ho about healing and radically change their diet. If they aren't accustomed to eating living foods and drastically change their diets too fast, the body starts dumping toxins and may cause them to become very sick and feel even worse. This is called a Herxheimer reaction, commonly known as a "Herx," when there is a massive die-off of bacteria, co-infections or yeast. The patient who doesn't understand what their body is doing may become frustrated and quit. They mistakenly conclude that natural healing doesn't work. The point is, if a 300-pound person who has been eating junk food his whole life suddenly stops poisoning his body and starts eating whole foods along with some liver- and kidney-detoxifying herbs, then his cells will automatically go into a cleanse mode. This is why some people who try to fast feel so terrible. Their body is cleansing! Cells are getting rid of stored toxins. Each person needs to go at his or her own pace. Be smart and remember, moderation in all things.

A major problem with modern medicine is that they split everything up and go to specialists. The body works as a whole, and if we want to heal, we must look at the whole body. As mentioned earlier, the thyroid needs iodine to function properly. Is your diet deficient in iodine or are you not absorbing it because you are taking an acid blocker? When the thyroid is deficient in iodine, then most likely the calcium levels will be out of solution too, because iodine controls calcium in the body. This leads to arthritis, cataracts in the eyes, kidney stones and bone spurs. A specialized medical doctor will rarely connect those dots and say your kidney stones, arthritis, cataracts and hypothyroidism were all caused from one thing, a simple mineral deficiency — iodine. And as Dr. David Brownstein explains, in medical school we were taught to never take iodine because it will make thyroid problems worse. As we have already discussed, iodine is one of many needed nutrients to reverse and prevent disease. Dr. Brownstein informs that over 96 percent of the population is deficient in iodine. No wonder we have so many sick people.

Healing The Cause Of Kidney Stones, Bone Spurs & Arthritis

> "The countless names of illnesses do not really matter. What does matter is that they all come from the same root cause ... too much acid in the body!"
> Theodore A. Baroody, D.C., N.D., Ph.D.

When we eat cooked, dead, processed or junk foods, the body becomes very acidic. Acids accumulate in the body and must be buffered or neutralized before being eliminated through the kidneys. In order to function, the body begins to neutralize the acids with our mineral reserves which include **sodium, calcium, potassium, magnesium** and **iron**.

> "Long-term, excess acidity leads to thinner bones and lower muscle mass."
> Anthony Sebastian, M.D., University of California

Magnesium Rich Foods		Calcium Rich Foods	
Spinach	Avocado	Kale	Egg yolk
Almonds	Kefir	Spinach	Fish
Swiss chard	Pumpkin seeds	Swiss chard	Irish moss
Broccoli	Black beans	Collard greens	Kelp
Banana	Chocolate (dark)	Mustard greens	Lentils
Apples	Apricots	Dandelion greens	Onions
Walnuts	Brazil nuts	Beet greens	Prunes
Cabbage	Cashews	Avocados	Cauliflower
Coconuts	Dates	Cabbage	Dulse
Dulse	Figs	Arugula	Walnuts
Fish	Grapes	Broccoli	Watercress
Hickory nuts	Lentils	Buckwheat	White beans
Okra	Parsley	Sesame seeds	Almonds
Peas	Peaches	Goat's milk raw	Butter raw
Kale	Pears	Cow's milk raw	Carrots
Pecans	Prunes	Figs	Parsnips
Spinach	Sunflower seeds	Sardines	Kefir
Turnip greens	Collard greens	Okra	Goat cheese

Through this buffering system, vital minerals are lost through the kidneys and bowels. When these minerals are not replaced, then our body begins leaching minerals, especially calcium from our own bones, to buffer the acids. This can cause muscles to break down to produce ammonia, which is strongly alkaline. The bones are our biggest calcium supply. The hips are our largest bone structure and a rich calcium source. This is where the body usually robs calcium from first to buffer the acids. In the meantime, we are being diagnosed with osteopenia and osteoporosis. One slip and fall and brittle bones fracture from the slightest trauma. The solution to reversing arthritis is to eat more alkalizing foods, especially vegetables and fruit in moderation. Supplementing the diet with minerals can be very helpful, and digestive enzymes ensure we are absorbing them. If you are taking an acid blocker or Tums, and neutralizing the required acid in the stomach, for proper digestion, you will have arthritic problems, because you're not absorbing your minerals. Acid blockers cause disease.

> **"There is one major cause of disease, and this is acidosis (low pH). Do you know that its major cause is putrefaction of fecal waste reabsorbed into your system? This causes toxemia, which means dirty blood ... The only way for your blood to become toxic is by reabsorbing your own toxic fecal waste from the large intestine."** Dr. Darrell Wolfe

Many sick people are so acidic that their alkaline reserves have been completely depleted. When there's no money in the bank, you can't make a withdrawal, and when there's no alkaline mineral reserves left, the body can't neutralize acids. With no minerals to buffer the acids, the body becomes saturated with acid wastes. The kidneys will then produce ammonia (9.25 pH) to buffer the acids, since the alkaline reserves have been exhausted. When someone complains of burning sensations when they urinate, then you know they are eliminating a tremendous amount of acids. This is the body's innate fire alarm, warning us to put the fires out with alkaline foods and minerals, before we burn up inside from acids.

After the body robs calcium from the bones to buffer acids, it turns to stone. If you deposit these stones at the joints, you'll develop arthritic knots on the fingers, spine (bone spurs), heels (heel spurs) and in the eyes in the form of cataracts. If the body deposits them in the kidneys, you will have kidney stones, and the sharp, razorblade-like edges will cause pain and possible bleeding. This is why calcium deposits or spurs can be so painful. When their sharp edges press against nerves, you will experience intense pain, like a sheriff did once as he hobbled in our office on crutches with gout so bad in his big toe, he couldn't wear a shoe. Once we neutralized the acids and put some minerals back in his bank account, he was pain free again and walking normally again.

> **"Nobody you know is 100 percent acidic. Nobody alive, that is! The fact is, 100 percent acidity is the very definition of death and decay!"** Michael Culter, M.D.

Organic plant-derived sodium is what keeps the joints healthy and limber. It also helps regulate fluid levels throughout the body. Spirulina is an excellent source of sodium to add in your diet as a supplement. Okra, celery, spinach, figs, raw goat's milk, chicken and turkey gizzards are all high in sodium.

The body was designed and usually does best to use minerals that have passed through the plant kingdom. Sodium chloride (table salt) is not used by the body because the sodium and chloride are held together by ionic bonds. This form of salt is toxic and cannot be used to buffer acids. That is why it can cause high blood pressure and fluid retention and medical doctors will recommend avoiding it. Pink Himalayan sea salt is an excellent alternative, because it contains 80 trace minerals and elements.

> **"After digestion, all foods report to the kidneys as being either acidic or alkaline. The kidneys are responsible for fluid balance and maintaining a relatively neutral pH in the body."** Loren Cordain, Ph.D.

Best Sources of Magnesium
- Chelate
- Citrate
- Glycinate
- Aspartate
- Threonate

Avoid: Magnesium Oxide & Calcium Carbonate

When our saliva pH hovers in the 6.8 to 7.0 area, our body can build back our mineral reserves and reverse dis-ease. The so-called "incurable diseases" like arthritis and fibromyalgia all of a sudden become reversible, because we have changed the environment that caused those dis-eases in the first place. Of course, if the foods we are eating are lacking in minerals, then we'll still have deficiencies. That is why most of us need to supplement our diets with a good mineral supplement. Plant derived and liquid are usually best because they are easier absorbed. Some of Mother Nature's best nutrient/mineral-packed foods are wheatgrass, barley greens, alfalfa and spirulina. They are loaded with health-restoring minerals. Supplementing with these greens is highly beneficial.

> **"You can trace every sickness ... and every ailment to a mineral deficiency."** Dr. Linus Pauling, Nobel Prize-Winning Scientist

Some of the best foods that are high in calcium are: all green leafy vegetables, raw nuts, seeds and beans. Keep in mind that the more cooked animal protein you consume, the more calcium you lose. This is why it is important to eat the majority of your food from the vegetable category.

When supplementing with minerals, avoid magnesium oxide. Getting too much magnesium, above 600 milligrams, can cause diarrhea. If you have kidney problems, use caution with magnesium.

Eat Right For Your Blood Type Diet

Some people do well to follow the *Eat Right For Your Type* or *Blood Type Diet* by Peter D'Adamo, N.D. He claims that people are healthier when tailoring their diets according to their specific blood types. For example, I had a woman who was eating two chicken salads a day, lots of vegetables and protein, trying to lose weight, but she kept getting headaches. She was a blood type B, and if you look below, you will see that chicken is poison in a blood type B body. It contains lectins that cause inflammation. Once she stopped eating the chicken, with her salads, the headaches ceased to exist. For some, these diet guidelines make a world of difference. I suggest everyone trying it for a couple of weeks or months to see how you feel. If the shoe fits, wear it.

The following information is a short, condensed version of the *Eat Right for Your Blood Type Diet* plan. For the complete list of beneficial foods, neutral foods and foods to avoid, go to www.dadamo.com.

Blood type As do best by avoiding most animal protein and dairy, while eating a more vegetarian diet with lots of fruits and vegetables. He advises them to stay away from dairy products, animal fats and meats. Beneficial foods for type As are ocean salmon, rainbow trout, black-eyed peas, pinto beans, flaxseeds, pumpkin seeds, olive oil, flaxseed oil, broccoli, carrots, onions, spinach, blueberries, blackberries, cranberries and prunes, to name a few.

Blood Type A – Foods to Avoid

Beef	American cheese	Sour cream	Olives	Ketchup
Pork	Cheddar	Swiss cheese	Peppers	Mayonnaise
Shrimp	Colby	Brazil nuts	Potatoes	Pepper, black
Catfish	Cottage cheese	Cashews	Tomatoes	Pickles
Garbanzo beans	Cream cheese	Pistachio	Bananas	Vinegar
Lima beans	Ice cream	Cabbage	Cantaloupe	Beer
Navy beans	Milk	Eggplant	Oranges	Sodas
Red beans	Provolone	Mushrooms	Wheat/white bread	Black tea

Blood type Bs have the ability to metabolize dairy. They do best to eat a balanced diet of fruits, vegetables, fish, dairy and meat while avoiding chicken. Chicken contains a lectin that can cause agglutination, leading to serious health problems. Beneficial foods for blood type Bs are ocean salmon, kidney beans, limas, navy beans, cottage cheese, feta cheese, goat milk, kefir, mozzarella cheese, ricotta cheese, yogurt, macadamia nuts, avocados, broccoli, cabbage, carrots, mushrooms, sweet potatoes, yams, bananas, grapes, kiwi, pineapple, plums, ginger and green tea.

Blood Type B – Foods to Avoid

Chicken	American cheese	Whole wheat
Pork	Ice cream	Cinnamon
Shrimp	Cashews	Ketchup
Black beans	Peanuts	Black pepper
Black-eyed peas	Peanut butter	Sodas
Garbanzo beans	Corn	Buckwheat
Lentils	Olives	Cornmeal
Pinto beans	Tomatoes	Flour

Blood type AB is the rarest blood type and does best consuming mostly a vegetarian diet, avoiding chicken, as it causes agglutination (clots) in the blood. Beneficial foods for blood type ABs are turkey, rainbow trout, ocean salmon, tuna, lentils, navy beans, pintos, red beans, cottage cheese, feta cheese, mozzarella, ricotta, sour cream, yogurt, flaxseeds, walnuts, olive oil, avocados, broccoli, celery, cucumbers, eggplant, mushrooms, sweet potatoes, yams, cherries, cranberries, grapefruit, grapes, kiwi, lemons, pineapple, plums, garlic and green tea.

Blood Type AB – Foods to Avoid

Bacon	Kidney beans	Kamut
Beef	Lima beans	Cornmeal
Chicken	American cheese	Corn
Pork	Ice cream	Olives
Shrimp	Milk	Peppers
Black beans	Provolone	Bananas
Black-eyed peas	Pumpkin seeds	Oranges
Garbanzo beans	Buckwheat	Ketchup
Black pepper	Pickles	Black tea
Sodas	Mangoes	

Blood type Os should eat a high-protein diet, including red meat, and restrict their carbohydrate intake, by avoiding whole wheat products, corn and dairy. Many Os are lactose intolerant and susceptible to celiac disease (inability to digest gluten). The nightshade vegetables (potatoes, tomatoes, peppers & eggplant) cause arthritic conditions in Type Os because their lectins deposit in the tissue surrounding the joints. Beneficial foods are beef, rainbow trout, salmon, black-eyed peas, pinto beans, mozzarella cheese, flaxseeds, macadamia nuts, pumpkin seeds, walnuts, olive oil, avocados, broccoli, okra, onions, sweet potatoes, spinach, plums, prunes and garlic.

Blood Type O – Foods to Avoid

Pork	Peanut butter	Milk	Corn	White flour
Catfish	American cheese	Monterey jack	Eggplant	Whole wheat
Kidney beans	Cheddar	Provolone	Mushrooms	Cinnamon
Lentils	Colby	Ricotta	Olives	Ketchup
Navy beans	Cottage cheese	Swiss cheese	Potatoes	Black pepper
Brazil nuts	Cream cheese	Yogurt	Blackberries	Pickles
Cashews	Ice cream	Whole wheat	Cantaloupe	Vinegar
Peanuts	Kefir	Cabbage	Oranges	Coffee

Mother Nature's Foods – Healing Light Energy

> "Man, the alchemizer, transfers **color and vibration** from his food to himself — and that is his aliveness, his vitality. A corpse has all the chemical elements, but you can't bring him back to life. The essential life of man is in the vibration that is man, and this life force is carried with the mineral elements in their response to the light of the sun." Bernard Jensen, D.C., Ph.D., N.D.

When light from the sun is refracted through a prism, it splits up into seven clear colors. Foods are nothing more than color materialized by the plant. Plants take sunlight, which is color, and through photosynthesis make food. Fruits, vegetables, nuts, seeds and flowers are manifestations of light energy transformed into physical edible matter. When we eat food and digest it, we break down the physical solid food material and change it back into light and color, which is energy to feed and nourish the body.

Dr. Oz's Green Drink
2 cups spinach
2 cups cucumber
1 head of celery
½ inch fresh ginger root
1 bunch parsley
2 apples
Juice of 1 lime
Juice of ½ lemon
Combine all ingredients in a juicer. Makes 30 oz.

A great way to alkalize your body and provide it with a tremendous amount of nutrition is by juicing. Fresh carrot, celery and one apple juiced is a healthy way to start your day. Another great juice recipe is Dr. Mehmet Oz's green drink recipe.

Restaurant owners understand how powerful colors are to increase appetites. Have you ever gone out to eat in a dark restaurant, except for the glow of red lights on the walls and tables? Red stimulates you to eat. It's important that we eat different colored foods to give us the energetic frequencies we need to be healthy.

> **"The power of meditation can be 10 times greater under violet light falling through the stained-glass window of a quiet church."** Leonardo da Vinci

Color is energy. The frequencies contained in colors make up life. Red, orange, yellow, green, blue, indigo and violet are the seven colors of life. We have seven energy centers in the body called the endocrine system. Ayurvedic medicine that originated in India over 2,500 years ago refers to these energy centers as chakras. This is our electrical system. Just as a wire can develop a short where electricity no longer flows, many health issues arise from blockages or imbalances in energy with specific chakras.

> **"Your physical (body) needs a minimum of 45 minutes of sunlight on the top of your bare head daily to fuel your pineal gland."** Jim Malcolm

Chakras

The **7th crown chakra** is located on the top of the head and involves the pineal gland. The pineal gland is a crystal that is activated by sunlight. It secretes melatonin to help us sleep, but also serotonin, to help us feel energized during the day. Take your hat off and stop putting on cancer-causing sunscreen. You need sunlight, in moderation, of course. The crown chakra relates to your connection to divinity or God. This area can be affected if you feel disconnected with source or a higher power. Migraines and headaches are common when out of balance.

The **6th brow chakra,** also known as your third eye, is where you receive intuition, purpose and direction in life. This area can be blocked when you lose your purpose in life. Headaches are also common when imbalanced.

The **5th throat chakra** deals with the self-expression and your ability to speak your truth. People who are afraid to speak up and voice their opinions may have problems with a sluggish thyroid, sore throats and a constant need to clear their throat.

The **4th heart chakra** is located in the center of your chest and relates to love, compassion and relationships. If you have been hurt, had your heart broken, and are afraid to open up and be in close relationships where you give and receive love, you may experience chest pain, heart problems, heart attacks and breast cancer. Conflict with family may manifest in the breast.

The **3rd solar plexus** is where we get our power and control. If you have been shamed, felt embarrassed, powerless or perhaps feel like a victim, you may experience stomach pains, anxiety and have gut feelings that something isn't right.

The **2nd sacral chakra** relates to our sexual organs. This is where we experience the joys of intimacy and sexuality. Money and guilt are associated with this chakra too. Problems can manifest here if you feel you are unattractive and question if anyone would ever desire you or have difficulty opening up in relationships. People who have been sexually molested may have problems here. Reproductive organ complications such as ovarian, cervical, testicular and prostate cancers are common when energy is blocked in this chakra.

The **1st root chakra** is located at the base of the spine and is associated with being grounded to Mother Earth and relates to our physical survival, safety, basic trust, security and will to live. People who hate their jobs or feel they are stuck in an unfulfilling career may experience eating disorders, fatigue, leg pains and colon problems.

Chakra	Endocrine Gland	Color	Emotion	Blocked By	Action	Sound	Note	Frequency
7 Crown	Pineal	Violet	Spirituality	Ego	I Know	ING	B - ti	936 Hz
6 Third Eye	Pituitary	Indigo	Intuition	Illusion	I See	MM	A - la	852 Hz
5 Throat	Thyroid	Blue	Truth	Lies	I Speak	EE	G - sol	741 Hz
4 Heart	Thymus	Green	Love	Grief	I Love	AY	F - fa	639 Hz
3 Solar Plexus	Pancreas	Yellow	Willpower	Shame	I Do	AH	E - mi	528 Hz
2 Sacral	Gonads	Orange	Pleasure	Guilt	I Feel	OO	D - re	417 Hz
1 Base	Adrenals	Red	Survival	Fear	I Am	OH	C - ut	396 Hz

"If you wish to understand the universe, think of energy, frequency and vibration." Nikola Tesla, Electrical Engineer 1856-1943

Sneezing rebalances the body's electrical system. Never suppress a sneeze. Another factor that can cause an imbalance of energy is when an upsetting emotional experience occurs and you wanted to express your feelings, possibly even scream or cry, but you suppressed it. Those emotional sound frequencies stay within the body, all bottled up. It is healthy to feel your feelings fully. Let the tones come out. Sound is energy. Sound is the foundation of the universe. Sound creates light. Many songs are written and sung to express how one feels. If you suppress your feelings with anti-depression/anxiety drugs what do you think is happening to your electrical system? You wouldn't want an electrical short in your house or car and certainly not your body's nervous system, right? Neurological diseases are becoming quite popular as more and more people take anxiety, depression and ADHD medications. Could drugs be causing a short in your neurological system, creating dis-ease?

According to Dr. Len Horowitz, 528 Hz frequency is the frequency of love and has the power to repair damaged DNA. It is the same frequency at which a blade of grass with radiant life containing chlorophyll resonates. The U.S. military uses 528 Hz sound frequency to tune the metal of their fighter jets. It is a healing frequency.

On the average, we humans as a whole are resonating at 67 megahertz. Cancer cells resonate at 43 megahertz. The emotion joy resonates at a rate 100,000 times greater than fear. Raising our vibrational level aligns us with healthy frequencies, while a low vibration leads toward disease and death.

> **"The spirit down here in man and the spirit up there in the sun in reality are only one spirit, and there is no other one."** The Upanishads

Cymatics is the study of how sound vibrations impact matter. Sand sprinkled on an electronic plate connected to a musical instrument forms geometrical patterns with each note. When exposed to classical music such as Bach or Beethoven, the sand amazingly forms beautiful symmetrical patterns. To the contrary, when exposed to a hard, acid rock style of music, the sand fails to form any sort of symmetrical pattern. What music do you choose to influence the vibrational frequencies of your body? Are they peaceful, invigorating and harmonious or sounds of agitation, pain and chaos?

> "It's the most important molecule you need to stay healthy and prevent disease — yet you've probably never heard of it. It's the secret to prevent aging, cancer, heart disease, dementia, and more, and necessary to treat everything from autism to Alzheimer's disease. There are more than 89,000 medical articles about it — but your doctor doesn't know how to address the epidemic deficiency of this critical life-giving molecule ... What is it? I'm talking about the mother of all antioxidants, the master detoxifier and maestro of the immune system: GLUTATHIONE." Mark Hyman, M.D.

Toxic Silver Dental Fillings

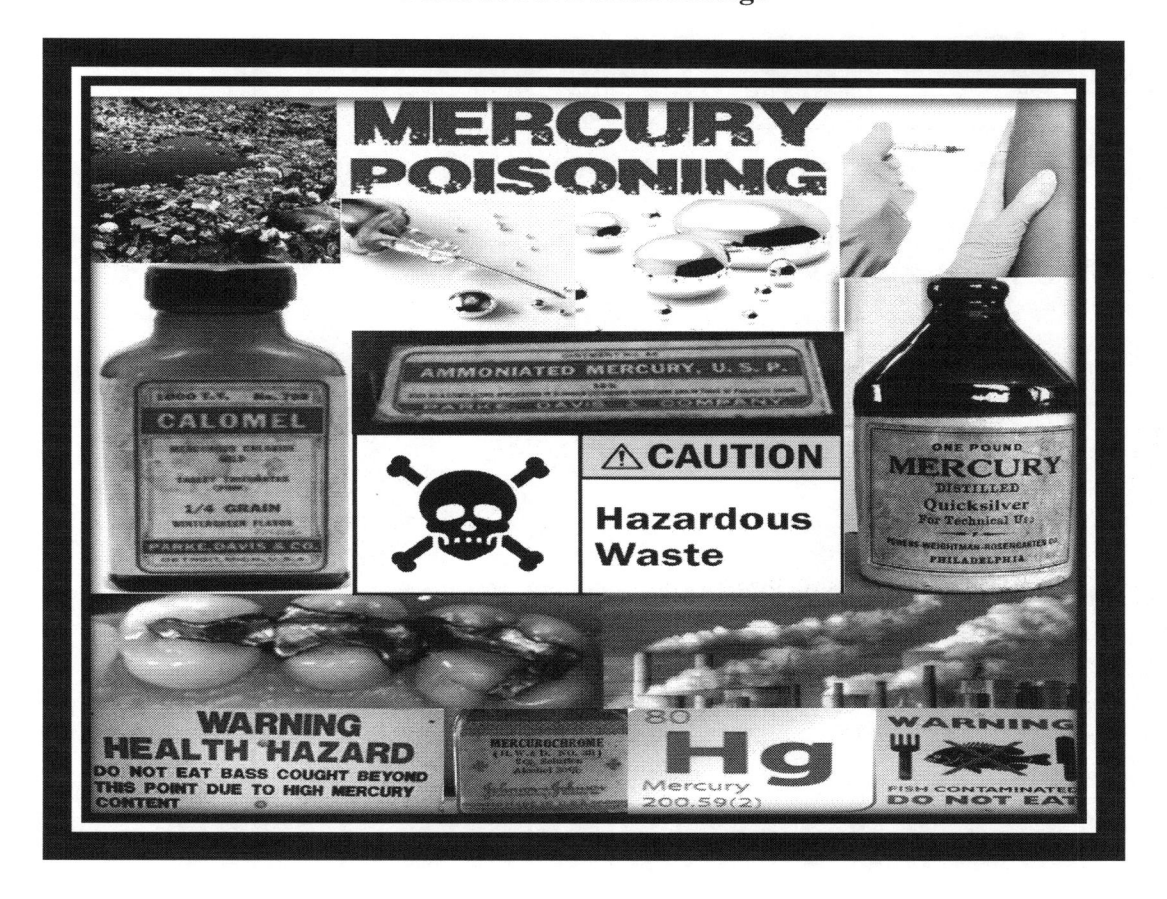

Our government estimates that one in six children being born is at risk of having developmental problems due to mercury contamination. Autopsy studies show that the level of mercury in brain tissue is directly proportional to the number of fillings in the mouth of the mother. (New England Journal of Medicine, vol. 349, Oct 30, 2003, pp. 1731)

In 1979, Dr. Hal Huggins began measuring electrical currents from metal amalgam fillings in the mouth. He also discovered that these electrical currents increase mercury release. Silver, amalgam dental fillings contain five metals: mercury, silver, tin, copper and zinc. When these metals are placed in your mouth, with the salt solution in your saliva, they create a battery that generates electrical currents or a flow of electrons. These minute electrical currents can wreak havoc on your health because they interfere with cellular function, especially the delicate nervous system and your brain. The renowned German physician Dr. Reinhard Voll estimated, after more than 40 years of research and observation, that nearly 80 percent of all illness is related entirely or partially to problems in the mouth.

Amalgam Dental Fillings Contain:
- 50% Mercury
- 15-30% Silver
- 10% Tin
- 3-30% Copper
- 1% Zinc

> **"It is interesting to note that cardiovascular disease has become widespread only since the 1920s, about the time of increased use of heavy metals in dental therapy but long after humans began consuming eggs, meat, milk, butter, and cheese, commonly thought to contribute to heart disease."** Daniel F. Royal, D.O., Medical Director of the Nevada Clinic and the Royal Center of Advanced Medicine, Las Vegas, NV

In 2004, dentists in the U.S. purchased 30.4 tons of mercury. In 2009, the FDA was ordered by a federal judge to change its content to read, *"Dental amalgams contain mercury, which may have neurotoxic effects on the nervous systems of developing children and fetuses."* Why? Because mercury is a poison! Mercury permeates all tissue and organs. Dr. Fritz Lorscheider from the University of Calgary School of Medicine demonstrated that mercury vapor from dental fillings placed in sheep traveled to various parts of the body, including the heart tissue of fetuses, the brain, pituitary, thyroid and adrenal glands.

> **"Mercury kills cells by interfering with their ability to exchange oxygen, nutrients, and waste products through the cell membrane. Inside the cell, mercury destroys our genetic code, DNA, leaving us without the ability to reproduce that cell ever again."** Hal A. Huggins, D.D.S., Founder of the Huggins Diagnostic Center

Mark A. Breiner, D.D.S., author of *Whole-Body Dentistry,* encourages you to ask your dentist why is it that before a silver (amalgam) filling is put into the mouth, it is considered a hazardous toxin? When it is removed, why must it be stored in a hazardous waste sealed container and taken away by a licensed hazardous waste company? The answer is obvious. Silver dental fillings are hazardous waste and according to the ADA, the only safe place to put them is in your mouth! Your mouth has become a toxic waste dump, and you paid to have the poison put in your teeth! So, according to the ADA, the fillings were safe to be put in your teeth, but once removed, magically become toxic. Does this make any sense?

> **OSHA mandates that a Materials Safety Data Sheet for mercury be present in every dental office. Here are the rules for handling scrap amalgam dental fillings:**
> 1. Store in unbreakable, tightly sealed containers, away from heat.
> 2. Use a no-touch technique for handling amalgam.
> 3. Store under liquid, preferably glycerin or photographic fixer solution.

The most commonly used amalgam is Dispersalloy, manufactured by Dentsply Caulk. On the box in large red letters it says: "DANGER VERY TOXIC TO AQUATIC LIFE WITH LONG-LASTING EFFECTS." "... DO NOT ALLOW MERCURY TO BE RELEASED INTO STREAMS OR WATERWAYS." Hmmm, if it's toxic to fish, how could it not be toxic to humans?

> **"I don't feel comfortable using a substance (silver dental fillings) designated by the EPA to be a waste disposal hazard. I can't throw it in the trash, bury it in the ground, or put it in a landfill, but they say it's OK to put it in people's mouths. That doesn't make sense."** Richard D. Fischer, D.D.S.

The U.S. Department of Health and Human Services lists mercury as the third most hazardous substance known to mankind, and the World Health Organization admits there is no minimum level of mercury that does not cause harm. It is so toxic that if a thermometer breaks in an elementary school, by law, the children are required to evacuate, and hazmat and OSHA are called in to clean up the toxic disaster. The area must be declared safe for children to re-enter. If inorganic mercury (the least toxic form) from a thermometer is so dangerous, then how could mercury in your silver fillings in your mouth be safe? They are not. We have been lied to about the safety of silver dental fillings.

A silver dental filling contains about 50 percent mercury. One molar mercury filling has about the same amount of mercury as a thermometer. The ADA and most dentists are under the impression that mercury and other metals are tightly bound and do not leak out; however, research proves otherwise. In 1986, the ADA finally admitted that mercury vapor does escape from amalgam fillings into a patient's mouth. Ironically, they then turn around and foolishly say it's safe to put in your mouth, despite researchers having demonstrated that a single amalgam filling releases as much as 15 micrograms of mercury per day!

Mercury vapor is considered the deadliest form of mercury because it is inhaled and passes through the lungs and into the blood stream, which carries mercury to all areas of the body, and adversely affects the nervous system and brain.

Researchers have even demonstrated that about 36 micrograms of mercury per cubic foot of air is released from the average amalgam filling with no stimulation, and 80 percent of the vapor is absorbed into the body.

More and more couples are having trouble conceiving. Why? Mercury has an affinity for sperm. If a woman has sensitivity to mercury, then she will produce antibodies that will target and kill mercury-laden sperm. Another problem is that mercury interferes with certain minerals such as selenium, zinc and manganese, which are necessary for sperm mobility. To make matters worse, mercury causes a loss of libido, which will guarantee a strike out in the pregnancy department if the home-run king never steps into the batters' box.

Years ago, mercury was used in contraceptive gels because it kills sperm. According to the CDC and EPA, one in 12 women of child-bearing age has unsafe levels of mercury. Mercury accumulates in the hypothalamus and pituitary, which secrete hormones necessary for pregnancy.

Is it coincidence that dentists who handle mercury fillings have the highest suicide and divorce rate among professionals? Dentists, according to insurance agencies, have one of the highest utilization rates of medical insurance as well. According to Joel Butler, Ph.D., professor of psychology at the University of North Texas, neuropsychological dysfunction was reported in 90 percent of dentists tested. These findings were reported at the ICBM conference in November 1988. Is it just coincidence that female dental personnel have a higher spontaneous abortion rate, a raised incidence of premature labor and an elevated perinatal mortality than any other profession?

Your work environment affects your health, and when you are around toxic metals all day, it has adverse effects. And for those who believe there is no harm in handling metals, try putting a piece of garlic in your shoe and walking around. In less than 10 minutes you'll taste the garlic in your mouth. Remember, anything you touch has the ability to pass through the skin and be absorbed into your blood.

An EDS scan checks for heavy metal poisoning. When metals show up, people always ask where they are getting them. Well, the average person consumes about 3-10 milligrams of aluminum daily from cookware, utensils, foil, deodorants, bleached flours, grated cheeses and prescription medications. Feminine hygiene products such as Massengill and Summer's Eve contain aluminum. Even fluorescent lights contain mercury. That's why LEDs are a better choice. They are mercury-free and more economical.

Industry mixes mercury with other substances to create ethyl or methyl mercury, which renders it more assimilable by your body, making it more poisonous. Coal plants and the combustion of fossil fuels fill the air with mercury vapors. Manufacturing plants dump mercury-filled wastes into our rivers, which make their way to the ocean, polluting the environment, and then we eat the fish. An article published in 2009 in USA Today showed that research done by the U.S. Geological Survey found every fish caught in a U.S. stream tested positive for mercury, and 27 percent of the fish caught had mercury levels high enough to exceed what the EPA considered safe to consume.

Another big culprit for heavy metal poisoning is tattoos. Tattoo ink contains a host of toxic and even carcinogenic ingredients, according to WebMD, so before you run out there to get your cool new tattoo, remember, tattoo inks, depending upon the manufacturer, may contain mercury, iron, lead, cadmium and aluminum. They can cause allergies and serious health problems.

In 1840, dentists here in the U.S. formed the American Society of Dental Surgeons. Members of this association were required to sign pledges promising not to use mercury in dental fillings. Some dentists were even suspended from the dental society for using silver mercury fillings in 1848. Mercury was referred to as "quicksilver" or "quacksalver." A "quack" is someone who pretends to cure disease, and a "salve" is medicine for a wound. It is interesting to note that the name "quack" was first given to anyone using mercury preparations on the skin claiming to "cure" disease. Ironically, many dentists are quick to label you a quack if you claim mercury fillings are harmful!

The old expression "mad as a hatter" refers to hat makers years ago who contracted mercury poisoning from processing hat felt using mercuric chloride. Those who were exposed to mercury as they made their hats often developed mental illnesses and became "mad as a hatter."

> **A truth's initial commotion is directly proportional to how deeply the lie was believed ... When a well-packaged web of lies has been sold gradually to the masses over generations, the truth will seem utterly preposterous and its speaker a raving lunatic."** Dresden James, British Novelist, 1931-2008

Various studies have demonstrated that small amounts of inorganic mercury cause high blood pressure, while larger amounts can cause low blood pressure. Russian researcher I.M. Trachtenberg revealed that mercury blocks acetylcholine, the neurotransmitter that allows nerve impulses to pass signals to organ tissues. It also damages the vagal nerve and constricts coronary arteries.

Mercury Detoxifying Support	
Glutathione	Selenium
Sulfur – (garlic, onions, eggs)	Chlorella
N-acetyl - L Cysteine	Methionine
DMSA – chelator	Vitamin C
DMPS – mercury chelator	Zinc
EDTA – chelator	Cilantro
Magnesium	Vitamin B6

R.P. Sharma and E.J. Obersteiner at Utah State University discovered mercury to be the single most toxic metal that they have investigated (even in such minute concentrations as 3.74×10^{-7} moles). Their research has proven that just a few micrograms disrupt normal cellular function. They inform that, *"Mercury is a strong protoplasmic poison that penetrates all living cells of the human body."*

At the Huggins Diagnostic Center, for patients in treatment or consultation for heavy metal toxicity, 1,320 patients reported the following symptoms.

Heavy Metal Toxicity Symptoms

1.	Unexplained irritability	73%	16.	Shortness of breath	43%
2.	Depression	72%	17.	Heartburn	43%
3.	Numbness and tingling	67%	18.	Itching	41%
4.	Frequent urination at night	65%	19.	Rashes, skin irritations	40%
5.	Chronic fatigue	63%	20.	Metallic taste in mouth	39%
6.	Cold hands and feet	63%	21.	Jumpy, jittery, nervous	38%
7.	Bloated feeling often	61%	22.	Death wish or suicidal	37%
8.	Loss of memory	58%	23.	Insomnia	36%
9.	Sudden anger	56%	24.	Chest pains	36%
10.	Constipation	55%	25.	Joint pains	36%
11.	Difficulty making decisions	54%	26.	Tachycardia	32%
12.	Tremors/shakes	52%	27.	Fluid retention	28%
13.	Twitching of muscles	52%	28.	Burning tongue	21%
14.	Leg cramps	49%	29.	Headaches after eating	20%
15.	Ringing in ears	49%	30.	Diarrhea	15%

Douglas Swartzendruber, Ph.D., experimental pathologist at the University of Colorado, explains that the accumulation of mercury from dental fillings in the central nervous system is an important connection to understanding neurological disorders such as multiple sclerosis. It has also been identified as a major contributor to ALS (Lou Gehrig's disease). The brain and central nervous system tend to attract mercury and other heavy metals.

> **"It is difficult to get a man to understand something when his salary depends upon his not understanding it."** Upton Sinclair, American Writer, 1878-1968

Your immune system has a group of marine-like soldiers who roam around looking for foreigners. They are the white blood cells. When they identify a cell that doesn't have proper identification to be in your body, their job is to destroy them. Each cell carries an I.D. card like a driver's license or passport. Healthy cells carry a five-protein I.D. card that allows them to exist in your body and escape harassment from white blood cells. Cells that have an altered code, such as ones with an atom of mercury attached to them, are ordered to be destroyed by the white blood cells. When doctors see the immune system attacking certain toxic cells, they misunderstand what is occurring and call it an autoimmune disease. Your intelligent immune system doesn't make mistakes; instead, it destroys foreign toxins. So, if cells are toxic with mercury, pesticides, a virus, Borrelia burgdorferi or a gluten molecule, the immune system attacks the toxic cells. The only way to truly stop the war is to remove the mercury or the toxins so cells can reveal themselves as "good guys." ALS is an example of this internal battle occurring.

In Dr. Masaru Emoto's book, *The Hidden Messages in Water*, he references toxic heavy metals that emit specific vibrational frequencies that resonate with certain emotions. When you understand how toxic metals are to delicate cells, it's a no-brainer that these toxins produce disease. A wise person avoids exposure to neurotoxic metals.

Metals Emit Emotional Vibrations	
Mercury	= Irritation
Lead	= Anger
Aluminum	= Sadness
Cadmium	= Uncertainty
Steel	= Despair
Zinc	= Stress

Mercury Facts

- Autopsies reveal a correlation between the amount of mercury found in brain tissue and the number and size of amalgam fillings in the mouth.

- Every time you eat food, chew gum, brush your teeth etc., mercury vapors come off the fillings. Drinking hot drinks and heated foods accelerates the release of mercury vapors.

- A 4-foot fluorescent light bulb contains about 8 milligrams of mercury and should be disposed of as hazardous waste. The average dental silver filling in your mouth contains about 1,000 milligrams of mercury. Place that much mercury in a 10-acre lake and the government says you cannot eat the fish from it.

- Multiple Sclerosis patients have been found to have 8 times higher levels of mercury in the cerebrospinal fluid compared to neurologically healthy controls (Eggleston, D.W., and M. Nylander, "Correlation of Dental Amalgam With Mercury in Brain Tissue." Journal of Prosthetic Dentistry, 58 (1987).

- Research has indicated that placement of amalgam fillings in monkeys has impaired kidney function by 60% in 60 days.

- Dr. Boyd Haley at the University of Kentucky has discovered that patients with Alzheimer's disease have higher than average levels of mercury in the tissue of their brains. When exposing rats to mercury vapors similar to what would typically be found in people with silver fillings, the rats developed changes in the brain that are similar to changes that occur in Alzheimer's patients.

- Pregnant women who have amalgam fillings run the risk of passing heavy metals to their unborn. In Canada, a study was done by Drs. Fritz Lorscheider and Murray Vimy, where they placed amalgam fillings in pregnant sheep. The mercury in the fillings was radioactively labeled so that the scientists could definitively trace the mercury to the fillings. After a few days, the sheep were examined and the findings were shocking. The amalgam-related mercury had spread to all the tissues of both the mother sheep and the unborn fetuses. Higher concentrations of mercury had accumulated in the kidneys, thyroid, intestines and jawbone.

- A German research team studied babies who died from SIDS (Sudden Infant Death Syndrome). Upon close examination, the research team found that mercury in the babies' brains was directly proportional to the number of fillings in their mothers' mouths. It is currently illegal to use amalgam dental fillings in Germany.

> **"Why is the ADA highly concerned about scrap amalgam while it preaches the safety of the amalgam in your mouth? It's the same stuff."** Hal A. Huggins, D.D.S.

Toxline is a search engine affiliated with the Agency for Toxic Substances and Disease Registry, a subdivision of the CDC. This search engine allows you to see the studies that have been done on toxicity issues such as mercury linked to cancer, heart disease, autism or Alzheimer's. For example, a search for "mercury and autism" pulls up 257 studies that reveal high mercury levels are associated with autism, while "mercury and cancer" pulls up 833 studies. People argue and say where's the scientific proof, or the CDC claims "the science is settled?" Well, here are thousands of published research articles that tell a different story if you want the science. As long as we are still alive and breathing, the science is never settled.

> Go to **TOXLINE or PubMed** search engine and look up any subject. This is the U.S. National Library of Medicine.

> **"Mercury may well be one of the biggest culprits in damaging DNA and setting the body up for various types of diseases."** Stephen B. Edelson, M.D.

Safe Dental Amalgam Removal
1. Wear a nose mask to breathe oxygen (avoid mercury vapors)
2. Use a rubber dam
3. Use large amounts of water
4. Use high-speed suction

When having dental work done, it is important to remember that anything placed in the mouth is toxic to some degree, and the important question is, which dental material is least toxic to you? Also, digital X-rays are much safer, because they greatly reduce radiation exposure.

> **"You should never put a gold crown in a mouth with amalgam (silver) fillings. The gold will speed up the release of mercury from the amalgams, so that your body burden of mercury will increase faster than it would with just amalgams alone."** Mark A. Breiner, D.D.S.

Are Your Root Canals & Cavitations Harboring Toxic Bacteria?

A root canal procedure consists of taking a dead tooth and scraping out the inner pulpal tissue, leaving the shell (dentin) and outer enamel, and keeping the dead tooth in the body. Once the pulp (the guts) has been removed, the dentist does what he can to disinfect the hollowed-out tooth. A tooth's dentin contains millions of microscopic, tiny tubules that transport nutrients from the center of the tooth to the enamel. It is estimated that if you laid out the tubules from end to end, from one small tooth, they would stretch about 3 miles long! These micro canals are so tiny that they are undetectable on X-rays. The problem is, it is impossible to completely sterilize these millions of tubules during a root canal procedure; however, most dentists have been trained that sterilizing the canal will kill any bacteria. Unfortunately, this is not true. The canal is then packed with a latex material called gutta-percha that is supposed to seal off the canal and render it a germ-free area; however, with the tooth canal area being closed off to the constant cleansing and oxygenating effect of the blood and lymph supply, it can become a breeding ground for infection. Dr. George Meinig explains in his book, *Root Canal Cover-Up*, when gutta-percha cools and hardens, it shrinks enough for bacteria to enter the teeth and provide a breeding ground for bacteria to thrive. Once the tooth is sealed at the top, any remaining bacteria locked within the dark, moist, low-oxygen environment is in an ideal atmosphere to thrive.

Odontoblasts (special cells that create dentin) extend into the tubules, and during the root canal procedure, they are left in the tubules and die. Like any living cell, once they die, they begin to decay and rot, just as the flesh of a putrefying corpse. As the biological terrain changes, these microbes and other pathological microbiota can migrate to other areas of the body, causing serious disease.

Research has shown that pathogenic bacteria from infected root canals destroy and kill white blood cells designed to eliminate them by your immune system. Another cause for infection is bacterial mimicry, when the bacteria mimics your body's own bacteria, causing your white blood cells not to attack. This can also lead to biofilms, where pathogens can hide out and are safe from the immune system.

> **"One third of all disease in this country can be either directly or indirectly traced to dental infections."** George E. Meinig, D.D.S., Author of *Root Canal Cover-Up*

Dr. Weston Price Proved How Toxic Root Canals Are

Many health problems will simply not clear up if there is an infected tooth as the cause. Extraction of the root-canaled tooth, in many instances, is the best solution, along with proper cleansing of the infected area (jaw). To demonstrate how toxic root-canaled teeth can be, Dr. Weston Price implanted root-canaled teeth from a heart disease patient under the skin of healthy rabbits. The rabbits soon developed heart disease and died. A rabbit's immune system is similar to a human. Dr. Price continued repeating this experiment with the same tooth on 27 different rabbits. Every rabbit died, even after autoclaving the tooth at high temperatures for 24 hours. To prove that these experiments with root-canaled teeth could be the culprits for disease and death, he performed other experiments to eliminate the possibility of coincidence. He took healthy teeth, non-decayed (wisdom) teeth and other sterile objects such as coins, pieces of glass and metal and sewed them under the skin of rabbits. No symptoms were reported and all rabbits appeared to be unaffected.

Dr. Price also demonstrated how deadly root-canaled teeth can be when he removed them from heart disease patients and ground them into a powder, which he sterilized and put through a filter to remove all bacteria. When a tiny amount of that powder was injected into rabbits, they died of heart disease. Dr. Price explains that bacteria from infected teeth can remain in the 3 miles of tubules, growing and multiplying and changing forms. These microbes produce toxic chemicals that many times cause illness. The bacteria in your mouth usually don't become a problem until they mutate into an anaerobic environment, like a root canal provides.

> **"Root canal treated teeth have now been proven to have a direct cause and effect relationship with the formation of the blood clots that acutely block off the blood flow in the coronary arteries and cause myocardial infarctions. Root canal treated teeth are the direct cause for the vast majority of heart attacks, period."** Thomas E. Levy, M.D.

Cavitations – A Breeding Ground For Infection

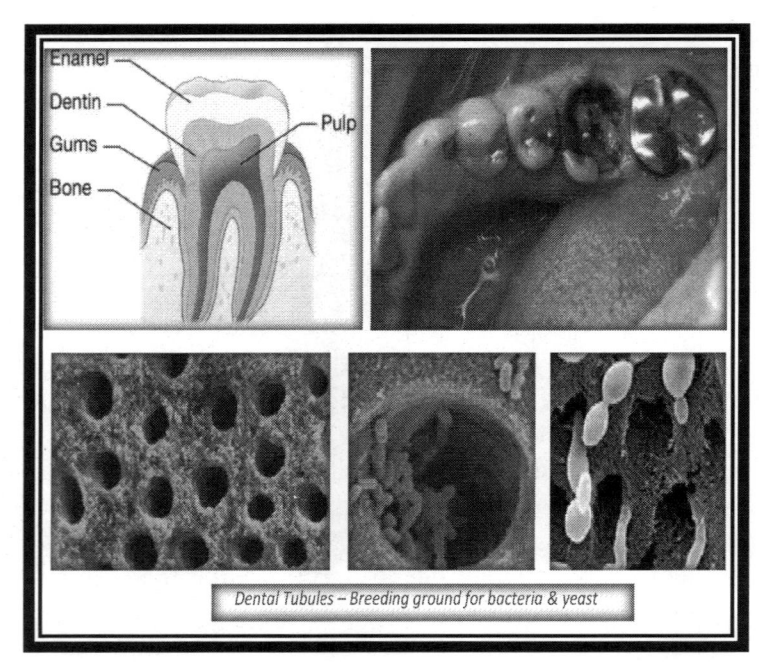

Dental Tubules – Breeding ground for bacteria & yeast

Your mouth contains more than 6 billion bacteria, with over 500 different species.

Cavitations, or holes in the bone from where teeth have been removed (wisdom teeth), are more often than not breeding grounds for anaerobic bacteria that continually seep into the system. If you have pain in the upper cheek, you may have an infection in a cavitation or root canal.

When a fluorescent dye was injected in the abdomens of rats, within 10 minutes, the dye was found in the dentinal tubules of the teeth. So, if you have an infection in a tooth or the gums, like periodontal bacteria, it can travel anywhere in the body. It has been shown that periodontal bacteria have been identified in atherosclerotic plaque. In fact, researchers in Finland analyzed blood clots that were aspirated out of blocked coronary arteries in individuals who had heart attacks. Using PCR testing, they identified that the same bacterial DNA in root-canaled teeth and gum disease was exactly the same as that found in arterial plaque and blood clots that caused the heart attack. They also found the same bacteria in the pericardial fluid that surrounds the heart. Could the majority of heart attacks be triggered by pathogens from infections located in the jaw or root-canaled teeth? As Dr. Robert Kulacz explains, "…the presence of oral bacteria from root canal teeth and gum disease in the arterial plaque and blood clots of heart attack patients points to direct causation, rather than correlation, between oral infection and cardiovascular disease."

> **"We dentists cause more ill health than any other profession; we just don't take proper credit."** Dr. Ed Arana, Founder of The Academy of Biological Dentistry

Dr. Mark Breiner tells his patients that if you suddenly have a drastic change in your health, the first things to check are root canals and implants. They may be harboring deadly bacteria that could possibly be the missing link to your health issues.

Just as bacteria from root-canaled teeth match the bacteria found in heart-attack-causing blood clots, the same researchers have identified matching bacteria from teeth that is found in ruptured intracranial aneurysms, linking dental infections as being a major culprit. Research continues to connect the dots of harmful bacteria from the jaw being associated with other problem areas in the body. For example, H-pylori bacteria, which causes ulcers in the stomach, many times originates from the bacteria in your mouth that is continuously swallowed.

> **One dot (.) this size in your mouth can contain 250,000 – 500,000 Anaerobic Bacteria**

When third molars (wisdom teeth) are removed, cavitations are left behind, which can become infected. Years later, if you experience tenderness, that is a possible indication of infection. Bacteria can get trapped in the cavitations and become anaerobic bacteria, giving off toxins. Many of the body's major organs, including the heart, are on the wisdom tooth meridian. Dr. Voll taught that cavitations in the wisdom tooth area are one of the leading causes of heart problems.

Cavitations have poor blood flow, so most antibiotics are ineffective in targeting infections in them. A biological dentist many times will open up the cavitation and cleanse out the infection, then re-pack it using platelet-rich plasma, which is a powerhouse of white blood cells and nitric oxide, to help regrow tissue and speed up healing. Ask your dentist if he or she uses platelet-rich plasma. Using ozone and high doses of Vitamin C are very beneficial as well.

> **Platelet Rich Plasma Therapy Helps Regeneration of Bone & Faster Wound Healing**

To identify infected cavitations, 3D X-ray imaging will reveal troubled areas. Dental Cone Beam is a special type of X-ray machine used when regular dental X-rays are not sufficient to identify infection. Also, most biological dentists agree that if an implant is needed, zirconium implants are usually safer (least toxic), because they do not contain metallic ions like titanium implants do.

Dr. Boyd Haley has proven that more than 90 percent of all root-canaled teeth are teeming with dozens of different pathogens and their toxic byproducts. Dr. Haley has also shown that some toxins removed from cavitations are even more toxic than deadly botulinum!

> **"My dental assistant once described an extracted root canal-treated tooth as smelling like a dead mouse that had been decomposing for a while."** Dr. Thomas Levy

Cancer can many times be caused from root canals, cavitations and mercury in the teeth, according to Dr. Vincent Speckhart, an oncologist in Virginia. There is a close relationship to pathogens such as Fusobacterium, found in chronically infected teeth, and cancerous breast tissue. Dr. Josef Issels of Germany, after treating cancer for over 50 years, has found this to be true as well. The tonsils are an indicator for the body's ability to deal with infections. He explains that the tonsils are part of the lymph system and act as filters, to help trap viruses, bacteria and toxins that can come from root canals and other infected areas. When India ink is placed in dental pulp, within 30 minutes it will show up in the tonsils. This is a clear indication that toxins from teeth drain into the tonsils. Hopefully you weren't a victim of the massive amounts of tonsillectomies that doctors performed in the 1970s because they perceived tonsils as "worthless."

The Cause Of Your Illness May Be In Your Mouth
- Root canals – harboring bacteria
- Infected teeth – Chronic Apical Periodontitis (CAP)
- Periodontal (gum) infection/inflammation
- Cavitational gangrene/bacterial infections
- Infected tonsils – draining root canals/infected teeth
- Infected dental implants
- Allergies to dental materials
- Toxic metals – mercury poisoning

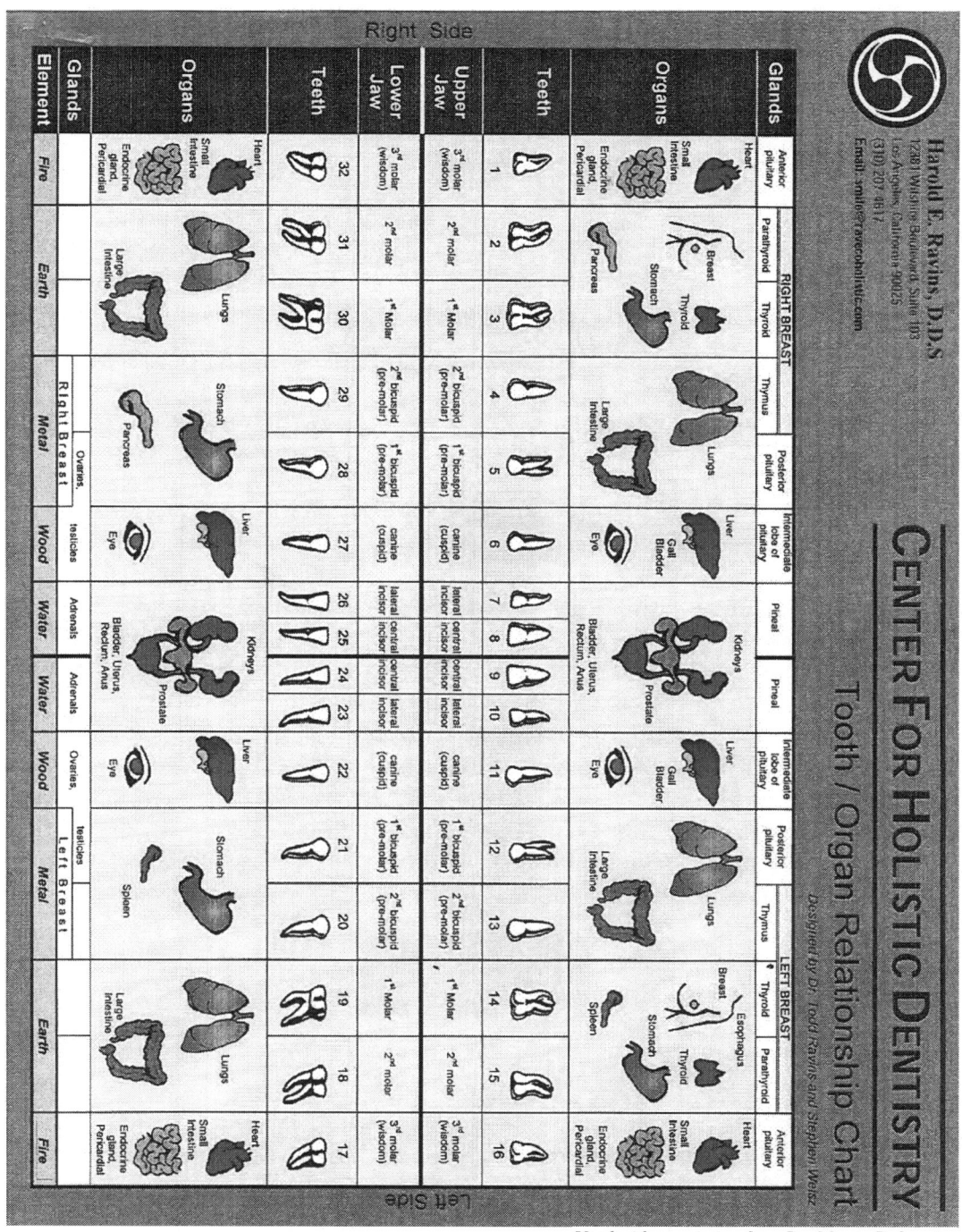

Used with permission from Dr. Mamta Dalwani

Dr. Issels reports that 97 percent of terminal cancer patients have root canals. Infrared imaging is used to identify hot spots associated with tumors. Dr. Thomas Rau, who operates the Paracelsus Klinik in Switzerland, claims that you cannot heal cancer until you treat mercury, root canals and cavitations. He finds that women with breast cancer usually have a root-canaled tooth on the meridian associated with the breast. Breast meridian connected teeth are Nos. 2, 3, 14, 15, 20, 21, 28 and 29. These teeth are your first and second molars on the upper jaw and first and second bicuspid on the lower jaw.

> "The vast majority of the adult population of the world has at least one significant tooth infection. Yet, these teeth nearly always go undiscovered and are rarely addressed. Never the less, it is these teeth along with infected tonsils and infected gums that cause the vast majority of heart attacks and cases of breast cancer." Thomas E. Levy, M.D.

Dr. Kulveer Mankia informs that research shows that rheumatoid arthritis (RA) associated antibodies are present well before symptoms occur, indicating that they originate from a site outside of the joint. He explains that periodontal disease and its bacteria may provide the primary trigger, the key initiator to systemic autoimmunity seen in RA.

Locate A Biological Dentist – Science-Based Dentistry

A biological dentist has been properly trained in how to remove mercury fillings in a safe and effective manner, with the least amount of metal toxicity exposure to the patient. Some dental materials, glue or cement may trigger allergies. A biological dentist can send off for a materials compatibility test, to look for possible allergies and what materials would be safest and least toxic to go in your teeth. Using materials that complement your immune system, instead of aggravating it, can have a huge impact on your overall health. To locate a biological dentist in your area, go to International Academy of Oral Medicine and Toxicology, (AOMT.org) and look for a Safe Mercury Amalgam Removal Technique (SMART) certified dentist.

> Locate A Biological Dentist
> **IAOMT.org** or **IABDM.org**
> 863-420-6373

Autism – A Symptom Of Heavy Metal Poisoning

We are bombarded with heavy metals in the environment, without the help of doctors injecting them into our bodies through vaccinations and silver amalgam dental fillings. Most autistic children lack the capability to detoxify mercury from the brain. When mercury accumulates and begins to interfere with neurological behavior, one of the most common symptoms is autistic behavior.

A recent study investigated 100 autistic children. Children whose mothers had six or more mercury fillings had a severe form of autism. Mothers who had five or fewer mercury fillings had children with a much milder degree of autism.

> **"There is NO CONTROVERSY! The failure of others to recognize facts does not change the truth."** Rashid A. Buttar, D.O. (Referring to Mercury Poisoning & Autism)

The Material Safety Data Sheet from Eli Lilly, June 13, 1991 (Section 5 – Health Hazard Information) clearly warns that thimerosal, (an ingredient in vaccines) which contains mercury, is a chemical known to cause birth defects, nervous system disorders, numbness in the extremities and even mental retardation.

> **"Mercury is the 'spark' that causes the 'fires' of autism as well as Alzheimer's. Autism is the result of high mercury exposure early in life versus Alzheimer's is a chronic accumulation of mercury over a life time. A doctor can treat ALL the 'fires,' but until the 'spark' is removed, there is minimal hope of complete recovery with most improvements being transient at best. However, once the process of mercury removal has been effectively started, the damage is curtailed and full recovery becomes possible and enhanced by utilizing various additional therapies including nutrition, hyperbarics, etc."** Rashid A. Buttar, D.O., FAAPM, FACAM, FAAIM (Vice chairman, American Board of Clinical Metal Toxicology)

Rashid A. Buttar, D.O., is the medical director of The Center for Advanced Medicine in Charlotte, North Carolina, where he has treated over 500 autistic children. By using the best of conventional, traditional and alternative medical treatments, his practice is highly successful in treating autism. He teaches that in order to heal autism, heavy metals, especially mercury, must be detoxified from the body. To learn more about his clinic and how he successfully treats autism, as well as cancer, heart disease and other chronic conditions, look him up at www.drbuttar.com or call his office at 704-895-9355.

Dr. Buttar explains that blood tests that check for mercury toxicity levels are useless. These metals are so toxic that the body pushes them out of the blood stream and stores them deep in the tissue. Lead is commonly stored in the bones, mercury in fat and the myocardium (striated muscle that makes up the heart).

> **"For the great enemy of truth is very often not the lie — deliberate, contrived, and dishonest — but the myth — persistent, persuasive, and unrealistic. Too often we hold fast to the clichés of our forebears. We subject all facts to a prefabricated set of interpretations. We enjoy the comfort of opinion without the discomfort of thought."** John F. Kennedy

Chapter 6
VACCINATIONS – WOLVES IN SHEEP'S CLOTHING

> "**The further a society drifts from the truth, the more it will hate those who speak it.**" George Orwell, English Journalist (1903-1950)

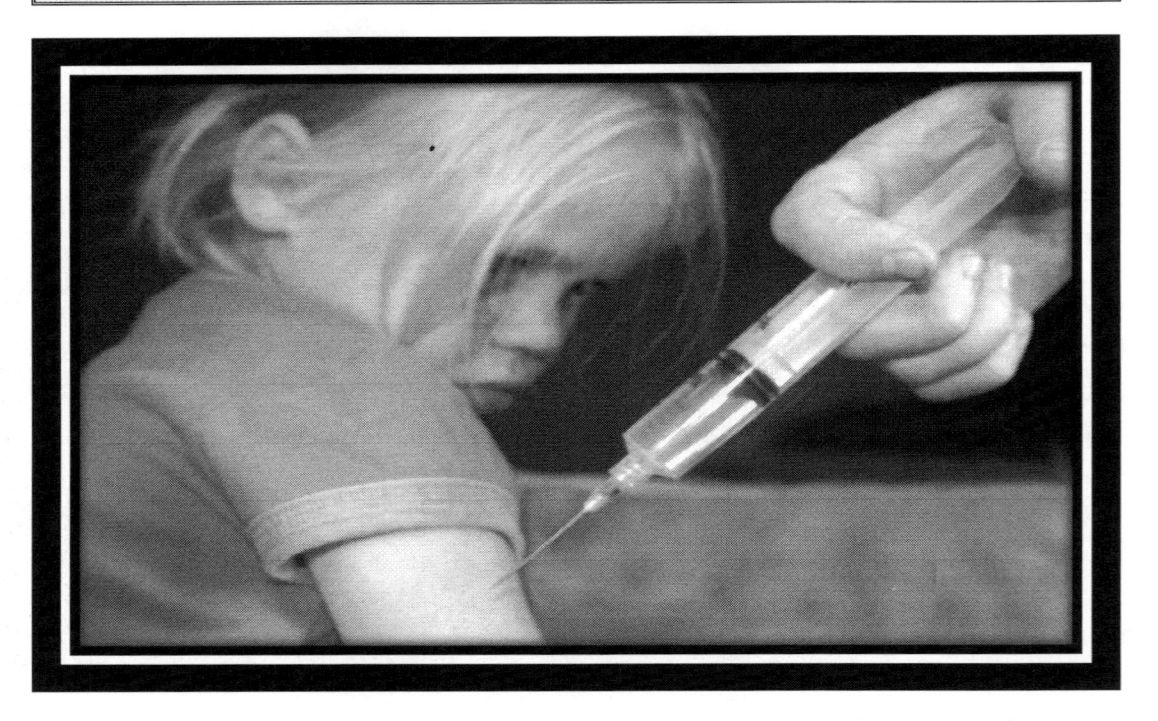

Michael Belkin was the proud father of a beautiful new daughter. Like most good parents, he wanted the best for her, so he trusted his doctors to give her vaccinations for disease prevention. When she was 5 weeks old, he took her in to get a second hepatitis B shot. That night, she began having tremors and was extremely agitated. Within 15 hours, his precious beautiful baby girl died. The autopsy report revealed a swollen brain, typical of vaccination toxicity.

> "**I am, and have been for years, a confirmed anti-vaccinationist ... I have not the least doubt in my mind that vaccination is a filthy process that is harmful in the end.**" Mahatma Gandhi, 1869-1948 (Political & Spiritual Leader of India)

Hepatitis B is a blood-transmitted or sexually-transmitted disease common among prostitutes and illicit drug users. So why are we vaccinating our children who don't use drugs and have multiple sex partners? Since the hepatitis B vaccine was licensed in 1996, there have been over 9,000 reports of adverse reactions, and those are just the ones actually filed. Interestingly enough, the hepatitis B vaccine was outlawed in France in 1998, after 15,000 citizens filed a class action suit against the government, after a launch to eradicate hepatitis B by vaccinating all age groups, including adults. Shortly after the mass vaccination campaign, an alarming number of citizens were being diagnosed with multiple sclerosis. Was it just coincidence? The government wants you to believe it was, but the people who were perfectly healthy before receiving the vaccine and then suddenly diagnosed with MS say otherwise.

> **"There are two ways to be fooled. One is to believe what isn't true, the other is to refuse to accept what is true."** Soren Kierkegaard, Danish Philosopher 1813-1855

Scientific research reports a different story than what the government claims. Studies have shown that the hepatitis B vaccine significantly increases the risk of multiple sclerosis and serious autoimmune disorders. Adults who received the hepatitis B vaccine were five times more likely than the control group to develop multiple sclerosis. The hepatitis B vaccinated group also had a significantly increased risk for rheumatoid arthritis. (Geier DA, Geier MR. A case-control study of serous autoimmune adverse events following hepatitis B immunization. Autoimmunity 2005 Jun; 38(4): 295-301) Another study done in France revealed that there was a 65 percent increase in adults being diagnosed with multiple sclerosis one to two years after the national campaign to vaccinate for hepatitis B. (Le Houezec D. Evolution of multiple sclerosis in France since the beginning of hepatitis B vaccination. Immunol Res 2014 Dec; 60(2-3): 219-25) Why does the government and CDC ignore this research? And why isn't the media reporting it?

> **"The hepatitis B vaccine has 250 mcg of aluminum. The adult daily max is 50 mcg of aluminum ... Five times the adult maximum, you are going to inject into a newborn ... birthday present?"** Paul Thomas, M.D. (Pediatrician, Portland, OR)

Tina took her beautiful, healthy, 3-month-old son, Evan, in to get a DPT shot. His body responded with a swollen leg, loss of head control, high-pitched screaming and then he collapsed and died in a seizure. SIDS (Sudden Infant Death Syndrome) was the diagnosis.

In 1994, Tina gave birth to another beautiful baby, this time a daughter, she named Miranda. When Miranda was 9 months old, she took her in for her second DPT shot. She trusted her doctor when he reassured her that vaccines were safe, and Evan's death had nothing to do with the DPT shot. The nightmare began all over again with little Miranda. She reacted with high-pitched screaming that could not be quieted, just as it happened with Evan. Within 48 hours, little Miranda died. This time the pathologist concluded and the coroner agreed that the cause of death was the DPT shot.

> **"There is a great deal of evidence to prove that immunization of children does more harm than good."** Dr. J. Anthony Morris, Former Chief Vaccine Control Officer & Research Virologist, FDA

> **WARNING:**
> 99% of doctors will tell you to vaccinate your child. 0% of doctors will accept responsibility when your child is injured by that vaccine!

Unfortunately, it took two dead babies for the truth to be told. If you were Tina, what would you do about your two dead babies that were killed from the shot your doctor gave them, and reassured you that they were safe? The truth is, no one knows how these vaccines are going to react in a child's body. No tests are performed to screen out high-risk children. The Center for Disease Control and Prevention (CDC) and most pediatricians say vaccines are safe, but do they really know? Children experiencing adverse reactions, acting strangely and then dying after receiving their shots is more than just purely coincidence. A mother, who carried that baby in her womb for 9 months and has been with him or her, night and day, knows when something's not right with her baby, despite what know-it-all health-care providers say. Intuition will tell you when something's not right. The truth is, vaccines have not been proven to be safe with double-blind placebo-controlled investigations like drugs or any other procedures must pass before entering the public market. In vaccine safety trials, vaccines are compared to other vaccines, and not compared to an inert substance. So, if the number of side effects caused by the new vaccine is found to be the same as the old vaccine, manufacturers declare the new vaccine to be as safe and effective. This is a huge red flag and any honest scientist will tell you this is unethical, completely unacceptable and ridiculously absurd. This is not science!

> **"Can you inject a foreign substance of any kind into a little baby and believe that in any way it will improve its health?"** William Howard Hay, M.D., The Congressional Record (Founder & Medical Director, Sun-Diet Sanatorium, New York)

UFC fighter Nick Catone and his wife Marjorie, a nurse, did everything they thought was best for their newborn baby boy, Nicholas. She nursed him for nearly 9 months and then fed him healthy organic foods and used essential oils. They took him into the pediatrician for regular visits and to get his recommended vaccinations. They noticed that he almost always got sick with typical cold symptoms shortly after each round of vaccinations and occasionally ran a fever. As usual, he was prescribed antibiotics. Following their pediatrician's recommendations, one week after being on antibiotics, Nicholas received the MMR shot. Another round of antibiotics was ordered, as he displayed more cold symptoms after the shot. On April 25, Nicholas went in for his 18-month well visit and received the DTaP vaccine and developed another cold. Shortly after, he developed a rash, and 12 days later he became extremely lethargic and ran a high temperature. On May 12, their beautiful, 20-month-old baby boy went to sleep in his crib and never woke up. When Marjorie went in his room the next morning, he wasn't breathing. Their precious baby died in his sleep. The autopsy report revealed mild cerebral edema (swollen brain), mild pulmonary edema and visceral congestion, typical signs of vaccine injury.

To have a happy, loving, innocent baby suddenly die rips a parent's heart in half. Nick and Marjorie hope others wake up to the dangers of vaccines, so others don't experience the same nightmarish hell they have gone through. "DTaP is the shot that killed my son. The truth must come out," exclaims Nick. The Catones have teamed up with "Learn The Risk," a group that educates people on the dangers of pharmaceutical products and vaccines. They have placed 32 billboards around the world.

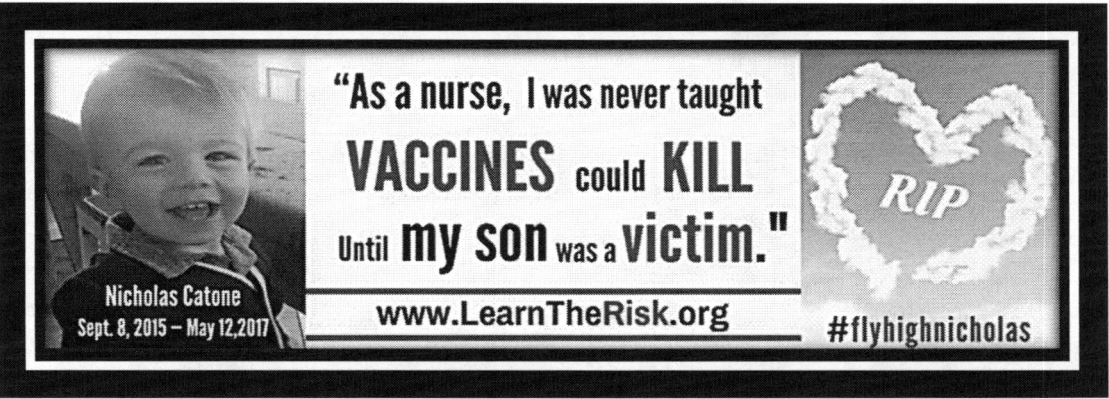

Used with permission from Nick Catone & Brandy Vaughan

> "Every day vaccine reactions happen, yet doctors won't report them and deny they exist. The very people who should speak the truth stay silent to protect their wallets, reputations, and practices. Their dishonesty betrays those they are supposed to protect. Vaccine-damaged families are treated so badly and exemptions are under threat because policy matters more than honesty."
> Suzanne Humphries, M.D.

Dr. Sherri Tenpenny pleads, "It continually breaks my heart that people have to personally experience a severe vaccine injury — or observe a serious reaction in someone they love — before they wake up to the absolute truth: vaccines can and do cause harm. They have heard the arguments and the stories from others. They ignored the pleas about risks and poo-pooed the concerns about vaccine reactions put forth by concerned friends. Instead, they trusted their uninformed pediatrician or caved under the pressure of their badgering RN mother-in-law."

> "When you give an injection like a vaccine, it explodes inside like a cluster bomb. All these diseases (diabetes, cancer, thyroid issues, etc.) use to be rare. Autism use to be 1 in 10,000. Now it's 1 in 50. Now, where is it all coming from? Vaccines are doing it." Dr. Shiv Chopra, Fellow of the World Health Organization

VAERS (Vaccine Adverse Event Reporting System)

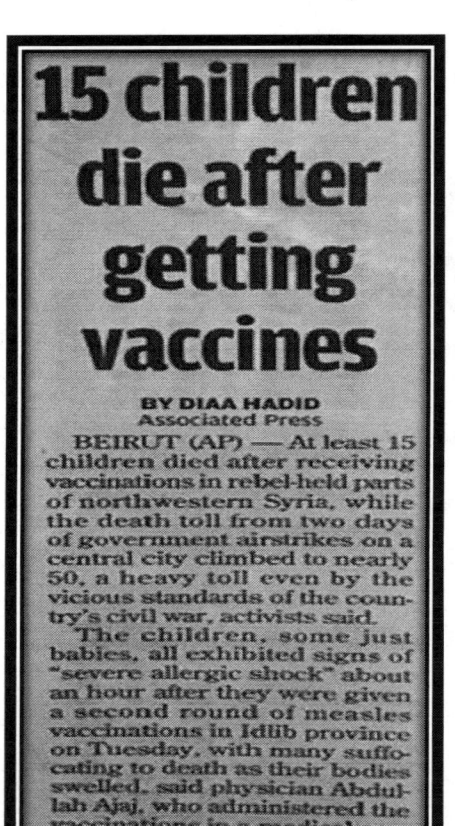

15 children die after getting vaccines

BY DIAA HADID
Associated Press

BEIRUT (AP) — At least 15 children died after receiving vaccinations in rebel-held parts of northwestern Syria, while the death toll from two days of government airstrikes on a central city climbed to nearly 50, a heavy toll even by the vicious standards of the country's civil war, activists said.

The children, some just babies, all exhibited signs of "severe allergic shock" about an hour after they were given a second round of measles vaccinations in Idlib province on Tuesday, with many suffocating to death as their bodies swelled, said physician Abdullah Ajaj, who administered the vaccinations in a medical center in the town of Jarjanaz.

2016 VACCINE ADVERSE EVENTS REPORTING SYSTEMS (VAERS)
59,117 Reports Filed in 2016:
432 Deaths
1,091 Permanent Disabilities
4,132 Hospitalizations
10,284 Emergency Room Visits

The fact that the government has a vaccine injury compensation program called VAERS (Vaccine Adverse Event Reporting System) is evidence in itself that vaccines are not safe and do cause harm; otherwise, there would be no need to offer such services to those who are harmed, right? From 1999 to 2004, a total of 128,035 adverse reactions were reported to VAERS, causing serious harm and 2,093 deaths. In 2016 alone, VAERS received 59,117 reports. If an adverse reaction occurs more than two weeks after a vaccine is administered, proving a connection is difficult; however, sometimes it takes a while before symptoms manifest, so the majority of incidences are never reported. Experts conclude that these figures are only a small percentage, because the system relies upon voluntary reporting and most pediatricians haven't been trained on what to look for with vaccine adverse reactions. Medical researchers like former FDA Commissioner Dr. David A. Kessler state that VAERS reports represent only a fraction of the serious adverse events. Many believe a more accurate number to be around 5 million adverse reactions a year, since it is estimated that less than 1 percent of adverse reactions are ever reported.

> "For over 20 years, the federal government has publicly denied a vaccine/autism link while at the same time, its Vaccine Injury Compensation Program has been awarding damages for vaccine injury to children with brain damage, seizures, and autism … Vaccines cause autism." Ken P. Stoller, M.D.

VAERS Has Paid Vaccine-Injured Families $3.7 Billion

President Ronald Reagan signed the National Vaccine Injury Compensation Act into law in 1988. Vaccine injury cases can sometimes end up going to a Vaccine Court. It may shock you to know that more than $3.7 billion has been paid to vaccine-injured victims, but only 20 percent of persons who apply receive compensation. If you're not guilty of wrongdoing, you don't pay $3.7 billion out to those victims who were harmed or killed from taking your product, right?

> "… it's troubling to me that in a recent Senate hearing on childhood vaccinations, it was never mentioned that our government has paid out over $3 BILLION through a vaccine injury compensation program for children who have been injured by vaccinations… at the same time it has claimed that vaccines do not cause injuries…" Bill Posey, U.S. Representative, Florida

CDC VACCINE SCHEDULE

1983	*2016*
24 doses	72 Doses
7 Injected	53 Injected
4 Oral	3 Oral

The U.S. has the highest vaccination requirements for infants in the world, at 26 doses, and we also have the highest amount of sick and chronically ill children, more than any other industrialized country. The CDC recommends an 8-in-1 vaccine combination to be given to infants at 2, 4 and 6 months old, but this combination has never been studied to see if it's safe. By the time a child is 6 years old, he or she will have received 49 doses of 14 vaccines.

> "There are 18 different ICD-9 codes that specify vaccine injury. Clearly, if there was no injury from vaccines, there would be no need to have an ICD-9 code." Irvin Sahni, M.D.

We Americans take pride in being good, many times even the best, but 33 nations have better infant mortality rates than we do. From the time our children are born until they are 18 years old, the CDC recommends 53 shots, which includes 72 doses in all, since some vaccines are multi-dose vials. If vaccines promote health and we get the most, why aren't our babies the healthiest in the world?

> **QUESTION: Has the vaccination schedule, with all these vaccines together, ever been tested?** "No, it has never been tested … **We are a global science experiment without a placebo.**" Dr. Lucija Tomljenovic

Mark Sibley, M.D., explains that he was taught that vaccine reactions like seizures, paralysis and SIDS were not ever possibly caused from vaccinations. He warns, "My older brother was an M.D. … He was an OB-GYN and took every vaccine and even 'extra' vaccines … He got leukemia at 50 and died within a few months … We were told it was not the 30 vaccines he took to be a 'safer' doctor … My baby brother was also an M.D. He did the same thing and got then a final annual flu shot at 56 and died a terrible death from Guillain-Barre paralysis and died in two months … We were told it was not from the flu shot … The vaccine court decided it was the cause of his death two years later and paid the family lots of blood money to hush them up."

> **"No one is more hated than he who speaks the truth."** Plato

Japan ranks at the top in highest life expectancy as well as having the world's lowest infant mortality rate. Babies born in the U.S. are

> **Merck's MMR Vaccine Package Insert, May Cause:** vomiting, diarrhea, anaphylaxis, ear pain, nerve deafness, diabetes, arthritis, myalgia, encephalitis, febrile seizures, pneumonia and **death.**

twice as likely to die in infancy as those born in Japan. The Japanese government banned the MMR (measles, mumps, and rubella) vaccine in 1993 after numerous children suffered adverse reactions including meningitis and death. Japan has also outlawed the hepatitis B vaccine at birth and is no longer actively promoting the HPV vaccine (Gardasil) either. According to the Japanese government in 2013, 1,968 adverse reactions were reported from the HPV vaccine, so their government did what any common-sense type of person would do, they banned it, before it could damage any more of their children. Why don't we do what is working for Japan?

> **"In 1975, when Japan stopped vaccinating children under the age of 2 years, dramatic improvements in their infant mortality occurred. Japan's place in the world scale of infant mortality went from 17, a poor position, to number 1, the best performance. It is quite clear that the shift of the lower vaccination limit to 2 years resulted in a dramatic decrease in SIDS, which dipped quickly from a very high, to the lowest rate of infant deaths in the world."** Dr. Mark Sircus

The injection of a virus along with chemicals and metals into the pure bloodstream of individuals does not prevent smallpox or any other disease; to the contrary, it increases disease epidemics and makes the disease deadlier. A healthy immune system is capable of handling the invasion of a single infection at any given time, like it occurs in nature; however, when we inject a child with many vaccines at once, they are bombarded with multiple diseases in one shot. Our immune systems were never meant to be bombarded with such devastating filth in one shot. No doctor knows how that onslaught of chemicals and pathogens will react in your body. You become a science experiment with each injection.

Does it make sense that God created babies in such a way that they would need foreign toxic matter injected into them to somehow magically make them healthy? Do you believe that God blundered when He created us and forgot to give us an immune system capable of resisting infections? Humans have been living on planet earth for thousands of years without vaccinations, and we've somehow managed to all get here. Yes, there have been disease epidemics in the past, but now we have sewer systems, drink sanitized clean water and have improved our living standards, which makes a huge difference in disease outbreaks. For every doctor who says vaccines are safe and effective, there is another one cautioning against them, from what they know and have seen. It's time to start investigating the scientific facts vs. fear-mongering lies.

> "40 years ago, when I started my practice, only 1 in 10,000 children had autism. Today it's 1 in 100. What is the only difference we have seen? The inordinate number of vaccines that are being given to children today. My partners and I have over 35,000 patients who have never been vaccinated. You know how many cases of autism we have seen. ZERO, ZERO. I have made this statement for over 40 years: NO VACCINES, NO AUTISM." Mayer Eisenstein, M.D.

Today we have fear of evil nuclear and biological war threats. North Korea threatens to fire nuclear missiles. We have school shootings that are causing mass hysteria. If someone threatened to drop a bomb in a school that exposed children to seven strains of streptococcus bacteria, three strains of influenza viruses, chickenpox, hepatitis B, hepatitis A, pertussis, diphtheria, tetanus, haemophilus influenza B, three strains of polio viruses, measles, mumps and rubella viruses, we would have our law enforcement agencies and the best SWAT team around called in to take on this extreme evil act of bioterrorism, right? Most mothers don't even want their kids around someone who is sick with a cold or the flu out of fear that they may catch it, but then we turn around and hold a small child down and inject all those toxic organisms right into their bloodstream through a needle and call it protection? Complete absurdity! Children have immature immune systems and underdeveloped kidneys. To roll the dice in hopes of this biological assault on their delicate little bodies will help achieve optimum health is as illogical and absurd as it is unscientific.

> **"No batch of vaccine can be proved safe before it is given to children."** Dr. Leonard Scheele, Surgeon General of the United States

Barbara Loe Fisher, president of the National Vaccine Information Center (NVIC), believed medical science was never wrong. She grew up in a family of doctors and nurses and trusted that vaccines were safe and effective. Her pediatrician never told her that her son was at high risk to receive another vaccine because he was recovering from the flu. The hot, red lump that developed at the site of injection from his third DPT shot was a warning sign that Barbara shamefully admits she ignored.

Four hours after taking her 2-year-old son in for his fourth DPT shot and oral polio vaccine, his face went pale and he sat lifeless in a chair for hours. She thought he had fallen asleep, but in actuality he was unconscious and having a seizure. High-pitched screaming followed by bizarre behavioral patterns were unexpected side effects from the shot. He was also unable to recognize the alphabet that he knew before that shot. Vaccinations left her son with multiple learning disabilities, delayed motor skills, attention deficits and subsequently a lifelong struggle with low self-esteem because he couldn't do what his peers could. *"I wish I could go back, as so many parents do, and instead of holding my child down on the table like a sacrificial lamb, I could take him in my arms and walk out of that doctor's office, and give him back the future that was his birthright,"* pleads Barbara, but she can't. What's done is done. Now she helps educate others on the risks associated with vaccinations.

> **"They don't teach us about the ingredients; they don't teach us about the studies. I almost feel like an ass. I just blindly followed through with vaccination with no real data, didn't know what was in them."** Rachael Ross, M.D., PhD (Award-winning talk show, The Doctors)

Dr. Rachael Ross explains how as a pediatrician she was not taught in medical school about vaccine ingredients, vaccine risks, what to look for when children experience adverse side effects and how to report it to VAERS. She believes every parent should have a choice and promotes **"My Baby - My Choice."** She encourages parents to find a new doctor if the one you currently use refuses to look at the data on vaccinations.

> **"I would challenge any colleague, clinician or research scientist to claim that we have a basic understanding of the human newborn immune system."** Dr. Bonnie Dunbar, Professor of Immunobiology, Baylor University

Vaccinations have been deliberately lied about through erroneous statistics, falsified data and faulty studies that have been funded by pharmaceutical companies and marketed to persuade Americans to believe that they are necessary to eradicate disease and keep us healthy. The CDC has disguised this wolf in sheep's clothing to be a harmless and safe blessing to the world. Nothing could be further from the truth.

> **"I have over 13,000 children in my pediatric practice and I have to say, as unpopular as this observation may be, my unvaccinated children are by far the healthiest."** Paul Thomas, M.D.

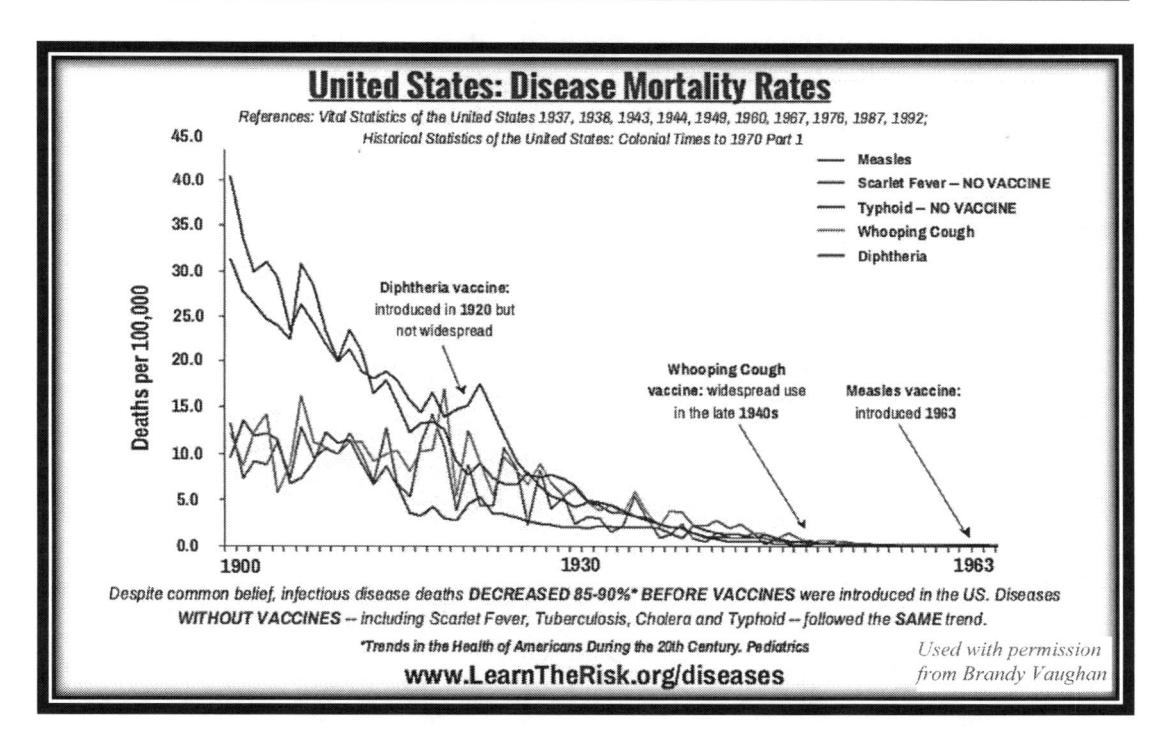

United States: Disease Mortality Rates

References: Vital Statistics of the United States 1937, 1938, 1943, 1944, 1949, 1960, 1967, 1976, 1987, 1992; Historical Statistics of the United States: Colonial Times to 1970 Part 1

Legend:
- Measles
- Scarlet Fever – NO VACCINE
- Typhoid – NO VACCINE
- Whooping Cough
- Diphtheria

Annotations on chart:
- Diphtheria vaccine: introduced in 1920 but not widespread
- Whooping Cough vaccine: widespread use in the late 1940s
- Measles vaccine: introduced 1963

Y-axis: Deaths per 100,000 (0.0 to 45.0)
X-axis: 1900 to 1963

Despite common belief, infectious disease deaths DECREASED 85-90%* BEFORE VACCINES were introduced in the US. Diseases WITHOUT VACCINES -- including Scarlet Fever, Tuberculosis, Cholera and Typhoid -- followed the SAME trend.

*Trends in the Health of Americans During the 20th Century. Pediatrics

www.LearnTheRisk.org/diseases

Used with permission from Brandy Vaughan

Most people, doctors included, are unaware of vaccination facts and history, and many don't have the foggiest idea of the toxic ingredients vaccines contain. The fact is, most diseases such as smallpox, polio, measles and pertussis (whooping cough) were already rapidly declining around the world before vaccines were ever introduced. For example, deaths from measles had already declined 95 percent before the measles vaccine was used, and historians conclude that better sanitation, hygiene, living quarters, health care, education and cleaner drinking water were responsible for ending most disease outbreaks. The vaccine manufacturers, who make $30 billion a year off their concoctions of toxins, want you to believe that vaccines are responsible for ending epidemics worldwide. This is an outright lie. Let's look at some facts.

> **"How often do we believe in something, not because we have in-depth research on it, but because authority figures tell us it is the truth? What if what we believe is just an illusion?"** Roman Bystrianyk, Co-author, *Dissolving Illusions: Disease, Vaccines, and the Forgotten History*

Unhealthy Living Conditions Cause Disease Epidemics

Overcrowded inner-city dwellings provided a perfect recipe for disease epidemics to flourish in big cities such as Chicago, New York, Boston and many cities in Europe in the 1800s and early 1900s. These unsanitary living environments proved to be breeding grounds for infectious diseases. Take into consideration the fact that in the Victorian era, in England, the average age of death among the urban poor was 15 to 16 years. Many people lived in overcrowded accommodations with inadequate ventilation. Horses instead of automobiles lined the streets, leaving manure and urine everywhere, which festered and drew flies and was a major source of typhoid fever infections. Along with horse manure in the streets came rat infestations. Posters to kill rats hung on city streets in an attempt to help protect people and property from rodent damage and destruction. It is estimated that in 1917, more than 2 million rats ravaged Boston, causing annual damages of $70 million and even higher figures in New York City!

In the mid-1800s, New York City had over 100,000 slum dwellers, where death was common amongst the poor. The lack of storm drains and septic systems for animal and human wastes created cesspools of disease-laden filth. Families often disposed of their slops and garbage in alleys, where it was consumed by scavenging pigs, dogs and rats. Heavy rains would spread pollution and flood food cellars, leading to food contamination and the spread of dangerous pathogens.

Before environmental laws were enacted in the 1800s, industries and slaughterhouses dumped animal carcasses and their wastes into any water source for disposal. The Chicago River and Lake Michigan were a soup of infection from industry, and as people freely poured their sewage into these waters, they would then turn around to obtain drinking water from the same source, until the 1900s, when a new drainage canal for wastes was finally opened. Until then, naturally infectious diseases stayed brewing constantly.

Chimneys in England spewed soot, and a smoky haze gave birth to the famous "London fog" that hovered over the city. Rotting corpses of dogs and horses in city streets were common. In 1858, the stench from dead animals, raw sewage and other rot was so horrendous in London that the British House of Commons was forced to suspend its sessions.

Hospitals were unsanitary and overcrowded, and often had infestations with rats. Contaminated milk that came from unhealthy cows that were fed whiskey slops and other rotten kitchen garbage were often the culprit for people getting sick. Cows drinking contaminated water were many times loaded with typhoid germs, and as Dr. Simmons reported, milk was the main source of typhoid infections. Before electricity and refrigeration, contaminated meat from diseased animals was sold in butcher shops. These harsh living conditions, minus refrigeration to keep food cold and fresh, provided the ideal breeding grounds for disease epidemics.

Harsh working environments proved fatal for many. People worked long, hard hours in factories, and young children labored in unsafe environments, to help feed families. Working conditions in mines, cotton mills, meat-packing plants, tanneries and glue and glass factories fostered many respiratory infections and disease. Lead and mercury poisoning contributed to lowered immune systems, making individuals more susceptible to disease and causing a deterioration of health. Many people, including children, died of typhus, a bacterium called Rickettsia prowazekii, spread to humans by lice, fleas and chiggers. Women had stillbirths due to stressful living and working conditions. These harsh and unsanitary conditions are the true culprits for disease epidemics. In 1920, an article in Good Housekeeping reported that 250,000 children died each year in the U.S. due to poverty! These were tough times; how could disease outbreaks not occur in such filthy living conditions?

> **"The evidence for indicting immunizations for SIDS is circumstantial, but compelling. However, the keepers of the keys to medical-research funds are not interested in researching this very important lead to the cause of an ongoing, and possibly preventable, tragedy. Anything that implies that immunizations are not the greatest medical advance in the history of public health is ignored or ridiculed. Can you imagine the economic and political import of discovering that immunizations are killing thousands of babies?"**
> William C. Douglass, M.D. (Honored twice as America's "Doctor of the Year")

Better Sanitation – The Eradicator Of Disease, Not Vaccinations

Once we began cleaning up our cities by installing indoor plumbing with municipal sewer systems and wastewater treatment facilities, waterborne diseases like dysentery, typhoid and cholera drastically declined. The flush toilet and electricity for the refrigeration of foods was a large contributor to improving health conditions and propelled us toward eradicating disease epidemics. By improving living conditions and cleaning up polluted environments, most diseases began to decline naturally. We eliminated the cause. To put into perspective how important proper sanitation is in preventing disease outbreaks, the Union Army during the Civil War (1861-1865) lost 186,216 men to disease, mostly caused by typhoid fever and dysentery, also known as the "Tennessee quickstep." This is twice the number of men killed in action! Yes, disease epidemics thrive in overcrowded camps and cities that lack clean water and sewers.

> "There is no question but that perfect sanitation has almost obliterated this disease (smallpox), and sooner or later will dispose of it entirely. Of course, when that time comes, in all probability the credit will be given to vaccination."
> John Tilden, M.D. (1851-1940)

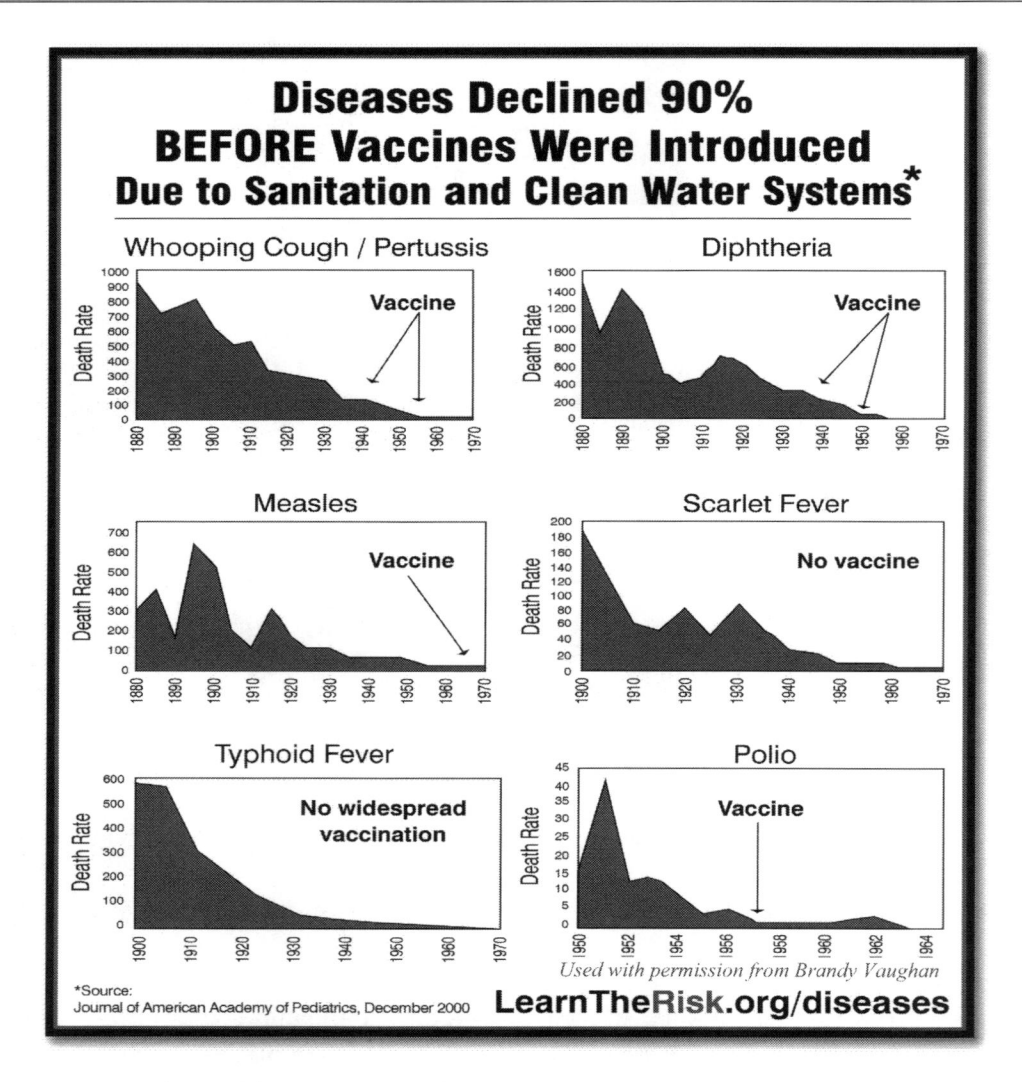

Diseases Declined 90% BEFORE Vaccines Were Introduced Due to Sanitation and Clean Water Systems*

*Source: Journal of American Academy of Pediatrics, December 2000

Used with permission from Brandy Vaughan

LearnTheRisk.org/diseases

From the mid-1800s and into the early 1900s, scarlet fever deaths plummeted nearly 100 percent. In fact, nearly all infectious diseases were declining during the late 1800s, and by the early 1900s, life had dramatically improved. Once again, better sanitation and improved living conditions are clearly responsible for this success. Keep in mind that scarlet fever outbreaks were virtually eliminated, way before antibiotics were available in the 1940s. Big Pharma likes to give antibiotics and vaccines the credit for eradicating disease, but any honest historian can look at disease outbreak records and dates, and clearly see that disease epidemics were virtually eliminated before vaccines and antibiotics were introduced. As Dr. William Osler, M.D., stated in the Maryland Medical Journal in January 1898, *"Three factors have been concerned in this extraordinary saving of life — the cleansing of towns, the purification of water supplies, and the introduction of good sewers."* Even Metropolitan Life Insurance stated "…the combined death rate of diphtheria, measles, scarlet fever, and whooping cough declined 95 percent among children ages 1 to 14 from 1911 to 1945, before the mass immunization programs started in the United States." (Bublin L, Health Progress, 1935-1945, Metropolitan Life Insurance Company, 1948, page 12)

> **"The most widespread and lethal diseases in the last 200 years were reduced due to cleaner drinking water, improved sanitation, nutrition, less overcrowded areas and better living conditions. Vaccines were introduced at the point where every single disease was already declining. To give vaccines credit for global reductions in disease is like giving a (bandage) credit for healing a wound that was already closing."** Dr. Dave Mihalovic

Today, the masses have fallen victim to the lie that vaccines are why disease epidemics have ended. "Mortality due to tuberculosis, diphtheria, scarlet fever, whooping cough, measles, typhoid, puerperal fever and infant gastro-enteritis started to fall long before the introduction of immunization and/or antibiotics." (Guberan, E., Schweiz. Med Wschr. 110, 1080, p. 574.) Dr. John Tilden predicted that in the future, corrupt vaccine manufacturers would try to convince the world that their vaccines are the reason disease epidemics ended, not better sanitation.

Vaccines are a business no different than selling cell phones or cigarettes. The problem is, when your pro-vaccination marketing plan has been sold to the masses like ice-cold Coca-Cola at a county fair, and is making your company billions of dollars, how are you going to stop the train going down the tracks? What would the doctors tell their patients? No one wants to admit that they were wrong or have been deceived. But an even greater incentive to keep on rolling down the tracks is the fact that this vaccination scandal is a $30 billion a year moneymaker. What kind of business would cut its own throat when that kind of money is lining its pockets? If there were no money to be made at vaccinations, the whole ridiculous hoax would be abandoned like rats leaving a sinking ship.

> "Up to 90 percent of the total decline in the death rate of children between 1860 and 1965 because of whooping cough, scarlet fever, diphtheria, and measles occurred before the introduction of immunizations and antibiotics."
> Archie Kalokerinos, M.D.

The Origin Of Vaccinations – Two Dead Boys

In 1796, Edward Jenner, a country apothecary who purchased his medical degree from St. Andrews University in Scotland for the sum of 15 pounds, inoculated an 8-year-old boy, James Phipps, with diseased matter that he believed to be cowpox from lesions on the hands of dairymaid, Sarah Nelmes. Cowpox is a disease that milkmaids occasionally caught from cows. For several days, he continued to inject the boy, and he never became ill. Then he injected the boy with smallpox and he became very ill, but after a few days he made a complete recovery with no effects from the smallpox inoculation. From this experiment, it was assumed that the cowpox vaccination was successful, and that it would provide lifelong protection against smallpox.

> "You may just as well try and stop a smallpox epidemic by vaccination as to prevent a thunderstorm with an umbrella." Dr. Druitte, late 1800s

What most medical historians fail to report is that James Phipps was revaccinated many times and died at the age of 20. Edward Jenner also experimented with vaccinations on his own son, and he, too, died, at the age of 21. Before these boys died, both of them contracted tuberculosis, which some researchers believe is directly linked to the smallpox vaccine. As the news commentator Paul Harvey used to say, "Now you know the rest of the story." Both of these boys died who received Jenner's vaccination experiment. If you were Jenner's neighbor and you witnessed two deaths after vaccinations, would you get in line to receive the vaccine? Unfortunately, most of the world stands in line to get their vaccinations, completely unaware that the father of vaccinations, Edward Jenner's track record started with two dead boys. This was the beginning of the vaccine industry.

> "It is nonsense to think that you can inject pus — and it is usually from the pustule of the dead smallpox victim; that is the basis of it; we used to think it was from cowpox, but the manufacturers deny that and say the most reliable form originates in the pustule of someone who had died from smallpox — it is unthinkable that you can inject that into a little child and in any way improve its health." Dr. William Howard Hay (1937)

Strict Vaccination Laws = Increased Disease Outbreaks

The implementation of vaccinating the masses for smallpox caused more people to die from it in the 20 years after strict compulsory laws than in the 20 years prior. In 1855, Massachusetts enforced the strictest vaccination laws ever in the U.S. They required all parents to vaccinate their children before the age of 2, and forbade the admission to public school of any child who had not been fully vaccinated. What were the results? No improvements in preventing or even declining smallpox outbreaks were seen. Even more shocking, there was a huge epidemic that occurred in 1872 to 1873, claiming the lives of 1,040 people. These repeat epidemics proved that strict vaccination laws actually did the opposite, and increased smallpox outbreaks, rather than reducing them! More people died of smallpox in the 20 years after strict compulsory laws than in the 20 years prior. These are official medical data facts and anyone can look them up. The smallpox vaccine failed to provide protection.

> **"Cancer was practically unknown until compulsory vaccination with cowpox vaccine began to be introduced ... I have seen 200 cases of cancer, and never saw a case in an unvaccinated person."** W.B. Clarke, M.D.

Chicago enforced strict vaccination laws too. By the end of 1868, more than 95 percent of Chicago residents had been vaccinated. In 1872, the smallpox epidemic hit the city, but failed to provide "herd immunity," with more than 2,000 people contracting smallpox. More than a fourth of them died, and the fatality among children under the age of 5 was the highest ever recorded. (Thomas Neville Bonner, Medicine in Chicago 1850-1950: Madison Wisconsin, 1957, p. 182.)

> **"What an act of insanity it would be to implant the infective products of undefined disease into the bodies of eight thousand healthy children in order to prevent the possible development of a very few mild cases of smallpox! Could absurdity go further than this?"** Dr. J.W. Hodge, 1911

Every soldier that entered the French army in the early 1900s was vaccinated; however, during the Franco-Prussian War, there were 23,469 cases of smallpox in the French army. The London Lancet, July 15, 1871, reports: "Of 9,392 small-pox patients in London hospitals, 6,854 have been vaccinated. More than 17 percent of those infected died."

After 10 years of incorporating a mass vaccination program in the Philippines, where 25 million vaccines were given against smallpox, over 170,000 got smallpox, and 75,000 deaths were recorded from 1911 through 1920. (Townsend Letter for Doctors, Feb/Mar 1994) Compulsory vaccination in the Philippines resulted in a death rate of 74 percent, the highest in history. If vaccines protect against disease, why did so many vaccinated individuals die of the disease?

> "You can't vaccinate believing that your children are protected and then feel that your children are not protected because somehow, some nonvaccinated child is carrying some secret organism that no one else is carrying. It just doesn't make any sense." Larry Palevsky, M.D. (Pediatrician)

Former British professor Vernon Coleman, M.D., explains that the smallpox vaccine caused so many deaths that the WHO abandoned mass vaccination programs and replaced them with surveillance, isolation and quarantine. He informs, "The myth that smallpox was eradicated through mass vaccination programs is just that — a myth."

> "I now have very little faith in vaccination, even as to modifying the disease, and none at all as a protective in virulent epidemics. Personally, I contracted smallpox less than six months after a most severe vaccination." R. Hall Bakewell, M.D., Vaccinator General of Trinidad

Mass vaccination programs were implemented in Germany, England, Italy, France and Japan as well. Dr. Charles Creighton, in 1888, reported in the Encyclopedia Britannica that despite having a strict vaccination rate, 60,000 people still died from 1870 to 1873 in the Prussian smallpox pandemic. Japan didn't do much better when it employed strict compulsory vaccination laws starting in 1872. Every infant in Japan had to be vaccinated within the first year of life. From 1885 to 1892, more than 25 million recorded vaccinations were on file, and revaccinations took place, yet official records show that 156,175 people came down with smallpox and 39,979 died! (Simon L. Katzoff, MD, "The Compulsory Vaccination Crime," Machinists' Monthly Journal, vol. 32, no. 3, March 1920, p. 261)

> "I was working in one of the oldest lung illness treatment centers in Germany, and just by chance, I looked at the files of those people who had fallen ill during the first German epidemic of smallpox, in 1947 ... We had always been told that the smallpox vaccination would protect against smallpox. And now I could verify, thanks to the files and papers, that all of those who had fallen ill had been vaccinated. This was very upsetting for me." Gerhard Buchwald, M.D.

The last reported case of smallpox in the U.S. was in Texas in 1949. Dr. Tom Mack, a smallpox expert with the CDC, reported, *"Even without mass vaccination, smallpox would have died out anyway."* In Leicester, England, Dr. Hodge reported, *"... an unvaccinated population has been far less susceptible to smallpox and far less afflicted by that disease since it abandoned vaccination than it was at a time when ninety-five percent of its births were vaccinated and its adult population well re-vaccinated."* (J.W. Hodge, MD, "How Small-Pox Was Banished from Leicester," Twentieth Century Magazine, vol. III, no. 16, January 1911, p. 342.)

> **"I have been a regular practitioner of medicine in Boston for 33 years. I have studied the question of vaccination conscientiously for 45 years. As for vaccination as a preventative for disease, there is not a scrap of evidence in its favor. The injection of virus into the pure bloodstream of the people does not prevent smallpox; rather, it tends to increase its epidemics, and it makes the disease more deadly. Of this we have indisputable proof. In our country (U.S.), cancer mortality has increased from 9 per 100,000 to 80 per 100,000, or fully 900 percent increase within the past 50 years, and no conceivable thing could have caused this increase but the universal blood poisoning now existing."**
> Charles E. Page, M.D.

The introduction of the diphtheria vaccine in 1895 failed to reduce diphtheria outbreaks; in fact, for the next five years, there was a 10 to 15 percent higher death rate than there had been for the previous 57 years, in Leicester, England. Diphtheria death rates in New York City from 1894 to 1920 had dropped by roughly 87 percent and vaccines are given the credit; however, when we look at the historical facts, like so many other disease-ending epidemics reveal, we find that diphtheria mortality rates had already started to decline long before the vaccine was introduced.

> **"A critical point which is never mentioned by those advocating mass vaccination is that children's health has declined significantly since 1960, when vaccines began to be widely used. According to the National Health Interview Survey conducted annually ... a shocking 31 percent of U.S. children today have chronic health problems ... In my medical career, I've treated vaccinated and unvaccinated children, and the unvaccinated were far healthier and more robust. Allergies, asthma, and behavioral and attention disturbances were clearly more common in my young patients who were vaccinated."** Philip Incao, M.D.

Polio Facts, Lies & The Rest Of The Story

Paralyzed kids in awkward leg braces and pitiful heads hanging out of iron lung machines in crowded hospital rooms terrorized the nation. After seeing heart-wrenching pictures of poor children crippled with deformities and hobbling on crutches, what normal person wouldn't want to do everything in their power to prevent such tragedies? These horrific images have imbued us with a fear of contracting the dreaded polio disease and have motivated most Americans to blindly jump in line to receive their polio-protection vaccine. Would you be completely shocked if the scientist who invented the polio vaccine confessed that instead of preventing polio, his vaccine actually caused it? Truth is stranger than fiction.

Polio is inflammation of gray matter in the brainstem and spinal cord caused from a chemical or virus that affects the muscles. According to the CDC, about 95 percent of polio is caused by a simple virus with no symptoms.

Polio Symptoms – CDC	
95%	No symptoms
4-8%	Mild flu like symptoms
1%	Permanent paralysis

About 4 to 8 percent of those infected will have what is perceived to be the flu with a headache, stiff neck, pain in the limbs, sore throat, cramping, diarrhea, mild fever and possibly vomiting, which usually resolves completely in 24 to 72 hours. It usually develops three to five days after exposure and once you recover, you have lifetime immunity from polio. Less than 1 percent of polio cases results in permanent paralysis of the limbs, usually the legs, and of those paralyzed, 5 to 10 percent die when paralysis strikes the respiratory muscles. The reality is, contrary to what we've been told, a very small percentage of the population ever has paralytic polio.

Polio can manifest in a wide variety of neurological symptoms, and at the time of introducing the polio vaccine, the definition of what polio is and who had it continued to change. This is why it is such a confusing topic. Wheelchair-confined president Franklin D. Roosevelt, along with the Rockefeller's medical men, launched a crusade with the "March of Dimes" campaign to eradicate polio, as he was said to have it. However, experts such as Dr. Armond Goldman from the University of Texas analyzed FDR's medical records and now believe that what he really had was Guillain-Barre Syndrome and not polio. (Goldman 2003 J Med Biog, 11:233-240)

Common Diseases Misdiagnosed As Polio Prior to 1958
- Aseptic meningitis
- Transverse myelitis
- Guillain-Barre syndrome
- Spinal meningitis
- Acute flaccid paralysis
- Enteroviral encephalopathy
- Traumatic neuritis
- Rey's syndrome
- Congenital syphilis
- Enteroviruses - Coxsackie or ECHO
- Limb paralysis from other vaccines
- Hand, foot, & mouth disease
- Lead poisoning
- Arsenic poisoning
- DDT poisoning

Before the introduction of the polio vaccine, many different diseases were grouped under the umbrella of polio. According to Dr. Bernard Greenberg, head of the department of biostatistics of the University of North Carolina School of Public Health, prior to 1954, laboratory testing was not pursued for polio diagnosis. In fact, all that was required to diagnose a patient with polio was for a physician to perform two examinations at least 24 hours apart, and detect partial or complete paralysis of one or more muscle groups. As a result, thousands of patients were misdiagnosed as having polio when they actually had aseptic meningitis, coxsackie virus, Guillain-Barre syndrome or one of the many other diseases listed in the box.

After 1955, when the polio vaccine was introduced, they changed the polio definition and began diagnosing aseptic meningitis and Coxsackie virus separate from polio. It is worth noting that all of these diseases still impact Americans today, the same as they did in the 1950s, during the polio epidemics. These diseases have not been eradicated, they have just been more carefully diagnosed and accurately named, instead of being all lumped together under the polio umbrella name, like they were prior to 1955. For example, in 1955, the year the Salk vaccine was released, the diagnostic criteria was changed, and it became much more stringent to diagnose, requiring paralysis to last at least 60 days, before diagnosing a case of polio. This drastically reduced the amount of people being diagnosed with polio, since the majority of them recovered within 60 days. Dr. Greenberg explained that the 1955 change in polio diagnosis meant that they were reporting a new disease, paralytic poliomyelitis, with a much longer lasting paralysis. They also refined diagnostic procedures and were no longer misdiagnosing and labeling Coxsackie virus and aseptic meningitis as polio, like they did prior to 1954. This alone eliminated a large portion of non-paralytic polio cases. Dr. Greenberg stated, *"... Thus, simply by changes in diagnostic criteria, the number of paralytic cases was predetermined to decrease in 1955-1957, whether or not any vaccine was used."* Of course, the vaccine was falsely given full credit for reducing polio. And to this day, the myth is still touted that the vaccine rescued the world from the death-grips of polio. Deception at its finest, however, the Chicago Tribune, in 1960, published an article exposing the lie. *"Several diseases which were often diagnosed as polio are now classified as aseptic meningitis or illnesses caused by one of the Coxsackie or ECHO viruses. The number of polio cases in 1961 (after the vaccine was introduced) cannot accurately be compared with those in, say 1952 (at the height of the polio epidemic), because the criteria for diagnosis have changed."* (Chicago Tribune 1960)

Medical literature explains that one cause for an increase in polio outbreaks was due to the DPT shot being introduced in the 1940s. According to the Lancet in 1949, "Researchers have known since the early 1900s that paralytic poliomyelitis often started at the site of an injection. When diphtheria and pertussis vaccines were introduced in the 1940s, cases of paralytic poliomyelitis skyrocketed." And the Journal of Infectious Diseases in 1992 stated that "Children who received DPT injections were significantly more likely than controls to suffer paralytic poliomyelitis within the next 30 days. According to the authors, 'this study confirms that injections are an important cause of provocative poliomyelitis.'"

A study published in JAMA documents a polio epidemic that occurred in Michigan in 1958, four years after introducing the Salk vaccine. Doctors took fecal specimens from 869 polio-diagnosed patients, and 401 of those yielded no virus. Poliovirus was found in 292, ECHO (enteric cytopathogenic human orphan) virus in 100, coxsackie virus in 73 and unidentified virus in three cases. *"In a large number of paralytic as well as nonparalytic patients, poliovirus was not the cause. Frequency studies showed that there were no obvious clinical differences among infections with Coxsackie, ECHO, and poliomyelitis viruses. Coxsackie and ECHO viruses were responsible for more cases of 'nonparalytic poliomyelitis' and 'aseptic meningitis' than was poliovirus itself."* (JAMA vol. 172, Feb 20, 1960, pp. 807-812) So, the real question is, how many people were misdiagnosed with polio and they didn't even actually have it? The reality is, polio has not been eradicated. It has just been renamed through accurate diagnostic procedures and to cover up the vaccine's failure in eradicating it. Many vaccine historians agree that this has been one of the biggest hoaxes in medical history.

> **"A lie told often enough becomes the truth."** Vladimir Lenin, Russian Communist, 1870-1924

As diagnostic procedures changed, so did the treatment, thanks to physical therapy pioneers such as Sister Elizabeth Kenny, a nurse who labored for 30 years to help reverse deformed polio patients with "the Kenny technique." Dr. John Pohl, an advocate of the Kenny technique, talks about how doctors would take children who were stiff and rigid with crooked limbs and, under anesthetic, straighten their limbs and put them in plaster casts for sometimes six months at a time. When they woke up, they would scream, he explains, as this was the wrong way to treat them. Physical therapy involving hot packs, muscle movement and stretching was a key to rehabilitating polio patients, unlike conventional medical practice that immobilized them. Sister Kenny's work helped many overcome their illnesses through muscle rehabilitation. Her opposing the medical status quo became the foundation for physical therapy in rehabilitation.

Iron Lung Or Transverse Myelitis?

Polio-Like Illnesses Are Still Diagnosed In The USA Every Year
- 1,400 cases of Transverse Myelitis
- 6,000 cases of Guillain-Barre Syndrome
- 75,000 cases of Aseptic Meningitis

People claim because of the polio vaccine we no longer have iron-lung machines. This is not true. We still have iron-lung machines, but they are called ventilators. When someone goes to the hospital with compromised respiratory muscles, instead of getting in a huge, full-body iron-lung machine like what was shown in the old 1950s pictures, we now use an up-to-date, modern ventilator, to help them breathe. In the 1950s, what would have been called polio is now called transverse myelitis, thanks to diagnostic improvements. Transverse myelitis, inflammation of the spinal cord, which damages nerves, causes some children to be permanently paralyzed and dependent upon a ventilator, which is the modern version of the iron-lung machine. There are about 33,000 people in the United States who suffer with transverse myelitis, and 1,400 new cases are diagnosed each year. So, once again, when the media shouts "hoorah for curing polio," be not deceived. Polio never went away. It was just renamed to cover up the vaccine's failure.

> "Polio has not been eradicated by vaccination, it is lurking behind a redefinition and new diagnostic names like viral or aseptic meningitis. ... According to one of the 1997 issues of the MMWR, there are some 30,000 to 50,000 cases of viral meningitis per year in the United States alone. That's where all those 30,000 to 50,000 cases of polio disappeared after the introduction of mass vaccination." Viera Scheibner, Ph.D.

Making The Polio Vaccine With SV-40 Virus

When live viruses are used to make a vaccine, a chemical such as formalin (formaldehyde derivative) is used to inactivate them, meaning they can no longer infect a cell. This process is not always 100 percent effective. Sometimes, viruses slip by, without being inactivated. When this happens, the vaccine actually causes the disease it's supposed to prevent. The vaccine batch, or lot of vaccines, is then referred to as being "hot."

A disturbing problem associated with the Salk vaccine, according to Dr. Stephen Chapman, is that once it passed safety requirements and showed that all of the virus was theoretically killed, the virus was reported to have the ability to resurrect after sitting for weeks and even months. Apparently, the safety testing didn't detect small amounts of the live virus. (Ratner, Herbert, "A Premature Salk Vaccine, April 19, 1956," Child and Family, vol. 20, 1988, pp. 255-263.) Dr. Wendell Stanley explained that formaldehyde in a vaccine can have a tanning effect upon the virus, where it can be held for days and even years and still be able to be reactivated at a subsequent time. Considering this, a troubling thought is the fact the SV-40 virus was, and still is, a possible risk in both the oral polio vaccine (OPV) and the inactivated polio vaccine (IPV) used today.

The IPV used today is still treated with formaldehyde, and we have known since 1961 that SV-40 virus has the capability to survive in formaldehyde longer than the 12-day minimum safety test required before vaccines are deemed safe. Dr. Edwin Lennette, director of the California State Department of Health, cautions that, in general, vaccines could test negative in the lab and in test animals, yet in humans something may go wrong. Just because the vaccine tests safe in the lab doesn't necessarily mean it's safe to be injected in humans.

Dr. Eddy Is Silenced & The Contaminated Polio Vaccine Infects 220,000 People

Bernice Eddy, M.D., Ph.D., was a bacteriologist and leading vaccine safety tester at the National Institute of Health (NIH) for the new Salk polio vaccine. In 1955, she discovered that many batches from Cutter Laboratory contained the live polio virus and that it was not inactivated or dead like it was supposed to be. In her laboratory testing with the polio vaccine on Rhesus monkeys, the results showed that it paralyzed them upon injection. Thank goodness she caught it in time before they released it to be injected in our children, right? Wrong! When she reported the startling research, proving the vaccine contained the live virus that caused paralysis upon injection, her vaccine superiors did the unthinkable. They silenced her! How could they ignore her findings and allow this to be injected in innocent children knowing that it would paralyze them?

With the incentive to market the polio vaccine and make huge money, her research screamed for America not to use the vaccine, but those in charge, with their power, greed and money, wouldn't listen, and the vaccine was released to the public. Dr. Alton Ochsner, a stockholder in one of the laboratories that produced the polio vaccine, was eager to inoculate the world. Disregarding Dr. Eddy's findings, he was determined to prove the Salk vaccine safe, so he publicly vaccinated his own grandchildren in front of the faculty at Tulane Medical School. His grandson died of polio within 48 hours and his granddaughter was crippled from it! Unfortunately, as ridiculous as it sounds, this too was silenced and the vaccine still went public! If only people standing in line for their shots knew what Dr. Eddy knew and could have seen the tragedy that took place after Dr. Ochsner vaccinated his grandchildren, they would have turned and run for their lives. Unfortunately, those with money manipulate the media and science to push their agenda, and the polio vaccine was released to the public. I imagine Dr. Eddy was screaming in protest, much like our own modern-day vaccine scientist, Dr. Judy Mikovits, is doing today after losing her job for reporting her data on identifying how our current vaccines are contaminated with deadly retroviruses. So, the toxic contaminated polio vaccine was launched and many fell sick to polio after vaccinations and enormous lawsuits were filed. The NIH director, Dr. William Sebrell, resigned, and the secretary of Health, Education and Welfare, Oveta Hobby, stepped down.

According to vaccine researcher Marco Caceres, if Dr. Eddy's supervisors would have listened to her, "40,000 children would not have been infected with polio, 200 would not have been severely paralyzed and 10 of them would not have died." With this polio vaccine backfiring fiasco, one must ask, do we have honesty in science anymore? Are our leaders so corrupt that the love of money rejects all scientific findings with our children's health and lives paying the price?

> **"What gives you the right to know a truth and not share it?"** Dr. Gilles LaMarche

In 1955, pharmaceutical companies Cutter and Wyeth were sued by Americans who took their children in to receive polio vaccinations and were later diagnosed with polio. According to Dr. Paul Offit from the CDC, at least 220,000 people who took the shot were infected with the live polio virus contained in Cutter's vaccine; 70,000 people developed muscle weakness, 164 were severely paralyzed and 10 were killed. Sadly, 75 percent of Cutter's victims were paralyzed for the rest of their lives. Further investigation revealed that two lots of the vaccine were contaminated with the live virus. (Am J Hyg. 1963; 78:29-60)

> **"Studies have shown that while the oral polio vaccine contains three strains of polio virus, a fourth strain can be cultured from the feces of vaccine recipients. This indicates that viruses have recombined and formed a new strain in the process of vaccination."** Virology 1993

SV-40, A Cancer-Causing Virus In The Polio Vaccine

In 1960, Dr. Eddy injected hamsters with the polio vaccine mixture cultured on monkey kidneys, and they developed tumors. When she reported her findings, that monkeys carried a cancer-causing virus, at a cancer conference in New York, she was demoted and lost her laboratory. Other research scientists like Dr. Maurice Hilleman (Merck's vaccine program developer responsible for over 36 vaccines) and Dr. Benjamin Sweet (Merck scientist who named the SV-40 virus) examined her research and found it to be accurate. They too, were able to isolate the virus, which was called SV-40, the 40th simian virus discovered. This virus has been present in the Salk polio vaccine that caused tumors to grow in hamsters. Dr. Hilleman admits Merck's responsibility in allowing this virus in the polio vaccine, but even more shocking is the fact that he admits the likelihood of importing and spreading the AIDS virus through vaccines as well!

> **"The greatest lie ever told is that vaccines are safe and effective."** Dr. Leonard G. Horowitz

In 1961, new federal law was passed that required no vaccines to contain the SV-40 virus; however, the previously made polio vaccines containing the SV-40 virus were not discarded. Instead, those contaminated vaccines continued to be injected into children up until 1963. Other experts claim that the SV-40 virus has contaminated batches of oral polio vaccine until the end of the 1990s. Dr. Hilleman later admitted that Merck knew the vaccines were contaminated and continued to dispense them to the public anyway.

> **"SV-40 infection is now widespread within the human population almost certainly as a result of the polio vaccine."** Dr. John Martin, Former FDA Virologist

In 1962, Dr. Eddy published her findings about the polio vaccine containing the SV-40 cancer-causing virus. Meanwhile, the existing vaccine batches were never re-called and it is estimated that 98 million children were injected from 1955 to 1963. Did she win a Nobel Prize for her research? No, in fact, just the opposite, as previously mentioned, she lost her labs, was denied permission to attend conferences and removed from further vaccine research. Is this how we reward our top scientists in this country when honest research is done to protect our children and they report the data?

> **"Had my mother and father known that the poliovirus vaccines of the 1950s were heavily contaminated with more than 26 monkey viruses, including the cancer virus SV-40, I can say with certainty that they would not have allowed their children and themselves to take those vaccines. Both of my parents might not have developed cancers suspected of being vaccine-related, and might even be alive today."** Dr. Howard B. Urnovitz, Ph.D.

According to the Lancet 2002, SV-40 from the African green monkey found in the contaminated polio vaccines has been detected in non-Hodgkin's lymphoma tumors and is responsible for up to half of the 55,000 non-Hodgkin's lymphoma cases being diagnosed each year. Even more shocking is the fact that 40 to 60 percent of children with brain tumors have the SV-40 virus. The law offices of Stanley Kops have proven that the oral polio vaccine has always been contaminated with SV-40, a known contaminant of polio vaccines grown on monkey kidney cells up through the 1980s. It has been linked by the FDA to be associated with cancers such as: mesothelioma, medulloblastoma brain tumors and bone, breast, colon and kidney tumors. Dr. Michele Carbone, a molecular pathologist at Loyola University Medical Center, discovered SV-40 genes and proteins in 60 percent of patients with mesothelioma (lung cancer) and in 38 percent of those with bone cancer. He has also identified the mechanism through which SV-40 turns a cell cancerous by switching off a protein that protects cells from becoming malignant. By 2003, more than 60 different labs have demonstrated a connection between SV-40 and cancer.

> **"One out of 200 people will have cancer directly caused by SV-40 virus."** Randy Tent, Ph.D.

CDC authorities have assured us that polio vaccines grown on the kidneys of the African green monkey did not contain this deadly contaminant. Stanley Kops has proven in the courtroom that not only is this not the case, but that the vaccine regulators who are responsible for keeping us healthy have known all along that SV-40 virus was never removed from vaccines. (S. Kops, Re: Debate on the Link Between SV40 and Human Cancer Continues," Journal of the National Cancer Institute, vol. 94, no. 3, February 6, 2002, pp. 229-230.) In 2002, at the Institute of Medicine conference, evidence was presented to prove that the oral polio vaccine has always been contaminated with SV-40 monkey virus, which has been linked by the FDA and other organizations with cancers such as mesothelioma and medulloblastoma.

If you think the CDC has your back, think again. Most doctors and healthcare providers get their information from the CDC. What they know and what they tell are two different stories. The corruption, deceit and lies are outrageous, to say the least. Choose wisely who you trust when it comes to a needle being jabbed into your skin containing who knows what kinds of viral fragments, dead or alive. It is interesting to note that it took about 40 years for scientists to link the SV-40 virus to human cancer. The question is, what will our scientists know 40 years from today about the vaccines we give our children now?

> "Many here voice a silent view that the Salk and Sabin polio vaccine, being made of monkey kidney tissue... has been directly responsible for the major increase in leukemia in this country." Frederick R. Klenner, M.D., F.C.C.P.

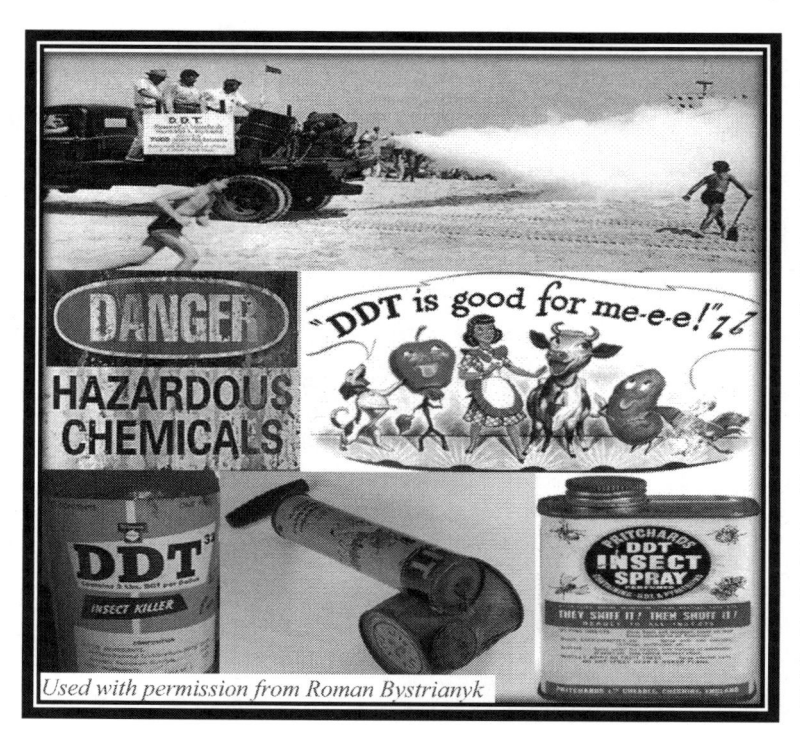

DDT – The Toxic Polio-Mimicking Insecticide

"DDT is good for Me-e-e!" was a slogan used to market the toxic cancer-causing insecticide and convince the masses that it was not only safe, but actually good for you. The more accurate slogan should have been "DDT Causes Polio-Like Symptoms in Me-e-e!" As I type these words, I can't help but wonder as we look back at our foolishness for poisoning people with the use of DDT some

> **Do you know why we don't spray kids with DDT anymore?
> BECAUSE SOMEONE QUESTIONED "SETTLED SCIENCE."**

75 years ago and thinking we were doing something great, is the same thing going to be said about our current vaccinations we are using today? In the year 2050, will our grandchildren shake their heads in disgust at how foolish and naive we were for using vaccines that caused the very disease they were supposed to prevent and leave us more susceptible to cancer and other dreaded autoimmune disorders? Time will tell.

> **Is Glyphosate the new DDT? Law suits are being filed for those diagnosed with cancer (Non-Hodgkin's Lymphoma).**

Like so many other toxic practices we have performed in the past, we now know DDT is a deadly poison that causes cancer. Our government banned its use in 1972. It was used in the 1940s and '50s by everyone from farmers and ranchers to moms and schoolteachers. It was sprayed on animals, inside houses and even on our foods like sandwiches and school lunchboxes. This tasteless and odorless insecticide was used in water to wash clothes, sprayed on beaches and directly sprayed all over your hair and face to kill typhus, malaria and all types of bugs. How does it kill bugs? DDT enters the nervous system and starts to paralyze the muscles and nerves until the insect finally dies. What is iron lung? Paralysis of the lung muscles, where the patient needs the assistance of a ventilator to breathe. Hmmm, could DDT poisoning be one of the largest contributors to polio epidemics, especially the notorious iron lung? By the 1960s it was discovered that DDT enhanced the release and intracellular multiplication of poliovirus. DDT was eventually phased out in the early 1960s, right at the same time polio was disappearing. The disturbing fact about DDT is, despite it being banned worldwide under the Stockholm Convention in 2001, it is still being used today in India, China and North Korea. You can buy it off the shelf in those countries. It is interesting to note that China is a heavy user of DDT and suffered a polio epidemic in 2011. If China, North Korea and India would stop using DDT, would polio epidemics cease worldwide like they have in North America?

> **DDT Still Used In:**
> - India
> - China
> - North Korea

Analyzing polio and DDT tonnage usage graphs from 1940 to 1970, one can see how DDT parallels with polio outbreaks. Researchers conclude that DDT toxicity disrupts mucosal immunity, which allows a previously benign virus to bypass the innate immune system and cause paralysis. Back in the 1950s, it would have been diagnosed as polio, but in today's modern diagnosis this would be labeled acute flaccid paralysis. With tons of DDT being used heavily, no doubt thousands of cases of what doctors thought was polio was nothing more than DDT poisoning causing paralysis.

> "Vaccines did not save humanity and never will ... Smallpox was not eradicated by vaccines as many doctors say it was. They say this out of conditioning rather than out of understanding the history or science. Polio virus was not responsible for the paralysis in the first part of the 20th century. Polio vaccine research, development, testing and distribution has committed atrocities upon primates and humanity. Bill Gates is not a humanitarian. Vaccines are dangerous and should never be injected into anyone for any reason. They are not the answer to infectious diseases. There are many more sustainable and benevolent solutions than vaccines." Suzanne Humphries, M.D.

Another terrible tragedy in medicine was the practice of doctors prescribing **arsenic** to treat lung problems such as asthma and cholera. It was also added to tobacco for smoking, and dentists used arsenic acid to kill nerve endings in decayed teeth. Farmers sprayed lead arsenate and calcium arsenate on fruits and vegetables as insecticides. It was used in paper, fabrics, paints and dyes. Paris Green and Scheele's Green (used as pigment in paints) contained arsenic-based ingredients that could produce polio-like symptoms when the toxicity levels affected the brain and nerves.

Congenital syphilis or tabes dorsalis is a slow deterioration of the nerves (demyelination) and gray matter of the spinal column. This crippling disease was sometimes mistaken for polio, since they are very similar. Morris Fishbein of the AMA approved arsenical Tryparsamide manufactured by Merck, under license from the Rockefeller Institute for Medical Research. Despite Tryparsamide being proven to be extremely dangerous, they allowed it to stay on the market contributing to ill health.

The drugs Neoarsphenamine and Neosalvarsan contained arsenic, and they were notorious for causing polio-like symptoms as well. Doctors misdiagnosing people with polio when they actually had heavy metal (lead and arsenic) poisoning caused from toxic chemicals and drugs was certainly another misleading factor in the polio outbreaks and diagnosis.

During the polio epidemics, the majority of middle- and upper-class people who could afford it, about 50 to 80 percent of children in the U.S., had their tonsils removed. Many studies revealed that bulbar polio was considerably higher in children who had tonsillectomies. In order for poliovirus to cause serious damage, it must make its way into the body through peripheral nerve damage, which occurs when doctors remove the tonsils. Numerous published studies show an increased risk of bulbar polio after tonsillectomies. (M. Siegel, M. Greenberg, and M.C. Magee, "Tonsillectomy and Poliomyelitis, II, Frequency of Bulbar Paralysis, 1944-1949, Journal of Pediatrics, vol. 38, no. 5, May 1951, pp. 548-558)

> "The live polio virus from the vaccine can remain in your throat for one to two weeks and your feces for up to two months. So not only is the vaccine recipient at risk of developing polio, but he or she can potentially spread the disease."
> Dr. Raymond Francis

Dr. Francis explains that those who are vaccinated can spread the disease. How ironic it is that people like to blame disease outbreaks on the those who are unvaccinated, not understanding that those who are vaccinated are carriers for the viruses and can spread the disease, completely the opposite of what is taught and certainly believed by most.

Polio Vaccine Maker Admits Failure — Media Claims Success?

We have been brainwashed to believe that vaccinations are the reason polio has virtually disappeared, which is a fabricated lie and perversion of the truth. Polio, as with so many other diseases previously mentioned, was on the decline before the vaccine was ever introduced. In 1953, before the polio vaccine was introduced, the death rate in the U.S. had already declined 47 percent. As a matter of fact, once the polio vaccinations began, the number of polio cases increased! For example, Rhode Island had a 450 percent increase and Massachusetts reported a 650 percent increase in polio after vaccines were given. In some countries, the polio epidemic ended without ever receiving the polio vaccine. In other countries, polio didn't even exist until people began receiving vaccinations! Idaho and Utah banned the polio vaccine because there had never been a reported case prior to use of the vaccine.

> "**Not only did the cases of polio increase substantially after mandatory vaccinations (a 50 percent increase from 1957 to 1958, and an 80 percent increase from 1958 to 1959), but the statistics were manipulated by the Public Health Service to give the opposite impression**." Dr. Bernard Greenberg, Head of the Dept. of Biostatistics for Public Health - 1962 U.S. Congressional hearings

The developer of the polio vaccine himself, Dr. Albert Sabin, publicly admitted that the vaccine had failed! How can the polio vaccine maker himself declare that the polio vaccine has been a failure while the media, CDC and most doctors say it's been a success at eradicating polio?

> "**Official data have shown that the large-scale vaccinations undertaken in the U.S. have failed to obtain any significant improvement of the diseases against which they were supposed to provide protection.**" Albert Sabin, M.D. (Developer of the Oral Polio vaccine)

At the same time the polio vaccine was causing outbreaks, the media was reporting a dramatic decrease in polio cases, a complete fabricated lie, to coerce Americans into believing the vaccine was safe and effective. And to this day, the masses give credit to polio vaccines for eradicating polio when Dr. Albert Sabin, the developer of the vaccine, admitted that his vaccine had failed. This is a powerful testimony of how corrupt the media is at selling a lie, the giant hoax that vaccines have eradicated polio. Is it possible that big pharma pays to fabricate the news they want the world to believe, regardless of the facts, so the masses keep coming in for their polio vaccines? Virologist Dr. Sven Gard declared that vaccinations in the United States caused as many cases of poliomyelitis as it prevented in 1955.

> **"Live virus vaccines against paralytic poliomyelitis, for example, may in each instance produce the disease it is intended to prevent; the live virus vaccines against measles and mumps may produce such side effects as encephalitis. Both of these problems are due to the inherent difficulty of controlling live viruses in vivo (once they are placed in a live person)."** Jonas & Darrell Salk, 1977 (Developer of the killed polio virus vaccine)

In 1976, Dr. Jonas Salk, creator of the killed-polio virus vaccine, made from monkey kidneys, testified before a Senate subcommittee that the live-virus vaccine had been the principal, if not the sole, cause of all reported polio cases in the U.S. since 1961. What more evidence do you need than for the creators of the polio vaccine to publicly admit their concoctions are worthless at preventing polio and actually caused it to increase? Why is it we don't hear these vaccine facts? Why is vaccine history lied about?

> **"In fact, all the polio cases in America (since 1979) came from the vaccine."** The Washington Post, January 26, 1988

Even the CDC admits that the oral polio vaccine, which has been used since 1965, has caused the only cases of polio in the U.S. since 1979. Between 1987 and 2001, the oral polio vaccine was the only cause of paralytic polio in the U.S., and 156 people received compensation from VAERS after becoming paralyzed from receiving the vaccine. The U.S. stopped using the oral polio vaccine in 2001. Are you OK with, "Oops, sorry for giving you the disease we were trying to prevent?"

> **"In Tennessee, USA, the number of polio victims the year before vaccination became compulsory was 119. The year after vaccination was introduced, the number soared to 386. In North Carolina, the figures are 78 and 313. There are similar figures for other states, and in the USA, as a whole, the incidence of polio increased by 50 percent after mass immunization was introduced. The**

> incidence of polio had, however, fallen dramatically before the first polio vaccine was introduced." Dr. Vernon Coleman

India has implemented an aggressive vaccination program. Some children under the age of 5 were reported to have received 15 doses of trivalent OPV, which has failed to eliminate childhood paralysis. With increased polio vaccination programs, there has been a correlating increase in acute flaccid paralysis (AFP). It's worth noting that India still uses DDT (a known carcinogen) heavily. Could the combination of DDT and high doses of polio vaccines be causing inflammation in the spinal column and nervous system, causing paralysis?

> "It is my firm conviction that vaccination has been a curse instead of a blessing to the race. Every physician knows that cutaneous diseases (including cancer) have increased in frequency, severity, and variety to an alarming extent. To no medium of transmission is the widespread dissemination of the class of diseases so largely related as to vaccination." B.F. Cornell, M.D.

According to The World Health Organization (WHO), 69 Nigerian children experienced vaccine-induced paralytic polio after being vaccinated. Russia and many other countries reported similar tragic cases of the vaccine backfiring and causing the very disease it was supposed to prevent. (Polio outbreak in Nigeria sparked by vaccine. Associated Press. Oct. 5, 2007) Even more disturbing is the fact that the National Institutes of Infectious Disease admits that, *"paralysis associated with oral polio vaccine is unavoidable as long as the oral polio vaccine is used for eradication of paralysis caused by poliovirus."* No wonder we can't eradicate polio worldwide. The vaccine keeps causing it!

> "The hiding of this Vitamin C secret in the cure of polio and similar thinking in the treatment of other infectious diseases has prevented the discovery of the treatment of most acute infectious diseases. This genocidal ignorance and flat-out murder has cost multi-millions of lives. These bastards have kept the newspapers, TV, radio, science reporters, lawyers, courts, etc., in line on all this. Let us see if they can stop the internet." Robert Cathcart, M.D.

According to WHO, the western hemisphere has been certified polio free since 1994 and no cases of wild polio have been reported in this region since 1991. So why are we vaccinating for it? The risk of imported polio is extremely low. Only six cases have occurred in the U.S. since 1980.

From 1955 to 1963, almost every dose of polio, injection or sugar cube, given to 200 million Americans was contaminated with the cancer-causing virus from monkey kidneys. Researchers estimate that there are now 15 cases of cancer for every one case of polio.

> **"Make yourself sheep and the wolves will eat you."** Benjamin Franklin

Measles

Many cases of measles are associated with a Vitamin A deficiency. Vitamin A, given in high doses, can greatly reduce measles complications and the risk of death. The World Health Organization and American Pediatrics recommend administering 200,000 IU of Vitamin A to children older than 1 year of age, and it is to be given immediately upon measles diagnosis with a second dose given the following day. Infants, 6 to 12 months old, should be given two doses of 100,000 IU of vitamin A. Infants younger than 6 months of age should be given two doses of two Vitamin A, at 50,000 IU.

Measles is a contagious viral infection transmitted by respiratory droplets (infected saliva or mucus) in the air spread through coughing and sneezing. It starts off like the flu, with a fever, muscle aches, cough, runny nose, inflamed or pink eyes, with white spots inside the mouth. Then two to four days later, a red, blotchy skin rash will spread over the body. Here in the U.S., for the most part, it's non-life-threatening. Measles outbreaks come in cycles about every two to three years, regardless of vaccination rates. Most people over the age of 70 have contracted measles in their life and overcome it without any serious complications. Elderly people know from experience that measles is just a routine illness that you contract in early childhood, and then have lifetime immunity. It's not a big deal like the media portrays it to be. Even the 1970s sitcom, "The Brady Bunch," had an episode where all six children got measles, stayed home from school and played games for a few days until the rashes and fever cleared up, and then they were done with it, voila, lifetime immunity, and back to school.

> **"We've got to stop calling chickenpox and measles diseases, because they're not. They're infections, and infections come and go in a week to 10 days, and leave behind a lifetime of immunity. A disease is something that comes and stays, and frequently can't be cured. So when you vaccinate to avoid an infection, what you potentially are doing is causing a disease."** Dr. Sherri Tenpenny

Throughout the 1800s, measles epidemics occurred about every two years. These were serious infections that filled the hospitals and roughly 20 percent of children who contracted them died. However, as previously mentioned, with healthier living conditions, measles death rates had declined by more than 98 percent by the time the measles vaccine was introduced in 1963. The disease was eradicated through healthier living conditions, not vaccinations. Let's take a look at vaccine historical facts. In 1920, 469,924 cases of measles were reported. By 1955, less than 3 in 10 million people had measles. The measles vaccine wasn't introduced until 1963, eight years after the epidemic had already ended naturally. Of course, Americans have been spoon-fed the lie that the vaccine was responsible for ending measles, but this is simply not true. Measles is most dangerous and can be fatal in underdeveloped countries with poor sanitation and malnourished children, especially those with Vitamin A and C deficiencies.

> **"In the United States, measles is generally a benign, short-term viral infection; 99.99 percent of measles cases fully recover. As it has not been proven that the MMR vaccine is safer than measles, there is insufficient evidence to demonstrate that mandatory measles mass vaccination results in a net public health benefit in the United States."** Dr. Shira Miller, PIC president

Most diseases had rapidly declined before the measles vaccine was licensed in 1963, and the measles death rate had plummeted to zero in Massachusetts and several other states. To prove how important proper sanitation is, it is interesting to note that measles death rates still remain as one of the leading causes of childhood death in underdeveloped countries where children are malnourished and live in poverty-stricken areas, lacking clean water and sewage facilities. It's interesting to note that statistics on measles mortality never distinguish between underdeveloped countries as compared to healthier, more advanced nations, where measles for the most part has been eradicated. The vaccine industry keeps Americans in fear mode of the next deadly disease pandemic, when the reality is, and history has proven, that large measles outbreaks clearly ended before vaccines were introduced.

> **"It was similar with the measles vaccination. They went through Africa, South America and elsewhere, and vaccinated sick and starving children ... They thought they were wiping out measles, but most of those susceptible to measles died from some other disease that they developed as a result of being vaccinated. The vaccination reduced their immune levels and acted like an infection. Many got septicemia, gastro-enteritis, etc., or made their nutritional status worse and they died from malnutrition. So, there were very few susceptible infants left alive to get measles. It's one way to get good statistics. Kill all those that are susceptible, which is what they literally did."** Archie Kalokerinos, M.D., Ph.D.

In 1984, in Sangamon County, Illinois, the CDC reported that 21 cases of measles occurred within a school population with a documented immunization level of 100 percent. People like to blame diseases on the unvaccinated, but this demonstrates that "herd immunity" from vaccinations has failed. (Measles Outbreak Among Vaccinated High School Students-Illinois, MMWR, CDC Control and Prevention, June 22,

1984, p.349.) After examining many schools that have high vaccination compliance records, the data reveals that measles outbreaks have become a disease of the vaccinated, reports Dr. Gregory Polond, M.D., and Robert Jacobson, M.D. They explain that "herd immunity" is not completely effective in preventing measles outbreaks. (Failure to Reach the Goal of Measles Elimination: Apparent Paradox of Measles Infections in Immunized Person," Archives of Internal Medicine, August 22, 1994, pp. 1816-1818.)

> "As measles immunization rates rise to high levels in a population, measles becomes a disease of immunized persons." Gregory A. Poland, M.D., Mayo Clinic, Vaccine Research Group

In a 1978 survey of 38 states, more than half of the children who contracted measles had been adequately vaccinated. The question is, if vaccines work, then why would you contract the disease after receiving the vaccination?

> "Decades of strict vaccination laws did absolutely nothing to improve the overall life expectancy of children in all age groups." Suzanne Humphries, M.D.

To blow an even bigger hole in the vaccination scandal, the WHO informs us the chances of you contracting measles are 14 times greater if you have been vaccinated for measles versus those individuals who have not been vaccinated! In 1985, our federal government reported that 80 percent of the 1,984 cases of reported measles occurred in vaccinated individuals! And when the measles outbreak occurred in Disneyland in 2015, only 14 percent of those affected were unvaccinated, according to JAMA Pediatrics, while the other 86 percent who contracted measles had previously been vaccinated. Any reasonable scientist would look at this data and conclude that vaccinations are failing us, right? The CDC, Fox News and most doctors fail to look at these facts.

The MMR vaccine is a live virus vaccine that can shed through the respiratory tract for several weeks after being vaccinated. Individuals who have recently been vaccinated carry the virus and can spread the disease! (Rosen JB, Rota JS, et al. outbreak of measles among persons with prior evidence of immunity, New York City, 2011. Clin Infect Dis 2014 May; 58(9): 1205-10.) When a pregnant woman is exposed to a child who has recently been vaccinated, the rubella virus can cause harm to the fetus. During the first 16 weeks of pregnancy, there is a risk that the fetus could develop congenital rubella, which may result in deafness, mental retardation and heart defects. (Lancet. 1982;781-784)

The CDC openly admits that 5 to 10 percent of vaccine recipients develop a rash and fever, which is one reason they started giving the immune globulin with it. CDC statistics also reveal that in the last 10 years, there have been 1,564 cases of the measles in the U.S. and ZERO deaths; however, there have been 83 deaths reported from the measles vaccine. Were those 83 deaths worth it? Wouldn't we be better off letting our children contract the wild measles instead of dying from the vaccine?

Dr. Anne Schuchat, the director of the CDC's National Center for Immunization and Respiratory Diseases, reported to Fox News in 2014 that there have been no measles deaths in the U.S. since 2003. However, according to VAERS database, 108 deaths occurred due to the measles vaccine. VAERS also reported that from 2013 to 2015, 694 reports were filed where the MMR vaccine caused disability.

Measles Deaths In The U.S. From 2004 to 2015
Deaths Caused From Measles - ZERO
Deaths Caused From Measles Vaccines - 108
Source: VAERS database

In a letter to Governor Edmund G. Brown of California, Eleanor McBean, Ph.D., states, *"I have uncovered some shocking data showing that our government, medical and military authorities know that vaccination has killed and crippled thousands of innocent people; but the facts have been suppressed. The vaccine business has continued to thrive in spite of its disastrous failure for the mere reason that it nets millions of dollars for the promoters, and this buys power with governments and propaganda control over* **the masses who don't know how to think for themselves."**

How does it make you feel to know that some of our so-called authorities label you as "someone who doesn't know how to think for yourself?" Are you ready to think and be responsible for your health, or do you want to just get in line with the masses and go down the loading shoot like lambs at a slaughterhouse?

> **"A critical point which is never mentioned by those advocating mass vaccination is that children's health has declined significantly since 1960, when vaccines began to be widely used. According to the National Health Interview Survey conducted annually ... a shocking 31 percent of U.S. children today have chronic health problems ... In my medical career, I've treated vaccinated and unvaccinated children, and the unvaccinated were far healthier and more robust. Allergies, asthma, and behavioral and attention disturbances were clearly more common in my young patients who were vaccinated."** Phillip Incao, M.D.

The MMR vaccine contains three live viruses: measles, mumps and rubella. It is also made with human fetal cells containing DNA fragments that may induce autoimmune reactions. These DNA fragments and retroviruses can provoke genetic mutations. Vaccines made with human fetal cell lines are exposing infants and children to human DNA and retroviral contaminants that are associated with rising cases of autism. (Deisher TA, Doan NV, et al. J public Health Epidemiol 2014 Sep; 6(9): 271-86). Research done in Norway, Sweden and the U.K. shows there is an association between reduced MMR vaccination rates and lower prevalence of autism spectrum disorders.

Wild Measles Protects Against Diseases In Adulthood

Medical journals are filled with research papers proving many problems associated with vaccines. Research done in Japan by Kubota and colleagues has shown that children who contract measles and mumps in childhood have a significantly higher protection against deadly heart attacks and strokes during adulthood. (Kubota Y, Iso H, et al. Atherosclerosis 2015 Jun 18;241(2): 682-86) A study done by Rosenlund and Bergstrom shows that children who contract measles are significantly less likely to ·develop allergies as opposed to children who are vaccinated. (Rosenlund H, Bergstrom A, et al. Pediatrics 2009 Mar; 123(3): 771-78) Data published in the Lancet in May 1999 by Alm and Swartz showed that children who never received the MMR vaccine had a significantly lower prevalence of allergies. A study published in JAMA in 2012 by Sun and Christensen shows a significant increase in the risk of seizures in children who receive vaccines. An earlier study in JAMA from July 21, 2004, by Vestergaard and Hviid showed that the MMR vaccine increases the risk of seizures by nearly three times during the two weeks after MMR vaccination.

> **"... a person's immune system and overall, long-term health are more robust if an illness such as chickenpox or measles is contracted and resolved naturally, as opposed to trying to avoid the infections through vaccination."**
> Dr. Sherri Tenpenny

Pertussis (Whooping Cough)

Whooping cough, or pertussis, is an infection that occurs every two to five years, regardless of vaccination rates. Pertussis is a mild infection with a lingering cough that usually resolves itself after a few weeks. Whooping cough had declined 99 percent by the time the vaccine was introduced in the mid-1940s and had been declining steeply for 70 years prior to administering the pertussis vaccine. Of course, the vaccine industry would have the world believe once again that their vaccines have come to the rescue for the whole human race, and without them, we would've all coughed ourselves to death.

> **"Every year, 35,000 children suffer neurological damage because of the DTP vaccine."** Edward Grant Jr., Former Assistant Secretary of Health, testifying before U.S. Senate Committee, May 3, 1985

Those who are vaccinated against pertussis can still spread the disease, making herd immunity and eradication unattainable, according to research published in the British Medical Journal. (2015 Jun 24; 13(1): 146.) Other research shows that high vaccination rates encourage the evolution of virulent pathogen strains that result in more severe disease-causing organisms and deadly infections. Interestingly enough, research has shown that 90 percent of whooping cough outbreaks occur in individuals who have already been vaccinated against whooping cough! If the vaccine works, why isn't it effective in providing protection? Oh, you want more science? In 2012, Dr. David Witt and colleagues showed that the majority of children with whooping cough had received their vaccinations. The highest incidence of the disease was found to be in 8- to 12-year-olds who had been fully vaccinated. Once again, the science shows that vaccines cause the very disease they are supposed to prevent. They are not effective in preventing disease!

> **"There is just overwhelming data that there's an association between the pertussis vaccine and seizures. I know it has influenced many pediatric neurologists not to have their own children immunized with pertussis."** Jerome Murphy, M.D., Former head of Pediatric Neurology, Milwaukee Children's Hospital

Scientific research has shown that when Bacillus Pertussis (whooping cough germ) is injected into animals, it leads to the secretion of insulin. In 1979, at the Fourth International Symposium on Pertussis, held in Bethesda, Maryland, it was shown that this same result occurs in those who have received pertussis vaccine. Drs. W. Hennessen and U. Quast reported in their publication "Adverse Reactions after Pertussis Vaccination," that the reactions after receiving the pertussis vaccine have a close relationship to the hypoglycemia syndrome.

> **"The rise in IDDM (juvenile onset diabetes) in the different age groups correlated with the number of vaccines given."** Barthelow Classen, M.D.; Former researcher, U.S. National Institutes of Health; Founder, Classen Immunotherapies, Baltimore

If your child has juvenile diabetes, it may be a result of the pertussis vaccine. After seeing blood sugar complications arise shortly after the pertussis (DTaP) vaccine, Dr. Robert Mendelsohn questions, *"Maybe it's time to investigate whether the pertussis vaccine has anything to do with the rapidly rising number of people with juvenile diabetes, adult diabetes, hypoglycemia and all disorders of insulin metabolism."*

Barthelow Classen, M.D., reported that juvenile diabetes increased 60 percent following a massive hepatitis B vaccination campaign for babies 6 weeks or older in New Zealand. He went on to further show that Finland's incidence of diabetes increased 147 percent in children under 5 after they received three new vaccines in the 1970s, and diabetes increased 40 percent in children from ages 5 to 9, after receiving the MMR and Hib vaccines, from 1988 to 1991.

> "Only after realizing that routine immunizations were dangerous did I achieve a substantial drop in infant death rates. The worst vaccine of all is the whooping cough vaccine ... it is responsible for a lot of deaths and for a lot of infants suffering irreversible brain damage. In susceptible infants, it knocks their immune systems about, leading to irreparable brain damage, or severe attacks or even deaths from diseases like pneumonia or gastro-enteritis and so on." Archie Kalokerinos, M.D., Ph.D.

Dr. Michael Odent reported in JAMA that children vaccinated for pertussis show a five times higher rate of asthma compared to non-immunized children. (JAMA. 1994 Aug 24-31;272(8):592-3 Pertussis vaccination and asthma: is there a link?)

Harris Coulter, Ph.D., explains that at least half of all U.S. children have had otitis media (ear infection) by their first birthday, and by age 6, 90 percent of children have had it. Roughly 1 million children are having tubes inserted in their ears each year. Otitis media, or "glue ear," was unheard of in American medical practice before 1940 or the early 1950s, before the pertussis vaccine was introduced. Is it purely coincidence that as soon as we started vaccinating for pertussis, all of a sudden, 90 percent of children started having "glue ear infections?"

> "My suspicion, which is shared by others in my profession, is that nearly 10,000 SIDS deaths that occur in the United States each year are related to one or more of the vaccines that are routinely given to children. The pertussis vaccine is the most likely villain, but it could also be one or more of the others." Robert Mendelsohn, M.D.

Silence Of The Scarlet Fever Streptococcus Vaccine Killer

Scarlet fever in the 1800s was an infectious disease that claimed more lives than whooping cough. It along with most other diseases was eradicated when we improved living conditions with better sanitation, purified our drinking water, and ate cleaner food, thanks to refrigeration. The nasty truth, that isn't talked about, is the fact that in 1912, a scarlet fever vaccine was developed from the strep toxin. By the 1930s, it was proving to have disastrous side effects when a group of student nurses received the vaccine and developed lupus. All nurses were healthy upon starting nursing school, but after receiving the vaccine, they began suffering with intense fevers, sore throats and joint pains. About one year after receiving the scarlet fever streptococcus vaccine, all these young nurses died. (M. Schaeffer and J. Toomey, "Immunization Against Scarlet Fever with Tannic Acid-Precipitated Erythrogenic Toxin," Pediatrics, vol. 1, 1948, pp. 188-194.) What a tragedy! The vaccine industry doesn't talk about the murderous scarlet fever vaccine. After killing the student nurses, an obvious disaster, it was hushed up and the vaccine was removed from the market.

Should we just forget about it along with the innocent lives it claimed? To the nurses who lost their lives due to vaccination tragedy, I hope this book gives something back to you, in the name of truth and justice, on behalf of your lives that were so wrongfully robbed from you, all in the false belief of immunization for health.

> **"You medical people will have more lives to answer for in the other world than even we generals."** Napoleon Bonaparte, French Military Leader & Emperor, 1769-1821

It is interesting to note that we do not vaccinate for scarlet fever, even though it claimed more lives than whooping cough did back in the 1800s, but somehow, without a vaccine program, the disease epidemic just cleared up on its own. Why is this not talked about? Because the fact that it cleared up on its own is a testimony in and of itself that improved sanitation is the true eradicator of disease epidemics, not vaccines. We would be a much healthier generation without the vaccination poisoning that has occurred and still continues, but the pharmaceutical lords want gullible people to believe in their sorcery. Fear-mongering in the name of disease prevention with toxic vaccinations generates billions of dollars for Big Pharma, and even more so by creating life-time customers with sick and immunocompromised individuals who will spend the rest of their lives treating symptoms with expensive drugs.

> **"Those who cannot remember the past are condemned to repeat it."** George Santayana

The terrible bubonic plague that swept through Asia, Europe and Africa in the 14th century killed an estimated 50 million people. Did a vaccine end it? No! Just as the scarlet fever plague was eradicated with better nutrition and improved sanitation, medical historians state that better nutrition finally ended the plague. The unspoken facts are the bubonic plague and scarlet fever plague resolved themselves without a man-made vaccine.

Flawed Vaccine Efficacy

> **"The great enemy of truth is very often not the lie — deliberate, contrived and dishonest, but the myth, persistent, persuasive, and unrealistic. Belief in myths allows the comfort of opinion without the discomfort of thought."** John Fitzgerald Kennedy, 1917-1963

Any honest scientist knows that in order to perform legitimate studies to test the safety and effectiveness of a product, there must be a control group. Scientific studies require controlled, double-blind, placebo trials. It is unscientific and completely ridiculous for the vaccine manufacturers to think that they are exempt from proving their products safe. The only studies done on vaccines compare new vaccines to old vaccines. The research that is needed but not done is finding out if receiving a certain vaccine is more effective than receiving no vaccine at all.

> **"Figures don't lie but liars figure."** Mark Twain

As we look at vaccine records for pertussis and measles outbreaks, it is apparent that the majority of children contracting measles and pertussis are the ones who have been vaccinated. Official vaccine records have proven that this is the case, time after time.

> **"There has never been a single vaccine in this country that has ever been submitted to a controlled scientific study. They never took a group of 100 people who were candidates for a vaccine, gave 50 of them a vaccine and left the other 50 alone, and measured the outcome. And since that has never been done, that means if you want to be kind, you will call vaccines an UNPROVEN REMEDY. If you want to be accurate, you'll call the people who give vaccines QUACKS."** Robert Mendelsohn, M.D.

The CDC uses words such as efficacy to confuse the public. They make the claim that vaccines effectively induce the production of antibodies and they are correct; however, that is only half of the equation. What they fail to honestly admit is that vaccines have not been proven to be clinically effective in protecting against disease. Many people who are vaccinated develop antibodies. That's a fact. However, they still end up contracting the disease. In other words, a vaccinated person with a high antibody titer can still contract the illness, so the vaccine is not effective in preventing the disease; however, the CDC labels it as effective because it produces antibodies. Who cares if the vaccine produces antibodies if you still end up contracting the disease?

> **"Vaccination at its core is neither a safe nor an effective method of disease prevention."** Tetyana Obukhanych, Ph.D., Immunologist

A similar twist of words occurs in the cancer industry with chemotherapy and radiation. The chemo or radiation may in fact kill the cancer cells and the establishment takes credit for curing cancer; however, they fail to mention that the patient's body is so weakened from the poison that they die two months later. So, the statistics record the cancer treatment effective for curing cancer, despite the patient dying shortly after treatment. Is this honest? Just as the cancer industry deceives us with cancer cure-rate statistics, so does the vaccination industry claim new vaccines are safe and effective as they compare new vaccines to old vaccines instead of those who receive the vaccine as compared to those who don't.

> **"Confuse the meaning of words and you confuse the mind."** Vladimir Lenin, 1870-1924 (Russian Communist)

What happens when children are killed or severely damaged from vaccinations? Who is responsible? The CDC claims that the vaccine, the doctor who administered it, the vaccine manufacturer and the government who mandated the shot are not responsible.

> **WHO IS RESPONSIBLE FOR VACCINATION DAMAGE?**
> - The vaccine is not responsible.
> - The doctor who gave the shot is not responsible.
> - The vaccine manufacturer is not responsible.
> - The government who mandates mass vaccinations is not responsible.
> - ✓ **The CDC states the genetically defective child is to blame.**

According to the CDC, when children are harmed or killed from vaccines, the genetically defective child is to blame. Who are these people that blame vaccine damage and death on the child? The CDC, with their devious tactics to cover up harmful vaccine side effects, has even warned that the DTaP shot will look like it causes seizures, SIDS, autism, etc., but states that it is not the vaccine. If it's not the vaccine, then what is it? It is absolutely appalling that the CDC muscles their way around to vaccinate every child and then weasels their way out of any responsibility for death and injury when it occurs. It's time that these officials take some responsibility for their actions and quit blaming innocent children as being genetically defective!

> **"Educated parents can either get their children out of harm's way or continue living inside one of the largest, most evil lies in history, that vaccines — full of heavy metals, viral diseases, mycoplasma, fecal material, DNA fragments from other species, formaldehyde, polysorbate 80 (a sterilizing agent) — are a miracle of modern medicine."** Andrew Baker

To demonstrate how powerful these elite groups (CDC, vaccine manufacturers and doctors) are, it is interesting to note that each of them is legally exempt and in no way held accountable for adverse vaccine reactions. In other words, if you choose to vaccinate and disaster occurs (SIDS, seizures, autism, etc.), then legal action against these groups is essentially impossible. You are just "out." Sadly, this may mean that you are taking care of a disabled child for the rest of your life or attending their funeral. Talk to a parent who had a perfectly healthy child, and then after a vaccination, they regressed into autism. Changing an adult, 20-year-old's diaper every day and knowing that they will never be able to function or live on their own is sad, frustrating and extremely expensive for the care they will need the rest of their lives. Educate before you vaccinate.

In the 1980s, thousands of children suffered from vaccine-caused adverse reactions and even death, and numerous lawsuits were filed, holding drug companies responsible for the safety of their products. Drug companies Merck, Wyeth, Lederle and Connaught blackmailed Congress by threatening to stop manufacturing vaccines unless a law was passed providing them with protection. In 1986, Congress passed the National Childhood Vaccine Injury Act (NCVIA), eliminating the potential financial liability of vaccine manufacturers due to vaccine injury claims. And in 2011, the U.S. Supreme Court gave drug companies complete immunity from all liability for harm caused by vaccines. Meanwhile, the federal government uses our tax dollars to pay billions of dollars to vaccine-damaged children. It's time to repeal immunity for drug companies against vaccine injuries.

> **"I did not find it difficult to conclude that there is no evidence whatsoever that vaccines of any kind — but especially those against childhood diseases — are effective in preventing the infectious diseases they are supposed to prevent. Further, adverse effects are amply documented and are far more significant to public health than any adverse effects of infectious diseases. Immunizations, including those practiced on babies, not only did not prevent any infectious diseases, they caused more suffering and more deaths than has any other human activity in the entire history of medical intervention. It will be decades before the mopping-up after the disasters caused by childhood vaccination will be completed. All vaccination should cease forthwith and all victims of their side effects should be appropriately compensated."** Viera Scheibner, Ph.D. (Principal Research Scientist, Author of 3 books, some 90 scientific papers & co-developer of Cot watch (a breathing monitor to prevent SIDS)

Some people argue that their children have received vaccinations and appear to be fine. Maybe your child will be one that is okay if you vaccinate and maybe they won't. We have many come into the office desperate for help. I have personally worked with vaccine-damaged children and their parents, and watching parents break down and cry out of frustration and desperation because their most prized possession in life, their child, has been permanently damaged or killed from vaccinations is disheartening. And what makes matters worse is that the parent chose to take the child in, and hold them still, to be injected with harmful toxins that affected the child for the rest of their life. Try consoling a mother and father burdened with guilt for choosing to vaccinate and seeing their beautiful, healthy, robust child experience neurological damage and regress into autism. The answer is always the same, "I wish I would have done some research before vaccinating." In some situations, depending upon how severe the case is, it is possible to detoxify the child, heal the gut and help improve the quality of life, but we cannot push rewind. The effects of vaccinations are many times permanent.

> "The CDC is not an independent agency. It is a vaccine company ... The CDC owns over 20 vaccine patents. It sells about $4.6 billion of vaccines every year."
> Robert F. Kennedy Jr.

Vaccinations Weaken Your Immune System

Increased levels of antibodies cause many allergies and respiratory illnesses. Science has identified five classes of antibodies, which include: IgG, IgA, IgM, IgE and IgD. Various chemicals found in vaccines can be a major cause for the development of IgE antibodies. Shots containing mercury (thimerosal), aluminum, acellular pertussis, rubella, DT vaccine and gelatin in the chickenpox vaccine have been reported to elevate IgE concentrations in the body, thus being a factor in many cases of allergies and asthma.

> "You'd think there would be loads of studies showing that vaccinated kids are healthier than non-vaccinated kids. There's not a single study showing that ... not one. There are increasing studies showing the reverse is true. It's the vaccinated kids with autism; with neurological problems; with weaker immune systems; with personality disorders; with cancer ... not the non-vaccinated children." Ted Koren, D.C.

All vaccines with the exception of the oral polio vaccine (OPV) are injected directly into the bloodstream. When God created you, He put in your body a mucosal immune system, also known as the secretory IgA. The secretory IgA is like a guard at a gate that prevents enemies from coming in and taking over. It filters microbes out, so that by the time an invading organism does get in the bloodstream, it is greatly reduced. So how does your body get rid of the microbes that do make it in? They are captured and taken right back out the gate, through the mucosal barrier by sneezing, coughing and sweating. That is why it is dangerous to take drugs that suppress your sneezing, coughing and sweating. The guards in your immune system are trying to take the illegal alien microbes back out, and you interfere with their work by suppressing your symptoms with cough syrup, Flonase, Sudafed and Tylenol. Sweating, coughing and sneezing are how the body eliminates toxins.

> "Every day new parents are ringing us. They all have the same tragic story. Healthy baby, child, teenager, usually a boy, given the DPT, MMR booster

> followed by a sudden fall or slow but steady decline into autism or other spectrums disorder." The Hope Project (Ireland)

Vaccines are injected straight into the bloodstream, through your body's first line of defense, the mucosal barrier, with no warning. God created us with a defense system to protect us against foreign invaders. They include your skin, mucus, tears, saliva and stomach acid. The guards in your immune system have no chance to sound the warning siren, to recognize, duplicate or defend itself against the vaccination attack. When these foreign substances, including antibiotics, preservatives, and chemicals that are designed to irritate the immune system, enter the body, bypassing all of your God-given natural barriers, then common sense cautions us to rethink what we are doing. It doesn't happen this way in nature. We are never bombarded with an onslaught of chemicals, mutated viruses and bacteria straight into the blood all at once. In a chaotic frenzy, wherever these toxins settle, the body in its quest to destroy them can sometimes begin to attack the organs and glands where the vaccine toxins lodge. This is called autoimmune. Some people and animals cannot withstand such an assault without sustaining damage and sometimes even death. We have been created with these defenses for a wise reason, and then a doctor comes along and figures out a way to bypass them with a needle brewing with live and dead toxins, and we wonder what went wrong when our baby won't stop screaming, runs a fever and is covered in a rash.

> "I am no longer 'trying to dig up evidence to prove' vaccines cause autism. There is already abundant evidence ... This debate is not scientific but is political." David Ayoub, M.D.

According to the CDC, one in six children has a developmental disability, while Health and Human Services (HHS) reports that 54 percent of children have chronic illness. Many of our children suffer from autism, seizures, autoimmune disorders, dyslexia, hyperactivity and other development disabilities. Doctors and nurses continue to give shots that they know very little about. The problem is, when your salary depends upon you not thinking for yourself but just merely following routine procedures blindly, you keep doing what your authorities tell you in order to keep a paycheck every week.

> "Autism may be a disorder linked to the disruption of the G-alpha protein, affecting retinoid receptors in the brain. A study of 60 autistic children suggests that autism may be caused by inserting a G-alpha protein defect, the pertussis toxin found in the DPT vaccine, into genetically at-risk children." Mary N. Megson, M.D.

Our immune systems have been battling microbes and infectious diseases since the beginning of time. How else could we have survived for all the centuries before man created vaccines? The fact that you are reading this sentence says that you are the best of the best, survival of the fittest. Your ancestors survived the disease epidemics of the past, without artificial vaccinations, and now you are here. Those who were weak didn't make it. That says a lot about your immune system. Congratulations, you are a winner, the best of the best.

> "What we forget is that millions of years of evolution have taken place on this planet, and up until the last 100 years, humans have lived in relative harmony with microbes. Yes, there have been epidemic infectious diseases in history, but they have always resolved themselves. I don't think there is any real appreciation for what we may be doing by using so many vaccines to try to eradicate so many organisms. If we stay the present course, will mankind be free from infectious disease but crippled by chronic disease? Will eradication of feared diseases, such as AIDS, through mass vaccination be one of man's greatest triumphs or will we live in fear of deadly mutations of microbes that have outsmarted man's attempt to eradicate them? We may look back at the crossroads we are at today and wish we had decided to make peace with nature instead of trying to dominate it." Richard Moskowitz, M.D.

Children who have been fully vaccinated were found to have a higher risk of asthma as adults. (Aust N Z J Public Health. 2004 Aug;28(4):336-8.) A New Zealand study revealed that 23 percent of vaccinated children develop asthma compared to zero in unvaccinated children. Another study of 450 children, 11 percent who had received the pertussis vaccination, suffered from asthma, as compared with only 2 percent of children who were not vaccinated. (JAMA. Aug 24-31; 272(8):592-3. 1994 "Pertussis vaccination and asthma: is there a link?")

> "The greatest threat of childhood diseases lies in the dangerous and ineffectual efforts made to prevent them through mass immunization." Robert Mendelsohn, M.D.

Research shows that children who receive vaccines are nearly eight times more likely to have epileptic seizures within 24 hours following the pertussis, polio and Hib vaccinations when compared to children who were not recently vaccinated. Convulsions are six times more likely to occur six to 11 days after being vaccinated with MMR. In 77 percent of the cases, onset of Guillain-Barre syndrome occurred within six weeks following the hepatitis B or influenza vaccine. (Souayah N, Nasar A, et al. J Clin Neuromuscular Dis 2009 Sep: 11(1): 1-6.) Hundreds of these red-flag-waving studies show that vaccines are dangerous, but our government ignores them and claims they are safe. Why is the science being ignored?

> "What is terrifying is that these pandemic vaccines contain ingredients, called immune adjuvants, that a number of studies have shown cause devastating autoimmune disorders. So, what is the deadly ingredient? It is called squalene, a type of soil. Squalene in vaccines has been strongly linked to the Gulf War Syndrome, Lou Gehrig's disease, multiple sclerosis, lupus, transverse myelitis, among other diseases. Studies of immune adjuvants using careful tracer techniques have shown that they routinely enter the brain following vaccination. One must keep in mind that once the vaccine is injected, there is little you can do to protect yourself — at least by conventional medicine. It will mean a lifetime of crippling illness and early death. The danger is the prolonged brain inflammation caused by activation of the brain's immune cells by squalene. In other words, your immune system may go in overdrive and start attacking your own body due to artificially heightened stimulation by squalene." Russell Blaylock, M.D.

In 1958, the American Academy of Pediatrics listed eczema as a contraindication for vaccination and warned, "Eczema vaccinatum is frequently iatrogenic (doctor/medication caused) and uniformly preventable. The following steps are recommended for prophylaxis:
1. No child with atopic eczema or other skin disorder should be vaccinated.
2. No child should be vaccinated if any member of his family has eczema or other skin disorder."

> "I've been practicing for 40 years, and in the past 10 years, the children have been sicker than ever." Doris Rapp, M.D., Founder of the Practical Allergy Foundation

Vaccinations – The Missing Link To Food Allergies

A hundred years ago, allergies were almost unheard of, but now over a million children carry around an EpiPen, just in case they have an allergy attack. We have always eaten peanuts, eggs, milk, wheat and corn, so what are we doing differently now to cause such an increase in life-threatening allergies? Could 72 doses of vaccines from birth to age 18 have something to do with it? Let the science speak.

According to the CDC, food allergies have risen by 50 percent between 1997 and 2011 in children under 17 years of age. About 15 million Americans suffer with life-threatening food allergies, and 300,000 of them are children who have reactions so severe it causes anaphylaxis shock, requiring emergency treatments. In society, police officers apprehend criminals who break the law and remove them from the public. Like police officers, the immune system removes criminals (illegal proteins) from the body that cause allergies. An allergy occurs when the body recognizes a foreign protein and begins an attack to expel it, since it is not recognized as a "good protein," with proper I.D., or as part of the body.

Allergy = Abnormal Recognition of a Protein

Food Proteins In Vaccines
- Peanut oil
- Eggs (ovalbumin)
- Milk (casein)
- Soy protein
- Wheat
- Corn
- Sunflower oil
- Yeast
- Polysorbate/sorbitol

Vaccines contain foreign food proteins: peanut oil, ovalbumin (protein in egg whites), casein (protein in milk), soy, wheat, corn, coconut, sunflower oil, sucrose, glutamic acid, gelatin, polysorbate 80 (sorbitol) and yeast proteins, to name a few. They're hidden ingredients, not listed on the vaccine label, so you really don't know what you are getting and how much in each vaccine, because according to the CDC, it is not regulated, and every batch is different. These foods, and especially peanut oil, were never meant to bypass the body's guards at the gate and be injected into a child's blood. Our digestive system was designed to break down proteins with strong stomach acids and digestive enzymes in the intestines. To bypass our digestive system and inject large food proteins through a vaccine directly into the muscle may be a major contributor of allergies. When these large undigested protein molecules enter the bloodstream, the immune system recognizes them as foreign invaders (illegal aliens without passports), and the immune system initiates a response to expel them, thus creating inflammation and an allergy.

> **"We are so constituted that we can never receive other portions into the blood than those that have been modified by digestive juices. Every time alien protein penetrates by effraction (vaccination), the organism suffers and becomes resistant."** Dr. Charles Robert Richet, 1913 Nobel Prize Winner

Dr. Charles Richet won the Nobel Prize in Medicine in 1913 for his work with anaphylaxis. He proved over 100 years ago that injecting a food protein into an animal or human causes immune sensitization to that protein. Subsequent exposure to the protein can result in allergic reactions or anaphylaxis. Why does the CDC ignore this science, and allow food proteins in vaccines? With our current vaccine schedule, children will receive 36 injections before the age of 18 months, when the immune system is still underdeveloped. By the age of 18, children will have received 72 doses of vaccines, containing massive amounts of food proteins, adjuvants and preservatives such as aluminum, mercury and formaldehyde. Do you think this may have something to do with our increase in allergies? This assault on the immune system increases your risk of developing allergies exponentially. Even the Institute of Medicine (IOM) confirmed that food proteins in vaccines cause food allergies. Many allergy specialists have demanded that food proteins be removed from vaccines; unfortunately, the CDC and vaccine manufacturers refuse. Why? The question is, do they want our children to be sick with allergies? It's as if the vaccine manufacturers own patents on allergy medications. Oh wait, they do. The EpiPen, manufactured by King, a subsidiary of Pfizer and marketed by Mylan, is $332 a pen at Walmart. Do pharmaceutical companies want our children to have allergies so they can sell millions of EpiPens and allergy medication?

Molecular Mimicry Again

> "If people let the government decide what foods they eat and what medicines they take, their bodies will soon be in as sorry a state as are the souls who live under tyranny." Thomas Jefferson

Adjuvants like aluminum are added to vaccines to aggravate the body and increase an immune response to whatever strain of virus or bacteria the vaccinations are attempting to produce immunity against. The dilemma is, aluminum can cause the body to overreact against germ proteins, which may be identical to our own body's proteins. This overreaction has been shown to stimulate IgE (allergies), inflammation and even trigger autoimmune disorders in mice and dogs.

Vaccine Proteins May Trigger Autoimmune Disorders
- Rheumatoid Arthritis – antibodies attack joints
- Lupus – antibodies attack body tissue
- Multiple sclerosis – antibodies attack nerve cells
- Type 1 Diabetes – antibodies attack insulin cells, pancreas
- Guillain-Barre – nerves controlling muscles are attacked
- Psoriasis – overactive immune, T-cells collect on skin
- Graves' Disease – antibodies stimulate thyroid
- Hashimoto's – antibodies attack thyroid
- Myasthenia Gravis – nerve cells unable to work muscles
- Inflammatory Bowel Disease – antibodies attack intestines

We are made up of proteins, just as bacteria and viruses have protein pieces too. Vaccines contain microbe proteins, which are similar to protein segments in the body. Many vaccines such as tetanus contain microbe proteins very similar to (or the same as) protein segments in your body. So, if you get a shot and those vaccine proteins attach to the cells in the joints, your immune system may initiate an autoimmune attack on the joints, and you develop rheumatoid arthritis. If they attach to the cells in the pancreas, you could develop diabetes, and if it's the thyroid, you may be diagnosed with Hashimoto's disease. When they attach to brain cells, you may have autism or seizures. Where the proteins attach is the part of the body your immune system may attack in an attempt to expel the foreign proteins.

Another red flag with vaccines is that when a child receives several doses, and the antibody levels soar into the hundreds and even the thousands (7,000 antibodies in some cases) with no wild measles or pertussis to attack, then those antibodies have the potential to attach to a similar protein molecule in any organ or gland. So, when you inject a child with aluminum to aggravate the immune system in conjunction with large food proteins, it is as risky as throwing matches into dry grass and hoping a fire (autoimmune disease) doesn't start. We are playing vaccine roulette, and just look at how many innocent children are losing.

> "It's been known for quite some time that injecting the body with Aluminum Hydroxide can trigger any kind of allergy, in animals, for instance. It now turns out that you can make mice allergic by feeding them apples or nuts together with medication for heartburn. These drugs contain Aluminum Hydroxide as an active substance and apparently, Aluminum turns the immune system against a simultaneously administered substance." Bert Ehgartner, Author of *Age of Aluminum*

Allergies and autoimmune disorders can both be triggered by foreign proteins being injected into the body and bypassing the digestive system. No one connects the dots, linking the vaccine as the spark that created a hypersensitive immune reaction, resulting in a fiery autoimmune response. If we want to prevent fires, we have to eliminate the sparks that cause them. Remember, the definition of an allergy is an abnormal recognition of a protein, and when we inject food proteins such as peanut oil, polysorbate 80 and aluminum into a muscle, we greatly increase our risks for allergies and autoimmune fires.

American Children - In Crisis
1 in 3 are overweight
1 in 6 have learning disabilities
1 in 9 have asthma
1 in 10 have ADHD
1 in 12 have food allergies
1 in 20 have seizures
1 in 36 have autism

Foreign proteins don't just end with vaccines. There are other factors creating allergies: genetically modified foods (GMOs), glyphosate herbicide, MSG, antibiotics, C-section births, failure to breastfeed newborns and prescription drugs. Mix all those together with vaccines, and you have a real witches' brew for your body to become a science experiment. It appears our science experiments are failing and our children are paying a heavy price.

Mercury (Thimerosal) In Vaccines

> "How is it that mercury is not safe for food additives and over-the-counter drug products, but it is safe in our vaccines and dental amalgams?" Congressman Dan Burton, Indiana

Mercury is the second most toxic metal known to man. The MSDS (Material Safety Data Sheet) on thimerosal

> **MATERIAL SAFETY DATA SHEET ON THIMEROSAL**
> - May cause damage to the following organs: kidneys, liver, spleen, bone marrow, central nervous system (CNS).
> - May cause **cancer** based on animal data. May cause adverse reproductive effects (female fertility-post implantation mortality, fetotoxicity) and birth defects. May cause genetic defects.

from Eli Lilly states on their own letterheads that thimerosal is a *"product containing a chemical known to the state of California to cause birth defects or other reproductive harm."* Despite this blatant warning, Lilly still continues using thimerosal in the manufacturing of vaccines.

We get mercury from vaccines, silver dental fillings, drinking water, fish, fluorescent lightbulbs, batteries, tattoo ink, coal plants and over-the-counter products, to name a few. Methylmercury, also known as organic mercury, is found in fish, with high concentrations in tuna, shark and swordfish. It is easily absorbed and difficult to eliminate. Inorganic mercury such as vapor from silver dental fillings accumulates in body tissue. Ethylmercury is an organic form of mercury found in petroleum hydrocarbons and vaccines. If a thermometer breaks in a school, by law you must call in the hazmat team and evacuate the building until the toxic spill is thoroughly cleaned and the building has been tested and considered safe. In 1982, the FDA made a recommendation that thimerosal (mercury) be banned as a topical, over-the-counter product because, well, it's toxic. Any medical product containing mercury can't be thrown in the trash, because it's toxic, but it is somehow safe to inject into pregnant women and 6-month-old babies with the flu shot? We are encouraged to take our babies in to the doctor and inject mercury straight into his or her bloodstream with a needle, and call it a well-baby visit? Have we lost our minds? Does this make any sense? The CDC says it's such a small amount that it is harmless. That's not what the majority of independent scientists with published studies in medical journals claim, those who aren't on a vaccine manufacturer's payroll. Let's take a look.

> **"You couldn't even construct a study that shows thimerosal is safe. It's just too damn toxic. If you inject thimerosal into an animal, its brain will sicken. If you apply it to living tissue, the cells die, if you put it in a petri dish, the culture dies. Knowing these things, it would be shocking if one could inject it into an infant without causing damage."** Dr. Boyd Haley, Professor & Chair, Department of Chemistry, University of Kentucky

Thimerosal, which is 49.6 percent mercury by weight, has been one of the most widely used preservatives in vaccines for many years. It is added to prevent bacterial contamination and kill organisms. All multi-dose vaccines must contain a preservative, usually thimerosal. Once in the body, it is metabolized or degraded into methylmercury.

> "So... let me get this straight: You break a mercury thermometer, you call hazmat. You remove mercury fillings and they become toxic waste the minute they leave your mouth. Pregnant women are warned of swordfish due to mercury toxicity. But put mercury into a syringe, and PRESTO! It's medicine, and it's safe for pregnant women and their fetuses." Jack Knight

Has mercury been removed from vaccines? Yes and no. Thimerosal, which contains mercury, is still added to seven vaccines; the flu shot, meningococcal, tetanus and diphtheria shots still contain mercury and never had it removed.

From 1999 through 2002, vaccine manufacturers discontinued putting mercury in most vaccines except for the flu shot and those mentioned previously. However, thimerosal is still used in the vaccine manufacturing process, so residual, trace amounts still end up in the vaccines. Since thimerosal is no longer added in the manufacturing process, it is no longer disclosed on the vaccine label; therefore, people believe vaccines are mercury free, but they are not. About 600 micrograms (mcg) or 600 parts per billion (ppb) of thimerosal is still in the so-called thimerosal-free vaccines.

Since 1997, the CDC recommended all pregnant women get the mercury-laced flu shot in their first trimester. Then in 2004, the flu shot was added to the list on the vaccine schedule for all babies 6 to 23 months of age. Vaccines that are 25 mcg of mercury, have 50,000 ppb of mercury. With this rigorous flu shot schedule, pregnant women and infants receive more mercury now than they did before 2002, when vaccines still added mercury and listed it as an active ingredient! And the ridiculous part about this is, uninformed doctors and parents argue out of ignorance that mercury has been removed from vaccines.

> "I think that the biological case against thimerosal is so dramatically overwhelming anymore that only a very foolish or a very dishonest person with the credentials to understand this research would say that thimerosal wasn't most likely the cause of autism." Boyd Haley, Ph.D.

Mercury is extremely toxic to the brain and nervous system at any dilution, explains Dr. Boyd Haley, one of the world's foremost experts on heavy metals. It can interfere with the immune system by altering the cytokine status, triggering autoimmune diseases and allergies. By continuing to inject this poison into our children, we are rolling the dice in hopes that no harm occurs. Thousands of parents of vaccine-damaged children plead for others to think twice before vaccinating. After watching his grandson be diagnosed with autism after a round of vaccinations, Indiana Congressman Dan Burton, during a congressional hearing in 2003, demanded criminal sanctions be brought against the head of the FDA and FTC and any other government agencies that knew about the dangers of thimerosal in vaccines and failed to protect American children by suppressing research information, proving how damaging it is.

A 2013 study was done to see if mercury in vaccines has any impact on a child's health. Infants who received the DTaP vaccines with mercury had twice the risk of autism compared to infants that received mercury-free DTaP vaccines. Infants who received 37.5 mcg of mercury from thimerosal-containing hepatitis B vaccines within the first six months of life were three times more likely to be diagnosed with autism, compared to those who received mercury-free hepatitis B vaccines. (Geier DA, Hooker BS, et al. Trans/Neurodegener 2013 Dec 19;2(1):25.)

> **"Thimerosal is the preservative in immunization shots, so anytime you get an immunization shot you are undergoing the same procedure that in the University Lab we used to give animals autoimmune disease — give a little tiny injection of mercury. And when you get an immunization shot you are getting a little tiny dose of mercury there."** Hal Huggins, DDS

165 Scientific Studies Link Mercury in Vaccines To:
- Neurotoxicity
- Brain Injury
- Neurodevelopmental disorders
- Autism
- Autoimmune disorders
- Kidney toxicity
- Hormonal imbalances
- Mitochondria toxicity
- Fetal toxicity
- DNA damage
- ADD

There are nearly 200 different studies providing evidence that thimerosal-containing vaccines are dangerous and unsafe for humans. Thimerosal-containing vaccines cause neurodevelopment disorders, including autism, ADD, and tic disorder. Pregnant women who receive thimerosal in vaccines significantly increase the risk of birth defects and fetal death. Thimerosal has also been proven to be toxic to human neuron cells in vitro. (Geier DA, King PG, et al. Thimerosal: clinical, epidemiologic and biochemical studies. Clin Chim Acta 2015 Apr 15;444: 212-20.)

The CDC chooses to ignore more than 165 scientific studies that show thimerosal is harmful in childhood vaccines, while basing their foundation that thimerosal is safe off six studies that were coauthored and sponsored by the CDC. Closer examination of why these six CDC-sponsored studies contradict independent scientific research over the last 75 years that consistently found thimerosal to be harmful revealed that three of the studies withheld important results from the final publication. Furthermore, a seventh study showed that infants who received thimerosal-containing vaccines were at a higher risk of developing autism, but the CDC conveniently failed to publicize or acknowledge that research. (Hooker b, Kern J, et al. Methodological issues and evidence of malfeasance in research purporting to show thimerosal in vaccines is safe. BioMed Research International 2014; article ID 247218.)

The CDC sponsoring research would be like taking someone who is convicted of murder and only considering evidence based upon the case from the suspect's friends and family while ignoring the evidence gathered from witnesses, nonfamily and law enforcement. Of course, the murderer is going to be found innocent if you only examine his side of the story and only listen to his family and friends. Obviously, they will only acknowledge evidence that supports him being not guilty, just like the CDC claims thimerosal is innocent from their own six studies, because they only look at evidence that provides them with what they want, not the honest, non-drug-funded, 165 research studies that show how harmful mercury is to the body.

> "He who doesn't take the time to learn the truth someday will suffer the consequences." J. Rueben Clark

According to an article in JAMA (Journal of the American Medical Association) 1999, by Dr. Neal Halsey (282) p1763, "Limiting Infant Exposure to Thimerosal in Vaccines," the EPA sets

EPA MERCURY TOXICITY LEVELS
2 ppb - Drinking Water Maximum
200 ppb - Liquid Waste = Hazardous
250 ppb - Tuna Fish

the limit at **0.1 micrograms of mercury per kilogram of body weight per day as a maximum "safe level" of exposure to mercury.** Then the CDC turns around and tells us to vaccinate our children with vaccines containing mercury levels that supersede way beyond the "safe level." By this standard a baby would have to weigh 550 pounds or 250 kilograms to safely receive one vaccine that contains 25 micrograms of thimerosal!

VACCINE	MERCURY IN VACCINE
FluLavel	25 mcg (50,000 ppb)
Fluvirin	25 mcg (50,000 ppb)
Fluzone	25 mcg (50,000 ppb)
Menomune	25 mcg (50,000 ppb)
Afluria	25 mcg (50,000 ppb)
Meningococcal	25 mcg (50,000 ppb)
Tetanus	25 mcg (50,000 ppb)

Did our so-called health experts flunk their mathematics courses in school? We are injecting a known poison (mercury) into our children, and to make matters worse, we ignore the safe level limit. Is it a mystery that childhood autism, ADD, cancer, asthma, diabetes, autoimmune disorders, etc., are skyrocketing each year when we ignore the EPA's safe limit? Even the FDA cautions pregnant women to reduce their fish consumption in order to reduce mercury exposure, but then turns around and completely ignores the massive amounts given in vaccines.

> **"Do you mean to tell me, since 1929, we've been using thimerosal and the only test that you know of is the one that was done in 1929? And every one of those people had meningitis and they all died?"** Congressman Dan Burton, questioning Dr. William Egan, FDA, at the June 6, 2002, Congressional Hearing

Children from 6 months to 35 months of age receive a half-dose of the flu shot, which is 12.5 mcg of mercury. This is 16 times over the safe level limit, according to the EPA! A 3-year-old child receives 25 mcg of mercury in the flu shot, which is almost 18 times the safe level. One dose of the flu shot contains 50,000 ppb of mercury. Multi-dose vials contain the highest amounts of thimerosal as opposed to single-dose vials. When a pregnant woman gets a flu shot, the tiny fetus is being injected with levels of toxic mercury that is hundreds of times above the "safe limit" as defined by the EPA. Six months later, after the infant is born, they give another dose and every year after that. We pump our babies full of known neurotoxic metals, and then wonder why 1 in 6 have learning disabilities and 1 in 36 are autistic. Doctors stand around scratching their heads, trying to figure out why their immune systems are attacking their brains, nerves and muscles. Hello, when you inject toxic mercury into the body, it's going to cause problems. How and where it manifests, is your guess.

MERCURY IN VACCINES
25,000 ppb - Infant Flu Shot
50,000 ppb - Flu Shot

> **"A single vaccine given to a 6-pound newborn is the equivalent of giving 180-pound adult 30 vaccinations on the same day."** Dr. Boyd Haley

Mercury causes brain neuron degeneration, which is linked to autism, Parkinson's disease, multiple sclerosis and many other neurological disorders. In 2007, Dr. Fritz Lorscheider and Dr. Naweed Syed of the University of Calgary, Faculty of Medicine, produced a stunning 5-minute video clip showing in vivid detail exactly what happens to your brain cells when they're exposed to mercury. I highly encourage you to watch it. It can be viewed on YouTube.

Watch on YouTube (5 minutes long)
How Mercury Causes Brain Neuron Degeneration – University of Calgary

The CDC states that ethylmercury in vaccines is cleared from the body more quickly than methylmercury, and is therefore less likely to cause any harm. This statement is based upon levels in the blood dropping because they assume it is being eliminated from the body and no longer poses a health threat. The fallacy of this statement is the fact that mercury is lipophilic, meaning that it concentrates in fatty tissues of the body, like the brain and nerves, which is made mostly of fat. Obviously, blood levels won't reveal an accurate measurement of mercury levels in the body, since it accumulates in fatty tissue and is not just circulating in the blood. This is one reason that metal toxicologist Dr. Rashid Buttar explains that blood tests are inaccurate for determining mercury toxicity. Ethylmercury, the kind used in vaccines, is not safer than methylmercury.

Dr. Stephanie Cave, author of *What Your Doctor May Not Tell You About Children's Vaccinations,* specializes in treating autistic children at her clinic in Louisiana. She explains that bile production is minimal in infancy, making it more difficult for metals to be cleared from the body. When added to a vaccine, the metals are even more dangerous, because the vaccines trigger immune reactions that increase the permeability of the GI tract and the blood/brain barrier.

Aluminum In Vaccines

> **"All these findings plausibly implicate Aluminum adjuvants in pediatric vaccines as casual factors contributing to increased rates of autism spectrum disorders in countries where multiple doses are almost universally administered."** Journal of Toxicology

When the CDC started removing mercury from some vaccines around 2000, they replaced them with aluminum. They swapped one neurological toxin for another. This is one reason we didn't see autism rates decrease. As previously mentioned, with more vaccines added to the schedule, especially the flu shot, we actually increased the amount of thimerosal children receive from vaccines as well.

Aluminum is an adjuvant used in vaccines to agitate the immune system, to create a response. The vaccine is injected into the muscle, and then white blood cells, macrophages, rush to clean up the toxic aluminum assault. These aluminum particles go to the brain, nerves, bones, kidneys and all over the body, which can trigger an autoimmune response to expel the toxic aluminum from areas of the body where it settles. Remember, the body is intelligent. It would never attack itself unless there is a toxicity issue, requiring an immune cleanup response. Your doctor then diagnoses you or your child with an autoimmune disease and prescribes an immunosuppressive drug such as Humira, a billion-dollar moneymaker for Big Pharma. Naturally, with a suppressed immune system from the drug, you know what comes next — cancer, the other big moneymaker.

Aluminum is a known neurotoxin, capable of destroying neurons necessary for proper cognitive and motor functions. When mice are injected with aluminum, with a dosage equivalent to what a human would receive in a vaccine, autoimmune and neurological disorders begin to manifest. Neuroscientist Dr. Chris Shaw's research shows a link between aluminum hydroxide used in vaccines and symptoms associated with Parkinson's, ALS (Lou Gehrig's disease) and Alzheimer's. He also found that nations with the highest prevalence of autism spectrum disorders (U.S., U.K., Canada, and Australia) require their children to receive the highest numbers of vaccines containing aluminum.

> "The aluminum in vaccines is not the same aluminum that you ingest or inhale. The aluminum in vaccines is in such a structure that it can easily pass into the brain and bring with it viruses and bacteria." Lawrence Palevsky, M.D.

Is it coincidence that the highest autism rates in the world occur in western countries that require the most aluminum-containing vaccines for preschool children? Researchers such as Dr. Masahiro Kawahara show similar findings on how aluminum causes neurological damage, leading to disease and cellular death by altering DNA and stiffening the myelin around nerves. Dr. Stephanie Seneff published a study in 2012 linking symptoms of autism to aluminum adjuvants in vaccines with a strong correlation to the MMR vaccine. She makes the following statement.

> "Our results provide strong evidence supporting a link between autism and the aluminum in vaccines." Stephanie Seneff, Ph.D., Senior Research Scientist, MIT

Dr. Seneff explains that the Tdap vaccine contains aluminum. Glyphosate, the main ingredient in Monsanto's Roundup weed killer, is synergistic with aluminum and is a powerful metal chelator. Chelators bind to metals and minerals, then deposit them in acidic environments. Virtually all of us have glyphosate in our bodies. So, the blood in the pineal gland, being located in the brain, near the end of the circulatory system, is naturally more acidic before returning to the lungs. It's the perfect opportunity for glyphosate to carry aluminum that's in the vaccine to the pineal gland and ruin it. This is one reason we are seeing so many neurological problems such as sleep disorders, multiple sclerosis, Alzheimer's, Parkinson's and Lou Gehrig's disease.

Today we are seeing one in six children suffering with neurodevelopment disorders, which is a huge increase from decades ago. When aluminum travels to the brain, it causes microglial activation and elevated IL-6 production, which is immune activation and brain inflammation. Dr. Tomoyuki Takano of Japan explains that any factor that activates or alters the state of microglia early in life can affect the neural development, thus triggering autism.

> "A major cause of the Roman Empire's decline, after six centuries of world dominance, was its replacement of stone aqueducts by lead pipes for the transport and supply of drinking water. Roman engineers, the best in the world, turned their fellow citizens into cripples. Today our own 'best and brightest,' with the best of intentions, achieve the same end through childhood vaccination programs yielding the modern scourges of hyperactivity, learning

> **disabilities, autism, appetite disorders, and impulsive violence."** Harris L. Coulter, PhD

The hepatitis B vaccine, given at birth, contains 250 mcg of

> **Maximum safe level of aluminum set by the FDA is 18.16 mcg for an 8-pound baby.**

aluminum. The safe limit is 5 mcg of aluminum per kilogram of body weight set by the FDA. A brand-new baby receives 14 times the "safe limit" as soon as they're born and we wonder why we are seeing such a rise in autism and neurological disorders? Official regulations set by the FDA state that aluminum should not exceed 4 to 5 mcg per kilogram of body weight; however, the CDC ignores this, just like they do with mercury, by recommending that we bring our children in to receive DTaP, hepatitis B, HiB and Prevnar shots all in the same day. At the 2-month-old visit, the shots they receive contain 50 times above the safe limit set for aluminum. By the time they reach the 18-month-old mark, the amount of aluminum they will have received from vaccines is 4,925 mcg, and the safe limit is 25 mcg aluminum! If children get all the CDC-recommended vaccines, they will end up receiving 6,150 mcg of aluminum! Hello, we have a serious mathematical problem with toxic metals from vaccines superseding way beyond the safe limit. Even if you believe vaccines are wonderful life-savers that never cause any harm, shouldn't you be alarmed that the heavy metal toxicity level of mercury and aluminum supersedes way beyond the safe level limit set by our own government? Why even have a safety limit, if we are just going to ignore it? Could this possibly be the reason we in the U.S. have the highest rate in newborn deaths, compared to any other country?

VACCINE	ALUMINUM IN VACCINE
Hib	225 mcg
Hepatitis B	250 mcg
DTaP	625 mcg
Pneumococcus	125 mcg
Hepatitis A	250 mcg
Gardasil (HPV)	225/500 mcg
Pentacel	330 mcg
Pediatrix	850 mcg

Aluminum is eliminated from the body through the kidneys; however, infant kidney function is low at birth, and doesn't reach full capacity until 1 to 2 years of age. According to medical literature, infants may not be able to excrete aluminum, and yet we turn right around and inject them with aluminum in the hepatitis B shot at birth!

Dr. Christopher Exley, professor at Keele University, with his research partners, found extraordinarily high levels of aluminum in the brains of deceased teenagers with autism. His research also shows that many neurological diseases are linked to aluminum toxicity. (Aluminum in brain tissue in autism, Journal of Trace Elements in Medicine and Biology, Volume 46, March 2018, pp.76-82)

> "The system is designed to create chronic disease. There's no money in being healthy. There's no money in being dead. All the money is in being chronically ill." Irvin Sahni, M.D.

Research shows that aluminum in vaccines stimulates the immune system to produce high antibody levels, which can lead to serious autoimmune and inflammatory disorders. When mice are vaccinated repeatedly similar to what our children receive, T-cells eventually produced autoantibodies. The overstimulation of the immune system eventually results in autoimmune injury similar to lupus.

Flu Shots – Proven To Be Toxic & Worthless

> "I would not take the flu vaccine. My wife does not take the flu vaccine. No one should take the flu vaccine. And in fact when I was head of CDC, I wanted to make that as a public statement and I refused to say that you should take the flu vaccine. That's why I'm now professor at Harvard." Dr. Alexander Langmuir (1910-1993) Former Chief Epidemiologist for the CDC

Unfortunately, it usually takes a serious adverse reaction or death of a loved one to get our full attention before we begin investigating questionable drugs and vaccines. Dr. Leonard Horowitz witnessed his mother developing Guillain-Barre syndrome and then dying shortly after receiving a flu shot. How many people must suffer and die? The flu shot is notorious for causing Guillain-Barre paralysis.

> "There is no evidence that any influenza vaccine, thus far developed, is effective in preventing or mitigating any attack of influenza. The producers of these vaccines know that they are worthless, but they go on selling them, anyway." Dr. J. Anthony Morris, Research Virologist & Former Chief Vaccine Control Officer at the U.S. Federal Drug Administration

At 1 ppb, Thimerosal Is Toxic To Developing Neurons

MERCURY LEVELS
Infant Flu Shot – 25,000 ppb
Adult Flu Shot – 50,000 ppb

Before you get your flu shot, you may want to know that most flu shots still contain mercury and that they are cultured on aborted fetal cells. A typical 0.5 milliliter flu shot contains 25 mcg of mercury or 50,000 parts per billion. The EPA classifies any liquid with 200 parts per billion of mercury as hazardous waste. The safety limit in drinking water is set at 2 ppb.

In addition to mercury and aborted fetal cells in the flu shot, there are other ingredients that pose serious health risks. More than two dozen scientific papers from 10 different laboratories have published how molecules of an oil-based adjuvant called MF-59, primarily made up of squalene, can cause autoimmune diseases in animals. When this squalene adjuvant contained in the flu vaccine is injected into the bloodstream at concentrations as small as 10 to 20 ppb, it can lead to self-destructive immune responses, like lupus and autoimmune arthritis. (Scan J of Immunology 54 (2001): 599-605 "Responses of the rat immune system to arthritogenic adjuvant oil.")

Tween 80, also known as polysorbate 80, used in the flu shot, has been shown to cause serious disruptions within the immune system. Research demonstrates that it can cause anaphylaxis, which is a sharp drop in blood pressure, hives and breathing difficulties that can be fatal. (Annals of Allergy, Asthma and Immunology. 95 (2005): 593-599)

> "If a person had five consecutive flu shots — their chance of contracting Alzheimer's disease is 10 times higher than the non-vaccinated person." Hugh Fudenburg, M.D., Ph.D., Author of over 80 research papers in Medicine, Biology & Immunology

Does the flu shot prevent the flu? In a review of 51 studies involving more than 260,000 children, Dr. Tom Jefferson, head of the Cochrane Influenza Review Panel, and researchers found, "No evidence that injecting children 6 to 23 months of age with flu vaccines is any more effective than placebo." They also concluded that flu vaccines do not prevent serious complications or death from influenza. (The Cochran Database of Systematic Reviews. "Vaccines for preventing influenza in healthy children." 1-(2006)

> "The vaccine doesn't work very well at all. Vaccines are being used as an ideological weapon. What you see every year as the flu is caused by 200 or 300 different agents with a vaccine against two of them. That is simply nonsense."
> Dr. Tom Jefferson, Cochrane Vaccines Field

When another study was conducted on healthy adults who take the flu shot, similar results were found. The Cochran Group reviewed 25 studies that involved more than 60,000 participants and found there was a very small reduction in contracting the flu and number of days missed from work. The study concluded, "Universal immunization of healthy adults was not supported by the results of this review."

> "Take all the profit out of manufacturing and administration of serums and vaccines and they would soon be condemned, even by those who are now using them." George Starr White, M.D.

When we artificially vaccinate against seasonal influenza strains, it prevents cross protection against lethal influenza strains. Studies on mice that were vaccinated against the flu, and then infected with avian influenza virus, as compared to mice who were not vaccinated, showed that the vaccinated mice had more severe disease and died. The unvaccinated mice survived. (Bodewes R, Kreijtz JH, et al. PloS One 2009; 4(5): e5538.)

> "I cannot think of anything more insane than vaccinating pregnant women."
> Russell Blaylock, M.D. - Neurosurgeon

For pregnant mothers who are being advised to get a flu shot, you may want to know that the flu shot given during pregnancy causes an increase in CRP (C Reactive Protein) which is a measure of inflammation. And what do you think inflammation in the womb is associated with? You guessed it, an increased risk of autism. Pregnant women vaccinated for the flu also have higher rates of spontaneous abortions. Of course, the CDC ignores this and claims the flu shot is safe.

> **Safety Data Sheet - Thimerosal (Influenza Vaccine Manufacturer)**
> Exposure in utero can cause mild to severe **mental retardation** and motor coordination impairment.

The safety data sheet on thimerosal contained in the influenza vaccine actually warns that exposure in utero can cause mental retardation! This is as plain and simple as it can get, a red-flag warning for those who can read.

Research has shown that the CDC policy to vaccinate pregnant women with thimerosal-containing influenza vaccines is not supported by science and should be discontinued. The 25 mcg of mercury exceeds

EPA safety limits. (Ayoub DM, Yazbak FE. Journal of American Physicians and Surgeons 2006 Summer; 11(2): 41-47.)

> "You can fool some of the people all of the time, and all of the people some of the time, but you cannot fool all of the people all of the time." Abraham Lincoln

Many other adjuvants in vaccines have been proven harmful to the body, such as formaldehyde, which is used to embalm bodies. It disrupts the nervous system and immune function and, according to NCI reports, may contribute to the cause of leukemia. Autoimmune diseases are becoming extremely popular with the onslaught of toxic vaccine ingredients.

> "Immunization programs against flu, measles, mumps and polio may actually be seeding humans with RNA to form proviruses, which will then become latent cells throughout the body ... they can then become activated as a variety of diseases including lupus, cancer, rheumatism and arthritis." Dr. Robert W. Simpson, Rutgers University

The ticking time bombs called vaccinations that we are injecting are creating diseases for tomorrow, and no one connects the dots. These "slow viruses" may take years or even 30 years to become virulent. Like dandelions in springtime, when the environment is right and they become active, then anything from autoimmune disease to heart disease and cancer can occur. And your "faulty genes" will get blamed instead of the real culprit, vaccination toxicity.

> "So what are flu shots really for? You won't like this answer, but I'll tell you what I now believe to be true: The purpose of flu shots is to 'soft kill' the global population. Vaccines are population control technologies, as openly admitted by Bill Gates, and they are so cleverly packaged under the fabricated 'public health' message that even those who administer vaccines have no idea they are actually engaged in the reduction of human population through vaccine-induced infertility and genetic mutations. Vaccines ultimately have but one purpose: To permanently alter the human gene pool and 'weed out' those humans who are stupid enough to fall for vaccine propaganda. And for that nefarious purpose, they probably are 60 percent effective after all." Mike Adams, The Health Ranger

Dr. Leonard Horowitz explains in his 544-page page book, *Emerging Viruses: AIDS and Ebola, Nature, Accident or Genocide*, that the deadly **AIDS** virus is undoubtedly "manmade" and has evolved from accidental vaccine contaminations, and then spread through vaccines to humans. Some theorized that the polio vaccine, containing hundreds of viruses, with the SV-40 virus being the

40th virus identified, was the original source, but that theory has been discredited. The hepatitis B vaccine was produced in chimpanzees during pilot testing among gay men in New York City and African villagers from 1972 to 1974, and this is the source of the AIDS virus, according to Dr. Horowitz. His book is packed with compelling, scientific documents, along with the National Institutes of Health's contracts, proving that chimpanzees, contaminated with many viruses, were used in the manufacturing of hundreds of hepatitis B vaccines, and then injected into central Africans and homosexual men in New York City. Even Dr. Gerald Myers, chief DNA sequence analyst for the U.S. government, explained that the origin of HIV began in the mid-1970s, and that some bizarre man-made (iatrogenic) procedure involving a swarm of variants (SIVcpz-infected chimpanzees) was most likely the culprit.

> **"The medical authorities keep lying. Vaccination has been a disaster on the immune system. It causes lots of illnesses. We are actually changing our genetic code through vaccination. Vaccination is the biggest crime against humanity."**
> Guylaine Lanctot, M.D. Canada

As the years go by, new things are proven and old things are disproven. What do we really know? Mother Nature operating under God's intelligence has been producing intelligent life for a long time. Man has basically been living in harmony with microbes since the beginning of time until the last several decades. In our feeble attempt to fix things, sometimes we create a monster worse than the original one. Some viruses can lay dormant in your body, and then marry another virus to become something completely different. When bacteria and viruses begin mutating, and new strains are created because of our vaccination experiments, then the Frankenstein monster we have created may be stronger than what we can handle. Autoimmune disorders and cancer are skyrocketing, and vaccines help provide the terrain to allow these diseases to flourish.

> **"Vaccines definitely carry a risk in every single person. Every time someone is injected with these heavy metals, environmental pollutants, or tissue from another animal or from another human, we are causing damage, every single time. It's just a matter of how that damage manifests."** Jack Wolfson, M.D., Cardiologist

Gardasil

Human papillomavirus (HPV) is a sexually transmitted virus that is spread through genital contact, usually by sexual intercourse. HPV is named for the warts, or papilloma, some of the viruses can cause. There are more than 100 subtypes of HPV and forms of the virus that can cause abnormal cell growth on the cervix, which may turn to cancer. Most cases are harmless and clear up on their own. Young teenage girls have almost no risk of dying from cervical cancer, but run a high risk of experiencing adverse reactions from the vaccine. HPV vaccine has been linked to autoimmune disorders, multiple sclerosis, (ALS) Lou Gehrig's disease, Guillain-Barre syndrome, lupus, paralysis, convulsions, chronic fatigue syndrome, anaphylaxis, and death.

Gardasil contains the highest concentration of aluminum of any vaccine on the market. After understanding how toxic aluminum is to the body, is it any wonder that as of December 2016, there have been 43,532 vaccine reactions and 250 deaths reported to VAERS from the Gardasil vaccine? Researchers state one in 10 people injected with Gardasil develop neurological issues, chronic Lyme disease and serious narcolepsy.

> **"Our children face the possibility of death or serious long-term adverse effects from mandated vaccines that aren't necessary or that have very limited benefits."** Jane M. Orient, M.D., Executive Director, Association of American Physicians and Surgeons

Disaster occurred in Carmen de Bolivar, Columbia, in 2013, when roughly 200 young girls, ages 9 to 16 years old, received the Gardasil vaccine at school without their parents' consent. Many were hospitalized after experiencing dizziness, fainting, numbness, nausea, vomiting and fatigue. Over 700 women throughout Columbia who were affected from the vaccine sued Merck for $160 million after the Gardasil vaccination nightmare. In June 2013, one month prior to the Columbian fiasco, the Japanese government withdrew its official recommendation for the HPV vaccine after thousands in Japan reported adverse reactions as well. How many children must suffer and die?

Dr. Diane Harper, the lead researcher for Gardasil, has admitted that Gardasil is more dangerous than the HPV (Human Papillomavirus) it was made to prevent, yet the CDC ignores her research and pushes our children to get the vaccine.

> **"The rate of serious adverse events is greater than the incidence rate of cervical cancer. The incidence of cervical cancer in the U.S. is so low that if we get the vaccine and continue PAP screening, we will not lower the rate of cervical cancer in the U.S. ... if you vaccinate a child, she won't keep immunity in puberty and you do nothing to prevent cervical cancer."** Diane Harper, M.D., Lead Researcher for Gardasil Vaccine Trials

This is a shining example, just one of many, of how the CDC ignores scientific research and continues to promote dangerous and worthless vaccines to the masses. Could it be that the pharmaceutical companies want to make billions off a product with no regard to our young girls' health? Clinical trials have not provided evidence that the HPV vaccine has prevented a single case of cervical cancer. In fact, HPV vaccines may actually enhance cervical disease in some young girls with pre-existing HPV-16/18 infections, according to Dr. Lucija Tomlijenovic.

> **"I predict that Gardasil will become the greatest medical scandal of all times because at some point in time, the evidence will add up to prove that this vaccine, technical and scientific feat that it may be, has absolutely no effect on cervical cancer and that all the very many adverse effects which destroy lives and even kill serve no other purpose than to generate profit for the manufacturers."** Dr. Bernard Dalbergue – former pharmaceutical industry physician

Autism

Many parents, nurses and doctors read the CDC information and take it as the gospel truth. They have no idea of the corruption and dishonesty that is involved in the vaccine industry. They often like to say there is no scientific proof that vaccines cause autism. Well, it just so happens that a top CDC scientist with a nagging conscience could no longer remain silent and has confessed that he and his colleagues destroyed evidence to cover up autism risks associated with the MMR vaccine.

> **"As a clinician, my current belief which guides my practice with these children is that any child given the HepB vaccination at birth and subsequent booster along with DPT has received unacceptable levels of neurotoxin in the form of the ethyl mercury in the thimerosal preservative used in the vaccine. In any child with a genetic immune susceptibility (probably about one in six), this sets off a series of events that injure the brain-gut-immune system. By the time they are ready to receive the MMR vaccination, their immune system is so impaired in a great number of these children that the triple vaccine cannot be handled by the now-dysfunctional immune system and they begin their obvious descent into the autistic spectrum disorder."** Jaquelyn McCandless, M.D.

CDC Whistleblower Admits MMR - Autism Link Cover-Up

> **"Our database includes thousands of cases of previously healthy children who began exhibiting autistic behavior soon after getting a routine vaccination."** Bernard Rimland, Ph.D.

Florida Congressman Bill Posey, in 2015, presented evidence to the House floor that whistleblower Dr. William Thompson, senior scientist for the CDC in 2014, admitted that the CDC was committing fraud, and that they knew the MMR vaccine was causing neurological disorders associated with autism. Rather than publishing the data so parents could be made aware of the risks linking thimerosal-containing vaccines to autism, they secretly destroyed it in a meeting in 2002. *"I regret that my coauthors and I omitted statistically significant information in our 2004 article published in the journal Pediatrics. The omitted data suggested that African-American males who received the MMR vaccine before age 36 months were at **increased risk for autism**,"* confessed William W. Thompson, Ph.D. Their research showed that there is a 340 percent increase in the risk for autism, with boys receiving the MMR vaccine on the CDC schedule, as compared to those receiving it later, and almost twice as high a risk with black children as compared to whites.

> **"Now that the draft has been abolished, mandatory vaccination remains the only time an American is asked to risk his life for his country."** Harris Coulter, Ph.D.

Dr. Thompson admitted that he and high-ranking CDC executives Coleen Boyle, Ph.D.; Frank DeStefano, M.D.; Marshalyn Yeargin-Allsopp, M.D.; and Tanya Karapurkar Bhasin, MPH, participated in the cover-up by destroying vital documents. *"... the (CDC) co-authors scheduled a meeting to destroy documents related to the (MMR vaccine) study. The remaining four co-authors all met and brought a big garbage can into the meeting room and reviewed and went through all the hard-copy documents that we had thought we should discard and put them in a huge garbage can."* Dr. Thompson, assuming that this was illegal, kept hard copies of all the documents in his office and computer files.

> **"The CDC knew about the relationship between the age of first MMR vaccine and autism incidence in African-American boys as early as 2003, but chose to cover it up."** Dr. Brian Hooker

This type of corruption at the CDC with vaccine research is unacceptable. The incriminating evidence within the CDC itself exposes the dishonesty used to cover up the truth and continue promoting vaccines as safe and effective. Why wasn't this huge fraudulent scandal blasted everywhere on the news? Could it be that the same elitists who control the CDC and Merck also control the news media? And the most disturbing question of all is, why aren't these scientists who participated in these crimes against children being prosecuted and locked up in prison? And why are they all still employed by the CDC? Is this not evidence enough of how corrupt the CDC is? Any other organization would have fired and prosecuted them, but for some strange reason our tax dollars continue to employ criminals, who are supposed to be there to protect our children and us! It's a classic example of the fox guarding the henhouse.

> "**The drug companies are lying, with the help of the CDC and FDA, about the role of vaccines in causing the autism epidemic ... The drug companies caused the autism epidemic and they, not the parents nor the public, must pay the costs. They are guilty, they are very profitable and can and should be held accountable.**" Bernard Rimland, Ph.D., Founder & Director, Autism Research Institute; Founder, Autism Society of America

| Smoking does NOT Cause Cancer – CDC 1958 |
| Vaccines do NOT Cause Autism – CDC 2012 |

YEAR	Vaccination Increase
1962 –	5 Vaccine doses given
1983 –	24 Vaccine doses given
2016 –	72 Vaccine doses given

Increased Vaccinations = Increased Autism

AUTISM RATES	
1970	1 in 10,000
1975	1 in 5,000
1985	1 in 2,500
2001	1 in 250
2004	1 in 166
2007	1 in 150
2009	1 in 110
2012	1 in 88
2013	1 in 50
2018	1 in 36

Whenever you hear, "The science has been settled," that's your first cue to investigate. Years ago, scholars claimed, "the science is settled, the earth is flat," and "the science is settled, smoking doesn't cause cancer." The science is never settled; otherwise, we would stop learning, improving and progressing. Time has a way of proving our ignorance, and we sometimes are slow learners. It took us 75 years to realize that lead in gasoline is extremely toxic before finally removing it. Looking back on how we used to spray DDT as an insecticide, we now understand how it caused polio-like paralysis and cancer, so we wisely banned its use. Back in the 1950s, the tobacco companies paid big money for smoking to be marketed heavily to Americans. Even doctors endorsed smoking, and often had ads showing them proudly smoking their favorite brands. The CDC even declared, *"Smoking does not cause cancer,"* in 1958. The science was there the whole time, proving smoking does cause cancer; however, millions of dollars were paid out by tobacco companies to silence the research, just as the CDC is doing now, by ignoring the science and declaring that "vaccines do not cause autism." It's just a matter of time before enough children are harmed and the masses wake up to this massive fraudulent practice that vaccines cause neurological disorders and autism is one of many symptoms that may manifest when neurotoxins are injected into our children.

> "Not in physics, astrology, astronomy, or astrophysics or any scientific body in the world does anyone say the science is settled! That'd be the least scientific thing you could say!" Del Bigtree

SYMPTOMS OF AUTISM IN CHILDREN	SYMPTOMS OF MERCURY POISONING IN CHILDREN
• Loss of speech	• Loss of speech
• Social withdrawal	• Social withdrawal
• Reduced eye contact	• Reduced eye contact
• Repetitive behaviors	• Repetitive behaviors
• Hand-flapping	• Hand-flapping
• Toe-walking	• Toe-walking
• Temper tantrums	• Temper tantrums
• Sleep disturbances	• Sleep disturbances
• Seizures	• Seizures

Mercury causes neurological and brain disorders. This is a known fact by any toxicologist who has done research. As Dr. Boyd Haley has proven in the chemistry labs, mercury in the smallest amount is toxic and should not be used in vaccines. Those who claim vaccines containing mercury don't cause autism are about as ignorant as someone who says tornadoes don't harm people, flying debris does. Yes, they are correct, but open your eyes and see the big picture. Tornadoes cause flying debris that harms people, just as vaccines contain mercury and other adjuvants and toxins that cause brain and neurological disorders that trigger autism.

> "We need to stop calling it autism and call it what it is! ---Vaccine Induced Brain Injury." Brian Hooker, Ph.D.

Autism / Childhood Disease Culprits
1. Vaccines – (72 doses) Increased Aluminum/Mercury
2. Glyphosate – Roundup Ready Crops
3. GMOs – (Genetically Modified Organisms) foreign DNA
4. EMFs – (Electromagnetic Fields) cell phones, Wi-Fi

The most effective way to determine if vaccines cause autism or not is to compare vaccinated children to unvaccinated children. Unfortunately, for some strange reason, the CDC refuses to do that study, and by now, you know the answer to that. The reality is, no study needs to be done, because many pediatricians such as Drs. Paul Thomas and Mayer Eisenstein, who have both vaccinated and unvaccinated patients, already know first-hand who the healthiest children in their clinics are: It's the unvaccinated children.

> "Autistic disorder change point years are coincident with introduction of vaccines manufactured using human fetal cell lines, containing fetal and retroviral contaminants, into childhood vaccine regimens. Thus, rising autistic disorder prevalence is directly related to vaccines manufactured utilizing human fetal cells." Journal of Public Health and Epidemiology Vol.6(9), pp. 271-286, Sept 2014

When performing an accurate scientific study, one needs to have a control group, unlike the CDC, which ignores standard scientific procedures and compares old vaccines to new vaccines to determine if they are safe and effective. Since the CDC isn't interested in doing studies to compare vaccinated children to unvaccinated children, let's look at the Amish, who do not vaccinate. Among the Amish, there are only four recorded cases of autism, and of those, three were adopted and had received vaccines prior to adoption. The other child lived near a coal-burning power plant, which is a big source of mercury exposure that can trigger neurological disorders. If autism was a genetic factor, like some argue that it is, and had no connection to vaccines, then we most likely would see autism in the Amish community, the same as we see in the U.S., which is one out of 36, but we do not.

> "Before vaccinations, there was virtually no autism and no sudden infant death syndrome. The main cause of sudden infant death syndrome is vaccinations. That has been established beyond a shadow of a doubt. Vaccinations do not work. They don't work at all." Lorraine Day, M.D., Former Chief of Orthopedic Surgery, San Francisco General Hospital

For those who have been told that there's no scientific proof that vaccines cause autism and disorders such as allergies, seizures, diabetes, neurological disorders and increased risk of cancer, I highly suggest reading Neil Z. Miller's book, *"MILLER's REVIEW of CRITICAL VACCINE STUDIES: 400 Important Scientific Papers Summarized for Parents and Researchers."* This book gives you 400 scientific studies, summarized to help parents, doctors, nurses and the general public become aware of the research that has been done but is ignored by the CDC and mainstream news media. Let's face it, most of us parents and doctors aren't going to take the time to read through three hours of research every night. Miller's book provides a nice summary of powerful research that has been done, if you want to see the science. The medical references are given so if you want to go online and read the whole study, you can. The problem is, most people only see what they want to see, one side of the story, not necessarily all the research. Neil Miller's book is a great resource for those who want scientific proof. The amount of

> Go to **Toxline** or **PubMed** search engine and look up any subject. This is the U.S. National Library of Medicine.

published research on the dangers of vaccines is a shocking wakeup. Be informed and make wise choices. For those who are interested, you can go online to Pubmed.com or TOXLINE and type in any medical subject and look at all the published research.

> **"The really sad thing is the amount of doctors that I've spoken to that say to me, 'Del, I know that vaccines are causing autism but I won't say it on camera because the pharmaceutical industry will destroy my career, just like they did to Andy Wakefield.' And that's where we find ourselves ... being bullied by an industry that doesn't actually care about the health of our children the way it should."** Del Bigtree, Emmy Award-Winning Medical Journalist

Chickenpox Vaccine - Creates Shingles

Chickenpox is not really a disease, it's an infection caused by the varicella-zoster virus. Once you get it, you break out in an itchy, blister-like rash that usually lasts five to 10 days. It's not a life-threatening disease for most people, unless you live in a third-world country in an unsanitary environment and are malnourished and suffer with Vitamin A deficiency. Many of us who grew up before 1995 (when chickenpox vaccine was licensed) remember getting chickenpox as kids. Mom wanted us to get chickenpox, the sooner the better, and let it run its course so we could be done with it and have lifetime immunity. But now, since most children get the chickenpox vaccine and aren't experiencing the wild chickenpox naturally, adults aren't being re-exposed, depriving their immune systems of a refresher course on chickenpox immunity. This is causing some older people to get shingles, and yes, you guessed it — now Big Pharma can save the day with their shingles vaccine.

If you have had chickenpox as a child, the varicella-zoster virus is dormant in your nerve cells. When you become overly stressed, sleep-deprived, eat too much junk food and your immune system is sluggish, then the virus can reactivate and surface as shingles, which manifests as a painful cluster of blisters that rupture and ooze and cause postherpetic neuralgia, which is severe nerve pain. If we would stop attempting to manipulate Mother Nature with vaccines and allow these mild, non-life-threatening infections to run their course, we'd have lifetime immunity and eliminate shingles outbreaks. But now, since we are trying to eliminate chickenpox with a vaccine, we have created the Frankenstein monster infection called shingles. Adults experiencing shingles outbreaks suffer much worse than the actual chickenpox infection that young children contract. According to the American Medical Association's Encyclopedia of Medicine, chickenpox is a "common and mild infectious disease of childhood" and "all healthy children should be exposed to chickenpox …at an age at which it is no more than an inconvenience."

> "Children must experience their symptoms and illnesses as a necessary rite of passage, thus allowing their immune and nervous systems to grow, mature, and develop appropriately." Lawrence Palevsky, M.D.

The CDC is expecting large outbreaks (50 million adults) who will experience shingles over the next 10 to 15 years due to the use of the vaccine. Wouldn't it be best to stop vaccinating children for chickenpox and just let children get it naturally so they become immune and re-expose adults to it, so we don't have to worry about shingles? Medical science fails to use logic when the opportunity to produce a drug or vaccine and make billions off treating the symptoms is a financial option.

Varivax (chickenpox) vaccine contains 1,350 viral particles, and the new chickenpox vaccine called Zostrix, which was approved in 2006, contains the same virus, but at a much larger concentration. More than 30 percent of vaccinated children still contract chickenpox. From 1995 to 1998, VAERS received 6,574 complaints of adverse reactions related to the chickenpox vaccine (Varivax), with 262 being very serious reactions, 30 anaphylaxis shock, and 14 deaths. (JAMA. Vol. 284 No. 10 September 13, 2000)

Research shows that those who received the shingles vaccine are more than twice as likely to develop arthritis as compared to an unvaccinated control group. (Lai YC, Yew YW. J Drugs Dermatol 2015 Jul 1; 14(7): 681-84) Other research has shown that chickenpox during childhood helps prevent coronary heart disease and supports normal development of the immune system. (Pesonen E, Andsberg E, et al. Dual role of infections as risk factors for coronary heart disease. Atherosclerosis 2007 Jun; 192(2): 370-75) Research done by Silverberg and Kleiman, published in 2012 in an issue of Pediatric Allergy Immunology, reports that children who contract wild chickenpox are significantly less likely to develop asthma and allergies than children who are vaccinated against chickenpox.

> "To all the pediatricians in the world, please show me the study that found 69 doses of 16 vaccines do not cause cancer, auto-immune disease, and brain injury." Dr. Jack Wolfson

Vaccinations Increase The Risk Of Diabetes

The pertussis toxin in the DPT shot is a known activator of the Islets of Langerhans in the pancreas that make insulin. Research published by Classen and Classen in Autoimmunity, July 2002, shows that the Hib vaccine significantly increases the risk of type I diabetes (Insulin-dependent diabetes), a common autoimmune disorder. Their extensive research has shown that the hepatitis B vaccine increases the risk of type I diabetes as well. Clusters of cases of type I diabetes occur two to four years post-immunization with the MMR, pertussis and

BCG vaccines. After analyzing 11 years of childhood vaccinations, and the development of diabetes, the research shows that all vaccines have the potential to induce diabetes, and the risk may even be greater in families with a history of diabetes. Even just one dose of MMR increased the risk of diabetes by 88 percent, and two doses of the oral polio vaccine doubled the risk of diabetes. (Classen JB. Open Pediatric Med J 2008; 2: 7-10.)

Vaccines are manufactured to stimulate an immune response in children with weak immune systems. Some children who have stronger immune systems may be over-stimulated, which increases the risk for inflammatory conditions and autoimmune diseases. Some children are even being diagnosed with double diabetes, meaning they have both type 1 and type 2 diabetes. Certainly, eating sugary junk foods is a factor for children having blood sugar problems, but when you throw gasoline on the fire like vaccinations do, no wonder we are seeing alarming rates of childhood diabetes.

> "... This ... forced me to look into the question of vaccination further, and the further I looked, the more shocked I became. I found that the whole vaccine business was indeed a gigantic hoax. Most doctors are convinced that they are useful, but if you look at the proper statistics and study the instances of these diseases, you will realize that this is not so ... My final conclusion after 40 years or more in this business (medicine) is that the unofficial policy of the World Health Organization and the unofficial policy of the 'Save the Children's Fund' ... (other vaccine promoting) organizations is one of murder and genocide .... I cannot see any other possible explanation ... You cannot immunize sick children, malnourished children, and expect to get away with it. You'll kill far more children than would have died from natural infection." Archivides Kalokerinos, M.D. (1927-2012), Awarded Australian Medal of Merit

Wild Measles, Mumps & Chickenpox Viruses Protect Against Cancer

Vaccines are designed to prevent infections, but not without a price. When children are denied the opportunity to experience natural infections such as measles and chickenpox by receiving artificial vaccinations, then their immune systems never reach maximum immune capacity. Natural diseases like measles, mumps and chickenpox help prime the immune system and serve as protection from diseases later in life. This reduction in exposure to common wild diseases inhibits optimal health. With an inexperienced immune system, due to vaccinations, research shows that vaccinated individuals are much more susceptible to cancer as compared to nonvaccinated individuals later in adulthood.

> **"The chief, if not sole, cause of the monstrous increase in cancer has been vaccination."** Dr. Robert Bell

Research done by Newhouse showed that women who contracted measles, mumps, rubella or chickenpox had a significant reduction in the risk of developing ovarian cancer. (Newhouse ML, Pearson RM, et al. Br J Prev Soc Med 1977 Sep; 31(3): 148-53) Kolmel found that those who contracted influenza, measles, mumps or chickenpox had a decreased risk of developing skin cancer. (Kolmel KF, Gefeller O, et al. Melanoma Res 1992; 2(3): 207-11) Children who contract wild chickenpox or influenza have a lower risk of developing brain tumors as adults. Numerous published studies conclude that childhood diseases contracted early in life provide beneficial protection against many different types of cancer later in life. (Albonico HU, Braker HU, Husler J. Med Hypotheses 1998 Oct; 51(4): 315-20) Infants with the least exposure to common infections have the greatest risk of developing childhood leukemia.

> **"Abolish vaccination, and you will cut the cancer death rate in half."** Dr. F.P. Millard

So many studies are published, and yet we never hear about them in the news. Natural diseases prime the immune system and serve as protection against cancer and other dreaded diseases. Research even shows that the MMR, DTaP and hepatitis B vaccines increase the risk of childhood leukemia. (Buckley JD, Buckley CM, et al. Leukemia 1994 May; 8(5): 856-64) Surprisingly, studies have even shown how measles infections can reverse cancer and that the measles virus may be used as a treatment. Scientists have found that the measles virus magnifies anti-tumor activity and kills cancer cells. (Donnelly OG, Errington-Mais F, et al. Measles virus causes immunogenic cell death in human melanoma. Gene Ther 2013 Jan; 20(1): 7-15.)

> **"Several of my personal friends now have cancer; some of them have died from it. I have inquired into the probable cause of the serious increase of this horrible disease. I believe, as do many other physicians, that cancer is due to impregnating the blood with impure matter, and it is obvious that the largest method by which this is done is vaccinations and revaccinations."** J.S. Preston, M.D.

Researchers Myers and Greiner published a study in 2005 in Cancer Gene Therapy showing that measles and mumps viruses killed malignant tumor cells, allowing treated mice to live longer than untreated mice. Research shows that common childhood diseases have anti-cancer benefits. Maybe God knew what He was doing after all by sending us these little immune system primers, such as chickenpox and measles, so we could prevent cancer? Man comes along and thinks he is smarter, and makes a bigger mess by attempting to manipulate Mother Nature's microbes, instead of allowing nature to run her course. Healthy people make peace with Nature, support their immune systems and give up the need to control and manipulate pathogens.

After understanding how beneficial contracting childhood diseases is to the immune, we can begin to see why so many doctors are opposed to all vaccines. Not only are the vaccine ingredients toxic, but they also deny the immune system the ability to be as effective as possible in preventing cancer and heart disease later in life. In this day and age, we need all the anti-cancer support we can get, and contracting childhood illnesses strengthens our immune systems to maximum capacity.

> **"Have we traded mumps and measles for cancer and leukemia?"** Robert Mendelsohn M.D.

Tetanus

We are told that mercury has been removed from vaccines, but the tetanus shot still contains 25 micrograms of mercury. Tetanus is a paralytic illness caused by a toxin released from the clostridium tetani bacteria, usually found in soils associated with animal feces. The neonatal tetanus in infants is the most common, and it can be deadly. However, the majority of these cases occur following childbirth and are the result of using non-sterile equipment to cut the umbilical cord. The cephalic tetanus, the one that causes muscle spasms in the face and "lockjaw," is least common, but recovery from such infection is usually complete. The British Medical Journal reports that tetanus can occur "despite adequate immunization and adequate levels of neutralizing antibodies." (British Medical Journal 320 (5 February 2000: 383) So, if you have had a tetanus shot, you can still contract the disease.

Most cases of tetanus occurred years ago, when people traveled on horses and animal feces was everywhere. We parked our horses instead of cars. This was also during a time when most doctors did not understand the importance of washing their hands and utensils thoroughly before delivering babies. As previously mentioned, Dr. Semmelweis was ostracized for claiming doctors need to wash their hands to stop spreading infections. The notion of hand washing with soap was laughed at by other doctors! Every doctor today knows how important it is to wash your hands and use sterile equipment to prevent infections. However, doctors in the 1800s used non-sterile utensils that many times spread disease, and this was the main cause for tetanus outbreaks.

Now, we are no longer cutting our baby's umbilical cords with rusty knives from the cow barn that weren't washed thoroughly after castrating a steer and then dropped in cow manure, thus harboring tetanus bacteria. With improved sanitation and using sterilized utensils, tetanus has, for the most part, been eradicated. Once again, the pharmaceutical companies want you to believe that the vaccine has been our savior, and without it, we'd all be suffering miserably with lockjaw.

> "Tetanus vaccine is probably one of the most ridiculous vaccines ever. Your chances of getting tetanus are about the same as walking out of here and getting hit by a meteor. If you get a cut or puncture wound and you put peroxide on it, your chances of getting tetanus are zero because tetanus organism is anaerobic. It cannot live in oxygen. Tetanus comes from the bowels of animals. As long as you don't have a sheep or a cow in your house, I don't think you're in any danger." Russell Blaylock, M.D.

What To Do For Deep Puncture Wounds (Tetanus)
1. Wash the wound thoroughly with warm, soapy water.
2. Allow the wound to bleed freely. This eliminates bacteria and brings infection-fighting white blood cells to the area.
3. Pour hydrogen peroxide over the wound. It kills germs, even anaerobic tetanus spores.
4. Use homeopathic remedy Hypericum 6x three times daily for 3 weeks, according to Dr. Andrew Lockie. When a wound is severe, it will help prevent tetanus (it has been used for more than a century). If muscle spasms occur, use Aconite 30c. If muscles of jaw and throat spasm and jerk, use Cicuta 6c. If puncture wound is sore and tender, use Hypericum 30c. If jaw is locked, use Oenanthe 6c.

As Dr. Blaylock points out, if you are not on a farm, around cow or horse manure, then your chances of contracting tetanus are very slim. If you are worried about tetanus, according to Dr. Tenpenny, a shot of tetanus immune globulin (TIG) can be administered for severe injuries. TIG will stay in the body for up to three weeks, providing immune support to neutralize any toxin that may exist by the tetanus-causing bacterium.

Dr. Carrel Produces Cancer In Chickens With Vaccine Ingredients

Remember Dr. Alexis Carrel, who kept a chicken heart alive for 29 years? He has done his own research to test vaccine ingredients. He took highly diluted poisons, similar to formaldehyde in the Salk vaccine, which was at 1:4000 concentration. Dr. Carrel wanted to see what would happen if he injected these ingredients at an even greater dilution, 1:5000 to 1:250000 in chickens. The results were shocking. Injecting these vaccine ingredients in chickens produced cancer. If we can produce cancer in animals with smaller dilutions of vaccine ingredients than the amount we give our children, then why are we still using formaldehyde?

> "Vaccines are the backbone of the entire pharmaceutical industry. The vaccinated children become customers for life." Dr. Sherri Tenpenny

If Americans are unaware, they'll just follow blindly, trusting the CDC, FDA and EPA to keep us safe and healthy. An honest person has to scratch their head and ask, how can the government, which we pay to protect us with our tax dollars, ignore this type of research? Medical journalist Del Bigtree answered that question when he pointed out that "Merck runs the CDC, Monsanto runs the FDA and Exxon runs the EPA — we have lost control of our nation!"

> - Monsanto controls the FDA
> - Exxon controls the EPA
> - Merck controls the CDC
>
>   Del Bigtree

"I am thoroughly convinced that the recent great increase in cancer is directly due to vaccination. I have written my report to several members of Parliament and invited them to the hospital to witness the dismal results of the Vaccination Act for themselves." William Forbes, M.D., Medical Director, St. Saviour's Cancer Hospital, Regents Park, London, England

VACCINE DOCUMENTARIES
- **The Truth About Vaccines** by Ty Bollinger (7 episodes)
- **Vaxxed: From Cover-Up to Catastrophe** by Del Bigtree

It's disturbing to witness beautiful, healthy children go in to receive vaccinations and instantly be diagnosed with neurological disorders like autism. When a famous person such as Robert De Niro, who has an 18-year-old autistic son, wants answers to vaccination information and things don't add up, then investigation begins. Two great vaccine documentaries are Ty Bollinger's seven-part, "*The Truth About Vaccines*" and Del Bigtree's "*Vaxxed: From Cover-Up to Catastrophe.*" Some episodes can be viewed on YouTube. I encourage everyone to treat the vaccine debate like a court case. If someone is accused of a crime such as murder, you lay all the facts out on the table. You listen to the prosecution and the defense, right? After careful investigation of the facts and hearing both sides, you make an informed decision and do what you feel is best for your child. I wish I could say our government and the CDC have our health's best interest, but as we've already exposed a rat's nest of corruption, they don't. They are heavily influenced by the pharmaceutical mafia. Don't take my word for it, do your own investigation. Remember, they once said the cancer-causing insecticide "DDT is good for me" and "smoking doesn't cause cancer." Most research that is done and publicized is bought and paid for by a higher power with an agenda. You being sick is part of the agenda. Healthy people do not generate income for their monopolistic empire.

> Congressman Dan Burton testified to other members of Congress the following:
>
> "How confident can we be in the recommendations with the Food and Drug Administration when the chairman (of Vaccines and Related Biological Products Advisory Committee) and other individuals on their advisory committee own stock in major manufacturers of vaccines? ...It almost appears that there is an 'old boys' network' of vaccine advisors that rotate between the CDC and FDA — at times serving both simultaneously..."

CDC Corruption

Danish researcher Dr. Poul Thorsen, employed by the CDC, authored and co-authored 21 of 24 studies that the CDC claims disprove any link between vaccines and autism. In 2011, Thorsen was indicted on charges of wire fraud and money laundering for stealing more than $1 million in autism research money. He went missing in 2013, tops the federal most wanted list and faces 260 years in jail. And this is the type person our tax dollars pay to do research at the CDC to determine if vaccines are safe for our children? If you can't trust him with research money, do we really want to trust him with autism research? If you still think the CDC has our best interest, read the book, *Master Manipulator – The Explosive True Story of Fraud Embezzlement and Government Betrayal at the CDC,* by James Ottar Grundvig. The corruption is overwhelming. Most people are afraid of this type of information because it exposes the fraud and corruption occurring in our government, and of course we would all like to believe that it doesn't exist. Like Dr. Boyd Haley explains, the CDC funds bogus research to take the blame off thimerosal while our children suffer.

> "Four scathing federal studies, including two by Congress, one by the U.S. Senate, and one by the HHS Inspector General, paint the CDC as a cesspool of corruption, mismanagement and dysfunction with alarming conflicts of interest suborning its research, regulatory and policymaking functions." Robert F. Kennedy Jr.

Dr. Julie Gerberding was the CDC director from 2002 to 2009, and oversaw many vaccine studies, many of which were deemed unreliable by the IOM. Shortly after the whistleblower, Dr. Thompson, admitted he and other researchers at the CDC omitted vaccine-autism data, she resigned. Did she really retire? No, in 2010, she became president of the vaccine division at Merck with a $2.5 million annual salary, while holding 31,985 shares of stock valued at roughly $2 million.

> **"I firsthand saw that certain government agencies and certain universities are manipulating the data in order to protect the sales of vaccines and to cover up any adverse effects."** Dr. David Lewis

Vaccine manufacturers sponsor research for their own products. Many authors of published research papers on the safety of vaccines are paid consultants and receive grant money from vaccine manufacturers. Professor of Medicine at Stanford University, Dr. John Ioannidis, a bias research expert, informs that most published medical studies provide false conclusions due to faulty study design, inaccurate data, manipulation in the analysis, and selective reporting of findings. (Ioannidis JP. Why most published research findings are false. PloS Med 2005 Aug; 2(8): el24.) Another study published in JAMA 2005 by Dr. Ioannidis claims that 31 percent of highly-cited original clinical research studies were either contradicted or shown to have exaggerated effects by subsequent studies. And research conducted by Faneli, published in Plos One in 2009, reports that 81 percent of research trainees in the biomedical sciences were "willing to select, omit or fabricate data to win a grant or publish a paper." It may also surprise you to know that the vaccine industry employs three lobbyists for every member of Congress, and many of the lobbyists are former members of Congress themselves.

> **"Never doubt that a small group of thoughtful committed citizens can change the world; indeed, it is the only thing that ever has."** Margaret Mead

Dr. Mikovits Discovers Disease-Causing Retroviruses In Vaccines

Dr. Judy Mikovits, Ph.D., a biochemist and molecular biologist with over 30 years of experience, has been the director of HIV, cancer, epigenetics and neuroimmune research studies. She has published over 51 papers in peer-reviewed journals and worked as a government scientist for many years, developing viruses and vaccinations. In 2009, she and her team were doing research on autism and neurological diseases. Many of the patients had motor-neuron disorders, chronic fatigue syndrome (CFS) and cancer. After careful examination, she was able to isolate a virus that came from mice that has adapted to humans. In 2011, she made the startling discovery that these retroviruses from mice were found in high numbers in children with autism and were being injected into humans through contaminated vaccines.

Retroviruses have a tendency to derange the immune system, allowing all sorts of viral, bacterial, and parasitic pathogens to rage out of control. Retroviruses from vaccines have the potential to mutate into new viruses, cancers and diseases that may take two months or two decades to manifest.

> **Watch on YouTube**
> **Whistleblower**
> **Dr. Judy Mikovits**

Like sleeping giants, they are quiet until a stressor activates them, and then like a shaken beehive, they create chaos in immune-deficient people. These retroviruses tear open your DNA, and insert their own DNA, to mutate your genetic makeup. These can be passed down to generation after generation. Dr. Mikovits reports that 67 percent of patients, and 4 percent of healthy controls, are infected with the retrovirus XMRV (xenotropic murine leukemia virus-related virus, a mouse retrovirus). This mouse-related virus can cause cancer, ALS, chronic liver disease, AIDS, ME/CFS, autism and many other neurological diseases. It affects your stem cells, the egg, the sperm and every cell in your body. She presented her research study to the National Institutes of Health, which revealed 14 out of 17 children with autism showed evidence of XMRV infection.

What is a retrovirus? Humans have a DNA genome; this is our blueprint. Retroviruses have an RNA genome, and their RNA is reverse-transcribed, or written backward, by an enzyme called reverse transcriptase. Basically, a retrovirus is a virus that contains RNA-encoded genes, rather than DNA. Using reverse transcriptase, the retrovirus is able to transform the single-stranded RNA into a double-stranded DNA. When the retrovirus infects a host, it integrates its DNA into the DNA of the host cell, which allows the retrovirus to replicate and spread. So, every time your cells replicate, so do the viruses. HIV virus, which can eventually result in AIDS, is a classic example of a retrovirus causing havoc in the body.

> **"God did not intend for animal viruses to be injected directly into the human bloodstream."** Judy Mikovits, Ph.D.

The first outbreak of chronic fatigue syndrome/ME (myalgic encephalomyelitis) occurred in 1934 to 1935 among 198 doctors and nurses at Los Angeles County Hospital after receiving a polio vaccine grown in mouse tissue and preserved with mercury (thimerosal). All staff members sued the hospital after getting sick from the vaccine, and settled for $6 million in 1939 (equivalent to over $100 million today). Fast-forward 60 years. In 1994, scientists reported that growing human viruses in animal tissue and then re-injecting that material back into humans could introduce new animal viruses into the human population. Dr. Mikovits reports that her research with XMRV retroviruses in 2011 showed that this has already occurred, and that millions of people are infected with these retroviruses from vaccines! Her full story is in her book, *Plague: One Scientist Intrepid Search for the Truth about Human Retroviruses and Chronic Fatigue Syndrome (ME/CFS), Autism, and Other Diseases.*

> **"Twenty-five million Americans are infected with the viruses that came out of the lab ... into the humans via contaminated blood and vaccines."** Judy Mikovits, Ph.D.

When she presented her data to the government, like honest researchers are sworn to do, government officials ordered her to destroy the data and claim that she made it all up. When she refused, she was arrested, thrown in jail and fired from her job. They told her if she didn't claim her research was a fraud, they would destroy her, and that is what they have done. They have discredited her and destroyed her reputation and career, just as they did Dr. Andrew Wakefield. Instead of winning a Nobel Prize for discovering contaminated retroviruses in vaccines, capable of harming and killing millions of innocent children, she has been kicked to the curb.

> **"MY PEOPLE ARE DESTROYED FOR LACK OF KNOWLEDGE."** Hosea 4:6

There are several retroviruses that are part of viral families, which include delta, lenti, beta and gamma. The human beta retrovirus is associated with biliary cirrhosis. We've already mentioned HIV and XMRV, but we also have a human T-cell leukemia lymphoma virus (HTLV-1) family, known to cause severe diseases as well. Dr. Mikovits warns by using murine leukemia viruses as vectors for gene therapy, they're causing cancer. The Gardasil vaccine is causing the disease it's supposed to prevent by using these retroviruses as vectors. And now Dr. Gary Owens has identified another strain of XMRV gamma retrovirus from mice, associated with cardiovascular disease. "This is just a nightmare that we've unleashed in our environment," explains Dr. Mikovits.

> **"The only safe vaccine is one that is never used."** Dr. James R. Shannon, Former Director, National Institutes of Health

The vaccine industry has known that since the 1960s, vaccines have been contaminated with avian leukemia virus, a retrovirus that infects commercially raised poultry. The influenza, measles, rabies and yellow fever vaccines are made by using chicken cells and eggs. These vaccines expose humans to the avian virus, which has the potential to activate cancer-causing genes called erbB and myc. When these genes are turned on, breast cancer can occur. Dr. Walid Heneine, a CDC virologist, warns that viral contaminants from animal tissues can replicate and cause disease in humans. Some viruses are known and some have yet to be detected. She explains that some of the unidentified viral strains in vaccines may be a contributing factor of many diseases and cancer. Dr. Heneine cautions vaccine recipients that we really don't know what are in these vaccines, besides disease-causing retroviruses, and what they are fully capable of doing. We already went through the horror of the polio vaccines from the 1950s being contaminated with the live SV-40 virus that infected 220,000 people. These retroviruses in today's vaccines could prove to be thousands of times more damaging. Time will tell. Do you want your child to be part of the experiment?

VACCINE INGREDIENTS

Mercury (thimerosal) 2nd most toxic substance known to man
Aluminum hydroxide, phosphate, sulfate – neurotoxin, notorious for causing Alzheimer's
Beta-propiolactone (considered a human carcinogen)
Gentamicin Sulphate & Polymyxin B (antibiotics)
Genetically modified yeast, potassium diphosphate, potassium monophosphate
Animal, bacterial and viral DNA
Glutaraldehyde (causes birth defects in animals)
Formaldehyde (formalin) embalming agent - Banned in Europe, causes cancer
Latex rubber – may trigger allergies
Human & animal DNA
MSG – banned in Europe
Inactivated virus from infected cattle tongue epithelium
Virus strains prepared in chick embryo cell culture
Polio vaccine (inactivated) contains VERO cells from African green monkeys
Rabies from duck embryo origin
Live virus prepared from duck embryo or human diploid cell culture
Dibutyl phthalate (endocrine disrupter)
Neomycin Sulphate (antibiotic)
Dried mouse brain infected with French neurotropic strain of yellow fever virus
Rotten horse blood (diphtheria toxin and antitoxin)
Macerated cancerous breasts
Pus from sores on diseased animals
Mucus from the throats of children with colds and whooping cough
Decomposed fecal matter from typhoid patients
HiB saccharides cultured on cow's brains
Live measles virus
Live mumps virus
Live rubella virus, VERO cells, monkey kidney cells linked to SV-40 virus known to cause leukemia
Monkey kidney cell cultures, human diploid cells from human **aborted fetal tissue**
Hepatitis A vaccine contains MRC-5. Obtained from **aborted fetal cell cultures**
Rubella MMR-II vaccine contains WI-38 created from tissue of an **aborted fetus**
Pig blood, calf bovine serum, fetal bovine serum, (cow's blood transmitter of Mad Cow Disease)
Influenza grown on retinal cells of **aborted fetal tissue**
Chickenpox (Varicella) is cultured on **aborted human fetus**
Phenoxyethanol (Antifreeze)
Polysorbate 80 & 20 – causes cancer
Tri(n) Butyl phosphate
XMRV (xenotropic murine leukemia virus-related virus, a mouse retrovirus)
Food proteins - ovalbumin (egg whites), casein (milk), gelatin, soy, coconut, palm, sunflower, wheat, corn, peanut oil, gelatin, bakers' yeast

> "It is difficult to imagine that the introduction of viruses, bits of bacteria, mercury, aluminum and more than 100 additional chemicals into the body of an infant can be considered harmless." Dr. Sherri Tenpenny

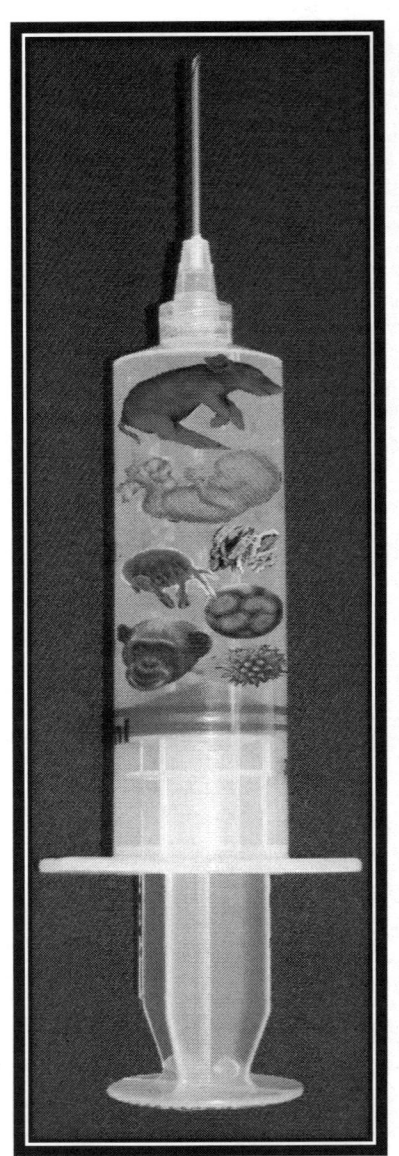

After reading the list of vaccine ingredients, do you really feel comfortable injecting those into your child? How many people will continue vaccinating their children when they know that some vaccine ingredients come from aborted fetuses? If I was ever introduced to something sketchy and dangerous, the ingredients in vaccines top the list. To put this filth into a brand-new healthy baby is as close to insanity, sorcery and witchcraft as you can get. Injecting toxic, foreign matter into their bodies is an outright sin against a beautiful child of God that has been given to us as our greatest gift, to love, nourish and cherish, and yet we turn around and defile the child with filth! These are known neurotoxins! Vaccinating their little bodies with these toxins in an attempt to make them healthier is a sheer mockery to God. The intelligence within just spent 9 months creating a mind-boggling and most amazing heart, lungs, kidneys, brain, nervous system and a self-healing immune system, and then we take that miracle of life and inject poison in it, in an attempt to make it healthier, as if it doesn't have enough sense to make it on its own? In case some of our highly

Nature's Immunizations
- Vitamin A/Cod liver oil
- Vitamin D
- Vitamin C
- Cinnamon
- Garlic
- Echinacea
- Homeopathic remedies
- Breast Milk

GEORGIA
Merck recalling doses of vaccine

ATLANTA — Merck & Co. is recalling about a million doses of a childhood vaccine, after testing showed a sterilization problem in a Pennsylvania factory.

The company is not aware of any harm to children who received the vaccine, known as Hib, which prevents meningitis and pneumonia. It is a three-dose shot recommended for all children under 5 and is usually given to infants starting at 2 months old.

The recall involves 10 lots of Hib vaccine and two lots of a combination vaccine for both Hib and hepatitis B, a Merck spokeswoman said.

She said the company did not find contamination in the vaccine itself, but in the plant where the vaccine is produced in West Point, Pa.

educated doctors have forgotten, children come into this world with an immune system far superior to anything an arrogant, know-it-all scientist can conjure up in a lab, to generate billions of dollars, to fill their deep pockets.

> **"Vaccination is not disease prevention — it's a particularly nasty form of organized crime in that it manipulates parents' protective instincts to get them to submit their child into getting poisoned for profit under the guise of disease prevention."** Erwin Alber

On January 29, 2001, Jack Doubleday, CEO of the California non-profit Natural Woman, Natural Man Inc., offered $20,000 to the first U.S. licensed medical doctor or pharmaceutical company CEO who would publicly drink a standard mixture of vaccine additive ingredients. In 2007, the offer was increased to $90,000 and will increase $5,000 per month, in perpetuity, until a doctor, pharmaceutical executive or any of the 15 current members of the ACIP agrees to drink a dose of chemicals that would be equivalent to the dose given to an infant. Guess what? Not one person was willing to drink the vaccine ingredients, but somehow, they claim it's OK to inject into our children? If you wouldn't consume it, why would you inject it?

> **"Fear can only prevail when victims are ignorant of the facts."** Thomas Jefferson

> **"The dissenter is every human being at those moments of his life when he resigns momentarily from the herd and thinks for himself."** Archibald MacLeish

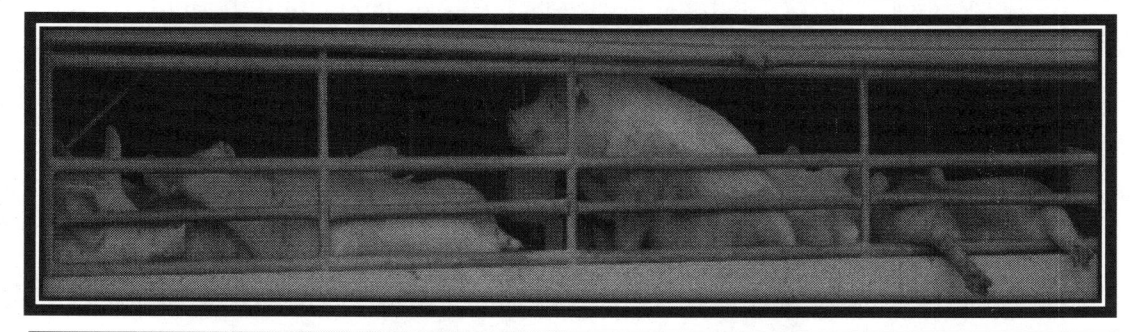

Are you like the hog at the slaughterhouse, following blindly down the shoot, because everyone else is doing it? Do your own research so you and your family can make wise, informed decisions for the things that are most important in life, like your children's health. Your innocent children don't have a choice. They depend upon you to love them and provide them with the best care possible. Every choice has a consequence. It has been estimated that 1 out of 200 children suffer severe reactions from the DPT shot. It has been reported that about 4,000 children die each year from the DTaP vaccine. Like Barbara Fisher said, *"When it happens to your child, then the risks are 100 percent."*

> **"Belief in immunization is a form of delusional insanity."** Dr. Herbert Shelton

Nature's Infectious Disease Busters

Research has shown that **Vitamin A** is extremely effective in preventing and reducing infections like pneumonia and measles. In the 1930s, doctors who understood how important Vitamin A is in fighting infections found that mortality dropped by 58 percent when children who were hospitalized with measles were given cod liver oil, which is high in Vitamins A and D and omega 3 fatty acids. Mother's breast milk is high in Vitamin A, and experts agree that breastfeeding is far more effective than vaccinations in preventing infections.

Viral respiratory infections occur in cold-weather months, particularly in fall and winter, and influenza epidemics do not occur in the summertime, even when the virus is freely circulating and large crowds gather. Why? Because a lack of sunlight lowers our Vitamin D levels, and low **Vitamin D** levels lower our immune systems, making us more susceptible to influenza, pneumonia and upper respiratory infections. Research done by Sabetta and DePetrillo showed that a higher level of Vitamin D significantly reduced the risk of developing an acute viral respiratory infection by 50 percent. Research has revealed that northern cities with the least solar radiation and Vitamin D had the worst death rates during the 1918 to 1919 influenza pandemic. Pregnant women who optimize their Vitamin D levels drastically decrease their risk of respiratory infections and pneumonia in their newborns. For those who choose to skip the flu shot but want added protection, supplementing with Vitamin D3 at 5,000 IU daily and in the winter months 10,000 to 20,000 IU daily adds immune support.

In 1953, Dr. Fred Klenner published a paper showing how effective **Vitamin C** was against measles and herpes zoster (shingles). The neutralizing power that Vitamin C has over bacterial and viral toxins works like an antibiotic, involving oxidative killing. Taking 1,000 mg of Vitamin C was used prophylactically, and all those who received 1,000 mg every six hours by vein or muscle were protected from the virus. Those who took 1,000 mg of Vitamin C by mouth every two hours, four to six times a day, would modify the (measles) attack, and if 12 doses each 24 hours were given, all signs and symptoms would disappear in 48 hours. Any immune support plan would be wise to enlist Vitamin C as a member on the team.

> **"Natural immunity is the only true immunity. Everything else is an artificial attempt to cheat nature, and nature is never cheated."** Dr. Ray Obomsawin

Numerous medical references include **cinnamon** as a treatment option for those with measles, cholera, influenza and malaria. Cinnamon contains Vitamins A and C, along with minerals zinc, magnesium, potassium and manganese, which are all very important for a strong immune system.

Garlic is king for fighting infections, and has been since the beginning of time. In 1901, garlic was used to treat 200 patients with tuberculosis in the city hospital of Venice, and every case reported improvement, especially early stages. In 1917, a hospital in New York experimented with 56 different treatments, and garlic came out on top against tuberculosis. It was also very beneficial for treating whooping cough. ("The Therapeutic Uses of Garlic," Medical Record, Sept 1, 1917, p.376.)

A 2003 study proved garlic to be effective against Methicillin-resistant Staphylococcus Aureus, also known as MRSA, which is now a deadly pathogen, resistant to many antibiotics. The study concludes that garlic, "inhibited the growth of, and killed MRSA…in a dose-dependent manner." (Journal of Antimicrobial Chemotherapy, Oct 2003, p.979.)

Echinacea has been made famous through the decades for its ability to fight infections and strengthen the immune system. Echinacea has been used for smallpox, blood infections, boils and a remedy for burns and anthrax.

> "There is no convincing scientific evidence that mass inoculations can be credited with eliminating any childhood disease … I urge you to reject all inoculations for your child." Robert Mendelsohn, M.D.

Homeopathy – An Alternative To Vaccines

Homeopathy has been used for over 200 years. Homeopathy is a safe, effective and inexpensive medicine that the pharmaceutical companies violently oppose because of the threat it poses to their billion-dollar monopoly on health care.

A homeopathic remedy, called a nosode, contains a diluted part or energetic frequency of the diseased pathological tissue to help support your body's immune system. The difference between a vaccine and a homeopathic nosode is that the nosode has been diluted to the point that it no longer contains the original substance of the diseased tissue, only an energetic frequency, but still stimulates your immune system with a response. This is why homeopathy is safe.

For example, a homeopathic nosode for **rabies** would be Lyssin (Hydrophobinum 30c) and then followed by Belladonna 6c. Thuja has been used to help with vaccination reactions. Samuel Hahnemann, M.D., the father of homeopathy, found that the homeopathic remedy Belladonna 30c prevented **scarlet fever** with a 90 percent success rate. It was so successful that regular physicians adopted its use and, by 1838, the Prussian government made its use mandatory. For more info, go to www.homeopathic.org.

If you are interested in homeoprophylaxis to strengthen the body to resist infections, look up immunizationalternatives.com. Dr. Isaac Golden conducted a 15-year clinical study in Australia that showed homeoprophylaxis to be 90 percent effective in preventing disease.

| **Dr. Andrew Lockie, author of The Family Guide To Homeopathy recommends** ||
INFECTION	*REMEDY*
Chicken Pox	Varicella 30c or Rhus tox 30c
Diphtheria	Mercurius cyan 6c
Influenza	Flu nosode 30c or Bacillinum 30c
Malaria	China sulph 6c or Arsenicum 6c two doses daily while visiting
Measles	Morbillinum 30c
Mumps	Parotidinum 30c or Rhus tox 30c
Rabies	Hydrophobinum 30c once a day for 7 days & then Belladonna 6c twice daily for 6 months
Rubella	Rubella 30c
Scarlet Fever	Belladonna 30c
Tetanus	Hypericum 6c three times daily for 3 weeks
Whooping cough	Pertussin 30c

What To Do For Pertussis (Whooping Cough)

1. Avoid all dairy products.
2. Drink plenty of fluids, especially water (coconut water is good).
3. Make soups, slow cooker chicken bone broth with vegetables, with lots of onions and garlic.
4. Use essential oils (lavender, eucalyptus, oregano, peppermint). Put lavender or eucalyptus oil in a diffuser where you sleep at nights. Drink 2 drops of oregano oil in water twice daily.
5. Take the Master tonic formula daily (garlic, onions, ginger, turmeric & vinegar).
6. Drink a hot lemonade, with raw honey, lemons, grated ginger & apple cider vinegar.
7. Take Vitamin C, Vitamin A and Vitamin D (cod liver oil is high in Vitamin A).
8. Take probiotics.
9. Licorice root, thyme, ginger & mullein are good.
10. According to Dr. Lockie, the homeopathic Pertussin 30c remedy is beneficial for preventing whooping cough. If coughing causes vomiting & is worse after midnight, use Drosera 6c. For a hard, dry cough that is worse around 3 a.m., use Kali carb 6c. When coughing is worse at night & vomiting mucus that is transparent and stringy, use Coccus 6x. If coughing turns the lips blue, cramps in fingers & toes & cold water seems to help, use Cuprum 6c. If stringy, yellow mucus is coughed up, use Kali bichrome 6c. If the child cries of stomach pains before coughing attacks with a severe headache, use Belladonna 6c. If the child feels sick most of the time & vomiting ends the coughing attack, use Ipecac 6c.

Caution: for infants do not use honey or essential oils.

> **What To Do For Measles**
>
> <u>Newborns</u> - Vitamin A at 10,000 IU (2 drops) added to breast milk or a bottle.
> Vitamin D at 2,000 IU daily, in a liquid form, added to breast milk or a bottle.
> <u>2 years or older</u> 15,000 IU Vitamin A (3 drops) added to water or juice.
> <u>2 to 5 years old</u> 20,000 IU Vitamin A (4 drops) added to water or juice.
> <u>7 years old to teenagers</u> 100,000 IU Vitamin A (20 drops) added to water or juice.
> <u>Adults</u> 200,000 IU Vitamin A (40 drops) added to water or juice.
>
> 1. Take Vitamin A and Vitamin D for 3 to 5 days for prevention and to help boost the immune system and speed recovery time. Adding in Vitamin C is good. Cod liver oil is high in Vitamin A.
> 2. Do not take acetaminophen (Tylenol). It shuts down the production of glutathione.
> 3. Fevers are good. They wake up the immune system and activate white blood cells — leukocytosis.
> 4. Keep fevers down, under 105, by sucking on ice chips, taking cool baths, etc.
> 5. Stay hydrated. Drink plenty of liquids.
> 6. Measles usually runs its course in about 10 days and provides lifetime immunity.
> 7. According to Dr. Andrew Lockie, Morbillinum 30c is beneficial. For cold symptoms and high fever use Aconite 30c or Belladonna 30c. For red, swollen, watery eyes, high fever & cold symptoms use Euphrasia 6c. For a feverish child with no thirst, very tearful and miserable, thick green mucus, light hurts eyes, dry cough at nights, lots of phlegm, upset stomach & diarrhea, use Pulsatilla 6c. If rash is slow to appear, use Bryonia 30c. If rash is slow to clear & spots turn purplish, use Sulphur 6c.
> 8. Licorice root and turmeric are good.
>
> **"Fevers below 105 do not pose a significant risk…"** Robert Mendelsohn, MD (Pediatrician)

For **mumps,** Dr. Lockie recommends the homeopathic remedy Parotidinum 30c and Rhus tox 30c during the incubation period. If testicles or ovaries are painful, use Pulsatilla 6c every 4 hours. For a high fever, swollen glands and redness in face, use Belladonna 30c.

> "There are studies now that show that there is an epidemic rise in allergies, asthma, and eczema in vaccinated kids. Diabetes is associated with certain vaccines. Autism almost always seems to follow vaccines …. For that reason, I encourage parents NOT to vaccinate their children. I don't call it immunization because the only REAL form of immunization is to get the wild disease." Robert Rowen, M.D.

Malaria

Malaria is a serious disease that can be fatal if left untreated. It is caused by a parasite contracted from infected mosquitos. The parasite grows in the liver and infects red blood cells. Common symptoms are fever, shaking, chills, vomiting, diarrhea, headache, muscle aches and fatigue. Symptoms usually begin 10 days to four weeks after becoming infected. However, symptoms may not develop until as much as a year later.

Archeologists discovered instructions for treating malaria in a 2000-year-old Chinese tomb. Upon investigation, they carefully studied the malaria remedy, isolated the active ingredient and called it "artemisinin." Researchers in China and Vietnam have confirmed that artemisinin is a highly effective remedy with close to a 100 percent success rate in treating malaria. Artemisinin is the active ingredient found in the herb called wormwood. Next time you travel to countries that recommend vaccines for malaria, you may want to pack the herb wormwood, since it has stood the test of time, being used for over 2,000 years, and is still effective to this day. Also, use a natural mosquito repellent made with essential oils and free of DEET (a toxic ingredient in insect repellents).

Natural Mosquito Repellent
- 80% Water in 8 oz. spray bottle
- 20% Isopropyl Alcohol
- 15 drops Rosemary
- 15 drops Peppermint
- 15 drops Lavender

According to Dr. Lockie, if traveling to a country known to have high rates of malaria, taking China sulph 6c or Arsenicum 6c, two doses daily while visiting, is good prevention. Use China 6c if sweating and weak, preceded by restlessness and pains in joints. For chills, fever and sweating, thirst or pains in spine, use China sulph 6c. If you have a burning fever, weakness, swelling and thirst, use Arsenicum 6c.

> "I sincerely believe that vaccines cause more harm to the health of the individual than the 'protection' and 'benefit' they are proclaimed to provide. Staying healthy without vaccines is not only possible, but being vaccine-free is the only way to maintain a lifetime of real health." Dr. Sherri Tenpenny

Traveler's Diarrhea

People go overseas on vacation or a cruise and often get sick with diarrhea. The culprit is usually found in contaminated water used to make ice cubes to go in a drink. Parasites, viruses and E. coli are the usual culprits. Take the antiparasitic herbs wormwood, black walnut, pumpkin, chaparral and fennel to clear up infections. We have the homeopathic Vermatox, Verma Plus and Para Plus to cleanse the body of parasitic infections.

> **"If an infant needs one vaccine that is 100 percent safe and effective – that would be breast milk."** Tetyana Obukhanych, Ph.D., Immunologist

Just because the school your child attends says you have to have your child vaccinated, does not mean there are not exemptions. You have the right to have a medical, religious, philosophical or proof of immunity exemption from vaccinations, depending upon the state in which you live. For health-care workers who do not want the hepatitis B vaccine, there is a federal exemption form online that you can download and give to your employer. Go to www.osha.gov to download it.

> **"If you believe a law is immoral, you have a duty to disobey it."** Pat McKay, Author of *Natural Immunity Why You Should NOT Vaccinate*

Know your constitutional rights. Freedom of religion is guaranteed to Americans. It is against my religion to violate the trust God has granted me when He sent me beautiful, healthy children. To risk putting foreign, toxic materials into their bodies violates that trust that has been given to me when I became a father. I am their guardian, and I have an obligation to give them the very best. Anything short of the best, I feel, is totally unacceptable and irresponsible on my part, and I do believe we are held accountable. Ignorance is not bliss. Do your homework, investigate the science on both sides, and then make an informed decision.

> **"When we give government the power to make medical decisions for us, we, in essence, accept that the state owns our bodies."** U.S. Representative Ron Paul, M.D.

I love my children too much to risk giving them something that has been proven in the past to harm and kill. God, The Almighty Creator, has entrusted me with these choice spirits, and I will not put toxic substances into their bodies. It is against my intuition, logic and religion. To do so would violate the trust given to me.

> **"Vaccination is not necessary, not useful, does not protect. There are twice as many casualties from vaccinations as from AIDS."** Gerhard Buchwald, M.D. (West Germany)

Vaccines Made From Aborted Fetal Tissue	
Mumps	WI-38
Measles	WI-38
Chickenpox	WI-38/MRC-5
Shingles	MRC-5
Hepatitis A	MRC-5
Tetanus	MRC-5
Pertussis	MRC-5
Polio	MRC-5
Rabies	MRC-5
Pentacel (DTaP)	MRC-5

MRC-5 cell line was developed from a lung tissue taken from a 14-week-old aborted human fetus and used in the following vaccines: chickenpox, tetanus, pertussis, Hib, hepatitis A and polio.

The WI-38 human diploid cell line (RA 273) was developed using the body of a 16-week-old female, human aborted fetus, and is used in measles, mumps and chickenpox vaccines.

When performing an organ transplant on a patient, doctors administer immunosuppressant drugs (Tacrolimus, Cyclosporine) to prevent the patient's immune system from rejecting and attacking the foreign body part. Vaccinations consist of injecting foreign DNA from aborted fetuses into our children. If our highly intelligent immune system sends the marines out in the body searching for foreign proteins to attack, like it does with an organ transplant, why would it choose to ignore foreign aborted fetal cell DNA fragments/proteins from vaccines? Could this be why we are seeing so many children diagnosed with autoimmune disorders like Type I diabetes, where the immune system destroys the pancreas, requiring a child to have to use an insulin pump the rest of their life? How can two parents with no history of blood sugar problems in their family have a perfectly healthy child and then the child suddenly becomes Type I diabetic shortly after a round of vaccinations? The DNA fragments of aborted fetal cells injected through vaccines into children are being taken up by stem cells and mutating, reproducing those mutations over and over again, leading to autoimmune diseases, encephalopathy and leukemia. It is estimated that 54 percent of our children suffer with disabilities now, the highest the world has ever seen.

> "The rise of mandatory and forced vaccination legislation should send a chill up every single American spine. That government can force you to accept any kind of medicine and inject you against your will is totalitarianism at its worst! This egregious form of state power is metastasizing." Ron Paul, M.D.

Some doctors, school nurses and county health department workers can get very pushy when you do not comply with what they have been instructed to do. You can request a religious exemption form from your county health department. When they ask why you choose to not vaccinate your child, a simple and firm, "It is against my religion," will suffice. Any other questions or harassment will usually cease if you simply respond by asking, "Do I need to have my attorney contact you?" Be kind and understand that they are simply doing their job. Here is a sample vaccine exemption form that may be used. If you choose to not vaccinate your child and want them to attend public school, simply fill in the blanks, have it notarized and present it to the county health department. Obviously, this sample form is for an Alabama resident. It can be altered for the state where you reside.

VACCINE EXEMPTION AFFIDAVIT

I (*Parent or guardian's name*) citizen of the State of Alabama and the United States of America affirm: Be it known to all courts, governments, and other parties that:

Being a person of strong Christian Morals, it is against my religious convictions to accept the injection of any foreign substance into my body or the body of my child. This includes, but is not limited to, any and all vaccinations, shots, tests for diseases, oral vaccines, epidermal patches, and in any other way that live or killed bacterium, viruses, pathogens, germs, or any other microorganisms, that may be introduced into or upon my body or any of my children's bodies.

This written statement to exempt my child from any immunizations, TB testing, and other shots/injections, because I hold genuine and sincere personal religious beliefs which are inconsistent with these medical procedures and experimentation. The practice of vaccination and the injection of any foreign substance is contrary to my conscientiously held religious beliefs and practices and violates the free exercise of my religious principles.

I (*Parent's name*), as the parent of (*Child's name*) am exercising my rights under the **First Amendment of the U.S. Constitution** and **C.R.S. 25-4-1704 (4) (b)** and (Alabama Government Code Section 16-30-3 and Alabama Code 22-20-3 Section 22-20-3) to receive religious exemption from vaccinations & testing.

Applicable law has been interpreted to mean that a religious belief is subject to protection even though no religious group espouses such beliefs or the fact that the religious group to which the individual professes to belong may not advocate or require such belief. Title VII of the Civil Rights Act of 1964 as amended Nov. 1, 1980; Part 1605.1-Guidelines on Discrimination Because of Religion.

SENATE BILL #942 SECTION 1 CHAPTER 7

3380 – IN ENACTING THIS CHAPTER, IT IS THE INTENT OF THE LEGISLATURE TO PROVIDE: EXEMPTION FROM IMMUNIZATION FOR MEDICAL REASONS OR FOR PERSONAL BELIEFS.

3385 – IMMUNIZATIONS OF A PERSON SHALL NOT BE REQUIRED FOR ADMISSIONS TO A SCHOOL OR OTHER INSTITUTION … IF THE GUARDIAN, PARENT, OR ADULT WHO HAS ASSUMED RESPONSIBILITY FOR HIS OR HER CUSTODY AND CARE IN THE CASE OF A MINOR, OR THE PERSON SEEKING ADMISSION FILES WITH GOVERNING AUTHORITY, A LETTER OR AFFIDAVIT STATING THAT SUCH VACCINATIONS ARE CONTRARY TO HIS/HER BELIEFS.

I affirm that vaccination & injections of any foreign substances and proteins conflict with my religious beliefs as stated above. Therefore, I would request that you accommodate my religious beliefs & practices by exempting my child from any vaccinations, injections, and testing of any kind.

Subscribed and sworn, without prejudice, and with all rights reserved, (Print Name Below)
_____,
Principal, by Special Appearance, in Propria Persona, proceeding Sui Juris.

_____
Signature of Affiant

                                    Acknowledgement

State of Alabama

County of_____:

On this_____ day of _____, 200____, before me

Personally appeared _____, to me known to be the person described in and who executed the foregoing instrument and acknowledged that he executed the same as his free act and deed, for the purposes therein set forth.

_____
(Notary Public)

My Commission Expires _____, 20____

For more vaccine exemption forms and specific information regarding each state's law, go to LearnTheRisk.org

> **"It is my opinion that no time is right or safe for any of the vaccines that the medical establishment promotes."** Dr. Sherri Tenpenny

Claiming religious exemption is a belief that the body is the temple of the Holy Spirit and to inject vaccines such as hepatitis A, rabies, rubella and chickenpox, that are manufactured from cells of aborted fetal tissue, defiles the Holy Spirit and is an abomination before God. If you believe abortion is evil, then why would you participate in a practice of culturing cells from aborted children? It's time to simply stand up for common sense and refuse this barbaric practice and claim vaccinations are against your religion, regardless of where you go to church or how you worship God, The Almighty Creator.

> **"Any action that is dictated by fear or by coercion of any kind ceases to be moral."** Mahatma Gandhi

---

Hepatitis B Refusal Form for Newborns at Hospital (Sample Form)
(Take this form to the hospital when you go to deliver)

DATE: _____

To all doctors, nurses and hospital personnel

This is to inform you that we are refusing the Hepatitis B shot for our new born baby. Thank you for honoring our choice to exercise this right.

We do **NOT** give consent for the vaccine or any others to be given to our child. If our child is vaccinated, we will take legal action.

Sincerely,

_____, Mother
_____, Father

_____   _____
Name of person who accepts letter   Date

340

> **"If you give up your rights now, don't expect to get them back."** Rand Paul, U.S. Senator, Kentucky

If you do choose to vaccinate, remember that antibiotics and cortisone suppress the immune system. So, if you have or are taking these, you don't want to vaccinate at that time. Dr. Boyd Haley teaches that you should never give a child a vaccine containing thimerosal (mercury) when sick and taking an antibiotic, because the glutathione levels drop, and you can't excrete the mercury. He believes, *"Anyone who vaccinates a sick child should be fined, it's criminal, very poor medicine."*

> **"Truth will ultimately prevail where there are pains taken to bring it to light."** George Washington (1732-1799)

As of today, only three states do not allow a religious exemption: California, Mississippi and West Virginia. Mississippi allows a medical exemption and also has an automatic exemption for home-schooled students. All other states allow parents to refuse vaccinations and claim "religious exemption" in order for their child to attend public school.

It's interesting to note that Mississippi has been declared "the unhealthiest state in America" while at the same time reporting the best vaccination rate in the U.S. at 99.4 percent among kindergarten children. Mississippi also has the highest infant mortality rate out of any state with 8.8 deaths per every 1,000 live births.

In 2015, a panel of 120 Italian doctors submitted a letter to the Higher Institute of Health (the Italian equivalent of the CDC) declaring that unvaccinated children are healthier overall and less prone to infectious diseases, including respiratory, neurological and behavioral disorders.

> **"The price of freedom is eternal vigilance ... Never trust your government. You need a revolution every 20 years, just to keep the government honest!"** Thomas Jefferson, 3rd President of USA & author of the Declaration of Independence (1743-1826)

Barbara Fisher explains that mandatory vaccination is the only law in this country that requires an American citizen to risk his or her life for their country. In times of war, when the draft was in effect, the young men being asked to take that risk were 18 years of age or older and could conscientiously object if they chose to. They were not 1-day-old infants. If you choose to vaccinate your child, simply ask your doctor what the health risks are. Most will reassure you that vaccines are safe and necessary for health. After they promise you how safe and effective they are, pull out a form such as the one below, and simply ask your physician to sign it, since he or she is so confident that vaccines are safe.

> **Physician Vaccination Signature Form**
>
> "I certify that the (*Name of Vaccine*) _____ vaccine being administered to (*Name of Child*) _____ is free from all known and yet unknown zoonotic or human viruses or viral fragments and will not cause acute or chronic illness in the recipient due to viral contamination or as a reaction to the components of this vaccine. As a physician I attest that this vaccine is safe and will not cause harm or damage to your child. (*Signature of Physician*) Date _____.

Most physicians will refuse to sign such a form, because they know that the vaccines are not safe and there are risks. If your physician refuses to sign such a form, then that is evidence enough to refuse a shot that he or she isn't willing to sign their name to.

> "**My honest opinion is that vaccine is the cause of more disease and suffering than anything I could name. I believe that such diseases as cancer, syphilis, cold sores, and many other disease conditions are the direct results of vaccination. Yet, parents are compelled to submit their children to this procedure while the medical profession not only receives its pay for this service, but also makes splendid and prospective patients for the future.**" Dr. Henry R. Bybee

Mandatory Vaccinations – A Violation Of The Nuremberg Code

> **The Nuremberg Code – August 19, 1947**
> 1. The voluntary consent of the human subject is absolutely essential.

After World War II, doctors who were found guilty of experimenting and forcing medical procedures upon humans, without their consent, were punished and some even put to death. To prevent medical procedures from being forced upon an individual without their consent, authorities set up the Nuremberg Code. This gives you the right to legally exercise free power of choice, voluntary consent, without the element of force, coercion, or constraint to make an informed decision on any medical procedure that may cause death or disabling injury. If you do choose a medical procedure, during the course of experiment, the human subject is at liberty to bring the experiment to an end.

These are our rights, and with over 30,000 VAERS reports being filed annually (the CDC states that only 10 percent of actual cases are ever reported), vaccines are a medical experiment that may cause harm and death. Under the

Nuremberg Code, we humans have the right to decline medical experimental procedures.

> "We are told, the science is settled on everything vaccine but as I compared the so-called evidence with the historical and scientific literature, it became clear that the education given to me and to doctors today, is an oppressive form of religion ... preached as gospel by the leading authorities who act as if their narrow truth is the only righteous belief." Suzanne Humphries, M.D.

Travel Vaccines

Nearly all travel vaccines are recommendations only and are rarely necessary or required. Yellow fever vaccine is the exception and sometimes can be required by International Health Regulations when traveling to some sub-Saharan African countries and tropical South America. Yellow fever is transmitted by mosquitoes, but is very rare. Also, the Saudi Arabia government for traveling during the Hajj requires the meningococcal vaccination. U.S. customs does not require a vaccination record to re-enter the country.

> "If you want the truth on vaccination, you must go to those who are not making anything off of it. If doctors shot at the moon every time it was full as a preventive of measles and got a shilling for it, they would bring statistics to prove it was a most efficient practice, and that the population would be decimated if it were stopped." Dr. Allinson

Healthcare Workers Reject Influenza Vaccines Because...
1. Fear of side effects
2. They had serious side effects from previous vaccinations
3. Belief that the vaccine will cause the disease
4. Little trust in vaccines' effectiveness

Nearly 10 percent of pediatricians and 21 percent of pediatric specialists admitted they do not follow the CDC vaccination guidelines for themselves and their own children. In England, 57 percent of healthcare workers reject the flu vaccine. In Germany, only 17 percent of nurses receive a seasonal flu shot, and in Brazil, only 13 percent of health-care workers get the flu vaccine. In Italy, 70 percent of physicians and 89 percent of nurses reject influenza vaccines. In China, only 13 percent of doctors receive the flu shot. If vaccines are safe and effective, why wouldn't every doctor and nurse around the globe be the first in line to get them?

> "As well consult a butcher on the value of vegetarianism as a doctor on the worth of vaccination." Bernard Shaw

The Vaccine Friendly Plan – For Those Who Choose To Vaccinate

If you choose to vaccinate, that is your choice and we respect people's right to choose. However, we expect the same courtesy to be extended to those who chose not to vaccinate. Many situations involve parents who are divided on the vaccine issue, usually from a lack of research. If you do choose to vaccinate, I suggest you follow Dr. Paul Thomas's vaccine-friendly plan, to help minimize possible adverse side effects. He recommends spreading the vaccines out over a longer period of time, and rejecting the hepatitis B vaccine at birth. Dr. Thomas is a pediatrician in Portland, Oregon, who advocates refusing certain high-risk vaccines and always getting the MMR vaccine by itself.

> **The Vaccine-Friendly Plan**
> By Paul Thomas, M.D. &
> Jennifer Margulis, Ph.D.
> www.drpaulapproved.com

> **"If you have autism in the family – don't do any vaccines."** Paul Thomas, M.D.

Never give acetaminophen before or after a vaccination, as it may cause the vaccine adverse reaction to worsen. Acetaminophen depletes glutathione, which is needed to help the detoxification process of foreign substances contained in vaccines. Without glutathione, serious vaccine injury is increased.

Autopsy reports of infants who died of SIDS were examined by Dawn Richardson and Karin Schumacher at the Austin, Texas, morgue, in which they compared the date of the child's death to when they received vaccinations. The data revealed that SIDS deaths clustered at 2, 4, and 6 months, the exact times when infants are recommended to receive their vaccinations. Is this just a coincidence, or did the vaccines cause it and no one connects the dots?

> **"Why do we have the highest infant death rate of 43 modern countries? If you can have the highest infant death rate and the highest childhood, that is 1-5 death rate, of all the modern countries that is the equivalent in the first year of 16,000 babies dying that wouldn't need to die if we had Sweden's infant death rate…What are the children dying of to make us have such a highest infant death rate? Are they dying of asthma-related diseases caused by vaccines? No one wants to look at that or even discuss it or even mention it. We have a sickness in this country, if you don't care for your children then you are in big trouble… when you can sit there and say we are satisfied that we spend all this money on medicine and still have the highest infant death rate in the world, your medical associations, your medical establishment is sick. It's either sick or it's criminal. Or both."** Boyd Haley, Ph.D.

Our founding forefathers fought a bloody battle to win the freedom of this great country. The spirit of America is all about the freedom to choose. Most of our ancestors left Europe to come to America so we could go to church where we want, homestead a piece of land and not be taxed to death. We wanted to be free of tyranny and unfair rulers. The powers that be are stepping on our toes, trying to take our rights away, by imposing on us mandatory vaccinations. We need to stand up and defend our constitutional rights, which grant us our liberties. Our health care, our choice to vaccinate or not, is ours, not the government's.

> **"America can only remain the land of the free as long as she is also home of the brave!"** Lynne Meredith, Author of *Vultures in Eagle's Clothing*

If you are interested in learning more about vaccine facts, go to YouTube and listen to Drs. Haley, Tenpenny or Humphries speak. When you stop listening to fear-mongering and look at facts, then you can make an informed decision about vaccines. I urge you to watch *Haley vs Offit: A Virtual Debate about Vaccines*. Dr. Offit claims that injecting a newborn baby with 10,000 vaccines at once would be perfectly safe. He and toxicologist Dr. Haley are interviewed, and it doesn't take long to find out who the honest researcher is. Listen and judge for yourself who makes the most sense. Educate before you vaccinate.

> Watch on YouTube
> **Vaccine Experts**
> Boyd Haley, Ph.D.
> Sherri Tenpenny, D.O.
> Suzanne Humphries, M.D.
> Del Bigtree – The High Wire

> **"Every pediatrician, family practitioner, or vaccine profiteer that isn't rising up against the corruption of the science of vaccines perpetrated by the CDC is betraying their oath to 'first, do no harm.' The blood of every vaccine-injured or killed child is on the hands of every pediatrician that parroted lies like 'vaccines do not cause autism' and 'the science is settled.' The vaccine industry will soon face the backlash as doctors, scientists, and parents across America become aware of your crimes, rise up to oppose your lies, and hold you accountable for the vaccine injury holocaust you've caused."** James Meehan, M.D.

Over 100 profound quotes by world-renowned doctors, researchers and experts on vaccinations and health are found in this chapter. Many have held some of the most prestigious positions at universities and in government health care. If a healthcare practitioner says to vaccinate for smallpox, polio and measles and you come down with the disease it's supposed to prevent, it doesn't take a genius to figure out that the vaccine has failed. We have a few not-so-good ideas occurring today, and the proof is in the pudding, like 1 in 36 children being diagnosed with autism.

> **IF YOU SUPPORT VACCINATIONS**
> **But have no problem with the following:**
> - No cumulative safety testing of the U.S. vaccine schedule prior to licensing.
> - No gold standard safety testing having been performed for ANY of the 70 currently licensed by the FDA vaccinations.
> - No carcinogenic or mutagenic capacity testing ever performed even though vaccinations contain animal DNA and carcinogens.
> - No route of exposure research to determine injected safe limits for vaccine ingredients.
>
> **THEN YOU ARE NOT PRO VACCINE FOR THE CHILDREN, YOU ARE PRO VACCINE FOR THE PHARMACEUTICAL COMPANIES' SALES.**
> Informed Citizens Against Vaccinations

What most people don't realize is that when a doctor discovers corruption and fraud in medicine and has the courage to speak up against it, they are usually ostracized, ridiculed and some may even lose their job, because Big Pharma will pay to destroy them and suppress the truth. For most, there is nothing to gain and much to lose by speaking out against corruption. Like in the days of prohibition, Al Capone paid for law enforcement, attorneys and judges to turn their heads and ignore their mafia dealings or suffer the consequences. We have a medical mafia that suppresses honest research and promotes harmful drugs and vaccines to keep the masses sick and diseased. They control the CDC with their money and power.

> **VACCINE REACTIONS - REPORT TO VAERS IF...**
> - High fever (over 103)
> - Skin reactions (hives, rash, eczema)
> - High pitched crying/screaming
> - Behavioral changes (mental/physical regression)
> - Vomiting or diarrhea
> - Respiratory distress (difficulty breathing)
> - Excessive sleepiness
> - Seizures
> - Brain inflammation (bulging fontanel)
> - Facial asymmetry (mouth palsy)
>
> Call 1-800-822-7967 or info@vaers.org To Report

The good doctors who have integrity to stand up to corruption and risk their lives and careers are the true heroes in medicine, not the phony ones who suppress honest research and go along with the agenda so they can keep their lucrative jobs and paychecks. To wield the sword of truth takes guts and courage, and I thank those who stand tall to make the world a better place. May God bless us all as we strive to make a difference in the world, not only for ourselves, but more importantly, for our children, grandchildren and future generations to come, so we can be healthy, free and prosperous.

> "Vaccinations will one day go the way of bloodletting. Doctors of tomorrow would be shocked that, without any good research showing any benefit and with much research showing harm, we continue using this bizarre 18th-century medical practice of injecting viri, bacteria, toxins and other chemicals into our children well into the 21st century. Don't follow advice blindly. Question authority, think for yourself, read, learn, don't do anything unless you are sure the benefits outweigh the risks. Remember, you can't fool mother nature." Dr. Andrea Brisson

Chapter 7
Healthy Living
Chiropractic Adjustments

> "The body is controlled by the nervous system, which is made up of your brain and spinal cord. The brain sends signals to the rest of your body via the spinal cord. These signals go to every organ, muscle and tissue of the body. If at any time there is an interruption to these signals due to a misalignment of one or more vertebrae, then not only will the body not receive the proper communication from the brain, but it cannot properly send messages back to the brain. This interruption of neurological signals is called a subluxation. The cause of the subluxation is stress. There are three kinds of stress: physical, chemical and mental/emotional.
>
> The primary purpose of a chiropractor's profession should be the detection and removal of subluxations. The chiropractor does this with what is called an adjustment. An adjustment is a very specific force put into the body. This force may be applied by the chiropractor using their hands, an instrument or even a very light touch. The purpose of the adjustment is to re-establish the communication between the brain and the rest of the body, thereby allowing the body the opportunity to heal itself." Dr. Jon Alan Smith, Albertville, AL

We humans, especially athletes, get knocked out of alignment. The neck, spine and hips greatly benefit from an adjustment periodically to realign our spine. Many headaches and pain subside once subluxations are corrected because the pressure is taken off the nerves.

> "Chiropractors adjust subluxations, relieving pressure from the nerves so that they can perform their functions in a normal manner. The Innate can and will do the rest." B.J. Palmer, D.C. – Developer of Chiropractic

Every house has a fuse box to keep electric wiring in a home safe. If a wire gets too hot or develops a short, it will trip the breaker. Just as your house has electrical wiring with fuses, so does the nervous system in your body. A short in your nervous system many times is caused by a subluxation, where pressure is placed on a nerve, thus short-circuiting the energy flow to an organ or gland. Lack of electricity flowing to your adrenal glands can cause chronic fatigue, dizziness, allergies and respiratory problems. All the medication in the world, including herbs, won't help until you fix the short by getting an adjustment.

> "It is useless to administer a powder, potion, or pill to the stomach when the body needs an adjustment." B.J. Palmer, D.C.

Competitive Athletes – What To Eat?

Game Day Energy Drink
½ cup blueberries
½ cup strawberries
½ cup raspberries
1 Tbsp. raw almond butter
1 Tbsp. pumpkin seeds
1 Tbsp. chia seeds
1 Tbsp. hemp seeds
2 raw walnuts
2 raw Brazil nuts
½ avocado
1 banana
1 raw egg
1 Tbsp. coconut butter
1 - 2 cups unsweetened almond milk or coconut milk
(1 scoop SEC Greens optional)
Mix in blender

Most of my life, I have competed in football, wrestling and powerlifting. A good workout makes you feel good, gives you energy, reduces stress, releases feel-good neurotransmitters and helps you sleep well at nights. I'm addicted to how it makes me feel. For some, going for a mile walk every day is good. For college and professional athletes who want to win a championship, the intensity levels increase to grueling workouts. Proper fuel and nutrition to repair and rebuild is foundational for success.

The question is, what is the best food to eat to get the edge over your opponent and perform at your very best, with maximum energy? First of all, I recommend staying away from sugary, high-caffeine energy drinks. Once the sugar and caffeine wear off, you crash. The same holds true for carb-loading before a competition or workout, where you eat lots of pasta, rice, bread, and sugary foods. This will spike your energy but leave you feeling more exhausted than before. This is not what you want come the fourth quarter.

Athletes need strength and stamina to last the whole game, match or competition. After athletes compete for any length of time, they begin to burn fats instead of sugars. This is why long-distance runners are loading up on fats and small amounts of proteins rather than carbs. Fats provide the best endurance fuel. High fructose corn syrup is junk. Avoid it.

Supplements – For Athletes
Bee pollen	Royal Jelly
Wheatgrass	L-Glutamine
Alfalfa	Rhodiola
Barley greens	Astaxanthin
Spirulina	Raw cacao
Chlorella	Whey protein
Suma	Maca
Probiotics	Chromium

Best Foods For Athletes
Avocado	Spinach
Coconut oil	Kale
Eggs	Broccoli
Raw nuts/seeds	Sprouts
Alaskan salmon	Berries
Chicken	Bananas
Beef	Watermelon
Grapefruit	Papaya
Olive oil	Mushrooms

Sugar weakens your body; a top athlete will have more endurance when avoiding it. If an athlete starts to cramp, then yes, an energy drink with electrolytes may be beneficial. Other than that, avoid them. Eating a piece of fruit, if possible, is usually a better option.

After a workout, muscles have been broken down and your body is depleted. Amino acids are needed to to help muscles recuperate and rebuild. Good sources of proteins are green leafy vegetables, crunchy vegetables (spinach, kale, arugula, broccoli, cauliflower, cucumbers, celery, carrots), wild caught Alaskan salmon, chicken, turkey, beef and eggs.

On game day, two to three hours before competing, some complex carbs may be beneficial, such as brown rice, sweet potatoes, eggs, almonds, walnuts and olive oil, which are all easy to digest and provide more sustained energy for the day.

> "If you are bored with life – if you don't get up every morning with a burning desire to do things – you don't have enough goals." Lou Holtz, Football Coach

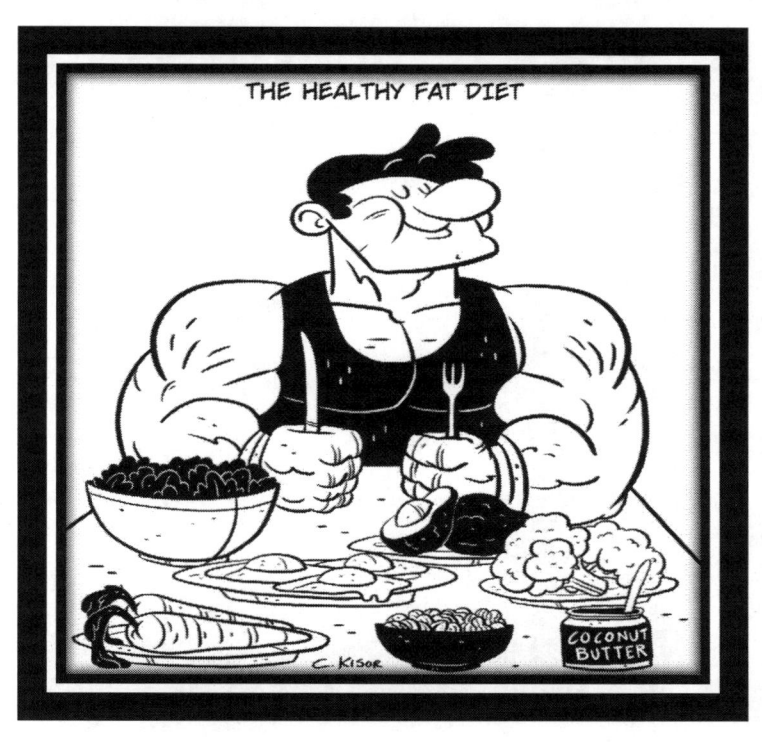

Dr. Jeff Volek, Ph.D., professor at Ohio State University and author of, *The Art and Science of Low-Carbohydrate Performance*, teaches that a low-carb, high-fat diet is ideal for athletes. He explains that athletes can only store roughly 2,000 kilocalories of carbs as glycogen, and so if you're exercising for more than a couple of hours, once you burn up the stored carbohydrates, you are going to hit a wall. Carb loading only provides you with about half an hour of energy, hence that's one reason it's not recommended. For athletes who eat fat and burn fat, they avoid hitting the wall and crashing. Fat-burning athletes have at least 2,000 to 30,000 kilocalories on their body in the form of adipose tissue that can be accessed during competition that provides enough energy to finish a 100-mile race.

Whey protein, high in the amino acid leucine, is a great fitness food. It helps build lean muscle. Consuming whey protein about 30 minutes before your workout, and within 2 hours after a workout, helps increase muscle building and fat loss. Bee Pollen is

Athletes Who Eat Low-Carb, High Fat Diets	
LeBron James	Dave Zabriskie
Ray Allen	Nell Stephenson
Timothy Olson	Ben Greenfield

another excellent supplement for athletes, because it is packed with nutrition and gives strength and stamina.

> **"If children gave up when they fell for the first time, they would never learn to walk."** Louise L. Hay

Enthusiasm for life is what keeps us healthy. Get out and get involved with something that motivates you. There are millions of possibilities out there. Do something that brings fulfillment into your life. Turn the TV off. It doesn't count as a hobby.

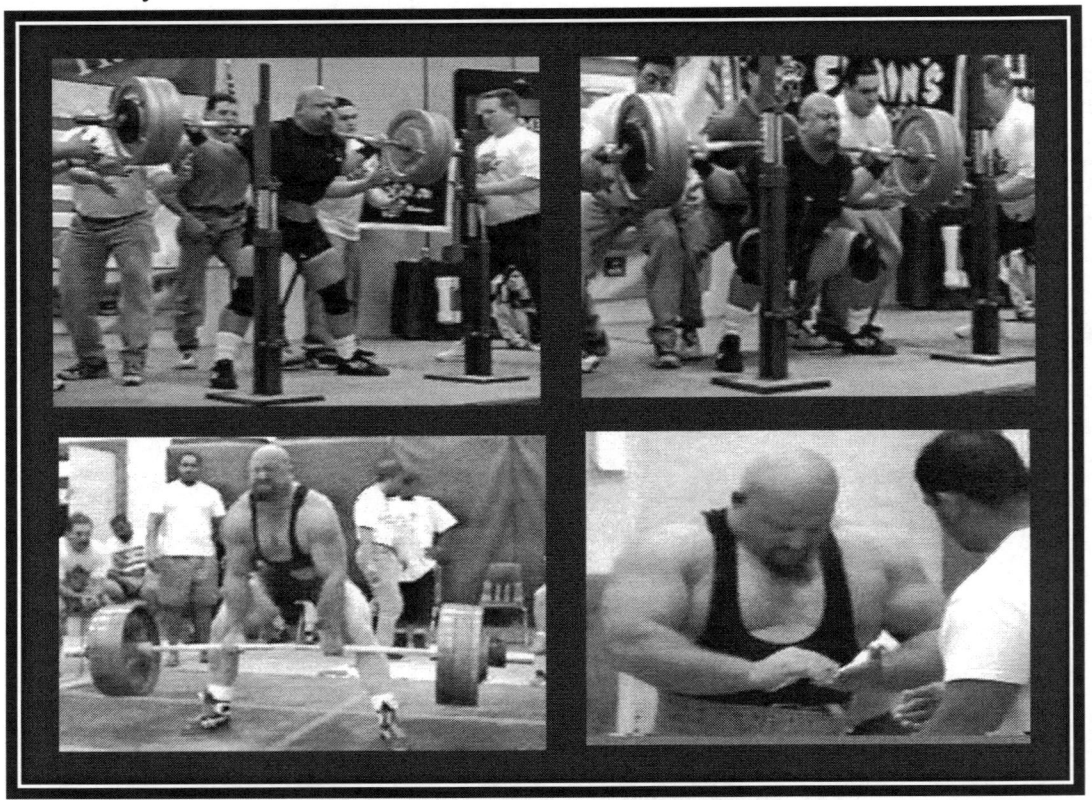

(Top two pictures) Reed Sainsbury competing in the 1998 USAPL Lifetime Drug Free National Powerlifting Championships in St. Louis, Missouri - 650 lb. Squat; (Bottom two pictures) Winning 1st place at The Rocky Mountain States Powerlifting Championships – 1998, Pocatello, Idaho

> **"Some people want it to happen. Some wish it would happen. Others make it happen."** Michael Jordan - NBA Basketball Player

Where Do Cows Get Protein?

If you look at a cow, what do they eat to get so big? They eat plants, such as alfalfa, grass and hay. If a farmer wants to fatten them up, they are fed corn or grains. How much milk does an adult cow drink? None, of course. Well then, how does she get protein to produce milk for her calf? Obviously, she gets all the protein she needs from a vegetarian diet. What about her calf, who gains 2.5 pounds a day? What does it eat? Mother's milk, and it contains less than 3 percent protein, and that calf gains 75 pounds a month. Within 9 months a 75-pound calf will weigh about 550 pounds by eating grasses with about 3 percent protein.

Some will argue that cows and humans are different and that it isn't a fair comparison, so we will look at a baby human. What is the newborn baby fed? Mother's breast milk, and that should be exclusively so for the first 6 months to one year of life, according to health experts. Now, how much protein is in mother's milk? Less than 2 percent, usually 1.6 percent, and that child doubles in size in about 5 months. So, if a child, who doubles in body weight every 5 months, has a diet consisting of less than 2 percent protein, how much do non-growing adults require? And how many adults are looking to lose weight and not gain?

What's the strongest animal in the world? Pound for pound, a gorilla is king. Gorillas are ripped and chiseled massive bodybuilders with physiques that would intimidate any NFL football player. A gorilla has a digestive system very similar to humans. As a matter of fact, if you take the intestinal tract from a gorilla and a human and lay them side-by-side, you cannot tell which one is which. A gorilla lives about 140 years and is a vegetarian. They consume fruits, vegetables and bamboo shoots. Where does the gorilla get all the protein to build massive muscles containing tremendous amounts of strength? Gorillas don't eat steak, chicken, milk, eggs, cheese and protein muscle-gainer powder-5000. They get all the protein they need from a vegetarian diet. A little piece of information that was probably never taught to you is the fact that protein is found abundantly in Mother Nature's perfect whole foods. Green vegetables, fruits and grasses contain protein, and it is easily absorbed and digested by the body, especially when compared to cooked animal meat.

I know many vegetarians who are healthy and vibrant. I know many meat consumers who are healthy and vibrant. Most Americans get way too much protein and eat too much sugar because we don't eat enough vegetables, which should be the staple of our diets. My point is, eat the diet that gives you an abundance of life-energy. There is no perfect one diet for everyone.

High-Protein Diets – Not So Healthy

A friend came to me excited about losing 40 pounds. He proceeded to tell me about how he cut carbs out and enjoys eating bacon, sausage and eggs for breakfast. He eats meats for lunch and more meat for dinner. By eating lots of meat and cutting out breads, pasta and sugar, he is losing weight. It is true that high-protein diets will help you lose weight; however, there is a price to be paid. Consuming large amounts of protein places the burden of removing nitrogen waste products from your blood through the kidneys. Too much protein is like too much sugar. Both lead to disease.

Eating a high-protein diet places a tremendous burden on the digestive system, not to mention all the nitrates, phosphates, steroids, antibiotics and other harmful chemicals put in as preservatives and fed to the animals so they grow bigger in a shorter amount of time. As mentioned earlier, meats are high in purines, which break down into uric acid. These acids accumulate in the joints. In order to buffer the acids, the body will use up its sodium, calcium, potassium, magnesium and iron reserves, thus leaving you depleted. These acids are what cause inflammation, joint pain, gout and arthritis. It also causes the pH to be very acidic, which creates the terrain for diseases to thrive. Remember, an alkaline terrain is where good health grows and an acidic terrain favors disease.

High-protein diets create a negative calcium balance in the body, which leads to arthritis. In other words, the more protein we eat, the more calcium is lost through the urine than is absorbed by the body from our food. This is why most arthritic people are heavy meat-eaters and dairy consumers. The body uses up its mineral reserves to buffer the acids created by the high-protein diet. When this happens, bone density decreases and osteoporosis sets in. Your medical doctor never addresses this cause, but you can rest assured that he has a bag full of prescriptions ready to prescribe to treat the pain.

You can't over-eat with raw fruits and vegetables. How many raw carrots, cucumbers and celery can you eat in one sitting? Once you eat what your body needs nutritionally, your body will let you know when you've had enough and you won't feel bloated like you can easily do with cooked, processed foods such as breads, pasta, dairy and meat. Even with sweet fruits like apples or grapes, you can only eat until you are satisfied, and then your body will let you know when you've had enough, and you stop eating before you feel full and bloated. This is how our bodies were designed to receive nutrition.

> "Ammonia, which is produced in great amounts as a by-product of meat metabolism, is highly carcinogenic and can cause cancer development. A high-protein diet also breaks down the pancreas and lowers resistance to cancer as well as contributes to the development of diabetes." Dr. Willard J. Visek, Cornell University

The following case study is an example of what happens to the body when an athlete consumes a high-protein diet for many years. The doctor told him there was no cure for arthritis and that pain medication and steroid injections were the only treatments available. After changing to an alkaline diet and getting his pH to a 7.0, Leon was feeling 85 percent better in two months.

Case Study

I'm a 60 year old Tool and Die Maker (machinist) by profession. For most of my life I have been very involved in athletics and fitness training. I am a 2nd degree Black Belt in Yoshukai Karate and was an instructor for 1 ½ years. I have also been an avid runner most of my life, running at least five miles a day.

Going to the gym every morning at 4:30 to train keeps me in shape but has taken a toll on my joints. For most of my life I have been in tip-top shape, able to do 500 push-ups and sit-ups without stopping. This I would do every day. When I was in my prime, I could do 200 consecutive pull-ups. I would spend four hours a day training in the gym.

In 2003, I tore my meniscus in my left knee kicking. Then in 2005, I had my left shoulder scoped. I had torn the rotator cuff completely loose and also the bicep tendon. In 2006, I was attacked by a cat and had to have surgery on my right arm and wrist. The cat bite got infected and actually did nerve damage to my arm and caused me to lose some of the cartilage in my wrist. I had a lengthy recovery and did not heal well. My injuries forced me to stop training. In 2007, I had my right knee scoped. I felt like my body was falling apart and my joint pains were becoming unbearable. Then I hit another brick wall, pleurisy in my left lung, not to mention my sinus trouble that had been plaguing me for the last 20 years.

My chiropractor, Dr. Hudgins, has helped me get off the steroid drugs I was taking for my sinuses. She recommended I see Dr. Reed Sainsbury, a naturopath, for my other complaints.

I was taking Darvocet for pain, but that wasn't enough so I started taking six to eight Aleve on top of that every day for joint pain. In the past I had been on Diclofenac, Celebrex, Loritab and massive amounts of Tylenol and aspirin. I was living on pain medication.

When I went to see Dr. Sainsbury, he did an EDS exam and identified what was causing my joints to be in so much pain. He checked my pH and found that I was very acidic and taught me that my high-protein diet was killing me and preventing me from healing. He told me that if I wanted to get well, I would have to get off the acidifying meats and get on an alkaline-vegetable diet. I was willing to do anything to get rid of this pain.

He found that my body had a tremendous amount of pesticides built up in my kidneys and liver, not to mention the pain medication-drug residue. He told me I was low on essential fatty acids and had a lot of calcium build-up in my body. He gave me some supplements to detoxify and nourish my body.

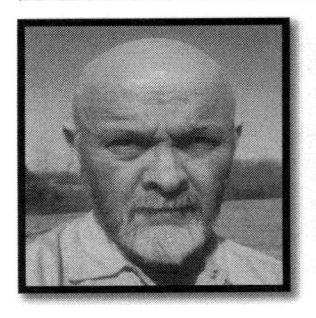

Once I got started on the detox program and began to juice vegetables every day (Dr. Oz's green drink), my pain began to subside. The silver dollar-sized calcium deposit (carbuncle) on my foot has shrunk down to the size of a nickel since I've been on this program, and all of my pain is gone. It's been two months now and I am feeling 80 to 90 percent better! I have come off all of my pain medication! I have turned things around and feel like a new person. I am amazed at how fast my body is healing. No drugs, no surgery, but lots of alkaline vegetables, herbs and nourishing supplements.

A. Leon Smith
Guntersville, Alabama

Mother Nature's Healers

Alfalfa is one of the most complete foods on the planet. It is actually higher in protein than beef, at 18.9 percent protein, while beef is 16.5 percent protein, eggs are 13.1 percent protein and milk is 3.3 percent protein. Alfalfa has been used for thousands of years to cure disease. It cleans, builds, strengthens and rejuvenates cells back to health. It is loaded with vitamins, minerals, amino acids and enzymes that are alkalizing agents to help neutralize acids that cause inflammation and pain. It has been used to heal just about every disease and is extremely beneficial for arthritis and gout. If you have arthritis, start eating fresh fruits and vegetables, along with large doses of alfalfa, so you can heal.

Wheatgrass and barley greens are two more of Mother Nature's greatest healers. If we incorporate these greens into our diet, the body receives the needed nutrients for cell regeneration. When cells are nourished and cleansed, then the acidic disease environment disappears, inflammation subsides and healing occurs.

Bee pollen is another complete nourishing food that is capable of sustaining life and healing disease. It is made from the flowering plant. Every little grain contains a powerhouse of nutrients. Scientists have discovered that the male sperm cells of flowering plants contain a miracle concentration of nearly all known nutrients. It is said that bee pollen contains the secret "ambrosia" eaten by the ancient gods to acquire eternal youth.

William Robinson, M.D., of the U.S. Department of Agriculture, demonstrated that bee pollen added to food could prevent or slow down the growth of cancerous mammary tumors in a unique strain of mice, bred to succumb to such tumors. Further research showed that existing tumors were reduced in size in the mice that were given bee pollen. The USDA published a report by the National Cancer Institute, in 1948, that bee pollen has a pronounced effect on malignant mammary tumors. Several other studies reveal that bees sterilize the pollen they harvest with a secretion that is anti-cancer. And according to French researchers, an antibiotic element has been identified in bee pollen. When salmonella and other harmful bacteria are exposed to bee pollen, it is destroyed. Could bee pollen be used as a natural antibiotic? Has Mother Nature already given us the greatest antibiotics and we just don't use them because they can't be patented by Big Pharma to make billions?

Who Are The Healthiest People In The World?

Five Long-Lived Healthy Cultures
1. The Himalayan Tibetans of Northwestern China
2. The Hunzakut of Eastern Pakistan near Mount Rakaposhi
3. The Russian Georgians of the Caucasus Mountains in Western Russia
4. The Vilcabamba Indians in the Andes Mountains of Ecuador
5. The Titicaca Indians in the Andes Mountains of Southwestern Peru

Where do the healthiest people in the world live? Researchers have identified five cultures where people live on the average of our human genetic potential of 120 years of age, with no major diseases. In the January 1973, issue of National Geographic Magazine these cultures were examined. They are all third-world countries with no modern-day medicine, antibiotics or vaccinations.

What do all these cultures have in common? Dr. Wallach lists the following in his book, *Rare Earths Forbidden Cures*.

1. The communities are found at elevations ranging from 8,500 feet to 14,000 feet in sheltered mountain valleys.
2. The annual precipitation is less than two inches.
3. Their water source for drinking and irrigation comes from glacial melt, and is known universally as "Glacial Milk," because the highly mineralized water is an opaque white or gray color from the presence of an enormous amount of suspended rock flour.
4. There is no heavy industry or modern agriculture to pollute their air, water, or food.
5. Only natural fertilizer including animal manure, plant debris, and "Glacial Milk" is applied to their fields.
6. Western allopathic medicine is not available to these cultures.

"The difference between the child prodigy (i.e. — music, art, math, physics, athletics, etc.) and the high school dropout is not genetics or income level of the parents, but rather the nutritional (and especially the mineral intake) competency of the child during pre and postnatal development." Joel Wallach, D.V.M., N.D.

According to Dr. Wallach's research, millions of people are born each year with unnecessary physical defects caused from mineral deficiencies. Allopathic medical doctors try to pin defects on genetics, but the research proves otherwise. For example, it is true that Down Syndrome or Trisomy 21 is a chromosomal defect in which there is an extra chromosome 21. However, Dr. Wallach has proven that Down Syndrome is not genetic. He explains, *"It in fact is the result of a preconception zinc deficiency which produces a chromosomal/DNA injury or defect similar in nature to the changes created by radiation. Nutritional studies in animals and cell cultures have demonstrated that Trisomy 21 or Down Syndrome can be created at will in the laboratory by preconception zinc deficiencies during the formation and development of the sperm and the egg – these facts underscore the critical nutritional needs for sexually active men and women. It has been clearly demonstrated in the laboratory animal, pet animal and agriculture experiments 98 percent of all birth defects are not 'genetic' in nature, but in fact are nutritional deficiencies of the egg, embryo and fetus and can be prevented by preconception nutrition."* Dr. Wallach continues to explain that in the animal industry, these tragic and expensive birth defects have been eliminated by giving correct nutrition to breeding animals.

"To understand how the developing embryo is so dependent upon a proper and adequate supply of vitamins, minerals, amino acids and fatty acids, we have to appreciate that embryonic tissues develop faster physically and biochemically than the most aggressive cancer cells; this rate of growth and development requires dizzying amounts of essential nutrients to complete certain biochemical and tissue maneuvers on time – the train only passes by once, if it is missed there is no going back and the child will be born with one or more biochemical, physical, mental or emotional defects." Supplementing our diets to ensure we are getting our necessary minerals for health is foundational for optimum health. Pregnant women should supplement to ensure the fetus is receiving all the nutrition he or she needs for optimal health.

"Those who now advocate eating natural foods as the only source of vitamins and minerals live in a dream world of yesterday. What was yesterday's law is today's folly. It really doesn't matter how well you balance your meals, or if you're a meat-eater, vegetarian, or a raw-foodist, you still run the risk of malnutrition if you try to get all your vitamins and minerals exclusively from the foods you eat." Paavo Airola, N.D., Ph.D.

> **U.S. Senate Document No. 264**
>
> "The alarming fact is that foods – fruits and vegetables and grains, now being raised on millions of acres of land that no longer contains enough of certain needed minerals, are starving us – no matter how much of them we eat! No man of today can eat enough fruits and vegetables to supply his system with the minerals he requires for perfect health because his stomach isn't big enough to hold them."
>
> "The truth is that our foods vary enormously in value, and some of them aren't worth eating as food.... Our physical well-being is more directly dependent upon the minerals we take into our systems than upon calories or vitamins or upon the precise proportions of starch, protein or carbohydrates we consume."
>
> "It is bad news to learn from our leading authorities that 99% of the American people are deficient in these minerals, and that a marked deficiency in any one of the more important minerals actually results in disease." U.S. Senate Document #264 published by the 2nd session of the 74th Congress (1936).

The fact that our soils are depleted of minerals and therefore our foods lack necessary minerals for health is one cause of disease. Farmers fertilize their fields with NPK (nitrogen, phosphorus and potassium). Why? Because these are the primary nutrients required by plants to give farmers a maximum yield with a minimum price. The other 57 minerals are many times lacking from the foods we eat because they are not put back in the soils.

Poison In Our Drinking Water

> **"When the well's dry, we know the worth of water."** Benjamin Franklin

Ever since the late 1990s, researchers have found that pharmaceuticals, especially oral contraceptives, are found in sewage water and are contaminating drinking water. Every year, 18 billion pounds of new pollutants and chemicals are released by industry into the atmosphere, soil and groundwater. Millions of prescription drugs taken by Americans are excreted in the urine and processed in city sewage treatment plants. Some city water is reprocessed sewer water, loaded with these chemical drug residues. Additional chemicals are added in the water that supposedly makes it FDA approved and safe.

> **"Don't assume that just because the water coming out of your tap is tested that it is safe. The EPA has cataloged over a quarter million unsafe water violations affecting over 120 million people on public water systems."** Lono Kahuna Kupua A 'O - Author of Don't Drink The Water

Chlorine

There's no doubt that chlorine kills bacteria and helps make our water supply safer than it was 100 years ago. However, now we have a new problem. If chlorine kills bacteria, what do you think it does to our "good" or "friendly" bacteria we need in the gut? We need these friendly bacteria in order to have a healthy microbiome for proper digestion and healthy immune systems. When chlorine kills off our good bacteria, this can be the start to many health challenges, including leaky gut and autoimmune disorders.

Most scientists will admit that chlorinated acids MX and DCA are two of the most dangerous chemicals you may be exposed to in our society. Both of these are in chlorinated drinking water. Chlorine is a powerful killer that harms delicate DNA in our cells. As a matter of fact, it has been linked to elevated Trihalomethanes (THMs) levels found in many cancer patients. (Joseph G. Hattersley, Journal of Orthomolecular Medicine vol. 15, 2nd Quarter 2000) The Journal of the National Cancer Institute reported a study that showed that drinking chlorinated water increases one's risks of developing bladder cancer by 80 percent. A Norwegian study, published in the International Journal of Epidemiology in 1992, claims that drinking chlorinated water increases the incidence of colon and rectal cancer 20 to 40 percent.

> **"During a hot shower, we inhale the steam, and the chlorine goes right through our lungs into our bloodstream."** Dr. Tom O'Bryan

Chlorine has been found to injure red blood cells, which can lead to anemia. Chlorine in our drinking water has been proven to cause scarring of the arteries. This may lead to heart attacks and strokes. Health-care professionals recommend drinking lots of water. Make sure you are drinking a healthy, purified water, free of chlorine, fluoride and other harmful chemicals.

Fluoride

> **"Fluoride is toxic to bones and increases risk of fracture at all levels of exposure including fluoridation at 1 ppm. Regardless of any other consideration, this is reason enough to discontinue fluoridation immediately."** John R. Lee, M.D. - Author of Natural Progesterone

Sodium fluoride (hydrofluosilicic acid) is an industrial pollutant, a waste byproduct of aluminum manufacturing, metal smelting and phosphate fertilizer companies. If you are a highly intelligent business owner, the best way to get rid of your manufacturing waste material is to convince someone else that it is highly beneficial for them and you'll sell it to them at a bargain price. Our taxes pay millions of dollars to put this deadly poison into our drinking water, and then we wonder why we have digestive problems and cancer!

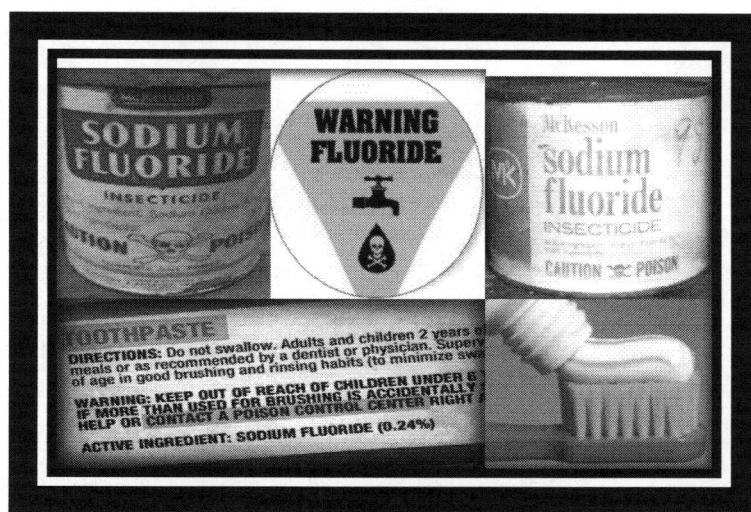

Sodium fluoride is rated more toxic than lead in chemistry indexes, and just a hair less toxic than arsenic. The Merck Manual lists it as a lethal poison. It's also a halogen that inhibits enzyme function and interferes with cellular functioning. There is enough fluoride in a standard tube of toothpaste to kill a 20-pound child. Fluoride is a deadly toxin used in rat poisoning products. It kills rats by destroying their digestive system. Harvard Medical School added fluoride to the list of top developmental neurotoxins in 2014. Many studies show how fluoride lowers the IQ of children.

According to John R. Lee, M.D., there have been eight reliable scientific studies done (and no reliable contrary ones) showing that fluoridation is associated with increased hip fractures. Furthermore, there is a significant association of fluoride and osteosarcoma. Dr. Lee points out that the chance of osteosarcoma for males, 10 to 19 years old, was 6.9 times higher in fluoridated municipalities compared to non-fluoridated areas.

Do Austria, Belgium, Denmark, Egypt, Finland, France, Germany, Greece, Holland, India, Italy, Luxembourg, Norway, Spain, Sweden, and Switzerland know something we Americans don't? What do they all have in common different than the United States? They have researched the fluoride myth and have banned the trash from being put in their drinking water. In western Europe, 98 percent of the population drinks non-fluoridated water. Why? Because there is no scientific research to prove fluoride in drinking water reduces

97% Of Europe Has Banned Water Fluoridation.
Why?
Because It's Toxic!

tooth decay. On the contrary, there is plenty of research to prove fluoride causes many health problems. Fluoride is nearly impossible to remove from the water, except by distillation or reverse osmosis.

In 1977, Dr. John Yiamouyiannis and Dr. Dean Burk (Former head of cytochemistry at the National Cancer Institute) conducted a study on cancer rates in 10 fluoridated American cities and 10 non-fluoridated cities over a 20-year period. Few Americans heard about this study because the results were counterproductive to aluminum manufacturing companies selling their waste products to be dumped in our drinking water. What the study revealed was a 10 percent increased mortality rate from cancer in those living in cities with fluoridated water, whereas there was no increase in cancer rates in the non-fluoridated cities.

When we ingest fluoride at levels as low as 1 ppm in drinking water, it causes chromosomal damage by interfering with the DNA's ability to repair itself. Hey, isn't that what cancer does? In this day and age with one out of every three Americans being diagnosed with cancer, isn't it about time we stay away from chemicals that have shown any possibility of increasing disease and harming our body?

The only difference between the fluoride in rat poison and your fluoridated toothpaste is the parts per million. In fact, it is documented that as little as one-10th of an ounce of fluoride can cause death. You'll notice that on your tube of toothpaste the FDA has a warning label to contact poison control or a physician if you accidentally swallow it.

A can of fluoride sold over the counter comes marked "poison," with skull and crossbones. Use a natural, non-fluoridated toothpaste. There is no way you can brush your teeth with fluoridated toothpaste and not absorb some of it in your mouth's sensitive cells. How much toothpaste do our children accidentally swallow each time they brush? Some kids swallow it on purpose because they are craving minerals, the same reason they eat their boogers, modeling clay, crayons, paint chips off the wall and put coins in their mouths. This is called pica.

> **"Let me state clearly and loudly that fluoridation of the water is the biggest hoax in medical history perpetrated on innocent people in the name of science."** Paavo Airola, Ph.D., N.D.

Fluoride Is More Toxic Than Lead

Calcium fluoride is what helps strengthen teeth, not sodium fluoride. We have been bamboozled into believing that by disposing of this pollutant into our drinking water, we can help prevent cavities in teeth. It is completely absurd to think that putting sodium fluoride in our drinking water is no different than using calcium fluoride because they're both fluoride. Dr. Richard Anderson explains, *"It would be like saying that the air we breathe is a gas (which it is), so therefore breathing Mustard Gas must be good also. Mustard Gas is good for killing just like sodium fluoride is good for killing."*

In 1938, Gerald H. Cox, a biochemist for the Mellon Institute (The Mellons were owners of ALCOA), presented the plan for adding fluoride to our drinking water. A big-shot attorney, Oscar Ewing, supported Cox's plan. Clever reports surfaced to convince government officials to put this toxic waste in our drinking water, while other reports that proved fluoride to actually increase tooth decay were buried.

> **"The great mass of people will more easily fall victim to a big lie than a small one."** Adolf Hitler - Mein Kampf (1925)

The fact is that there were no animal studies, nor any double-blind, controlled studies done to prove fluoride safe. They just went ahead and subjected 40,000 humans to the left-over trash from aluminum. Before they began the studies, there were no thorough dental examinations, no X-rays performed, on the people in the experimental area. How were they expecting to find out if fluoridation was harmful, safe or effective? Why would we accept fluoride being put in our drinking water, without proof that it was safe and effective?

The Grand Rapids-Muskegon, Michigan, study is supposedly the one study that proved fluoride acceptable to be put in our drinking water. Muskegon was considered the non-fluoridated control city. This was to be a 10-year study. However, five years into the study, things weren't turning out how the fluoride pushers had hoped. Tooth decay in non-fluoridated Muskegon was decreasing at the same rate as the fluoridated Grand Rapids. So, what was their solution? They just decided to drop Muskegon from the study. What kind of scientific study can just drop their control group in the middle of a 10-year study, and then later come out with their conclusive report that tooth decay dropped in Grand Rapids after putting fluoride in the drinking water? From this and other phony reports like it, most of the U.S. now drinks fluoridated water.

> **"For cartilage to repair, the system must be fluoride free. Fluoride in all forms, including toothpastes, should be avoided by everyone."** John R. Lee, M.D.

Another flaw in the fluoride hoax is that fluoride can't actually penetrate teeth because they both carry a negative charge. No study has ever been able to prove that fluoride prevents cavities. The U.S. public health service shows no difference in tooth decay statistics between fluoridated areas and low fluoridated areas.

The World Health Organization conveniently voted on fluoridation when only 60 out of 1,000 delegates were present. It just so happened that it was a day when those 60 who were present were the ones who favored fluoridation. Do you think it was a coincidence?

In 1990, the National Cancer Institute publicly announced that fluoride was carcinogenic. Scientists at Seibersdorf Research Center in Austria have concluded that as little as 1 ppm of fluoride slows down the activity of the immune system. To hammer another nail in the fluoride coffin, U.S. geneticists have demonstrated that the degree of chromosomal damage increases proportionally in direct relationship to the amount of fluoride in the water. In fact, at the Nippon Dental College in Japan, studies show that putting the same amount of fluoride commonly found in U.S. water supplies into drinking water causes normal cells to mutate into cancer cells. In 1982, researchers at the Japanese Association of Cancer Research in Osaka reported, *"Last year at this meeting, we showed that sodium fluoride, which is being used for the prevention of dental caries (cavities), induces chromosomal aberrations in the irregular synthesis of DNA. This year, we report findings that show malignant transformation of cells is induced by sodium fluoride."*

Statistics prove that in every city where fluoride is used in the drinking water, disease increases, tooth decay increases, births of mongoloid children increase and crime rates are higher. Of course, these reports are never mentioned in the media because we get "fake news."

Fluoride speeds up the aging process by inhibiting enzyme production. Dr. J.A. Albright and colleagues from Yale University report that as little as 1 ppm of fluoride decreases bone strength and elasticity, which leads to osteoporosis. It breaks down collagen, which weakens tendons, bones, cartilage, connective tissue, teeth and skin. Dr. Wolfgang Klein teaches that the smallest amount of fluoride inhibits the essential DNA repair enzyme by 50 percent, causing chromosomal damage. It causes genetic damage to the immune system and can trigger autoimmune disorders. Research demonstrates that white blood cells' ability to fight infection is hindered in the presence of fluoride. Fluoride also displaces iodine, which is needed for proper thyroid function.

Research has also linked fluoride in drinking water with early puberty. We are seeing girls at the age of 7 reach puberty now! Fluoride accumulates in the pineal gland, which secretes melatonin. Melatonin is believed by many doctors to control the onset of puberty.

The pesticide cryolite contains fluoride. It is used abundantly on grapes and potatoes. California wines can contain very high amounts of fluoride, due to pesticide application on grapes. I have had patients tell me they get headaches after drinking a glass of wine. Is it the wine, pesticides or high fluoride content? Take your pick.

You may be shocked to know that many prescription drugs contain fluoride: Levaquin, Lipitor, Diflucan, Prevacid, Celebrex, Flonase, Decadron and Avodart. It's not just in drugs, it's also found in baby foods and baby formulas, table salt and dry cereals.

> "In point of fact, fluoride causes more human cancer death and causes it faster than any other chemical." Dr. Dean Burk, Chief Chemist Emeritus of the National Cancer Institute

Dr. Phyllis Mullenix, a leader in the field of neurotoxicology, investigated fluoride in drinking water. When she published her findings that fluoride causes cognitive deficits, retarded behavior and lowering of IQs in 1994 in the Journal of Neurotoxicology and Teratology, she was fired. Another expert, Dr. William Marcus, senior toxicologist in the Office of Drinking Water at the EPA, reported how toxic fluoride is and how it's responsible for causing cancer, birth defects and osteoporosis in areas where fluoride is added to the drinking water. He too was fired. Another coincidence?

Children who have had excessive exposure to fluoride will many times have mottling (white spots) teeth. Some will try to blame it on having fevers when they were younger, but the chalky white or brown areas on teeth are the result of fluorosis, which is the first sign of weak teeth, caused from fluoride.

Fluoride can be a major problem for people with insomnia due to its calcifying effect on the pineal gland, which secretes melatonin for sleep. Researchers studying cadavers show how fluoride deposits in the pineal gland and, as we age, it leads to calcification, which has been associated with Alzheimer's, Parkinson's, schizophrenia, hormone imbalances, strokes and bipolar disorders.

> "Fluoride makes your body absorb extra aluminum, and where does the aluminum go? Your brain. And what metal shows up alarmingly in the brains of Alzheimer's victims? You guessed it." William Douglass, M.D.

It's time to demand that we quit poisoning our water. Start drinking purified water that does not contain chlorine and fluoride. If you'd like to learn more about getting involved to remove fluoride from American water supplies, join the Fluoride Action Network at FLUROIDEALERT.ORG.

Antidepressant Drugs Cause Abnormal Behavior

> "In my talks, I show how the molecules of emotion run every system in our body, and how this communication system is, in effect, a demonstration of the bodymind's intelligence, an intelligence wise enough to seek wellness, and one that can potentially keep us healthy and disease-free without the modern, high-tech, medical intervention we now rely on." Candace B. Pert, Ph.D.

Doctors prescribe Prozac even with the FDA warnings of 575 side effects. As of October 1993, there were 28,623 complaints of adverse side effects filed with the FDA, including 1,885 suicide attempts and 1,349 deaths.

Many of the violent acts committed in our society and schools are committed by those who are on antidepressant or psychiatric drugs. These mood-altering drugs may cause bizarre behavior. We were meant to feel emotions. Hormones are released in tears. When we take a drug, it dulls our God-given senses, and suppresses our natural feelings, putting us in zombie-mode. Suppressing these emotions and tears produces toxic grief hormones.

> "In my mind, both kinds of user — the one who gets the drugs from a doctor and the one who buys them from a dealer — are doing the same thing: altering their chemistry with an exogenous substance that has widespread effects, many of which are not fully understood, in order to change feelings they don't want to have." Candace B. Pert, Ph.D.

Dr. Joseph Glenmullen, a Harvard psychiatrist and author of *The Antidepressant Solution,* explains that the reason Prozac causes behavioral disturbances is because it is similar to cocaine in its effects on serotonin. Since the 1950s, it has been known that serotonin is a stress neuro-hormone. It is so disruptive, it can cause docile animals like rabbits to become aggressive in laboratory experiments. Ann Blake Tracy, Ph.D., explains how serotonin drugs such as Prozac, Zoloft, Paxil and Effexor are extremely dangerous. And then we wonder why kids bring guns to schools, and go on killing sprees, after their doctor prescribes a mood-altering drug to interfere with serotonin levels similar to cocaine.

> "The modern medical system, officially known as allopathic medicine, is the most dangerous system in terms of the survival of the human race. In number of casualties (total U.S. casualties during all four years of WW 11 equal 234,874, as compared to 392,556 medical casualties in 1996 alone), it has outranked war by many times. Yet, the vast majority of people in the Western World adhere to it like glue, support it like it was their friend, trust in it like it was God, and like cattle walking to the slaughterhouse, become weaker, maimed and often, dead long before their time." Richard Anderson, N.M.D.

Headaches

Causes Of Headaches
- Dehydration
- Constipation
- Liver/Gallbladder toxicity
- Subluxations/pinched nerve
- Stress/tight muscles
- Poor circulation/oxygen
- Hormonal imbalance
- Metals/chemicals/pesticides
- Magnesium/minerals low
- Food allergies (gluten, dairy)
- Blood sugar imbalances
- Poor digestion, low enzymes

What causes headaches? If a person isn't having regular bowel movements (two to three per day), then backed-up fecal matter is reabsorbed into the portal vein that wraps around the intestines. This toxic waste travels up to the liver. If your liver and gallbladder are toxic and fail to process the waste materials out of the blood fast enough, then these toxins can travel to the brain and inflame blood vessels and capillaries, causing pressure and inflammation — and then you have a throbbing headache. What do most Americans do? They take an aspirin or pain medication. Is your headache caused by a deficiency of aspirin? Of course not. Headaches aren't caused from a lack of aspirin.

The dangerous part of taking aspirin is that we have done nothing to fix the cause of the problem. It is equivalent to you driving your car home and suddenly, the red engine oil light comes on the dash. Only a fool wouldn't stop their car and put oil in it to avoid burning up the engine. God created your body with red engine oil light warning signs, called pain. The wise person heeds the warning signs and fixes the problem. Taking acetaminophen for reoccurring headaches is equivalent to sticking duct tape over the engine oil light.

> "My general philosophy is the fewer drugs people take, the better off they are."
> Jere Edwin Goyan, San Francisco Pharmacist, Former head of FDA

High doses of popular painkiller produce abnormal liver tests

BY CARLA K. JOHNSON
Associated Press

CHICAGO — Healthy adults taking maximum doses of Tylenol for two weeks had abnormal liver test results in a small study, researchers found, raising concerns that even recommended amounts of the popular painkiller might lead to liver damage.

In the study, 106 participants took four grams of Tylenol — equivalent to eight extra-strength Tylenol tablets — each day for two weeks. Some took Tylenol alone and some took it with an opioid painkiller. Dummy pills were given to 39 others.

There were no alarming liver test results among the people who took the placebos. But nearly 40 percent of people in all the other groups had abnormal test results that would signal liver damage, according to the study that appears in today's Journal of the American Medical Association.

"I would urge the public not to exceed four grams a day. This is a drug that has a rather narrow safety window," said a study co-author, Dr. Neil Kaplowitz of the University of Southern California.

Heavy drinkers should take no more than two grams daily, Kaplowitz said.

Another co-author, Dr. Paul Watkins of the University of North Carolina, said he's less worried than Kaplowitz, noting that acetaminophen, the active ingredient in Tylenol, has been used for 50 years and has a good safety record.

The maker of Tylenol, McNeil Consumer & Specialty Pharmaceuticals, said its own research found much lower rates of abnormal liver results. The company's studies tracked high-dose users over longer periods than did the new study.

"It doesn't lead to liver disease and it usually resolves as patients continue to take acetaminophen," said Dr. Edwin Kuffner, senior director of medical affairs at McNeil.

PLEASE SEE PAINKILLER | A7

Aspirin

Americans consume more than 30 tons of aspirin per day. Since 1852, when the German chemist Charles Frederic Gerhardt formulated it in a lab, aspirin has been no stranger in American households. Many people can't make it through a day without aspirin. Aspirin is dangerous. It alone causes over 3,000 people every year to go to the hospital and die from gastric bleeding. Aspirin poisons more children every year than any other toxic substance.

If you are an aspirin pill-popper, you might want to know that aspirin is a form of salicylic acid, which is also the basis for an anticoagulant used in rat poisons. How does it work to kill rats? The poison causes internal hemorrhaging and the rodent bleeds to death on the inside. When you take it, it causes internal bleeding which eases the pressure off of your capillaries, thus allowing pain to subside. So, you trade your headache in for gastric bleeding. In the process, it also destroys the natural mucous lining in the stomach, which leads to bleeding ulcers, while leaving you depleted of electrolytes.

Acetaminophen causes more than 56,000 emergency room visits each year. Of course, your doctor never tells you that the reason your liver has damage and your kidneys are on the verge of needing dialysis is caused from all the aspirin, painkillers and other drugs he prescribed for you to take for the last 20 years. But don't worry, because once again they have you covered. Dialysis centers are being built all over, to treat your drug-damaged kidneys.

Natural Birth = Healthy Baby

Dr. Lewis Mehl of the University of Wisconsin Infant Development Center researched some 2,000 births. Half of the births took place at home and the other half in the hospital. The study reported that there were 30 birth injuries among the hospital born children and none among those born at home. Fifty-two of the babies born in the hospital required resuscitation, while only 14 of those born at home did. Six hospital babies suffered neurological damage, compared to 1 born at home.

A hospital is where sick people go. Why would a healthy pregnant woman want to go where sick people are gathered to have a healthy baby? Exposing your newborn baby to sick people with staph infections, pneumonia and bronchitis is not what I recommend. Millions of pathogens are circulating through the heating and cooling system's ductwork, blowing in on you and your brand-new baby. Is this what you want on the first day of life?

> **"After working in hospitals for most of my life, I can assure you that they are the dirtiest and most deadly places in town. ... 5 percent of all hospital patients contract new infections that they didn't have when they arrived."** Robert Mendelsohn, M.D.

The first mistake doctors make when a woman is in labor is laying her flat on her back. The woman should be up and walking or in whatever position feels most comfortable to her. Lying flat on her back makes unnecessary work to bring the baby uphill, against the force of gravity. Using gravity to assist the birth, such as squatting, is a very natural and effective way to deliver.

The next mistake is made when the doctor breaks the water. Labor should start on its own, and it will, when the mother's body and the unborn child are ready. When the doctor goes in and breaks the water, Mother Nature is out of control and the doctor is in control. Think about it. The pregnant woman's body was intelligent enough to grow a new life. Do you think it somehow gets confused at the end and suddenly is not smart enough to know when to break the water and let the baby come down the birth canal?

Childbirth should be as natural as possible, to ensure good health and wellness for your baby. Robert A. Bradley, M.D., in his must-read book for pregnant couples, *Husband Coached Childbirth,* explains how most doctors interfere with the natural birthing process that leads to unnecessary pain and suffering. With the help of the husband, Dr. Bradley has delivered over 23,000 babies and concludes that only 3 percent need Cesarean sections, and another 3 percent require medicated births. The remaining 94 percent should deliver fine, with the husband doing most of the work. The doctor is there as a lifeguard, in case further assistance is needed. Dr. Bradley's statistics are astounding when compared to how many women are coaxed into drugging themselves in hospitals and going into surgery for a C-section in order to pull the child out when it convenient for him or her.

Coming through the birth canal is a natural and healthy experience to prime the child's immune system. When a baby is born naturally (vaginal birth) they inherit the microbiome from mother. Toward the end of pregnancy, the mother's body starts colonizing the vaginal tract with massive amounts of Prevotella bacteria. Yes, this is good bacteria! When the child comes through the birth canal, covered in these bacteria, a message is sent for the baby's gut to start manufacturing digestive enzymes, to break down breast milk. Babies who are born by C-section are robbed of this important immune-system jump start in life. Numerous studies show that vaginal births produce healthier children with a lower risk of disease throughout life. This is far more beneficial than an artificial vaccine!

Mothers pass some degree of immunity to their babies through the placenta and breastmilk. Breastfeeding infants borrow immunity from the mother's innate immune system and memory immunity from previous natural infections. Vitamin A and a host of other viral-neutralizing agents such as interferon, cytokines, myoepithelial progenitors and stem cells come from mother's breast milk and are extremely beneficial in measles prevention and other infectious diseases. Colostrum, which is secreted from the mammary glands immediately following delivery, is loaded with antibodies (T lymphocytes) that prime the immune system, fight infections and give protection against disease. (J. Schlesinger et al., "Evidence for Transmission of Lymphocyte Responses to Tuberculin by Breast-Feeding," The Lancet, Sept 1977, pp. 529-532.)

In the U.S., 35 percent of births end up with doctors pulling the child out by C-section. That is saying that one-third of our women are abnormal and are not capable of a natural God-designed vaginal birth. This is ridiculous, especially if you look at Third World countries where the masses can't afford surgery. Strangely, women there seem to deliver babies fine. Money is certainly an incentive, because the doctor makes a whole lot more by performing a C-section, and then of course it is done when convenient for him, so he can schedule you and the baby around his schedule, instead of him being available when you and your child are ready.

A lactating woman's milk from the right breast has a predominate potassium composition, while the left breast has a high sodium composition. The baby may prefer one side to the other based upon which nutrients he or she needs most at that particular time.

A natural form of birth control, according to American Indians, is to eat wild yam roots every day. After eating those for two months, conception will not occur. When Indians wanted to become pregnant, they simply stopped eating wild yam roots.

> **"The safest place for a healthy mother to have her baby is not in a hospital, but at home. ... I tell all healthy women, including my own daughters, that they should refuse to have their babies in the hospital."** Robert Mendelsohn, M.D.

Chapter 8
MASTER OF PUPPETS

How Much Do Your Drugs Actually Cost?

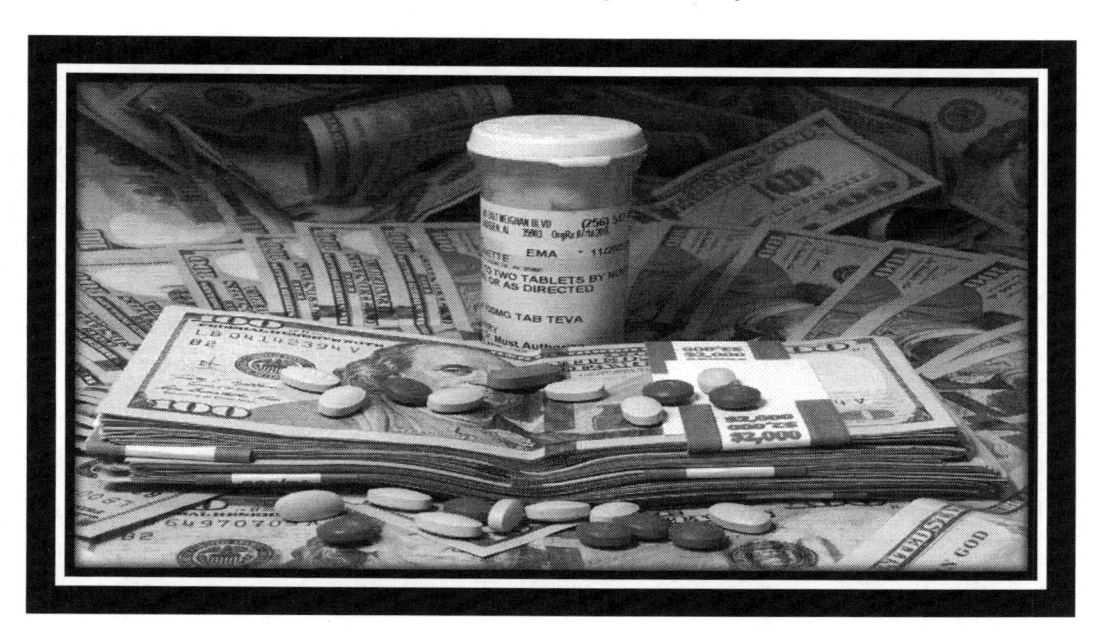

The following drug cost statistics are from Federal Budget Analysts in Washington, D.C. According to Sharon Davis and Mary Palmer of the U.S. Department of Commerce and the Bureau of Economic Analysis:

DRUG	RETAIL COST		ACTUAL COST	% OF MARKUP
Xanax	$136	100 tabs	.24 cents	569,958 %
Celebrex	$130	100 tabs	.60 cents	21,712 %
Claritin	$215	100 tabs	.71 cents	30, 306 %
Keflex	$157	100 tabs	$ 1.88	8,372 %
Lipitor	$272	100 tabs	$ 5.80	4,696 %
Norvasc	$188	100 tabs	.14 cents	134,493 %
Paxil	$220	100 tabs	$ 7.60	2,898 %
Prevacid	$44	100 tabs	$ 1.01	34,136 %
Prilosec	$360	100 tabs	.52 cents	69,417 %
Prozac	$247	100 tabs	.11 cents	224,973 %
Tenormin	$104	100 tabs	.13 cents	80,362 %
Vasotec	$102	100 tabs	.20 cents	51,185 %
Zestril	$89	100 tabs	$ 3.20	2,809 %
Zithromax	$1,482	100 tabs	$ 18.78	7,892 %
Zocor	$350	100 tabs	$ 8.63	4,059 %
Zoloft	$206	100 tabs	$ 1.75	11,821 %

Considering that spending on prescription drugs has tripled from 1990 to 2001 to over $140.6 billion, according to Kaiser Family Foundation, it would be accurate to say that prescription drugs are a profitable business.

Who finances the medical schools in this country? Cynthia Crossen, from the Wall Street Journal, in 1996 published a book called, *Tainted Truth: The Manipulation of Fact in America.* Her book exposes the corruption of lying with statistics. She goes on to reveal that, in 1981, the drug industry gave $292 million to colleges for research to ensure that every medical university around promotes disease maintenance through the use of pharmaceuticals. In 1991, the pharmaceutical industry gave universities $2.1 billion. If a homeopathic or herb company were to give $2 billion to colleges, do you think they would be promoting the benefits of these natural remedies? Like the old German proverb says, *"Who eats my bread dances to my tune."*

The pharmaceutical industry, with its generous financial contributions, has a monopoly on health care in this country. Very little research is done on anything natural, because if they cannot patent something and make millions, they are not interested.

> **"To achieve world government, it is necessary to remove from the minds of men their individualism, loyalty to family traditions, national patriotism and religious dogmas."** Brock Chisolm (Director of the U.N. World Health Organization - SCP Journal 1991)

After reading the above quote, hopefully, every American who cherishes their family traditions, national patriotism and religion will realize that some of our leaders apparently have a different agenda for us.

> **"Researchers are like prostitutes. They work for grant money. If there is no money for the projects they are personally interested in, they go where there is money."** Dr. Sydney Singer

Rockefeller Oil Interests & I.G. Farben

John D. Rockefeller Sr. (1839-1937) was a wealthy businessman who founded Standard Oil of New Jersey and, later, OPEC (Organization of Petroleum Exporting Countries). OPEC functions as a cartel by maximizing profits from crude oil. An elite group of very wealthy businessmen pool their resources for the strict purpose of limiting competition by price-fixing the market. By squashing out all competition, you can create a monopoly and thus set any price you want on your products. So, if you like to complain about high gas prices, you can thank Rockefeller oil interests.

By the 1860s, Rockefeller owned the world's largest refinery and was consolidating most oil refining into one giant corporation. By 1879, he owned 90 percent of America's oil refining capacity, and owned stock in 41 other corporations. So, what does Rockefeller's oil have to do with your health? If you want to unwind the noose and trace it back to its roots to understand why medicine is the way it is, then we find it goes way back to a deal Rockefeller made with a German chemical/drug company, I.G. Farben.

I.G. Farben (Interessen Gemeinschaft) means, "Community of Interests." This German-based company controlled nearly the entire German drug and chemical industries during the 1930s. It gained ownership of the technology for producing synthetic fuels from coal, a process called hydrogenation. In the late 1920s, I.G. Farben became a threat to Rockefeller's oil empire by offering a less expensive synthetic substitute. Rockefeller, a clever, money-driven businessman, came up with a solution.

> **"I used to have a drug problem but now I make enough money."** David Lee Roth (Van Halen)

The Big Drug Deal

If you can't beat them, join them. I.G. Farben met with John Rockefeller and made possibly the biggest drug deal in the world. They shook hands on a deal that would allow Rockefeller to sell oil, but not drugs, and have the hydrogenation patent for use outside of Germany, while I.G. Farben would sell only chemicals. In 1930, these two super-powers established a joint company to develop the oil-chemical field. By 1940, I.G. Farben's operations were in 93 countries and were the world's largest chemical manufacturer. It controlled 380 companies, many of them pharmaceuticals, such as Bayer, Proctor and Gamble, Monsanto, Dow Chemical and Hoffman-LaRoche Laboratories. The Rockefeller/I.G. Farben cartel was well on its way to being in control of most of the world's manufactured chemicals, including drugs, that require coal tar or crude oil as a component in the manufacturing process.

> **"Power tends to corrupt, and absolute power corrupts absolutely."** First Baron Acton

Restructuring Medicine In The USA

In 1900, there were more than 15,000 homeopathic practitioners here in the U.S., one-sixth of the entire medical profession! We also had 22 homeopathic medical colleges training doctors. By 1923, only two homeopathic schools remained, and by 1950, all schools teaching homeopathy were closed. By 1940, over 1,500 chiropractors were prosecuted for practicing "quackery." What happened to our health care?

At the turn of the century, the AMA had established a council on medical education in the U.S. The objective was to reform U.S. medical schools. In 1910, Abraham Flexner, a layman, produced "The Flexner Report," while being employed by Andrew Carnegie, John D. Rockefeller and Simon Flexner. He was paid to produce a report that would discredit homeopathy, naturopathy and other natural healing modalities so that the drug/oil cartels could control the future medical market.

Our medical schools here in the U.S. were restructured by a nonphysician, Abraham Flexner, while being financed by Rockefeller oil interests. They began re-forming medical schools, and for obvious reasons would not license hundreds of schools teaching natural healing methods. Fourteen of America's homeopathic colleges suddenly didn't meet "criteria." So, after our homeopathic/naturopathic colleges were denied licensing, the only medical schools left were those schools that favored drug-oriented medicine. Do you think this was coincidence?

> **"No one should approach the temple of science with the soul of a money changer."** Dr. Thomas Browne, English Physician

Over 100 years later, many people are enslaved into America's disease maintenance system by being hooked on prescription drugs. We pump $3-per-gallon gas in our cars, and many can't even afford the co-pay on their prescription drugs. Whether you believe it or not, you are a slave to the drug and oil business unless you don't use drugs and don't drive a vehicle. Maybe the Amish have it figured out?

In 1987, the American College of Surgeons, the American College of Radiology and the American Medical Association were convicted of conspiracy to prevent chiropractors from practicing in the U.S. Judge Susan Getzendanner described the conspiracy as "systematic, long-term wrongdoing and the long-term intent to destroy a licensed profession."

> **"The reality, therefore, is that government becomes the tool of the very forces that, supposedly, it is regulating."** G. Edward Griffin, Medical Historian

Why Don't Insurance Cover Natural Health Care?

To understand why insurance does not cover holistic health care, we need to look at the cause. By 1974, Rockefeller owned a large portion of stock in the largest and third-largest insurance companies in the U.S. In the years following, the Rockefeller monopoly muscled its way around, buying many more insurance agencies. Owning and controlling drugs, oil and insurance companies could ensure residual income and cinch the knot for eliminating competition.

> **"The FDA and the drug companies are doing everything they can to prevent you from learning about these safer, gentler (yes, and much cheaper) ways to heal and help yourself."** Earl L. Mindell, Ph.D. – Author of the Vitamin Bible

For financial business purposes, naturopathy and homeopathy were ridiculed and unfairly represented in clinical trials, and still are to this day. You don't have to have a Ph.D. to figure out why. Creating a health-care system that would only allow a licensed medical doctor (no homeopaths or naturopaths in most states) to treat disease using the I.G. Farben/Rockefeller expensive, addictive, patented drugs would allow them to control the health-care market. Of course, only allowing insurance to cover prescription drug costs would also ensure a lucrative financial payoff.

> **"In the specialized field of drugs and pharmaceuticals, the Rockefeller influence is substantial, if not dominant."** Edward Griffin

Dr. Ralph Moss was fired from Memorial Sloan-Kettering in the 1970s for refusing to play ball with these pharmaceutical boys. Laetrile (Vitamin B17), which comes from apricot or fruit pits, was then and still is effective for healing cancer. When he refused to cover up the research proving it to be an effective treatment for cancer, he found himself without a job. Since so many of our insurance and government agencies are intertwined and controlled through this cartel, they hold tight reins on the market. Cancer treatment in this country is organized around a medical monopoly that ensures a continuous flow of money to the pharmaceutical companies, medical technology firms, research institutes, and government agencies such as the FDA and the NCI, and quasi-public organizations such as the American Cancer Society (ACS). This is "the cancer industry," exhorts Ralph Moss, Ph.D.

> **"… For the truth is that the medical industry is far less than optimal. It is basically controlled by those who support the drug companies. The drug companies are owned by those who control the banking industries. They manipulate nations and war. Enough said. If anyone does not believe me, I say: Seek truth with an open mind and you will find all the proof of that which I have said. We all need to know the truth, and the sooner, the better, if we want to save the freedom and health we still have."** Richard Anderson, N.M.D.

The FDA — A Pawn In The Game

Is it coincidence that about half of our high-ranking FDA officials have previously been employed by major pharmaceutical companies immediately before coming on board with the FDA? Studies show that another half of those employees take executive jobs in pharmaceutical companies when they leave the FDA. An article in USA Today in September 2000 showed that 54 percent of the experts on advisory committees had a direct financial interest in the drug or topic they were asked to evaluate.

> "The FDA is supposed to regulate the pharmaceutical industry, but instead they are teaming up to work on an antifraud campaign against an industry that some could construe to be an economic competitor." Mark Blumenthal, Executive Director, American Botanical Council

In 1974, FDA scientists testified before Congress that the FDA is nothing more than a pawn for the pharmaceutical company. Of course, things of this nature never receive much media attention. However, it is interesting to note that during that same investigation, Congress identified 150 FDA employees who owned stock in 27 of the companies they were supposed to regulate.

Money Handlers

> "Some even believe we are part of a secret cabal working against the best interests of the United States, characterizing my family and me as 'internationalists' and of conspiring with others around the world to build a more integrated global political and economic structure — one world, if you will. If that is the charge, I stand guilty, and I am proud of it." David Rockefeller

The Rothschilds, who are worth more than $500 trillion, own nearly every central bank in the world, and they have seven business partners who control our currency in this country. Most Americans think we live in a free country, but when you understand that both sides of every war since Napoleon have been financed by these international bankers, for hundreds of years, you come to realize how powerful their monopoly is. Presidents and leaders of countries are merely puppets whose strings are pulled to keep them dancing to their tune. When a president like Abraham Lincoln refuses to borrow money at an astronomical interest rate from these bankers to finance the Civil War, they have him assassinated. Years later, president John F. Kennedy started talking about how he was going to do away with the Federal Reserve and take back our country. Unfortunately, once again, the elitists eliminated him, end of story. To cover their tracks they had Jack Ruby (who was in bad health and knew he would soon die) murder Lee Harvey Oswald, the original assassin suspect. If you don't want a murder trial with an investigation, you destroy the suspect and evidence, and that is what they did, to avoid the truth behind John F. Kennedy's assassination.

> "Permit me to control the currency of a nation and I care not who makes its laws!" Baron de Rothschild - Rothschild Banks of London and Berlin

International Bankers – Owners Of The Federal Reserve
1. Rothschild – Banks of London and Berlin
2. Lazares Brothers – Bank of Paris
3. Israel Moses – Sieff Banks of Italy
4. Warburg – Bank of Hamburg, Germany and Amsterdam
5. Lehman Brothers – Bank of New York
6. Kuhn, Loeb and Co. of Germany and New York
7. Chase Manhattan (Rockefeller) – Bank of New York
8. Goldman Sachs – Bank of New York

The following is a list of very wealthy people who have enough money and power to "care not who makes the laws."

These eight international bankers are the owners of the phony Federal Reserve System set up by Paul Warburg of Kuhn, Loeb and Co., who used President Woodrow Wilson as a puppet to sign this corporation into existence in 1913. The privately-owned Federal Reserve is no more federal than Federal Express.

> "Because the Federal Reserve Bank of New York sets interest rates and controls the daily supply and price of currency throughout America, the owners of that bank are the real directors of the entire system. These shareholders have controlled our political and economic destinies since 1913."
> Eustace Mullins, *Secrets of the Federal Reserve*

If I started the Bank of Sainsbury today, bought my own printing press and began to print money without it being backed by gold and silver, then loaned the money out to millions of people at a high interest rate, it wouldn't take long before I became very wealthy. This is what the Federal Reserve has been doing since 1913. They make a fortune off the interest paid from phony currency that is not backed by gold or silver, and we Americans are slaves to this debt. It is such a debt that we can't even pay the interest!

> "If the people understood the rank injustice of our money and banking system, there would be a revolution before morning!" Andrew Jackson, 7th U.S. President (1767-1845)

The hard-working American middle class has been paying for it dearly ever since, as we struggle to make ends meet. Many families have both spouses working to make a living, while we pay high taxes. The IRS is their collection agency.

> **"Whoever controls the volume of money in any country is absolute master of all industry and commerce."** President James Garfield

Medical Ghost Writing

According to Erica Johnson of CBC News, medical ghostwriting is the practice of hiring Ph.D.s to come up with clever drug reports, purposely leaving out negative side effects, for drug companies to get their poisons on the market. Next, they recruit doctors to put their names on the reports as the authors. Once they have dishonestly manufactured their golden goose, they submit it to be published in prestigious medical journals, such as the Lancet or the British Medical Journal. It is reported that these devious ghostwriters can receive up to $20,000 for every falsified report they publish.

> **"It appears that money can't buy you love but it can buy you any 'scientific' result you want."** Carolyn Dean, M.D., N.D.

More and more of these frauds are being exposed in our disease maintenance system. It is appalling that the New England Journal of Medicine has admitted that deceitful ghostwriters have written 50 percent of the drug reviews in its journal! Dr. Jeffrey Drazen, the New England Journal's editor, explains that pharmaceutical money muscles its way in and around everything to the point that he simply can't find experts to write for him that do not have pharmaceutical connections. So, what does this mean? There's a good chance your doctor is reading falsified drug reports that leave out negative side effects while making the drug look better than it actually is.

> **"The relationship between medical journals and the drug industry is somewhere between symbiotic and parasitic."** Richard Horton, Editor of the Lancet

Dr. M. Michael Wolfe, a medical expert, received an unpublished drug review on Celebrex from the editors of JAMA. He read it and was impressed because it appeared to be superior to two other arthritis drugs, not causing as many ulcers. Dr. Wolfe and colleagues promoted the product by submitting a highly favorable editorial of their own to accompany the newly released findings in JAMA. Consequently, doctors began prescribing Celebrex to millions of arthritis sufferers.

Over time, most drugs show their true face, riddled with harmful side effects. Celebrex was no exception. Dr. Wolfe continued to investigate why Celebrex was not as the report had endorsed it to be. As more and more data were located on Celebrex, he quickly came to realize the initial report he had received was a product of ghostwriting. Numerous discrepancies were found between the first report and his newly found data, such as reports of ulcers developing six months later. This was deliberately left out of the first report. Further investigation found that Celebrex was no better than the other two drugs, but once again, the drug companies deceived medical experts, medical journals, doctors and the patients taking the drug.

> **"We are being hoodwinked by the drug companies. The articles come in with doctors' names on them and we often find some of them have little or no idea about what they have written."** Editor of the British Journal of Medicine

Digging a little deeper into the rat's nest, Dr. Wolfe came across some more interesting dot-connecting information. He found that the initial report he was given included 16 authors who were faculty members of eight medical schools, and every single author was either an employee of Pharmacia (Manufacturer of Celebrex) or a paid consultant of the company. As a matter of fact, between 1990 and 1997, nearly all clinical trials performed on non-steroidal anti-inflammatory drugs (NSAIDS) such as Vioxx, aspirin, Motrin, Aleve, Bextra, etc., were sponsored by pharmaceutical companies, who buy and pay for whatever they want.

> **"Scientists should always state the opinions upon which their facts are based."** Author unknown

Paying To Squash Competition

Mark Fisherman, in his book, *Manufacturing the News*, explains that under the current system of journalistic reporting, a favorable support will always be given to the status quo, regardless of what the true facts might. Money can buy almost any report to show virtually anything you want. One example of this appeared in a national newspaper with a study entitled, "Saint John's Wort Not Effective for Treating Depression." This deceiving article failed to report that the study was done on both Prozac and St. John's wort, but the article led you to believe that it was only about St. John's wort. The results, after giving depressed patients Prozac and St. John's wort, revealed that neither the drug nor the herb had any effect on the patients. Of course, the headline news was claiming St. John's wort to be ineffective for treating depression, while conveniently leaving out mentioning that Prozac failed to show any improvement either.

> **"The deception going on in the media is appalling."** Bill O'Reilly

The article also failed to mention that there are lots of other scientific studies that have proven St. John's wort to be extremely effective for depression. The media will twist and distort reports so you hear what they want you to hear. So next time you are reading or watching the news, it may be just a little biased. So much of history, especially World War II, has been lied about. Remember, there are always two sides to every story, and those who win the war write the history books. The international bankers have written the history they want you to believe. Our younger generation is beginning to forget what our forefathers fought for. Capitalism is what gives people incentive to work hard and be rewarded for their efforts. It's what made this country great. Socialism rewards you for being lazy. Our younger generation is beginning to embrace socialism because that is the ideology being taught. Remember the words of the Russian communist Vladimir Lenin, *"The goal of socialism is communism."* He also said, *"Atheism is a natural and inseparable part of Marxism, of the theory and practice of scientific socialism. Our program necessarily includes the propaganda of atheism."*

> **"Accuse your enemy of what you are doing, as you are doing it to create confusion."** Karl Marx, Author of The Communist Manifesto 1818-1883

Miasms

A miasm is a genetically inherited energetic change (glitch) in the DNA that causes you to become more susceptible to disease. Dr. Samuel Hahnemann introduced his theory of miasms and chronic disease in 1816. He taught that these miasms made dents or breeches in the physical and mental health of a person in which the debilitated life force could not repair. Many of us have miasms, inherited weaknesses from our ancestors. The three most common miasms are tuberculosis, gonorrhea and syphilis. These diseases leave an energetic glitch or dent in the DNA that is passed down from generation to generation, thus leaving you susceptible to certain diseases. Most doctors refer to this as genetics. Hahnemann called them miasms. The three most common miasms are:

Miasms
1. Psora
2. Sycosis
3. Syphilis

The **PSORA (PSORINUM) MIASM** – Tuberculosis (Tuberculinum). It is degenerative in nature and is the oldest, most universal, least-known chronic miasm.
- Affects the upper respiratory system, lungs and skin.

- Chronic cough – asthma, bronchitis, pneumonia, emphysema
- Breathing complications
- Skin rashes – psoriasis, eczema, dermatitis
    - ❖ *Remedy – homeopathic Psorinum formula*

The **SYCOSIS MIASM** – Gonorrhea (gonococcinum, medorrhinum). This miasm is destructive in nature and very common.
- Causes excessive growth and hyperactivity in certain organs, glands and systems.
- Warts, moles, cysts, skin tags and tumors
- Hyperactivity
- Diabetes
- Hypertension
- Cancer (Tumors)
    - ❖ *Remedy – homeopathic Sycosis formula*

The **SYPHILIS (SYPHILINUM) MIASM** – (Syphilis, luesinum) A destructive and degenerate miasm that deteriorates the body and mind.
- Affects mostly the nervous system.
- Tics
- Seizures
- Multiple sclerosis
- Muscular dystrophy
- Alzheimer's
- Psychological disorders
    - ❖ *Remedy – homeopathic Syphilinum formula*

"Modern medicine is not scientific, it is full of prejudice, illogic and susceptible to advertising. Doctors are not taught to reason, they are programmed to believe in whatever their medical schools teach them and the leading doctors tell them. Over the past 20 years, the drug companies, with their enormous wealth, have taken medicine over and now control its research, what is taught and the information released to the public." Abram Hoffer, Ph.D., M.D.

Chapter 9

HEALTH SECRETS YOUR DOCTOR NEVER TOLD YOU

> "Orthodox medicine has not found a cure for your condition. Luckily for you, I happen to be a quack." Author unknown

ACNE
- Many skin issues are caused from an overgrowth of candida yeast. Do a candida yeast cleanse (see candida protocol).
- Most acne is caused from toxins built up in the liver, spleen, kidneys and intestinal tract. Get the bowels moving two to three times a day. Cascara sagrada, senna, aloe vera and psyllium are good for the bowels.
- Rebuilding the microbiome with probiotics is important.
- Colostrum and fish oil are good.
- Many times with acne we find the lymphatic system to be sluggish. Dandelion, nettles, burdock and red clover are good lymphatic, liver and spleen cleansers.
- Blood sugar spikes may cause acne. Avoid carbs such as breads, cereals, potatoes & sweet fruits. Eat a gluten-free no-grain diet. Avoid, wheat, rye, corn, rice & oats.
- Eat vegetables & healthy fats: avocados, eggs, olives, nuts, seeds, butter & coconut oil.
- Hormonal issues can also be a factor. Evening primrose oil can help.
- Acne in teenagers can sometimes be a potassium and zinc deficiency.
- Niacin and Vitamin A can be beneficial.
- Holy basil may help.
- Essential fatty acid deficiency can trigger acne. Flaxseed oil, borage oil or black currant oil are good.
- Eliminate trans fats (partially hydrogenated oils) such as margarine, shortening, French fries, microwave popcorn, breakfast pastries & most packaged foods such as crackers and cookies.
- Mix 4 drops of tea tree oil with 1 tsp. of raw honey (Manuka is good). Rub on skin for 2 minutes and rinse off.
- Vitamin D (20,000 I.U.) daily can help.
- *I recommend KLS-Enviro Plus, Trifolo Plus, Alpha E Spleen, Omega Complete & Diadren Forte*

ADD/ADHD
- Get off junk food (sugar, flour and chemicals). Many children have gluten and dairy allergies, and what does the average child eat for breakfast? Cold cereal, processed grains in a bowl of milk that spikes the blood sugar sky high. Cold

cereals are one of the worst foods you can eat. Most ADD kids are sensitive to sugar. Avoid breads, cereals and milk. Don't skip breakfast. Start the day off with a healthy breakfast shake or eggs, omelet with vegetables and healthy fats to stabilize blood sugar levels and feed the brain throughout the morning. Healthy fats are eggs, avocados, butter, coconut oil, olives, nuts and seeds. You can't hype a child up on sugar-laced gluten cereals and other junk foods and expect them to sit still and concentrate all morning long in school. Feed them a nongrain breakfast. A smoothie breakfast shake is good.

Breakfast Shake Recipe
½ cup blueberries
½ banana
1 tbsp. raw almond butter
1 tbsp. pumpkin seeds
1 tbsp. chia seeds
1 tbsp. hemp seeds
2 raw walnuts
2 raw Brazil nuts
¼ avocado
1 egg (optional)
½ tbsp. coconut butter
1 cup unsweetened almond or coconut milk
1 scoop SEC Greens (optional)
Mix in blender until smooth
*Adding stevia will sweeten drink

- Eating a bowl of vegetable/beef stew for breakfast is a great way to start the day with a healthy, low-glycemic, high-fat, high-protein meal to help sit still, concentrate and learn.
- Many kids don't have ADD. They are being poisoned by consuming a diabetic, brain-destroying diet high in sugars and grains. Change their diet and watch the improvements with their moods and ability to study, focus and learn. Research done on prisoners fed junk foods (high in grains & sugar) vs. healthy foods shows huge behavioral differences for those on healthy diets. Gluten and sugar are poisons. They cause brain deterioration.

Most children need 12 hours of sleep each night.

- Run an EDS scan to check for food allergies and heavy metals.
- Supplement the diet with minerals, amino acids, essential fatty acids and B vitamins.
- The adrenal glands may be out of balance. Norepinephrine can be very effective.
- Check for blood sugar issues. Chromium is good.
- Thyroid dysfunction may be a factor. Kelp is important.
- Dopamine is nature's Ritalin.
- Phosphatidyl serine can be very beneficial.

WARNING: ADD/ADHD drugs may cause permanent Tourette's syndrome.

- Probiotics taken on an empty stomach are good.
- ADD kids usually have an inability to break down fats. Supplement their diets with digestive enzymes. The enzyme lipase breaks down fats. Alpha Zyme II or Diadren Forte are good.
- GABA, valerian, kava, passionflower and chamomile help calm and relax.
- Ginkgo is good support for the nerves and brain.
- Fish oil (DHA) and glutathione are beneficial
- Eat 1 tablespoon of coconut oil a day or cook with it. It's brain food.
- Resveratrol, turmeric, alpha lipoic acid, zinc & Vitamin D are good.

- Essential oils vetiver and lavender can help improve focus. Rub it on the temples, behind the ears and on the wrists.
- *I recommend ADD/ADHD, intraMAX, Dopamine, Brain Formula, Clear Mind, Nerve Formula & Diadren Forte*

ADDICTIONS

- Emotions: feelings of self rejection. Feeling a void in the soul. Wanting to avoid feeling.
- Avoid gluten. Eat healthy fats.
- For caffeine withdrawal, start by reducing your caffeine intake by half. Every two days, cut it in half again until you are down to zero. Drink plenty of water to reduce headaches, and take Vitamin C. Some light exercise is important to move toxins through the body.
- Most addicts, according to Dr. Billie Sahley, have a deficiency of GABA, serotonin, glutamine and other neurotransmitters.
- ACC (Acetylcholine chloride) can help with cravings, fatigue and depression and lowers blood pressure.
- Acetaldehyde helps with alcoholism, chemical sensitivities, allergies & yeast.
- The phenolic Salsolinol helps reduce cravings for alcohol, chocolate and certain foods.
- Vitamin D, magnesium, valerian, tyrosine Rhodiola, fish oil, lemon balm, hops, ginseng, periwinkle & St. John's wort are good.
- Alcohol accelerates the excretion of magnesium through the kidneys, causing most alcoholics to have severe magnesium deficiencies.
- Essential oils lemon, bergamot & lavender help to calm the mind and enhance mood.
- *I suggest Neuro Balance, Irie, Endo Glan Plus, Diadren Forte, Herbal & Mineral Complete*

Support To Quit Smoking
- Calcium/Magnesium – 600 mg
- Vitamin C – 1,000 mg
- Chromium – 100 mcg
- Niacin – 50 mg
- Soybean Lecithin
- 5-HTP – 200 mg

CRAVINGS – Open a 500 mg capsule of L-Glutamine and pour the powder under your tongue. You can also do this several times a day to prevent cravings for alcohol and sweets.

AIDS

- Emotions: feeling defenseless & hopeless, nobody cares.
- Eat a gluten-free diet. Support the immune system. Follow the same protocol for cancer.
- Una de Gato (Cat's Claw) and olive leaf are good to help stop viruses from replicating and help balance the immune system.
- *I suggest Immu C, Arco Plus, Allibiotic, Complete Probiotics & Alpha E Spleen*

ALLERGIES

- Emotions: Suppressed weeping. Who are you allergic to? What is irritating you?
- When your immune system reacts to a foreign protein, you have allergies. Allergy classifications include IgE, IgG, IgA, IgM & IgD.
- If you eat something and your lips go numb and you break out in hives 20 minutes to two hours after consumption, this is known as an IgE (Immunoglobulin E) food allergy, which can be identified with the RAST test or skin allergy test.

Allergy Busters
▪ Fermented vegetables
▪ Bone broth
▪ Apple cider vinegar
▪ Hot & spicy foods
▪ Pineapple
▪ Spirulina
▪ Probiotics
▪ Royal Jelly
▪ Raw local honey

- A food sensitivity is a non-IgE reaction, which is a delayed hypersensitivity reaction that may take four hours to four days for symptoms to manifest after consuming the offending food.
- Allergy shots contain aluminum. Aluminum is a neurotoxin. Do you want that in your body? An EDS scan can check for allergies.
- A toxic liver, according to Dr. Royal Lee, causes many allergies. I would add the intestinal tract (leaky gut) as well.
- Do a colon cleanse and get the bowels moving two to three times a day.
- Do a liver cleanse. Milk thistle, dandelion, nettle, red clover and barberry are good liver cleansers.
- An imbalance in the digestive system can be a big factor. Take enzymes.
- The stomach needs potassium and zinc in order to produce hydrochloric acid to break down foods correctly. Undigested fats and proteins get in the bloodstream and cause allergies, acidosis and inflammation. If they settle in the sinuses, you have sinus issues. If they go to the brain, you will have a headache. If they go to the joints or muscles, you will have aches and pains (fibromyalgia).

Common Allergies
▪ Wheat
▪ Dairy
▪ Corn
▪ Peanuts
▪ Soy
▪ Shellfish
▪ Strawberries
▪ Eggs

- When we are acidic, we become highly sensitive to many foods and substances.
- Sodium deficiency can trigger many allergies. Spirulina, alfalfa and celery juice are high in sodium.
- Avoid eating wheat and dairy. Milk and dairy products are mucus-forming. Mucus causes many allergies.
- Most people with allergies have an overgrowth of candida yeast, which increases sensitivities. Do a candida yeast cleanse.

- Mannan and Acetaldehyde help alleviate sensitivities to yeast.
- Have an EDS scan done to determine food or inhalant allergies. A custom phenolic (desensitizer) or homeopathic remedy can be imprinted to desensitize you for specific allergies.

> No human has the enzymes to fully digest proteins of wheat, barley & rye.

- The sycosis miasm can be causing hyperactivity in the organs and glands, thus creating allergies.
- Many times, you crave what you are allergic to. When working with children, I always ask what their favorite food is. Most will say macaroni and cheese or pizza. That is my first clue that they have a gluten and dairy allergy. Many will crave it. We crave what we are allergic to. If you take them off those foods, they will pitch a fit, because it's their crack-like drug, lighting up the gluten receptor sites in the brain like a pinball machine.
- Dark circles around the eyes indicate allergies.
- Bee pollen, royal jelly and spirulina can be beneficial.
- Hista Plus is nature's Benadryl. It dries up drippy sinuses by supporting the liver in producing antihistamines. Myrrh Plus works well with it to clear out any infections.
- Mix 3 drops of frankincense oil with water and drink twice daily.
- Mixing ¼ cup of olive oil with ¼ cup of coconut oil and adding 10 drops of peppermint oil and 10 drops of eucalyptus oil will provide a vapor rub formula.
- *I recommend Alrgy/Sin, Myrrh Plus, Licro Plus, Cat's Claw, Hista Plus & Diadren Forte*

(ALS) LOU GEHRIG's DISEASE

- Emotions: unwillingness to accept self-worth.
- Lyme Disease is usually the culprit. Lyme bacteria causes inflammation in the muscles, joints and nerves.
- Gluten sensitivity is usually a major factor causing inflammation. Eat a gluten-free diet.

> **Overcoming Lyme Disease**
> - Cat's Claw   1 capsule 3 x a day
> - Olive Leaf   1 capsule 3 x a day
> - Ashwagandha 1 capsule 3 x a day
> - Teasel Root   40 drops 3 x day
> - Colloidal Silver   1 tsp 3 x day
> - Protease 2 between meals 3 x a day

- Heavy metals, especially mercury, are usually a culprit. High iron levels and a copper deficiency cause free radical and tissue damage.
- *I suggest the Lyme Protocol, KLS Enviro, Omega Complete, Circu Plus, Gota Plus, Alpha Oxzyme & Soybean Lecithin.*

ALZHEIMER'S DISEASE

- Emotions: Tired of coping, can't face life anymore. Feeling hopeless.

- Also known as Type 3 Diabetes. Avoid sugar and grains. A ketogenic diet is ideal. Paleo or Mediterranean diets are good.

> **Avoid eating GRAIN to boost your BRAIN.**

- Your brain is 60 percent fat, and 25 percent of your body's cholesterol is in the brain. Fats are brain food. Fat-free diets and statin drugs are detrimental to the brain and cause memory loss!
- Feed your brain healthy fats such as avocados, olives, eggs, butter, nuts, seeds & coconut oil. WE NEED HEALTHY FATS FOR HEALTH!

Healthy Fats (Brain Food)
- Coconut oil
- Olive oil
- Avocados
- Eggs
- Olives
- Butter
- Nuts & Seeds

- Black-, blue- & purple-colored fruits and berries such as blueberries & blackberries contain antioxidants, which are excellent for brain health.
- An EDS scan will check for heavy metals. Mercury and aluminum poisoning are notorious memory destroyers. Remove toxic silver dental fillings.

> **"The brain needs cholesterol to thrive."** David Perlmutter, M.D.

- Glutathione, turmeric, garlic, chlorella, cilantro and parsley bind to metals, thus helping the body to detoxify.
- Increase circulation, especially to the brain. Ginkgo biloba, ginseng, capsicum, rosemary, cinnamon and gotu kola are good.
- Exercise is very important to increase blood flow and oxygen to the brain. Get out and walk, swim or ride a bike.
- Studies show that taking Advil and Aleve for two or more years increases your risk of Alzheimer's and Parkinson's disease by 40 percent.
- Intestinal health is crucial for reversing Alzheimer's. Probiotics support a healthy microbiome.
- Phosphatidyl serine and lecithin can be beneficial. Vitamins B-12 & D-3 are good.
- Acetylcholine can help with memory and mental alertness. Acetyl-L-carnitine (ALCAR) is beneficial.
- Unfortunately, drugs such as night-time pain relievers, antihistamines and sleep aids block acetylcholine. Dr. Malaz Boustani tells older adults not to take these anticholinergic drugs because they are notorious for causing cognitive impairment and memory loss.
- Glutathione helps mop up heavy metal poisoning.
- Fish oil is good.
- Serrapeptase may be beneficial.
- Frankincense and bergamot oil are very beneficial.

> **Gluten is a mild to moderate toxin.**

- Vitamin D3 (5,000 – 10,000 IU a day) is a brain hormone and very beneficial.
- CoQ10 is important. Statin drugs paralyze your cells' ability to make it.
- *I suggest chlorella, Circu Plus, Gota Plus, Brain Formula, Clear Mind, Vitamin D, Alpha Oxzyme, Dopamine & Phosphatidyl-Serine*

AMENORRHEA
- Absence of menstrual cycle. Many times, stress is the culprit, causing hormonal imbalances. Mental stress, emotional stress, physical stress and chemicals can all drain your hormones. Many of us worry about things we can't control. This is why there are so many hormonal imbalances. A woman's menstrual cycle has four phases it goes through each month and a normal cycle ranges from 26 to 32 days.
- Women who are obsessed with working out can deplete hormone levels to the point that they stop menstruating. Women should avoid working out the week of their cycle. This is a time to relax and de-stress.
- Blessed thistle is good, as it helps stop bleeding and is good for blood clots too.
- If you get stressed out or experience an emotional upset and skip a cycle or two, that indicates that your adrenals are exhausted. The adrenal glands manufacture sex hormones necessary for a normal cycle. Take Adrena Plus, MG/K Aspartate & Licro Plus.
- Black cohosh, zinc and flaxseed oil are good.
- Progesterone cream can be beneficial.
- *I suggest Her Formula, Female Formula, Female Balance, FHS Formula, Endo Glan F, Ovary Uterus Plus & Evening primrose oil*

ANEMIA
- Women shed 500 ml of iron each year through menstruation.
- Eat more raw vegetables. Eat fruit in moderation. Chives are high in iron. Bananas are good. Juice green vegetables and beets. Kelp, nettles, dandelion, comfrey, yellow dock, parsley, alfalfa and blackstrap molasses are good.

Herbs High In Iron
• Chickweed
• Comfrey root
• Licorice root
• Golden seal
• Peppermint

- Dairy products (milk & cheese) can reduce iron absorption as much as 60 percent. Tannic acid in tea reduces iron absorption as well.
- Iron deficiency can cause you to crave certain nonfood items, such as chewing on paper, called pica.
- A piece of red meat or organ meat like liver is good to consume a few times a week.
- Make sure zinc and copper levels are balanced. A zinc or copper deficiency will cause the body to reject iron. When red blood cells are broken down,

normally the body will store the iron to use later. If you have a copper deficiency, the iron, as well as iron from the diet, cannot be properly utilized by the red blood cells, causing iron to build up in storage areas of the body. Anemia develops, and adding more iron supplements into the body will not correct the problem. Supplementing with copper is required to correct the anemic situation. The excess iron buildup often is deposited at the joints, causing rheumatoid arthritis.

- Vitamin B12 is important, as well as a B complex.
- The stomach has to be acidic to use iron. Iron has a positive charge and so does the lining in your intestinal tract. Like repels like, so iron and other positive-charged minerals may pass through the digestive system without being absorbed if the hydrochloric acid levels are low in the stomach. Acid-blocker medications prevent you from absorbing your nutrients! This is why people who take antacids develop iron deficiency. Get off of them and heal your gut. When the stomach produces sufficient amounts of acid, then this allows iron to bind with a protein. The protein is absorbed and carries the mineral into the later stages of digestion and into the blood. If you have acid reflux or heartburn, take Alpha Gest to help support proper digestion.
- Liquid Iron by Natrol is a good supplement for anemia.
- If the sycosis miasm is affecting the spleen, it can cause iron imbalances.
- If prescription iron causes constipation, you most likely have an overgrowth of candida yeast. If it turns your stool black, you're not absorbing it.
- Probiotics can help.
- Too much iron causes health problem. Alcohol is known to increase iron absorption, which can contribute to cirrhosis of the liver. Dark beers and red wine are high in iron, which may be why so many experience headaches after consumption.
- Sickle Cell Anemia is usually associated with a zinc deficiency, causing excessive calcium to accumulate in the red blood cells, resulting in the cells becoming rigid and deformed.
- *I recommend Liquid Iron, Scrofulara Plus, Alpha E Spleen, Alpha Gest III & intraMAX*

ANGINA

- Calcium & magnesium is required for muscle contraction and relaxation, allowing valves to open and close properly.
- Magnesium is the mineral that nourishes the heart. When we get low in magnesium, we have chest pains. MG/K Aspartate is good.
- Vitamin E has proven to be very valuable.
- L-Carnitine, L-Arginine and coenzyme Q10 can help.
- *I recommend MG/K Aspartate, Cardi Plus, Heart Formula & Hawthorn Plus*

ANXIETY

- Emotions: feeling unable to "call the shots" in life. Bach flower, Rescue Remedy is good.
- Many times, there is a magnesium/potassium deficiency causing the nervous system to be out of balance. MG/K Aspartate is good to help calm and relax.
- Valerian, passion flower, chamomile, ashwagandha and kava are good.
- Serotonin levels may need balancing. Tryptophan is responsible for producing serotonin, which relaxes the brain and nerves.
- Norepinephrine can help, especially with children.
- GABA can help calm and relax.
- B vitamins are important.
- CBD oil can help.

Relaxing Oil Blend
▪ Sweet almond oil 2 oz
▪ Lavender oil 5 drops
▪ Lemon oil 5 drops
▪ Marjoram 1 drop
▪ Sandalwood 1 drop
Massage on neck & head

- The autonomic nervous system has two parts, the sympathetic dominant mode (fight or flight) when we are keyed up, and the parasympathetic dominant mode (rest and digest) when we are relaxed. Phosphorus is needed for the parasympathetic nervous system when we are in "rest and digest," slow gear and sluggish. When we are in sympathetic dominance mode, "fight or flight," keyed up and jittery, stressed out, we burn up our minerals, especially magnesium and potassium.

Hot Epsom Salt Bath
▪ 2 cups Epsom Salt
▪ 1 cup Baking Soda
▪ 20 drops lavender oil
Soak for 20-30 minutes.

- Get on a gluten-free diet, as gluten causes inflammation of the nervous system.
- Eat healthy fats: coconut oil, eggs, butter, olives, nuts and seeds. Your brain and nerves need healthy fats.

Unresolved emotions from the past are the seeds of disease.

- Emotional issues from the past can throw the body out of balance into a chaotic frenzy creating anxiety. Do an emotional release (RFA) to heal the trauma. Many people walk around in their adult bodies with a young child (inner child) re-living a traumatic emotional event from the past, constantly replaying it. If you have been molested or abused or felt unwanted or unloved, there is most likely an emotional wound that still needs to be healed. Talking with a counselor doesn't heal it. We can't change the past, but we can change how we feel about it. Bach Flower remedy, Hibiscus is good for those who have been sexually abused.
- *I recommend Kava Kalm, Valeri Plus, Clear Mind, Irie, GABA, Dopa Mucuna & MG/K Aspartate*

ARTHRITIS

- Emotions: feeling unloved & criticized. Rigid thinking, inflexible. Repressed anger eating eating you up inside. Resentment causes stiff joints, especially in formerly injured areas.
- Rheumatoid arthritis may be triggered by allergies, Lyme disease and heavy metal poisoning. Cat's claw and olive leaf are good to balance the immune system and stop viruses from replicating.
- Chronic bacterial infections (most common is a dental abscess or root canals) can deplete the body of copper, creating an imbalance with iron (infectious anemia). When the extra iron is deposited in the joints, rheumatoid arthritis can occur. If you are anemic (low iron), you may need to supplement with copper. This is why some people who wear copper bracelets, get relief, most likely they are low in copper.
- Word to the wise: Too much copper can cause calcium accumulation around the joints, creating sore, stiff achy joints. Balance is the key.
- If you are one who can predict the weather, you can tell when it's going to rain because your joints start to ache, that is a likely indication that you have an issue with mold or fungus, which thrives in damp environments. The moisture activates mold and fungus spores, and you feel worse. Some individuals feel better after leaving wet, humid areas and moving to warm, dryer climates such as Arizona because of this.
- Most arthritis is caused by an imbalance in the digestive system.
- Your diet needs to be mostly vegetables, healthy fats and fruit in moderation. Test for allergies to make sure you are not allergic to citrus.
- Balance your pH. Your saliva should be around 6.8 to 7.0. Juicing vegetables nourishes the body, flushes acids out and alkalizes the body. Carrot, celery, and red beet juice are very effective for melting stiffness away. Raw potato juice helps arthritis. Alfalfa, comfrey, carrot tops, beet tops, wheatgrass, and any other edible greens are healing foods for inflamed joints. Dr. Oz's green drink can help.

Inflammatory Infections
- Borrelia burgdorferi
- Babesia
- Brucella
- Chlamydia
- Coxiella
- Epstein-Barr virus
- Escherichia coli
- Hepatitis C
- Mycotuberculosis
- Mycoplasma
- Neisseria
- Parvovirus B19
- Staphylococcus Aureus
- Streptococcus

- Some people don't do well with raw vegetable juice. In that case, make lots of slow cooker vegetable meals with a smaller portion of chicken or beef.
- Drinking bone broth is very healing and anti-inflammatory as well as balancing your pH.

- A majority of arthritis is caused from eating too much protein in the form of meat. High-protein diets cause arthritis because they create an acidic condition in the body. The body draws upon sodium, calcium, potassium, magnesium and iron to neutralize or buffer the acids. This leaves the body depleted of minerals, and without sufficient organic plant sodium, crystallization takes place.
- Knots on the fingers, spurs and gout are warning signals by the body to get sodium into the cells. Sodium (from vegetables, not table salt) keeps the joints limber.
- Supplement with enzymes and hydrochloric acid so you properly digest your foods and get nutrition to the cells.
- Most arthritis sufferers have indigestion, so they take acid blockers like Prilosec, Prevacid and Tums. These only make arthritis worse because they shut down the secretion of digestive juices or neutralize them in the stomach so you don't absorb your minerals.
- Do a colon cleanse so that the small intestines can absorb nutrients. BR-SP Plus is good.
- Limit your consumption of meats and avoid dairy products. The more milk you drink, the more calcium deficient you'll become. Pasteurized milk drains the body of alkaline minerals. It takes more calcium to digest it than it gives back. Milk does not do a body good. It does it a lot of harm unless you can get it raw from a farmer. Fermented dairy, like kefir and homemade yogurt, is fine.
- Iodine controls calcium in the body and nourishes the thyroid. Get the thyroid gland balanced. Calcium, magnesium, phosphorus, Vitamin D, manganese, sodium and potassium are important. Take large amounts of alfalfa, comfrey and bee pollen. They are loaded with nutrition.
- Arthritis pain on the left side of the body can be caused from a sodium deficiency. Take spirulina. It is rich in sodium. Juicing celery is very beneficial.
- Arthritis pain on the right side of the body can be caused by a potassium deficiency. Take bee pollen, burdock and alfalfa. They are rich in potassium.
- Cod liver oil is good.
- Lecithin will dissolve calcium deposits in the body.

Dr. Oz's Green Drink
2 cups spinach
2 cups cucumber
1 head of celery
½ inch fresh ginger root
1 bunch parsley
2 apples
Juice of 1 lime
Juice of ½ lemon

Combine all ingredients in a juicer. Makes 30 oz.

Carbonated drinks block calcium absorption in the body.

- Orthophosphoric acid (Alpha Ortho Phos) will help dissolve calcium plaquing in the arteries, kidney stones and bone spurs. It will lower blood viscosity, so it shouldn't be used with blood-thinner medication. It is also good for swelling.
- Dr. Norman Childers healed himself of arthritis by eliminating nightshade vegetables from his diet. They contain an alkaloid that inhibits normal collagen repair in the joints. They can trigger joint pain (especially in blood types A and O).

Nightshade Vegetables
▪ Tomatoes
▪ Potatoes
▪ Eggplant
▪ Peppers
▪ Tobacco

- Candida yeast can cause inflammation in the joints.
- Weak knees, where the muscles give out, are usually caused from exhausted adrenal glands.
- CBD oil (Cannabidiol) is medicinal marijuana without making people feel "high." It is very beneficial for pain and inflammatory conditions.
- Fish & borage oil is good. Turmeric, Vitamin C, Vitamin D, glucosamine and MSM are good. The late Tommie Bass recommended wild cucumber tree bark & prickly ash. He also recommended swallowing three ripe pokeroot berries three times a week.
- A hot Epsom salt (2 cups) bath with 20 drops lavender oil and 20 drops of peppermint oil can help stiff joints. Frankincense and ginger oils help reduce inflammation, and wintergreen is good to rub on topically.
- Vitamin D3 needs K2 to help absorb calcium into the bones.
- *I recommend Alpha Green II, R Plus, Arnica Plus, Liga Plus, Omega Complete, Alpha Flavin, Alpha Gest III & Relieve Joint Pain*

> **"Sodium was named the 'youth' element due to its properties of promoting youthful, limber, flexible, pliable joints."** Dr. Bernard Jensen

ASTHMA

- Emotions: reliving childhood fears. Feeling stifled, suppressed sorrow & breathing.
- Weak adrenal glands will trigger respiratory issues. The adrenals need pantothenic acid, potassium and sodium. Royal jelly is high in pantothenic acid. Alfalfa is rich in potassium and sodium.
- Check for mold and fungus. They are the culprits behind many respiratory issues.
- Licorice root is good for the adrenals.
- Lime juice is good.
- Bee pollen can help. Mullein and ginger are good for the lungs.

- Lobelia is a bronchial dilator. It helps you breathe easier. It also helps relax the body and is antispasmodic.
- Asthma may be allergy induced. Check for food and inhalant allergies.
- Get off wheat and dairy products.
- Mix a drop each of eucalyptus oil, ginger, peppermint and thyme with a little coconut or olive oil and rub on chest. This will help you breathe.
- The Psorinum (tuberculosis) miasm may be a factor. Did any of your ancestors have tuberculosis?
- *I recommend Mullein Plus, Licro Plus, Pneumo Plus, Mold X, Vit D & Adrena Plus*

ATHLETE'S FOOT
- Is a form of ringworm caused by the fungus Tinea pedis. In order to clear fungal (yeast) forms out of the blood stream, we must change the terrain of the body and get it alkaline. Fungus thrives in an acidic atmosphere. Thyme oil, tea tree oil, pau d'arco, garlic, oregano, caprylic acid, grapefruit seed extract, olive leaf extract and colloidal silver are all antifungal.
- Tea tree oil, oregano or lavender oil can be used topically to help kill nail fungus.
- A good probiotic (acidophilus) is important.
- Get off sugar, breads and pasta. Sugar feeds yeast. Even fruit sugar will feed yeast.
- Raw onion juice rubbed between the toes will kill fungus. Apply two to three times daily.
- Make your own 3 percent hydrogen peroxide formula from 35 percent food-grade hydrogen peroxide by adding 1 ounce to 11 ounces of distilled water. Store leftover in refrigerator. Soak your feet in ¼ cup of your 3 percent hydrogen peroxide mixed with warm water in a foot tub.
- *I suggest Lapacho Plus, Arco Plus, Mold X, Alpha Green & Complete Probiotics*

ATRIAL FIBRILLATION
- An irregular, often rapid heart rate that can cause poor blood flow.
- When discs shrink in the back due to degenerative disc disease, they can press on nerves corresponding to the heart. Get a chiropractic adjustment and supplement with minerals.
- Calcium, magnesium, selenium, CoQ10, L-Carnitine, Vitamin D & C, fish oil, turmeric, garlic, ginger and Hawthorn are good.
- *I suggest MG/K Aspartate, Cardi Plus, Heart Formula, Hawthorn Plus, Omega Complete & intraMAX.*

AUTISM

- Detoxify the body of heavy metals, especially mercury. If you do a hair analysis for heavy metals and no metals show up, that is an indication that the individual is a non-secretor of metals. It does not mean they don't have heavy-metal poisoning; it means that the cells are holding on to it and the body can't get rid of it!
- Dr. Boyd Haley explains that autism is not caused from "bad genes." It is the inability to excrete metals, especially mercury, from the body.
- Vaccinations contain mercury (thimerosal) and aluminum, both neurotoxins.
- A gluten-free diet is crucial.
- Almost all autistic children have an overgrowth of candida yeast. Sugar and grains feed yeast. Follow the candida yeast protocol diet.
- Drinking warm bone broth is very antifungal and beneficial. Doing a three-day bone broth fast starves out the yeast and can improve brain function exponentially.
- Supplement the diet with liquid minerals/vitamin supplement. Magnesium and Vitamin B-6 are important.
- Probiotics and fish oil are beneficial.
- Ginkgo, dopamine and malvin may help. The phenolic Taurine can help with environmental toxicities and autism.
- Glutathione is a good antioxidant and mops up heavy metals.
- Dental fillings are another big source of heavy metal poisoning. Dr. Rashid Buttar has successfully treated over 500 children with autism in North Carolina by detoxifying them for heavy metals.
- *I recommend Clear Mind, Brain Formula, Chlorella, Alpha Oxzyme, Circu Plus, Omega Complete, Complete Probiotics, Dopamine & intraMAX*

Heavy Metals
- Arsenic
- Antimony
- Tin
- Nickel
- Mercury
- Aluminum

AUTOIMMUNE DISORDER

> "Epstein-Barr is responsible for an overwhelming number of so-called autoimmune conditions, including CFS; fibromyalgia; eczema and psoriasis; psoriatic arthritis; hepatitis A, B, C and D; MS; RA; and lupus." Anthony William

- Emotions: deep-seated grief, feeling totally helpless.
- The immune system does not make mistakes. It is highly intelligent and does not attack itself, unless there is some type of toxicity issue in the cells, causing the immune system to recognize them as foreign toxic (nonself) cells. So, if you have an autoimmune disease, it's not

Stop Guessing & Start Testing EDS

bad genes or bad luck. There is a toxicity issue causing your immune system to do exactly what it's supposed to do, attack foreign proteins. If mercury,

Possible Toxins Causing Autoimmunity		
Heavy Metals	Mercury	Aluminum
Food Allergies	Gluten	Milk
GMOs	Mold	Parasites
Lyme Disease	Pesticides	Chlorine
Epstein-Barr virus	MSG	Fluoride

Lyme disease or Epstein-Barr virus is in your thyroid gland, the marines of your immune system will identify those toxins and declare war on them. The toxins must be removed in order to restore balance and health. An EDS exam will identify what toxins are causing disturbances, and what homeopathic remedy will be best to detoxify the body.

- 80 percent of the immune system resides in the gut. The microbiome in the gut must be healthy in order to balance your immune system so that it stops attacking your own cells.
- Stop eating poisons causing the body to attack. A gluten-free/grain-free diet is a must. Gluten causes inflammation, which triggers allergies and autoimmune attacks.
- Usually a stressful event occurs to put you in fight-or-flight mode, which exhausts the adrenals, thus triggering an autoimmune disorder. The adrenal glands control the white blood cells.
- Autoimmunity in Ayurvedic medicine is undigested anger. Do some emotional release work to clear out your internal conflict (yes, the one you think you have already healed).
- The ketogenic, Mediterranean or paleo diets are very beneficial.
- Eat healthy fats, vegetables and meat in moderation. Soups and slow cooker vegetables with bone broths are very healing and anti-inflammatory to the gut.

Gut Healing Foods
▪ Bone broth
▪ Kefir (from goat's milk)
▪ Fermented vegetables
▪ Steamed vegetables
▪ Omega 3s (salmon)
▪ Coconut oil

- Probiotics from fermented foods are best. Adding beneficial bacteria into the gut builds up the microbiome which supports almost every system in the body. Take a multi-strain (10 or so) with about 70 billion CFUs per every 2 capsules along with your fermented foods.
- Cat's claw and olive leaf are great for autoimmune issues because they help balance the immune instead of stimulating it.
- Vitamin D3 helps heal intestinal permeability, thus preventing allergies.
- Glutamate (amino acid) is fuel for the epithelium cells & helps to absorb nutrients. It helps boost the immune system. (Do not take if you have yeast infections – may increase yeast growth).

- Fish oil – omega 3 fatty acids turn on and off genes to produce an anti-inflammatory effect. Very beneficial for brain health & the cardiovascular system.
- Zinc Carnosine helps heal the GI tract. It's very beneficial for healing ulcers and reversing damage caused from drugs such as aspirin and other pain medications.
- Colostrum – comes from breast milk, the first three to five days after childbirth. It contains antibodies newborns need for immunity against bacteria, viruses, fungus, mold & parasites. It is excellent for healing the gut & repairing damaged villi.

Gut Healing Support
- Probiotics
- Colostrum
- Vitamin D
- Glutamine
- Fish oil
- Turmeric

- Lyme disease can be a major contributor to autoimmune disorders. Follow the Lyme detox protocol.
- Drink 3 drops of Frankincense oil in a glass of water twice daily.
- *I suggest Omega Complete, Allibiotic, BR-SP Plus, Arco Plus, Immu C & Complete Probiotics*

BACK PAIN

- Emotions: low back = fear of money. Middle back = guilt. Upper back = feeling unloved, no support.
- Chiropractic adjustments can help tremendously if you have subluxations or pinched nerves. The adjustments may not hold if you have nutritional deficiencies. Manganese is disc food. Low back pain and headaches are usually caused from a manganese deficiency. Take 2 capsules of Liga Plus with each meal and many times your chiropractic adjustments will hold.
- Pain between the shoulder blades (a burning sensation) is usually the result of a liver/gallbladder issue. Take 3 capsules of Beta Plus with each meal. A couple of Alpha Gest III with your meals helps you break down your fats, carbs and proteins. Undigested fats and proteins, poor digestion, causes inflammation and pain in the body.
- Middle- to low-back pain can be caused from exhausted adrenal glands, especially if you wake up at nights from 3 to 5 a.m. The adrenals affect the lungs, so coughs and respiratory problems are associated with weak adrenals.
- Massage therapy is effective for relaxing tight muscles that are pulling vertebrae out of alignment.
- Calcium is required for muscle contraction, and magnesium is required for muscle relaxation. Many Americans are depleted of magnesium, thus not being able to relax, feel good and sleep well. Take 2 capsules of MG/K Aspartate with each meal.
- Inflamed and toxic kidneys can trigger back pain.

- Backed-up fecal matter in the colon (constipation) can put a tremendous amount of pressure on nerves, causing back pains and sciatica. Do a colon cleanse with Fiber Life. Make sure your bowels are moving two to three times a day.
- The phenolic Phloridzin can help with back and joint pains and blood sugar issues.
- *I suggest Arnica Plus, R Plus, Liga plus, Alpha Flavin, Alpha Gest III & Relieve Joint Pain*

BELL'S PALSY
- Partial or total weakness or paralysis of the facial nerves cause drooping on one side of the face, impaired speech or other stroke-like symptoms.
- Is believed to be caused by a virus. May be linked to Epstein-Barr, herpes simplex or zoster (shingles), Coxsackie virus or Lyme disease. Cat's claw and olive leaf are anti-viral.
- Calcium and magnesium are important.
- Zinc, Vitamin D3, Vitamin B12 and ginseng are good.
- *I suggest Cal Lac Plus, Omega Complete, Brain Formula, Clear Mind & Arco Plus*

BIPOLAR (MANIC DEPRESSION)
- Emotions: feeling hopeless, it's no use, or "I'll never be enough."
- Eating a gluten-free diet is important. Gut inflammation causes severe mood disorders, since more serotonin is produced in the gut than the brain. If you want healthy plants, treat the roots, not the leaves. If you want a healthy brain, treat the gut, not the brain.
- A ketogenic diet is optimum. Healthy fats are brain food. Coconut oil and avocados are excellent.
- Pygnogenol, Damiana, ginkgo, ginseng, gota kola, ashwagandha & soybean lecithin can help.
- Vitamin D3 & K2 are important. Get out in the sunlight for at least ½ hour every day.
- Diffusing holy basil oil, vetiver and chamomile oils is good. Rub it on your temples or consume 2 drops of each in water twice daily.
- *I suggest Irie, Clear Mind, Brain Formula, Omega Complete, Chola Plus, Pygnogenol, Alpha Oxzyme & intraMAX*

BLOOD CLOTS (DEEP VEIN THROMBOSIS)
- Hot, painful, swollen skin around affected area with difficulty walking may be a sign of a blood clot, especially after inactivity due to an injury. Sitting all day at a desk or riding in a car or on a plane can cause clots to form.
- Exercise is important to keep blood moving. If traveling, stop every couple of hours and walk around to circulate blood in legs. If you work at a desk,

- get up and move every hour. Sitting all day increases your risk for clots to form.
- Compression socks can help.
- Using aspirin to thin your blood is dangerous and may cause kidney and liver failure. Regular aspirin use is notorious for causing stomach ulcers, tinnitus and bleeding in the brain (hemorrhagic stroke).
- Factors that can cause clots are being overweight, too little exercise, birth control pills/hormone changes, pregnancy, high stress, recent infections, surgery, smoking & drug use.
- Vitamin E (natural complex, not synthetic) can help prevent and dissolve blood clots. Sunflower seeds are high in Vitamin E.
- Nutritional deficiencies caused from certain medications like Metformin can trigger clots because they deplete Vitamins B12, B6 & folate.
- Natural anticoagulant foods include papaya, berries, pineapple, garlic, ginger, turmeric, raw honey, apple cider vinegar, green tea, wild caught fish (fish oil), evening primrose oil, nuts, seeds, sunflower seeds, avocados, beans, most fruits & vegetables.
- Serrapeptase may be beneficial.
- Hawthorn is good for busting clots, high blood pressure & strengthening the heart.
- Nattokinase breaks down and dissolves fibrinogen, a component of blood clots, and lowers blood viscosity for improved circulation and lowered blood pressure.
- If you are taking a prescription blood thinner, use caution with the 3-Gs (ginkgo, garlic & ginger), as they thin the blood as well.
- *I suggest Vascutin, Veno Plus, Circu Plus, Heart Formula & Omega Complete*

Natural Aspirin (Blood Thinner) Alternatives
- Gingko biloba
- Ginger
- Garlic
- Cayenne
- Turmeric
- Bromelain
- Cinnamon
- MSM
- Vitamin E
- Nattokinase
- Magnesium
- Evening primrose oil
- Fish oil

BREASTFEEDING DISORDERS
- Alfalfa, dandelion, fennel, red raspberry leaf, nettle, fenugreek, anise and blessed thistle can help produce milk supply.
- Avoid yarrow, sage and black walnut, as they decrease milk production.
- Supplement with vitamins and minerals. It's hard to produce milk if you are deficient in nutrients.
- For low milk supply, mix one drop of fennel, clary sage and basil oils with 1 tsp. of coconut oil and apply it to breasts twice daily.
- *I suggest Alpha E Spleen, Alpha Green, Trifolo & intraMAX*

BRONCHITIS
- Emotions: disharmony in family or home
- Mullein and lobelia are good.
- When we support the adrenal glands, we strengthen the lungs. The adrenal glands secrete anti-inflammatory steroid hormones to help us breathe. Royal jelly and bee pollen are good.
- The Psorinum miasm may be present.
- Mold and fungus can be causing inflammation. Oregano oil is good.
- Get off dairy products and check for other possible allergens.
- *I recommend Mullein Plus, Licro Plus, Mold X, Pneumo Plus & Adrena Plus*

BURNS
- Aloe Vera (99 percent pure) is good.
- Taking Vitamin E, 400 IU daily is good.
- Eat lots of eggs & avocados. The skin needs cholesterol to heal.
- Mix 25 drops of lavender oil with 2 Tbsp. of olive oil and 2 Tbsp. of raw honey. Apply to burn daily.
- *I suggest Omega Complete, Evening primrose oil & MB Builder*

BURSITIS
- Inflammation of the bursa.
- Rest the inflamed area and apply ice packs to reduce inflammation for 20 minutes three times daily. Hot castor oil packs can help.
- Enzymes are very anti-inflammatory, especially when taken on an empty stomach. They clean up debris in the blood stream.
- Fish oil, calcium, magnesium, Vitamin D, collagen and glucosamine can help.
- Wintergreen, peppermint & lemongrass rubbed on topically can help with pain and inflammation.
- *I suggest Alpha Green, Alpha Flavin, Liga Plus, R Plus, Arnica Plus & Alpha Zyme III.*

Castor Oil Pack
1. Soak a flannel or cotton cloth in castor oil and place on skin.
2. Cover fabric with a piece of plastic.
3. Apply a hot water bottle over the plastic to heat the pack.
4. Cover with towel & leave on for 1 hour.

CANCER
- Most cancer (breast & prostate) takes seven to 10 years to grow to the size of a pinhead before it can be detected.
- Without sugar, cancer cannot survive. Stop eating sugar and you starve cancer cells to death. This is why fasting is so healing, as is a ketogenic diet.

- We all have cancer cells. However, a properly functioning immune system will destroy cancer cells before they spread out of control. When cells begin to mutate and the immune system is unable to stop them, then cancer is diagnosed. Instead of trying to kill, poison or radiate cancer, we build up and balance the immune system so that it can effectively do what God created it do, naturally – seek and destroy cancer cells.

  > More than 200 studies link Vitamin D deficiency to cancer. Optimizing Vitamin D levels can reduce the risks of 16 different cancers in half, including breast cancer.

- Supplementing with Vitamin D can cut cancer risks by half. Get out in the sunshine half an hour a day.

- Bloodroot was listed as a cancer remedy in the *United States Pharmacopoeia* from 1820 to 1926. German researchers found that bloodroot added to animal feed was more effective and much safer than antibiotics at preventing infections.

  > **Dr. Joel Wallach has proven that 200 mcg of Selenium a day will reduce these cancers:**
  > - Breast Cancer by 82%
  > - Prostate Cancer by 69%
  > - Colon-Rectal Cancer by 64%
  > - Lung Cancer by 39% (even if you smoke)

- Dr. James Morré from Purdue University taught that cancer cells produce a specific protein called Enox2. He developed the Capsol-T formula to stop the protein from replicating. When apoptosis (cell death) occurs, the lymphatic system needs drainage support to eliminate dead cancer cell toxicity. Insufficient lymphatic drainage will cause swelling. Detoxify the body, especially the lymphatic system, liver, spleen and kidneys.

  > **Cancer Toxins**
  > - Heavy Metals
  > - Yeast/Fungus
  > - Mold
  > - Pesticides
  > - Chemicals
  > - Miasms
  > - Epstein-Barr
  > - Radiation
  > - Parasites
  > - Acidosis

- Cancer cells have a protective coating (protein-based cell membrane) that doesn't allow the immune system to recognize the cancer. Taking proteolytic enzymes (protease) on an empty stomach between meals can help break down the protective coating so the immune system can target cancer cells.

- All tumors grow from hormones. Estrogen feeds cancer. Birth control pills and synthetic hormone replacement increase estrogen levels in the body, which feed cancer.

  > **Immune Support**
  > 1) Capsol-T
  > 2) Immu C
  > 3) KLS Enviro

- Increase circulation. Ginkgo biloba, ruscus and ginseng are good for circulation.

- Dr. Otto Warburg, Nobel Prize winner, proved that cancer cannot live in a high oxygen alkaline environment. Increase circulation and we increase oxygen to the cells. Deep breathing exercises are good.
- Rebounding on a mini-trampoline is beneficial. Dr. Morton Walker states that rebounding 30 minutes every day will reduce your risk of cancer by 90 percent.
- Stop using microwave ovens. Heating foods and drinks with a microwave oven is eating and drinking radiation poison! We have "CAUTION RADIATION" signs on doors of X-ray rooms and put radiation shields over our body at the dentist office but then turn around and radiate our food? Think before you eat.
- Do an emotional release. What's eating you up inside? Are you subconsciously looking for an escape route? Cancer patients always have emotional issues on a subconscious level. Holding on to deep resentment, hate, revenge, guilt, hurt & unforgiveness are common. Who hurt you? Who are you angry at? If you don't heal the emotional scars from the past, the physical body will lack the vital force needed to heal cancer. Letting go and healing emotionally empowers your immune system with healing energy.
- Get the pH of the body more alkaline, 6.8 to 7.0. Acidosis and sugar feed tumors. Stop feeding the cancer. Change the terrain and cancer cannot exist. If it is white, don't put it in your mouth with the exception of cauliflower, garlic and onions. Eat green leafy vegetables. Asparagus, carrots and berries (camu, acai, goji, & blueberries) are good. Parsley and cilantro are good.
- Turmeric is one of the best cancer fighters in the world. Garlic, ginger, onions, green tea, ashwagandha, holy basil, chlorella and spirulina are excellent as well.

Dr. Oz's Green Drink
2 cups spinach
2 cups cucumber
1 head of celery
½ inch fresh ginger root
1 bunch parsley
2 apples
Juice of 1 lime
Juice of ½ lemon
Combine all ingredients in a juicer. Makes 30 oz.

Unresolved Emotions Are The Seeds Of Disease

Emotional Conflict – The Root Cause of Cancer
- **Anger** weakens the **liver**
- **Grief** manifests in the **lungs**
- **Worry** affects the **stomach**
- **Stress** exhausts the **heart & brain**
- **Fear** debilitates the **kidneys**
- **Anger & anxiety** conflict with family, cripples the **pancreas**
- **Feeling Powerless** manifests in the **thyroid**
- **Conflict with child**, home or mother, affects the **Left Breast**
- **Conflict with your partner** or others affects the **Right Breast**

Essential Oils Immune Support
- Frankincense oil   2 drops
- Myrrh oil   2 drops
- Turmeric oil   2 drops

Mix with 4 oz of water and drink twice daily.

- Medicinal mushrooms like maitake and reishi are good.
- Drinking bone broths is very healthy and immune boosting, especially for the gut, which is where 80 percent of the immune system resides.

> **Medicinal Mushrooms**
> - Shiitake
> - Reishi
> - Cordyceps
> - Lion's mane
> - Turkey tail

- Eating fermented foods like kefir and kimchi is good.
- Take a probiotic to help build up the microbiome.
- Eating a ketogenic diet (healthy fats, no carbs) for 3 months at a time will starve out cancer cells. Cancer has to have sugar to live. Avocados, coconut oil and salmon are good.
- Graviola, Una de Gato (cat's claw), Essiac tea, laetrile and elderberry are good anticancer agents.
- Remove silver (amalgam) fillings from teeth and replace them with composite materials. Locate a biological dentist who has been trained on how to remove them safely at IAOMT.org or call 863-420-6373.
- Beryllium toxicity is associated with lung cancer.

> **Resentment Is Fuel For Cancer Cells**

- An EDS scan identifies the nails compromising the immune system. Most of the time there are several layers of toxins to the onion that must be detoxified to generate a healing response. Remove the nails and heal the cause.
- CBD oil is beneficial
- *I suggest KLS Enviro, Immu C, Graviola, Capsol T, Essiac Tea, Amygdalin B-17, Alpha Green II, Circu Plus & intraMAX*

CANDIDA YEAST

- Emotions: frustration and anger multiplying inside, blaming others.
- Every human has naturally occurring fungus in the intestinal tract that helps you break down and digest food. It aids in the absorption of nutrients. When the microbiome is out of balance from antibiotic use, too many grains and sugar, then the yeast can become systemic. To bring an overgrowth of yeast back into balance calls for a strict diet.
- If you have a white coating on your tongue, you most likely have a candida yeast overgrowth.

> **What Causes Candida Yeast?**
> 1. Antibiotics
> 2. Birth control pills
> 3. Sugar
> 4. Grains
> 5. Heavy metals
> 6. Food allergies
> 7. Low stomach acid
> 8. Acid reflux medication
> 9. C-section births
> 10. Chlorine & fluoride

- If you were delivered by C-section at birth, you were deprived of being coated with beneficial bacteria from the birth canal that primes the immune system and helps prevent yeast overgrowth. If you weren't breast fed for at least 6 months, your immune system was short-changed again. This leaves

FOODS TO EAT			FOODS TO AVOID		
FRUIT	green apples*	berries* avocados	**SUGAR**	fruit juices	honey
	grapefruit*	lemons limes	molasses	maple syrup	soft drinks
			sports drinks	diet drinks	alcohol
	fresh coconut		coffee	tea	
MEAT	fish	salmon tuna	**GRAINS**	bread	wheat
	beef	steak wild game	corn	rice	quinoa
	chicken	lamb venison	millet	oats	oatmeal
	turkey	duck pheasant	pasta	crackers	chips
DAIRY	yogurt - plain	butter cream cheese	**STARCHES**	potatoes	beans
	sour cream	kefir	peas	mushrooms	hot dogs
EGGS			breaded meats		
VEGETABLES	broccoli	carrots spinach			
	cabbage	onions garlic	moldy cheese	Roquefort	
	cucumbers	celery okra			
	collards	radishes asparagus	egg substitutes	dried fruits	raisins
	string beans	tomatoes	processed meats	prunes	dates
BEVERAGES	herbal teas	bone broth	figs	melons	
	water w/lemon/lime				
OILS	coconut oil	flaxseed grapeseed	pickles	salad dressing	soy sauce
	olive oil	apple cider vinegar	green olives	malt products	beer
NUTS/SEEDS	almonds	pecans walnuts			
	macadamia	cashew hemp seeds	hydrogenated oils		
	pumpkin	Brazil nuts	peanuts	pistachios	peanut oil
*Eat sparingly					
***Most vegetables are fine					

you more susceptible to yeast overgrowth problems.
- Antibiotics kill off beneficial bacteria in the gut, upsetting the balance of the microbiome, leaving naturally occurring yeast to rapidly multiply and become systemic.
- Oral contraceptives (birth control pills) feed yeast.
- If you are taking a PPI (proton pump inhibitor) drug such as Prevacid or Prilosec, you are decreasing acid in your stomach, which is needed to sterilize and kill fungus, viruses and bacteria. This invites infection into your body because the front door (stomach acid) is wide open. These medications are dangerous because they upset the natural balance of the digestive system, allowing yeast to multiply and circulate into other areas.
- Heavy metals in the body favor the growth of yeast.
- Yeast and fungus thrive in an acidic body, just like mold does in a warm, dark, humid shower.
- Sugar feeds yeast. Get off sugars and starches, including fruit, juices, soft drinks, potatoes and honey.

- Eat a grain-free diet. Breads, pasta and anything made with flour, wheat, barley, rye, corn & rice feed yeast. How do you make beer or whiskey? Soak a grain like barley or corn in hot water and it releases sugars that feed yeast during the fermentation process to produce alcohol.
- Eat healthy fats, vegetables and meats. Bone broth is very healing and anti-fungal.
- Coconut oil contains caprylic acid, which is antifungal. Consuming 1 to 4 tablespoons a day is very beneficial. It's also brain fuel and gives you energy!
- Slow cooker recipes with lots of vegetables, especially garlic and onions, are very beneficial.
- Fermented vegetables are beneficial for the microbiome.
- Eat warming foods that are bitter and very antifungal, such as ginger, garlic, turmeric, black seed, cinnamon, Swiss chard and green leafy vegetables like kale and spinach.
- Vitamin B12 feeds yeast.
- Get the bowels moving three times a day. Take a multi-strain probiotic formula to balance good bacteria in the intestinal tract.
- For vaginal yeast infections, douche with white vinegar. Applying some coconut oil mixed with manuka honey is very antifungal.
- Turkey tail, reishi and chaga mushrooms are excellent for eradicating yeast.
- Most vaginal yeast infections occur after a round of antibiotics, eating a lot of sugar, breads, grains or consuming alcohol. Pau d'arco (taheebo tea), echinacea, goldenseal, black seed turmeric and thyme are antifungal.
- Probiotics are very important.
- Iron and zinc deficiencies are common in individuals with yeast and fungal conditions. Too much copper will feed yeast.
- Enzymes such as cellulase break down and digest the cell wall of candida.
- The phenolic Mannan can help desensitize the body to itching candida infections.
- Bentonite clay can help.
- Research has proven that clove oil is just as effective as the drug Nystatin in combating yeast infections. Drink 1 drop of clove oil daily in a beverage to help eradicate yeast.
- Cinnamon and grapefruit oils are helpful for eliminating fungus as well.

Mold & Fungus Killer
- Oregano Oil - 2 drops in 4 oz of water.
- Drink 3 times a day.

Eradicating Candida Yeast With Bone Broth
Do a three-day bone broth fast to starve out the yeast, heal the gut and balance your pH. Adding a tablespoon of coconut oil to the bone broth is antifungal and gives you energy.

Antifungal Essential Oils

Oregano	Clove
Tea tree	Lemongrass
Cinnamon	Thyme
Lavender	Geranium
Chamomile	Cassia

- *I recommend Lapacho Plus, Arco Plus, Mold X, Candida Clear, Complete Probiotics & Alpha Green.*

CANKER SORES

- Occur inside the mouth, on the tongue or inside the cheek. Is usually an autoimmune disorder caused by a gluten, dairy, citrus or chocolate sensitivity. Avoid peanuts, peanut butter, nuts and sweets. Do an EDS allergy scan to check for sensitivities.
- Swishing apple cider vinegar in your mouth eliminates harmful bacteria that can be causing sores.
- Applying hydrogen peroxide with a cotton ball directly on the sores can help.
- L-Lysine, Vitamin B12, folic acid, iron, myrrh, zinc, goldenseal & licorice root are good.
- *I suggest Immu C, Camu Plus, Complete Probiotics & Alpha E Spleen*

CARPAL TUNNEL

- Compression of the median nerve in the wrist triggers carpal tunnel.
- Vitamins C and B6 can help.
- Calcium and magnesium may be beneficial.
- Serrapeptase may be beneficial.
- Mix 2 drops each of wintergreen, lemongrass, helichrysum, peppermint and cypress oils and apply to painful area twice daily. May be diluted with coconut or olive oil.
- *I suggest Arnica Plus, R Plus, Liga Plus, Alpha Flavin, Pain Relief Plus & Omega Complete*

CELIAC DISEASE

- Gluten sensitivity, 97 percent of people don't know they have it. Most have dairy sensitivities as well, along with a Vitamin B12 deficiency.
- Avoid wheat, barley, rye oats, kamut, corn, rice, millet, breads, pasta, malt vinegars, malt beer, caramel colors, soy sauce, lunch meats.

Signs of Gluten Intolerance

1. Digestive issues – gas, bloating, diarrhea, constipation
2. Brain fog after eating
3. Headaches – migraines
4. Joint pains (fibromyalgia) – hands, knees, hips
5. Keratosis – chicken skin on back of arms
6. Adults still have pimple outbreaks like teenagers
7. Fatigue — wake up feeling tired – never feel rested
8. Mood issues – anxiety, depression, ADD
9. Hormone imbalances
10. Autoimmune disease – colitis, lupus, MS, etc.
11. Dizziness – feeling off balance

- Eat vegetables, nuts, seeds, meat, fish and legumes. The paleo, keto or Mediterranean diets are good.
- Coumarin can help desensitize allergies to wheat and dairy foods.
- *I suggest BR-SP Plus, Complete Probiotics, Colostrum, Omega Complete, Immu C & Arco Plus*

Celiac Gut Healers
▪ Probiotics
▪ Colostrum
▪ Vitamin D
▪ Glutamine
▪ Fish oil
▪ Turmeric

CHICKENPOX
- A mild infection (it's not a disease) that causes an itchy, blister-like rash that lasts for usually about a week. Avoid scratching.
- Echinacea, elderberry, astragalus, calendula, Vitamin C & garlic are good.
- Applying vinegar, baking soda or raw honey on itchy skin can help. Taking an oatmeal bath can be beneficial.
- Mixing 2 drops each of lavender, tea tree, oregano and lemon oil with 2 Tbsp. of coconut oil and applying to skin twice daily can help soothe itching and speed up healing. Neem oil is good.
- According to Dr. Andrew Lockie, author of *The Family Guide to Homeopathy*, the homeopathic remedies Varicella 30c or Rhus tox 30c given once a day for 10 days is a good preventative. For chickenpox infection with low-grade fever, take Aconite 30c or Belladonna 30c, or Ferr phos, every 2 hours, up to 10 doses. If large blisters develop, child whines and doesn't want to be left alone, use Antimonium tart 6c. If child has rash, fever, and is very restless use, Rhus tox 6c. If child is very clingy, fearful, not thirsty in spite of high temperature, use Pulsatilla 6c. If child has rash, fever, very thirsty and hungry, but refuses to eat, use Sulphur 6c. If temperature is down, rash is beginning to heal, but some infected, use Mercurius 6c.
- *I suggest Echinacea Complex, Alpha Flavin & Allibiotic*

CHRONIC FATIGUE SYNDROME
- Support the endocrine system, especially the adrenal glands.
- Sodium feeds the adrenal glands. Use pink Himalayan salt.
- Low energy in the morning is usually a thyroid issue. Kelp is good for the thyroid.
- Low energy in the afternoon indicates sluggish adrenal glands. Magnesium is the spark plug for the adrenal glands. Royal jelly is good for the adrenals. Norepinephrine can be beneficial.
- DHEA — take on empty stomach. Testosterone can help.
- Lyme disease can trigger low energy.
- The CDC states that 90 percent of Americans carry Epstein-Barr virus (EBV). It flares up when we get stressed out, not enough sleep, and eat too many sugars & grains.
- Cytomegleo virus is a common energy-zapping infection.

- Yeast (candida) can cause low energy. An EDS scan identifies the energy-zapping culprits.
- Vitamin B12 is the "energy vitamin" found only in animal sources of foods.
- *I recommend Adrena Plus, Endo Glan Plus, Ginseng Plus, Licro Plus, Clear Mind, Diadren Forte, Royal Jelly & intraMAX*

CIRCULATORY PROBLEMS
- Ginkgo biloba, ginseng, butcher's broom, gotu kola, cayenne, ginger, garlic and parsley help increase circulation.
- Calcium plaque build-up can restrict blood flow. Calcium binds to heavy metals, which can interfere with circulation. Alpha phosphoric acid dissolves calcium plaquing in the arteries.
- When the pH of the body is acidic and those acids meet calcium, it turns to stone. Blockages in the arteries, kidney stones and bone spurs are results.
- Cold hands and feet are common complaints. Magnesium and potassium help circulation.
- EDTA (chelation) therapy can be beneficial for increasing circulation and detoxifying heavy metals.
- *I suggest Circu Plus, Chola Plus, Veno Plus, Alpha Ortho Phos, Vascutin, Omega Complete, Gota Plus & Brain Formula*

CIRRHOSIS
- Chronic liver disease causes scarring and liver dysfunction.
- Avoid alcohol, smoking, caffeine and fried foods.
- Eat plenty of dark green, leafy vegetables.
- Liver cleansing herbs include milk thistle, dandelion, ginger & burdock. Turmeric, spirulina, chlorella, wheatgrass & alfalfa are good.
- An EDS scan will check for environmental pollutants such as chemicals, pesticides, heavy metals, radiation & pathogens.
- *I suggest KLS -Enviro, E Plus, Beta Plus, Hepachol & Alpha E Spleen.*

COLDS
- Emotions: too much going on at once.
- Cold and flu season hits in the winter, usually around the holidays, because: 1. Lack of sunlight = low Vitamin D levels 2. Consumption of lots of sugars and gluten 3. Confined to indoors, lack of fresh air and 4. Stress, yes, the holidays are stressful for most people.
- Taking 50,000 IU a day of Vitamin D3 and K2 (MK7) 500 mg is a great immune booster.
- The adrenal glands control the susceptibility to viral infections. This is why we usually get sick after an emotional upset or lots of stress and not enough sleep. Adrena Plus and Licro Plus support the adrenals.

- The common cold is a good old-fashioned house cleaning party. When trash and mucus accumulate in the body and the dumpsters (lymph nodes) are so full and inflamed that your cells can't do their jobs, then they have a special cleanup party. The sinuses become inflamed and the mucus is discharged from the nose. Coughing up phlegm is another way to help rid the body of these wastes. We want the waste to come out, not stay in!

- Any medication you take to suppress what your body is cleaning out is as foolish as you bringing your kitchen garbage sack back into the house after mom just threw it away. She doesn't want the garbage in her house and neither do your cells want infected mucus interfering with cellular activity.

- Make sure your channels of elimination are open. Are you constipated? Get the bowels moving two to three times a day with herbal laxatives like aloe vera, cascara sagrada, psyllium, senna leaves, etc.

- Do a garlic enema to get your bowels moving. Remember, 80 percent of your immune system resides in the gut. Eating fermented vegetables and using probiotics are beneficial.

- Drink lots of water and hydrate those mucus-filled areas of the body.

- Get out in the fresh air and move. Go for a walk or bike ride. Rebound on a mini-trampoline and pump the lymphatic system so the garbage can circulate out of your body.

- Do a dry-brush massage to stimulate the skin. Then lie down and rest.

- When you are sick, it's good to sleep as much as you can for two days. Sleep is healing. It's important to go out and get some fresh air, sunshine on the skin and exercise in moderation to pump the lymphatic system. Have you noticed how you usually feel better after exercising? Too much lying around the house can make you feel worse.

- A hot sauna bath with essential oils (peppermint & eucalyptus) can help eliminate toxins. Don't pour chlorinated/fluoridated tap water over your hot rocks in the sauna, unless you want a gas chamber! Use purified water. If you can't get in a sauna, boil some water on the stove and then remove from heat and add 10 drops of peppermint and 10 drops of eucalyptus oil. Put a

Cold & Flu Busters
- Echinacea
- Elderberry
- Goldenseal
- Ginger
- Garlic
- Oregano oil
- Zinc
- Vitamin C
- Vitamin D
- Olive Leaf
- Cat's claw
- Colloidal Silver

Master Tonic Immune Formula
¼ cup chopped garlic
¼ cup chopped white onions
¼ cup grated ginger
2 Tbsp. grated horseradish root
2 Tbsp. turmeric powder
1 habanero pepper or
1 tsp. cayenne (optional)
24 oz. apple cider vinegar
  Fill a 1-quart Mason jar with dry ingredients and mix well. Pour in vinegar and shake daily for 2 weeks. Strain, squeeze well and drink. Take 1 Tbsp. up to 6 times a day.

- towel over your head and breathe in the steam for 5 minutes. Other beneficial oils are lemon, ginger and thyme.
- Fruits and vegetables should be your main foods. Get off dairy products. They are mucus-forming foods. Cook homemade, slow cooker vegetables, and chicken soup with fresh garlic, ginger and onions.
- Bone broth is very anti-inflammatory and healing. Drink several cups a day. A tablespoon of coconut oil in it is beneficial. Use sea salt for desired taste.
- Eat three cloves of fresh garlic daily. Garlic is a natural antibiotic.
- Colloidal silver, beta glucans, reishi mushrooms, vitamin C and zinc help fight infection and boost the immune system.

Cough Syrup Remedy
- Peppermint oil   1 drop
- Frankincense oil 1 drop
- Lemon oil   1 drop
- Ginger oil   1 drop
- 1 spoonful honey

Mix in 4 oz of water and drink

- EDS testing will determine which immune supplements are best for your body at this specific time.
- Colds can also be triggered by nutritional deficiencies.
- Stuffiness in the right nostril indicates a potassium deficiency. The best sources of potassium are bee pollen, alfalfa and burdock.

Cold & Flu Support
Immutox II - 10 drops 2 x a day
Arco Plus - 50 drops 2 x a day

- Stuffiness in the left nostril indicates a sodium deficiency. The best sources of sodium are spirulina, celery, watercress, Irish moss and dulse.
- Stuffiness in both nostrils can be helped with royal jelly, which is high in pantothenic acid and nourishes the adrenal glands.
- A nasal spray called Sinu Orega containing sea salt, oregano oil, clove bud oil, sage & bay leaf is good for sinus infections.
- A sore throat and swollen tonsils can be caused from a sulfur deficiency. The tonsils are the sulfur sacks of the body, and they help purify the blood. Eat eggs, onions, garlic and apricots, as they are high in sulfur.
- Nasal drip can be triggered by an excess amount of mucus in the pituitary. Gota kola and wood betony can help. The phenolic Indole can help enhance the immune system.
- *I suggest Arco Plus or Echinacea Plus, Camu Plus, cat's claw, Olive Leaf, Allibiotic, Immune Formula & Adrena Plus*

COLD SORES
- Caused from the herpes simplex virus I.
- L-lysine is very beneficial. Other important nutrients include Vitamin C, Vitamin B complex, zinc, niacin, calcium, magnesium and acidophilus.
- Lemon balm, garlic & aloe vera are good.
- *I recommend H-S Formula, Arco Plus, Camu Plus, cat's claw, Olive leaf, Alpha E Spleen, L-lysine, Immune Support & Complete Probiotics.*

CONSTIPATION
- Emotions: unwilling to release old feelings, ideas & beliefs. Stuck in the past.
- First thing upon arising, drink 16 ounces of water and hydrate the body. Just as a toilet cannot flush without water, neither can the bowels move when dehydrated. Many Americans are dehydrated and don't know it. The difference between a prune and a plum is water content.
- Exercise helps tremendously. Get moving!
- Beneficial bacteria (flora) in the intestinal tract is important. Antibiotics kill this "good bacteria" off. Many drugs are constipating, especially pain medication.
- Magnesium is the mineral that helps you relax so that the muscles in the colon can move.
- High doses of Vitamin C can be beneficial.
- An enema can help get the bowels moving.
- Parasites can be an issue.
- Psyllium husk, cascara sagrada, aloe vera, rhubarb and Senna are good bowel movers.
- *I recommend Intestinal Formula, BR-SP Plus, Cape Aloe, Complete Probiotics & Fiber Life*

COUGH
- Chronic coughs are an indication that the body is trying expel microbes, mucus and other irritants. We want the toxins out. Taking cough suppressant medication keeps the toxins in.
- Coughs that won't clear up are usually caused from mold. Arco Plus & Mold X are good.
- Coughs or lung issues are usually symptoms of sluggish adrenal glands. Licro Plus & Adrena Plus are good.
- Calcium lactate, B12, wild cherry & boneset herbs can help.
- Echinacea, cat's claw, elderberry and Vitamin C are good.
- *I suggest Mullein Plus, Licro Plus, Arco Plus, Mold X, Pneumo Plus & Adrena Plus*

CRAMPS
- Researchers estimate that 80 percent of Americans are not getting enough magnesium.
- Muscle cramps, "charley horses" and twitches are usually caused from calcium and magnesium deficiencies. Calcium allows a muscle to contract. Magnesium allows it to relax. In our high-paced lifestyle, we get stressed out and burn up our magnesium reserves and then wonder why we can't sleep at nights and have cramps, high blood pressure, heart palpitations, constipation, headaches, nausea, indigestion & hormonal issues.

- Vitamin K2 is good for nighttime muscle cramps.
- Take a hot Epsom salt bath. Epsom salt contains magnesium, a natural muscle relaxant that is absorbed through the skin. Add 2 cups of Epsom salt and 20 drops of lavender oil in your hot bath and soak 30 minutes before bed. It is also very good for stress and anxiety.
- *I recommend Cal Lac Plus or MG/K Aspartate, Herbal & Mineral Complete, Alpha Green II & intraMAX*

CROHN'S DISEASE

- Did you have a "gut feeling something was wrong?" or is "he or she a real pain in your rear end?" Emotional stress can manifest in the gut. Do an emotional release (RFA) so the trapped emotions can move out and your physical body can heal.
- Heavy metals and parasites can cause inflammation in the intestinal tract.
- Mainstream medicine claims Crohn's is incurable. Dr. Jordan Rubin, founder of "Garden of Life," cured himself of Crohn's disease. The Primal Defense formula is a blend of homeostatic soil organisms, fermented whole foods and 12 probiotics (good intestinal bacteria). This blend helps restore proper intestinal balance in the gut, rebuilding the microbiome and thus eliminating symptoms.
- Avoid gluten and grains, which cause inflammation in the gut.
- Slow cooker vegetables with chicken or beef bone broth is very healing.
- Sangre de Drago is a powerful antioxidant and intestinal/ulcer healer.
- Essential oils ginger and peppermint are very healing. Take 2 drops of each in water or coconut oil twice daily.
- Vitamin D, glutamine and turmeric are good.
- *I recommend Immu C, Arco Plus, Para Plus, BR-SP Plus, Omega Complete, Complete Probiotics, & Colostrum*

CUTS

- Wash the cut with warm, soapy water and allow it to bleed profusely, to cleanse germs.
- Hydrogen peroxide is a good disinfectant. It kills even tetanus spores. Keep this in the house and use it on cuts after washing the wound.
- Cayenne pepper (capsicum) sprinkled on cuts will stop the bleeding.
- Table sugar sprinkled on cuts will also stop bleeding.
- Sangre de Drago (Liquid Stitches) is a sap from a tree from the Amazon rainforest that you can pour on the cut that fights infection and seals the cut. Natives in the jungle use it for large cuts when stitches aren't available. It's a very powerful antioxidant and helps knit the skin back together. It can be taken internally to help heal sore throats & gastric ulcers.
- *I recommend hydrogen peroxide topically and Sangre de Drago for cuts to stop bleeding & fight infection*

CYSTS

- Hot castor oil packs are good to help shrink cysts.
- The sycosis (gonococcinum & medorrhinum) miasm is usually the culprit that causes cysts.
- Ovarian cysts can be caused from hormonal imbalances. Natural progesterone helps balance excess estrogen in the body. Kelp is high in iodine for thyroid health.
- Maca, black cohosh, dong quai, milk thistle and yarrow are good.
- Avoid eating soy products, as they are endocrine disruptors.
- *I suggest Sycosis, Female Formula, Female Balance, Endo Glan F & Evening Primrose oil (for ovarian cysts)*

Castor Oil Pack
1. Soak a flannel or cotton cloth in castor oil and place on skin.
2. Cover fabric with a piece of plastic.
3. Apply a hot water bottle over the plastic to heat the pack.
4. Cover with towel & leave on for 1 hour.

DEMENTIA (SEE ALZHEIMER's DISEASE)

- Emotions: feeling hopeless & helpless, tired of struggling with life.
- A brain disorder that causes a long-term, gradual decrease in the ability to think and remember.
- Check for pesticide and heavy-metal poisoning.
- Avoid artificial sweeteners, as they are neurotoxins.
- Avoid sugar, carbs and grains, as they cause brain degeneration. A ketogenic diet is ideal. Mediterranean and paleo diets are good too.
- Your brain is 60 percent fat. Fat-free diets and statin drugs cause memory loss! Feed your brain healthy fats. They are brain food. We need healthy fats for health. Statin drugs are linked to dementia and memory loss.
- Dr. Dale Bredesen, of the Buck Institute for Research on Aging, reports eating a low-carb, low-glycemic, low-grain and high-fat diet reverses dementia.
- High blood pressure medications restrict blood flow to the brain, decreasing oxygen and nutrient nourishment, which may lead to brain degeneration.
- Get up off the couch and move! Exercise is important for blood flow and oxygen to the brain.
- Alpha lipoic acid is good.
- Phosphatidyl serine and lecithin can be beneficial. Vitamin B12 & D3 are good.
- Acetylcholine can help with memory and mental alertness.

Healthy Fats (Brain Food)
■ Coconut oil
■ Olive oil
■ Avocados
■ Eggs
■ Olives
■ Butter
■ Nuts & Seeds

- Glutathione helps mop up heavy metal poisoning.
- Vitamin D is a brain hormone and very beneficial.
- CoQ10 is important. Statin drugs paralyze your cells' ability to make it.
- *I suggest chlorella, Circu Plus, Clear Mind, Gota Plus, Brain Formula, Vitamin D, Alpha Oxzyme, Dopamine & Phosphatidyl-Serine*

DEPRESSION/ANXIETY

- Emotions: hopelessness, feeling boxed in. Feeling, "I'll never be enough."
- Exercise is the best treatment for depression. It releases the feel-good endorphins like serotonin, dopamine, glutamate and GABA. Physically active people are usually less likely to have depression. Get up, get dressed and go do something to make the world a better place. Find a way to contribute to a good cause and, in the process, you just may find happiness. When you focus your energy on what you can do to help someone else, this disperses depression.

NEUROTRANSMITTERS	
Serotonin	moods/depression
Dopamine	mental processing
GABA	anger outbursts
Acetylcholine	mental alertness

- Visit a children's hospital and make friends by reading funny story books to those who are sick. This or similar acts of kindness help depression. Why? Because you are giving. And we only have what we give. So, staying at home, focusing on yourself, causes depression! The Dead Sea is dead because it receives water, but it doesn't give. Be a giver.
- HCL in the stomach breaks proteins down into amino acids. Pepsin breaks amino acids into peptides, which are needed for neurotransmitters to keep us free from depression. If you experience heartburn or acid reflux, your digestive system may be the cause of depression. The older we get, the less HCL we produce, which causes indigestion. Supplement with digestive enzymes and HCL. Alpha Gest III is good.

Hot Epsom salt bath
▪ 2 cups Epsom Salt
▪ 1 cup Baking Soda
▪ 20 drops lavender oil
Soak for 20-30 minutes

- Your gut is your second brain. It produces more neurotransmitters than your brain! In fact, 90 percent of serotonin is made in the gut! Many people who are depressed have a gut issue.
- A sluggish thyroid can bring on depression. Kelp is high in iodine that nourishes the thyroid. Kelp Complex & Thyro Plus are good.
- Statin drugs are notorious for getting cholesterol too low, and then the body can't manufacture hormones, which may cause depression. Cholesterol below 150 is dangerously low. Your brain needs cholesterol for health!
- Dr. James Greenblatt informs that low cholesterol is associated with depression and higher suicide attempts.

- Dr. Jazayeri published in the Australian and New Zealand Journal of Psychiatry that EPA (omega-3 fatty acids) are as effective as Prozac in treating major depressive disorders.
- Essential fatty acids, magnesium and potassium are important.
- Get on a gluten-free diet. Gluten from flour (breads & pasta) causes inflammation and leaky gut. Use almond or coconut flour in place of regular flour.
- Bach flower remedies are good.

Healthy Brain Foods	
Avocados	Ghee
Eggs	Olives
Nuts	Butter
Seeds	Salmon
Coconut oil	Walnuts
Olive Oil	Blueberries
Dark Chocolate - (70% cacao)	

- We store memories and emotions like a virus on a computer's hard drive. RFA (Relaxed Focused Attention) is an emotional release to clear out these emotional glitches causing depression and anxiety.
- Emotional Freedom Technique is a method of tapping on specific meridians to redirect the mind to release negative emotions.
- Dr. David Bresler recommends giving long, tight hugs for pain. Being held is enormously therapeutic. Dr. Robert Rynearson says, "I'm convinced that a tender embrace can prevent and cure a host of different problems." People who are hugged and touched can often stop taking medication in order to sleep at nights.
- Essential oils lavender, ylang ylang, bergamot, rosemary and orange are good to breathe in deeply. Diffusing the oils is good, or rub some on your temples and feet.
- L-tryptophan, 5-HTP, Phenylalanine, tyrosine, SAMe, lion's mane, zinc, folate, Vitamins C, B, D and fish oil are good.
- St. John's wort, skullcap, valerian, kava, passion flower, ashwagandha, zinc, dopamine, L-dopa, serotonin and norepinephrine can help with depression.
- CBD oil is good.
- Rhodiola and maca can help.
- Dr. Russell Blaylock explains how over 75 million Americans suffer with depression and neurodegeneration caused by chronic brain inflammation after the age of 50. To reduce brain inflammation, he recommends avoiding vaccines (the flu shot), MSG & pesticides.
- Dr. Gary Null, Ph.D., lists Camu Camu as the second most potent known plant for obtaining natural antidepressant compounds. Clear Mind formula contains Camu.
- Postpartum depression is usually a sign of exhausted adrenal glands. Licro Plus & Adrena Plus are good.
- Walking barefoot on wet grass or a sandy beach is very grounding (earthing). Try 15 minutes a day and see how you feel.

- *I suggest Clear Mind, Brain Formula, Kava Kalm, Irie, Endo Glan Plus, Kelp Plus, Omega Complete, MG/K Aspartate, Alpha Gest III & Vitamin D*

DERMATITIS
- Irritants such as heavy metals, pesticides and chemicals can inflame the skin.
- Test for allergies. Many household cleaners, bug sprays and detergents can trigger symptoms.
- Vitamins D and C, fish oil & evening primrose oil can help.
- Lavender and geranium oils, 2 drops each, are very good to rub on skin topically, mixed with ½ tsp of coconut oil.
- *I suggest KLS Enviro, Hepachol, Omega Complete, Vitamin D & Complete Probiotics*

DIABETES
- Emotions: obsessed with a need to control. Deep sorrow, no sweetness left. Worry, anxiety, anger, conflict with family members.
- Fasting blood sugar, first thing in the morning, should be between 70 and 80 mg/dl. Measuring your blood sugar 2 hours after a meal should never go over 120 mg/dl. Anything over 140 mg/dl is pre-diabetes, and if you go over 200 mg/dl, you have type 2 diabetes.
- Hemoglobin A1C measures your average blood sugar over the past 6 weeks. Anything over 5.5 is considered elevated, and over 6.0 is diabetes.
- Diabetics have high blood sugar because their body cannot transport sugar into the cells, also known as insulin resistance.
- Avoid eating grains, as they spike your blood sugar more than eating straight sugar or candy. Cold cereals are the worst!
- Avoid potatoes, fruit juice, soft drinks, diet drinks, candy & desserts.
- Some people can't tolerate beans because they contain enough starch to spike the blood sugar.
- Eat healthy fats: avocados, olives, eggs, butter, coconut oil, nuts & seeds; lots of vegetables; and baked meats in moderation.
- Statin drugs are linked to diabetes.
- The adrenal glands, pancreas and liver regulate blood sugar levels.
- Chromium, vanadium and zinc are important.
- Increase circulation throughout the body. Ginkgo, ginseng and butcher's broom are good vessel dilators.
- Ashwagandha, holy basil and juniper berries are good.

Foods To Avoid
- Wheat/Flour
- Rice
- Corn
- Oats
- Breads
- Pasta
- Cereals
- Crackers
- Potatoes
- Chips
- Watermelon
- Raisins
- Sports drinks

- Heavy metals, especially mercury, can affect the pancreas and cause blood sugar issues.
- Many diabetics get gout, caused from high uric acid. Brewer's yeast from alcohol, wheat & corn produces uric acid. Yeast (fungus) secretes poisonous byproducts called mycotoxins. Ochratoxin, Patulin & Aflatoxin create insulin resistance, cause kidney damage and oxygen disruption and interfere with the breakdown of sugar.
- In Type 1 diabetes, Dr. Isogai of Japan discovered that the fungus Cryptococcus will destroy pancreatic islet cells, which are responsible for producing insulin. Most grains, wheat, corn & peanuts are contaminated with fungal mycotoxins. Cryptococcus mycotoxins produce uric acid and alloxan. Alloxan is used to make white flour, and it destroys beta cells in the pancreas, triggering diabetes. Stop poisoning your body with contaminated grains. Doing a candida yeast/mold cleanse can be very beneficial. See candida section.
- Dandelion is an antidote for excess sugars and supports healthy liver and bile production as well as being a diuretic.
- Alpha Lipoic Acid and Vascutin are good support for diabetic neuropathy.
- Chromium is utilized to help blood sugar enter your cells. Lacking chromium, blood sugar cannot enter your cells, so it is converted to fat and stored in fat cells.
- The sycosis miasm affects the isles of Langerhans in the pancreas.
- Essential oils cinnamon, ginger & coriander are great to help balance blood sugar levels.
- See chapter on diabetes for more details.
- *I suggest Dia Plus, Dia Zyme, Circu Plus, Licro Plus, Metaba Plus, Ginger Plus II, Diabetic Formula & Cinnamon 6*

Healthy Foods To Eat
Most Vegetables
Avocados
Eggs
Coconut oil
Olive oil
Butter
Nuts & seeds
Salmon
Trout
Chicken
Turkey
Beef

DIAPER RASH
- Usually caused by yeast or infrequent diaper changes.
- Pau d'arco is antifungal.
- Probiotics are important.
- Mix 2 drops each of lavender & tea tree oil with 1 tsp. of coconut oil and apply to rash.
- *I suggest Pau D'Arco Plus, Candosolve & Complete Probiotics*

DIARRHEA
- Emotions: running away from a situation. Obsessed with order.

- Diarrhea is many times constipation in disguise. The body is cleansing itself of infection. We want the infection to come out, not stay in. Stay hydrated. Drink lots of liquids.
- A grated raw apple with skin and 3 raw grated carrots is good.
- Shepherd's purse will stop diarrhea if needed. Other beneficial herbs include bayberry, cayenne, chamomile, Sangre de Drago and ginger.
- Take 2 drops each of peppermint oil with a 1 tsp. of honey mixed in 2 oz. of water.
- *I recommend Universal Complex & Complete Probiotics*

DIVERTICULITIS
- Intestinal cleansing is needed. Psyllium husk powder will help cleanse built-up fecal matter, which causes inflammation and feeds infection.
- Stop eating breads, pasta and dairy. Slow cooker vegetables are good. Reduce your red meat consumption.
- A raw fruits and vegetables diet can help.
- Bone broth and coconut oil are anti-inflammatory foods.
- Add more fiber to the diet, such as flaxseeds and spinach.
- Probiotics and fermented foods are beneficial.
- Aloe vera, slippery elm and licorice can help.
- Parasites, heavy metals and emotions can all contribute to diverticulitis.
- *I recommend Verma Plus, Universal Complex, BR-SP Plus & Fiber Life*

EAR INFECTIONS
- Get off all dairy products, especially milk and cheese.
- Children respond well to homeopathic remedies for ear infections.
- Garlic, echinacea, zinc, Vitamin D3 and acidophilus help boost the immune system and fight infection.
- A warm roasted onion placed directly on the ear can be used for a poultice for ear infections.
- Putting a couple of drops of Wally's Ear Oil, (almond oil, tea tree oil, eucalyptus, garlic, mullein and echinacea) on the skin, and gently massaging the oil all around both ears and down under the cheek bones, where the lymph nodes are, is very effective.
- Rub 1 drop of basil oil and 1 drop of frankincense oil around the ears and on the bottom of the feet. May need to be diluted with coconut oil or olive oil for infants.
- *I suggest Otalga Plus, Echinacea Complex & Complete Probiotics. Red Root Combo for small children.*

Infant Ear Infections
Immutox 1 drop in ear
Otalga   2 drops in ear

ECZEMA
- Emotions: oversensitive, irritation, mental eruptions, unresolved hurt feelings.
- Allergies and toxins like heavy metals, pesticides and chemicals can be major factors. Skin issues are usually caused from the liver, spleen and kidneys not filtering out the wastes sufficiently, so the body pushes toxins out through the skin. KLS Enviro is good.
- Leaky gut may be the culprit. Rebuild the the microbiome.
- Low levels of HCL can trigger allergies. When we aren't breaking down our fats and proteins, allergies arise. Alpha Gest III with each meal is good digestive support.
- Evening primrose oil, fish oil, Vitamin D3 and probiotics are good. Lavender oil may help.
- The Psorinum miasm may be a cause.
- *I suggest KLS Enviro, Arco Plus, Alpha E Spleen, Omega Complete & Complete Probiotics*

EDEMA
- Swelling occurs when the lymphatic system becomes sluggish.
- Many times, the kidneys are overloaded with toxins. Kidneys regulate fluid levels in the body. When the kidneys aren't able to remove enough sodium and water from the body, swelling occurs.
- Venous insufficiency occurs when the veins aren't able to transport the blood from the feet and back to the heart. This causes swelling. Veno Plus is good.
- Drink lots of water. Cells will hoard water if they have been deprived of water in the past.
- The adrenal glands secrete hormones that regulate salt and water balance. Cortisol helps reduce inflammation.
- Renin is a hormone secreted by the kidneys and released into the bloodstream that results in the formation of angiotensin. Angiotensin acts upon the adrenal cortex, causing it to increase the production of the hormone aldosterone, which is the major hormone affecting sodium retention. When sodium is low, aldosterone production increases, causing the kidneys to conserve sodium. This hormone causes you to crave salt. The adrenal hormone (ACTH), secreted by the pituitary, will also cause you to crave salty foods. When the sodium levels are normal or high, aldosterone levels decrease, resulting in lower sodium levels being reabsorbed by the kidneys.
- Water balance in the body is affected by sodium, potassium and chloride.

> **Eczema Oil Formula**
> - 15 drops Geranium oil
> - 1 Tbsp. Coconut oil
>
> Mix together and rub onto skin twice daily

- A lack of potassium can cause swelling. Bodybuilders use potassium before a show to help shed extra water weight.
- Switch from table salt to sea salt.
- Start juicing carrots, parsley and celery or Dr. Oz's green drink recipe to get mineral levels balanced.
- Diuretics burn up your kidneys and may cause you to need dialysis treatments.
- Exercise is crucial to drain fluids. The lymphatic system relies upon movement to regulate fluid levels. Bouncing on a mini-trampoline is very beneficial.
- A lymphatic massage can help.
- Cadmium toxicity will cause sodium retention, which can cause swelling.
- *I Suggest Lymphatic Drainer, Solidago, Rena Plus, Alpha Green II & Alpha Flavin*

> **"The greatest crime physicians are guilty of is administering diuretics (water pills). These pills not only take the fluid out of the body, but also the sodium, potassium, and minerals that might be in the solution, therefore starving the body of essential nutrients!"** Donald Lepore, N.D.

ENDOMETRIOSIS
- Emotions: unresolved sadness, feelings of insecurity or a lack of self-love, blaming others.
- When the tissue that lines the inside of the uterus begins to grow outside of the uterus, this creates a lot of pain. Something is causing an imbalance. An EDS exam helps us identify the culprit. Hormonal imbalances such as too much estrogen and low progesterone can cause this. Heavy metals, pesticides and chemicals are common hormone disrupters.
- The liver helps balance hormones and protects against harmful chemicals and pesticides. A liver cleanse is usually beneficial. KLS Enviro & Hepachol are good.

Castor Oil Pack
1. Soak a flannel or cotton cloth in castor oil and place on skin.
2. Cover fabric with a piece of plastic.
3. Apply a hot water bottle over the plastic to heat the pack.
4. Cover with towel & leave on for 1 hour.

- Fish oil or evening primrose oil is beneficial.
- A few drops of clary sage oil applied to the skin over the abdomen can help. Applying a warm compress to the area helps the oil penetrate deep into the body. Taking 2 drops each of sandalwood and frankincense oils twice daily can help.

- Chasteberry, B vitamins, pygnogenol and progesterone cream are beneficial.
- *I suggest Female Formula, Female Balance, Her Formula, KLS Enviro, Endo Glan F, progesterone cream & Evening primrose oil*

EPILEPSY
- Emotions: feeling a need to persecute self. Rejection of life.
- Heavy metal poisoning is the No. 1 culprit. Mercury & aluminum cause neurological interference.
- Remove metals from teeth. Locate a biological dentist.
- Avoid sugar and grains. A very high-fat ketogenic diet is ideal. Fats are brain food.
- Eggs, onions and garlic are high in sulfur. Sulfur helps detox metals.
- Support the pituitary gland and nervous system. Valerian root, passion flower, skullcap and chamomile can help balance the nervous system.
- Vitamin B-6 and taurine can help.
- Magnesium and potassium can be beneficial.
- CBD oil can help.
- Serotonin, dopamine and malvin are neurotransmitters that need to be balanced for health.
- Emotional issues can be the root of epilepsy. The RFA process can heal emotional issues and subsequently heal physical ailments.
- The syphilinum miasm is usually a cause in epilepsy.
- Phosphatidyl serine can be beneficial.
- *I suggest Valeri Plus, Clear Mind, Brain Formula, Circu Plus, Chola Plus, Omega Complete & MG/K Aspartate*

ERECTILE DYSFUNCTION (IMPOTENCE)
- Emotions: guilt, conflicting ideas about sex. Spite against mate or unresolved fears toward mother.
- The inability to achieve an erection many times is caused from poor circulation bringing blood to the muscles of the penis. Circulation support includes gingko, ginseng, kola nut, cayenne, ginger and garlic. Gota Plus, Male Formula, His Formula & Circu Plus are good.
- Suma, maca, ginseng, sarsaparilla, damiana, saw palmetto, yohimbe, oat straw and ginger help nourish the reproductive organs.
- Calcium, magnesium, zinc, Vitamin E, flaxseed oil, amino acids and selenium are important.
- Avoid soy, as most of it is derived from genetically modified organisms (GMOs). Soy contains plant-based estrogens, which interfere with hormone balance, and most of us are exposed to a plethora of xenoestrogens, from plastic water bottles to synthetic estrogens in pharmaceuticals, lowering testosterone and causing feminization of males.

- Arginine converts into nitric oxide within the penis, which triggers the erection process, according to Dr. Sahley. Dr. Ronald Katz gives 2800 milligrams of arginine for two weeks for renewed sexual performance.
- Cholesterol is needed for hormone production, especially testosterone. Statin drugs will sabotage your sex life. You can't drug the body and expect things to stand tall when called upon.
- Eat healthy fats like avocados, eggs, coconut oil, nuts & seeds.
- Many sex hormones are manufactured in the adrenal glands. Stress will weaken the adrenals, which leads to chronic fatigue and E.D. Licro Plus and Adrena Plus are good.
- Vitamin D3 is actually a hormone and supports testosterone production.
- Pine bark is good.
- Patchouli, sandalwood, jasmine & ylang ylang oils increase testosterone and help increase libido.
- Cardamom oil applied topically can have an arousing effect. Breathing in the oil is beneficial too.
- Marijuana, coffee & alcohol can cause erectile dysfunction.
- *I suggest His Formula, Male Formula, Gota Plus, Adrena Plus, Endo Glan M, Omega Complete & testosterone.*

EYE DISORDERS (CATARACTS)
- Emotions: not liking what you see in life, not wanting to see life as it is.
- Cataracts are usually a warning sign that calcium is out of solution in the body. The body will disperse extra calcium in the eyes.
- If you are too acidic or deficient in calcium, the body will leach calcium from your own bones (the hips – largest source in the body) to buffer the acids, and then drop the calcium at the joints (which forms spurs) or in the kidneys (as stones) or in the eyes (as cataracts). This leads to osteoporosis. Cataracts, bone spurs, heel spurs, arthritic knots and kidney stones form when we become too acidic.
- For eye floaters (black spots), eat two medium carrots each day. Hemp seeds are good too.
- Eat more vegetables to alkalize the body, and take plant-derived liquid minerals (all 60).
- Get the calcium levels balanced. Iodine (kelp) helps keep calcium in balance.
- Sodium from vegetables like celery, dulse, olives, spinach, okra and strawberries help balance calcium levels.
- Chicken liver, elderberries, beef, butter, eggs, kale, turnip greens, collard greens & broccoli are excellent foods for the eyes.

- The sycosis miasm may be the culprit, causing hyperactivity in the parathyroid gland, which regulates blood calcium levels. Elevated parathormone tells the brain the body needs more calcium.
- Vitamin E, B complex, Vitamin D, Vitamin C, Vitamin A, zinc, selenium, alpha lipoic acid and L-glutathione can be beneficial.
- Heavy metals may be culprits, especially mercury.
- Bilberry is good for night blindness & nearsightedness.
- Collagen Complete is good for dry eyes.
- Bilberry, eyebright, bayberry, cayenne, comfrey, holy basil and golden seal can help.
- *I recommend Bilberry Plus, Kelp Complex, Eye Therapy, Alpha Green II & Veno Plus*

Eye Drop Formula for Styes, Burning or Pink Eye
- Take a saline bottle and empty ¼ of it
- Add 25% Immutox II (homeopathic formula)
- Shake well – Place 2 drops in both eyes
- Apply 2-3 times a day

FATIGUE
- Emotions: feeling "burned out" in one's job or relationship. Lack of love for what you do.
- People taking high blood pressure medication like Atenolol need to be aware that it causes extreme fatigue.
- Exhausted adrenal glands will cause low energy. Stress depletes the adrenals. Take Licro Plus and Adrena Plus.
- If you perspire all the time, your adrenals are revved up too high. If not controlled, this will lead to a lack of sweat caused by adrenal exhaustion.
- Low potassium levels can indicate adrenal exhaustion. This can cause low blood sugar and cause you to crave sugar.
- Magnesium is the spark plug for your adrenals. MG/K is good.
- Sluggish adrenals will cause you to crave salty foods. If you crave sweets, that's an issue with the pancreas.
- Marijuana exhausts the adrenal glands, leaving you feeling tired all the time.

Adrenal Exhaustion Signs
- Tiredness
- Dizziness/Lightheaded
- Allergies/Coughs
- Dark circles under eyes
- Headaches
- Low sex drive
- Blood pressure problems
- Joint pain
- Depression
- Dry skin
- Weight gain
- Loss of muscle tone

- Middle- to low-back pain can be caused from exhausted adrenal glands, especially if you wake up at night from 3 a.m. to 5 a.m. The adrenals affect the lungs, so coughs, asthma and respiratory problems are usually caused from sluggish adrenals.

> **Chronic Fatigue Support**
> - CFS A Plus 10 drops three times daily
> - Licro Plus 50 drops three times daily
> - Ginseng 50 drops three times daily
> - Adrena Plus 3 capsules three times daily

- Test for heavy metals and the sycosis miasm that can affect the adrenal glands. High copper levels decrease adrenal activity.
- Check for Epstein-Barr, mono virus and Lyme disease, as they are common nails in the tire zapping your energy.
- If you are a night person or get your second wind around 10 p.m., that is a sign you are running on adrenalin.
- DHEA is good.
- Vitamin D, magnesium and zinc are good.
- Vitamin B12 and ashwagandha can be beneficial.
- *I suggest Licro Plus, Ginseng Plus, Clear Mind, Neuro Balance, CFS A Plus, Adrena Plus, MG/K, Endo Glan Plus, Ashwagandha, Rhodiola, Holy Basil & DHEA*

FEVER

- Leukocytosis is when the body heats up to increase immune function and fight infection. Let a fever run its course. Your body is intelligent and knows what it's doing. Do not suppress it with drugs unless temperatures reach 104 degrees.
- Stay hydrated by drinking lots of fluids, and stay off solid foods. Fresh fruit and vegetable juices are good.
- Cyprus oil is good.
- Holy basil may help. Boneset is good for a fever & cough.
- Kids with fevers respond well with coffee enemas (4 cups warm coffee in enema bag with 1 squeezed lemon). Make sure water is warm, not too hot. Usually works best to do in morning hours.

> **Fever & Flu Formula**
> *Children's Composition Plus*
> - Yarrow
> - Peppermint
> - Elder Flower
> - Lemon Balm
> - Chamomile

- For children, rub 1 to 2 drops of diluted peppermint or frankincense oil on the bottoms of the feet.
- Calcium lactate can help.
- *I suggest Children's Composition Plus, Echinacea Plus and Camu Plus*

FIBROCYSTIC BREAST DISEASE

- Emotions: unresolved hurts, nursing a hurt from a partner. A blow to the ego.

- Women develop cysts in their breasts and ovaries when they have (1) an iodine deficiency and (2) excess estrogen. Iodine decreases excess estrogen. Take Kelp Complex and Kelp Plus.
- Too much estrogen will cause weight gain in the hips, thighs and sometimes in the arms.
- Sea kelp protects against estrogen dominance.
- The best way to balance hormone (estrogen) levels is to eat 7 cups of cruciferous vegetables a day. This would include kale, spinach, broccoli, Brussels sprouts and collard greens, etc.
- If you have tender breasts, you need more iodine.
- Iodine is needed for the thyroid, breasts, uterus and ovaries. Women need to eat sea vegetables often and supplement with kelp.
- Test for the sycosis miasm. It can be a contributing factor as well.
- Turmeric and Lion's mane mushroom can help.
- Avoid soy – it causes tumors.
- Avoid birth control. Most of the time you need less estrogen, not more.
- *I suggest Kelp Complex, KLS Enviro, Evening primrose oil, Hepachol & Kelp Plus.*

FIBROMYALGIA

- Usually chronic fatigue, joint pain and rashes are a result of the body being too acidic, accompanied with heavy metals, which favors candida yeast.
- Get on a high vegetable diet to alkalize the body. Start juicing Dr. Oz's green drink. Slow cooker vegetable, chicken or beef soups are good, especially drinking the anti-inflammatory bone broth.
- Detox the metals out and clean up the blood.
- Get silver dental fillings removed.
- Take enzymes to help metabolize interstitial fluids that accumulate in certain areas and cause pain.
- Consume a grain-free, dairy-free diet such as ketogenic, paleo or Mediterranean diet. Food sensitivities to wheat, dairy, corn, soy, citrus or sugar can be the main culprit for inflammation in the muscles and joints, causing pain. Check for allergies.

> **Muscle Pain Relief**
> - Peppermint oil 5 drops
> - Lavender oil 5 drops
> - Lemongrass 5 drops
> - Wintergreen 5 drops
>
> Mix with 1 Tbsp. coconut oil and massage on muscles.

- Vitamins C and D and turmeric are good.
- Lyme disease may be the culprit.
- Peppermint, wintergreen and lemongrass oils help reduce pain and inflammation.
- *I suggest Arnica Plus, R Plus, KLS Enviro, Alpha Flavin, Liga Plus, Alpha Green II, Kelp Plus, Diadren Forte and Omega Complete*

> **"I have found that hypothyroidism is a primary cause of fibromyalgia in at least 80 percent of patients with fibromyalgia."** David Brownstein, M.D.

FLU (SEE COLDS)
- Build up the immune system by eating mainly fruits and vegetables. Slow cooker meals with chicken vegetable soup are beneficial, especially drinking the bone broth.
- Eat garlic, onions, ginger and turmeric, as they are mother nature's most powerful infection fighters.
- Drink plenty of water, and get fresh air and direct sunlight if possible.
- Echinacea, elderberry, astragalus, olive leaf and cat's claw are good.
- Vitamins C and D and zinc are good.
- Star anise oil is anti-viral, a powerful remedy for flu bugs. Tamiflu uses star anise to obtain shikimic acid, a major ingredient. What the pharmaceutical companies don't reveal is that pure star anise oil is much more effective for eradicating flu viruses than their concoction with adverse side effects.
- Essential oils eucalyptus, oregano, lemon and thyme are good. Rub peppermint and frankincense oil on your temples, neck and bottoms of the feet.
- The homeopathic remedy Oscillococcinum can help recovery from the flu.
- *I suggest Echinacea Complex, Immu Flu, Flu Stop, Immune Formula & Allibiotic*

FOOD POISONING
- Charcoal helps absorb toxic poisons in the body.
- Garlic and goldenseal are good.
- Drink lots of water to flush poisons out.
- Peppermint oil can help with nausea.
- *I suggest taking 6 charcoal tablets every six hours & Echinacea Complex*

FREQUENT URINATION
- For men this usually occurs from a swollen prostate. See Prostatitis
- *I suggest, K/B Plus, Juni Plus & Rena Plus. For men use, Male Formula, Flaxseed oil and Prosta Plus.*

GINGIVITIS
- Oil pulling (swishing 1 tsp of coconut oil in your mouth with 2 drops of clove or myrrh oil) for 5 to 10 minutes a day is good. Spit it out, after. Cinnamon oil is good too.
- Vitamin C is very important.
- *I suggest Otalga Plus, Myrrh Plus, Camu Plus, Alpha Flavin & intraMAX*

GALLBLADDER DISORDERS
- Emotions: feelings of bitterness & anger, refusing to forgive. Who are you mad at? Who's the person you won't forgive? Do an emotional release (RFA).
- Gallstones can be dissolved with the herb boldo. Stonebreaker Plus, Hydrangea Plus and E Plus all contain boldo and are excellent gallstone and kidney stone eliminating formulas.
- Many people have their gallbladders removed and then they bloat and swell because they aren't breaking down their fats. Supplement with digestive enzymes, especially lipase to break down fats. Diadren Forte is good.
- Parasites can cause liver/gallbladder issues. Black walnut hulls, wormwood, cloves, pumpkin seed powder, pink root and male fern cleanse parasites from the body.
- Stop eating pork. Meat from swine is a risky source of contracting parasites.
- Avoid fried foods, vegetable oils, hydrogenated oils and processed foods.
- Drinking bone broth and eating slow cooker vegetables are good. Green apples are beneficial.
- Lecithin and flaxseed oil help break down fats.
- See chapter on gallbladder/liver flush for stones.
- Milk thistle, dandelion root, artichoke leaf, blessed thistle, turmeric, and lemon oil are good.
- *I suggest L/GB-AP, Stonebreaker Plus, Alpha Gest III & Beta Plus*
- *For a gallbladder attack take 50 drops of Stonebreaker Plus or Hydrangea every ½ hour.*

> **Gallstone Eliminator**
> - Stonebreaker Plus - 50 drops every hour

GOUT
- Emotions: the need to dominate, anger, judging others harshly.
- Stop drinking soda and diet drinks, as they have a pH of about 2.
- Get off the high-protein, sugar, dairy and grain diet. Stop eating meat and dairy. A vegetarian (lots of vegetables) diet for two weeks will clear out high uric acid levels that cause crystals to form in the joints, creating pain and inflammation. Kidney stones may form from eating too much protein.
- Avoid antibiotics, as they are very acid-forming.
- Get on a fruit and vegetable juice diet to get the pH of the body alkaline. Dr. Oz's green drink recipe is good. Leave off the spinach since it's a high purine and oxalate-rich food along with beans, peas, beets and nuts.
- Eat lots of red sour cherries. They neutralize uric acid. Black cherry juice is good.

- Drinking chicken vegetable bone broth is very soothing and anti-inflammatory.
- Burdock, nettles, dandelion, alfalfa, comfrey and parsley are good to flush out uric acid.
- Celery seed extract or celery juice is good.
- Vitamin C, turmeric, magnesium and fish oil are anti-inflammatory.
- Take digestive enzymes to metabolize acids in the tissue.
- Mix 3 drops each of holy basil, turmeric and peppermint oil with 1 tsp. of coconut oil and rub on painful areas.

> **Gout Eliminator**
> - Alpha Green II 2 capsules every hour
> - Alpha E Spleen 2 capsules every hour
> - KLS Enviro   50 drops every hour
>
> Take until symptoms subside

- *I recommend KLS Enviro Plus, Arnica Plus, R Plus, Alpha E Spleen, Alpha Green II, & Alpha Zyme III*

GRAVE'S DISEASE
- An autoimmune disorder affecting the thyroid, causing it to enlarge and over produce thyroid hormones, which may cause anxiety, trembling sensations and a racing heart.
- Get on a gluten-free diet.
- Test for allergies that may trigger autoimmune issues.
- Heavy metal poisoning, Epstein-Barr virus and Lyme disease may be factors.
- Mycoplasma bacteria may be a culprit.
- Aspartame poisoning can trigger this, so stop using artificial sweeteners.
- Vitamin D3 and K2 is good.
- Cat's claw, olive leaf & ashwagandha are good.
- Consume 2 drops of frankincense, myrrh and holy basil oil in water twice daily.
- *I suggest Arco Plus, Immu C, Kelp Plus, Endo Glan Plus & Complete Probiotics*

HAIR LOSS (ALOPECIA)
- You can spend hundreds of dollars on hair-care products or you can nourish the roots of your hair so it's shiny, healthy and not coming out in clumps.
- Dihydrotestosterone (DHT) is a hormone that shrinks hair follicles, thus causing hair loss. Saw palmetto and pygeum (bark from the African plum tree) helps block DHT, helping to regrow hair.
- Stress is the major culprit that causes hormonal imbalances, which increases adrenaline and cortisol, secreted by the adrenal glands. If we constantly stay in high-stress, fight-or-flight mode, this creates an imbalance in the endocrine system that eventually leads to adrenal exhaustion, blood-sugar issues and can affect the thyroid and hair loss.

- Hypothyroidism can cause hair loss. Kelp is high in iodine, and it nourishes the thyroid. Kelp Plus or Thyro Plus formulas are good. Take digestive enzymes so you absorb the nutrients you are taking.
- Decreasing stress levels and supporting the adrenal glands is crucial. Ashwagandha and rhodiola help your body deal with stress. Adrena Plus and Endo Glan Plus are good endocrine support formulas to help balance hormones.
- An essential fatty acid deficiency can cause the hair to fall out. Evening primrose oil, fish oil and flaxseed oil are good.
- Pumpkin seed oil is high in zinc, so it can be helpful.
- Drinking bone broth, which is high in collagen, can help.
- Antibiotics and prescription drugs (even thyroid medication) can cause hair loss.
- Radiation and X-rays (even dental) can cause hair loss.
- Hair that falls out in chunks can be an indication of parasites.
- Vitamin E, zinc, copper, biotin and B complex are important.
- Ginseng and probiotics can help.
- Rosemary and lavender oils can be used with olive oil to put in hair and massage on scalp. These oils help prevent hair loss and stimulate new hair growth.
- Consume foods high in essential fatty acids such as salmon, tuna, pumpkin seeds, chia seeds, hemp seeds and flaxseeds.
- *I recommend Juni Plus, Universal Complex, Omega Complete, Evening primrose oil, Chola Plus, Ashwagandha, Rhodiola & Endo Glan Plus*

HASHIMOTO'S DISEASE
- Autoimmune thyroiditis causes the thyroid to under-produce hormones.
- 43 percent of people diagnosed have gluten sensitivity, and by eliminating gluten from the diet, nearly 50 percent can reduce their thyroid medication.
- Eat a grain-free diet and consume lots of vegetables and healthy fats. Bone broth is very anti-inflammatory and healing.
- Test for food allergies.
- Test for heavy metals, candida yeast, Epstein-Barr virus and Lyme disease, as they cause thyroid disruptions.
- Selenium, Vitamins D and B complex, cat's claw, olive leaf and ashwagandha are good.
- Consume 2 drops each of frankincense, myrrh and holy basil oil in water twice daily.
- *I suggest Arco Plus, Immu C, Kelp Plus, Thyro Plus & Endo Glan Plus*

HALITOSIS (Bad Breath)

- Supplement with enzymes to ensure proper break down of proteins so that the fecal matter stench doesn't come out of your mouth when you speak.
- Floss your teeth after meals to remove food particles that decompose and produce foul-smelling breath.
- Add 2 drops of peppermint oil to your toothbrush/toothpaste.
- Get your bowels moving two to three times per day.
- Probiotics and fermented vegetables are good.
- Drink lemon water. Eating parsley can help.
- *I recommend Otalga Plus, BR-SP Plus & Alpha Zyme II*

Bad Breath Eliminator
- Oregano oil — 2 drops
- 1 tablespoon coconut oil

Mix together and swish in mouth for 2 minutes, spit out.

HEADACHE

- Emotions: self-criticism, hurt feelings going unexpressed, unable to control.
- We spend over $31 billion a year treating headaches.
- In 2012, Dr. Alexandra Dimitrova and researchers at Columbia University Medical Center in New York concluded a study showing that 56 percent of people with chronic headaches were gluten sensitive and 30 percent had celiac disease. Eat a grain-free diet.
- Check for allergies. Gluten and dairy are the worst offenders.
- Charcoal-grilled meats contain large amounts of tar and may trigger headaches. Avoid eating barbecue from charcoal.
- Magnesium helps relax tight muscles and relieves stress. MG/K is good.
- A massage can help relieve tight muscles causing pressure and pain.
- A chiropractic adjustment can instantly relieve the pain if caused from a pinched nerve.
- Blood sugar issues can trigger headaches. Diadren Forte & Licro Plus are good.
- Poor circulation and oxygen deprivation can be a factor. Ginkgo is good. Brain Formula & Circu Plus are good.
- If headaches occur around menstrual cycle, hormones may be a trigger. Endo Glan Plus & Her Formula are good.
- B vitamins are beneficial along with spirulina. Carrot & celery juice can help.
- Dehydration, not drinking enough water to flush out toxins, can cause pain. Drink half of your body weight in ounces of water a day. A 200-pound person should consume 100 oz. daily.

Headache Eliminator
- Lavender oil   2 drops
- Peppermint oil 2 drops

Rub on base of neck, forehead and temples.

- Toxins in the liver and kidneys and a sluggish gallbladder can cause pain. KLS Enviro & Beta Plus are good cleansers.
- Holy basil may help.
- Many people have digestive imbalances due to a lack of HCL acid and digestive enzymes.
- 90 percent of headaches are caused from liver/gallbladder problems. If you take acid reflux medication or have had your gallbladder removed, you probably need support to digest fats. Undigested fats and proteins get absorbed into the bloodstream and cause pain and inflammation. Hydrangea Plus, L/GB-AP Plus & Diadren Forte are good. If you do not have a gallbladder, Beta Plus is good to help break down fats. Right shoulder blade pain is an indication of liver/gallbladder congestion.
- If you have a headache, try pressing on the right side of your abdomen on the gallbladder area and hold for 2 minutes. If headache subsides, then you probably have an issue with fat metabolism triggering it.
- Constipation, failing to eliminate two to three times a day can put pressure on nerves that manifest in a headache. Take Intestinal Formula or Cape Aloe
- *I suggest Hydrangea Plus, E Plus, Universal Complex, MG/K Aspartate, Veno Plus, Diadren Forte, Alpha Flavin & Circu Plus*

HEART ATTACK

"Most modern heart disease is caused by magnesium deficiency." Mildred S. Seelig, MD

- Emotions: in a relationship that hurts. Violating the laws of love, knowingly or unknowingly. Wanting release from responsibility. Lack of joy.
- The heart has 40,000 neurons that can sense, feel, learn and remember. Statistically, more people die of heart attacks on Monday mornings than any other time. Why? Because they hate their jobs and can't face going in to work one more time.
- In an emergency heart attack, drinking a teaspoon of cayenne pepper in a cup of hot water has helped stop the attack and save lives.
- Dr. Andrea Frustaci studied the relationship between heart disease and heavy metals. Heart biopsies showed levels of mercury were 22,000 times higher than those in biopsies of other tissues in the body.
- Increase circulation. Calcium deposits and plaque build up in the arteries, restricting blood flow. Alpha Ortho Phos dissolves calcium deposits and blockages in the arteries. It's Roto Rooter for your circulatory system. It also dissolves bones spurs and kidney stones.
- Exercise is important. I recommend burst training.

Healthy Heart Support	
Infection V	5 drops 2 x a day
Hawthorn Plus	50 drops 2 x a day
Cardi Plus	2 capsules 2 x a day
MGK	2 capsules 2 x a day

- Avoid trans fats, vegetable oils, margarine, shortening, Wesson oil, soybean oil, refined carbohydrates and conventional dairy. Eat fresh vegetables, fruit in moderation, healthy fats and organic meats like wild-caught Alaskan salmon.
- Hawthorn berry, garlic, turmeric, potassium, magnesium, copper, L-carnitine, L-taurine, Vitamin E, Vitamin B complex, Vitamin C, selenium and coenzyme Q-10 are good.
- All muscles, including the heart, run on potassium. Do not use elemental potassium. Plant-derived or potassium aspartate are good.
- Check for the Coxsackie virus. It can cause sudden heart attacks. Most heart complications are caused from this destructive virus that can be deadly. The homeopathic remedy Infection V detoxifies viruses from the body.
- Essential oils ginger, lemongrass & helichrysum are good. Diffuse them and rub them on your skin.
- *I suggest Heart Formula, Hawthorn Plus, Circu Plus, MG/K Aspartate, Omega Complete & Cardi Plus*

Circulatory Support
- Ginkgo Biloba
- Ginseng
- Hawthorn
- Butcher's Broom
- Ginger
- Cayenne
- Vitamin C
- Alpha Ortho Phos

> "Vitamin C is the cement of the blood vessel walls and stabilizes them. Animals don't get heart disease because they produce enough endogenous Vitamin C in their livers to protect their blood vessels. In contrast, we humans develop deposits leading to heart attacks and strokes because we cannot manufacture our own Vitamin C and generally get too few vitamins in our diet." Matthias Rath, M.D.

HEARTBURN (ACID REFLUX)
- Emotions: feeling everyone is against you, gut-level fear.
- Is usually caused from a deficiency of hydrochloric acid. The esophageal sphincter closes tightly, preventing acid from coming up into the throat when hydrochloric acid (HCL) levels are optimal. Burping is caused from acid being produced by fermenting proteins in the digestive tract. In order to produce hydrochloric acid, the body needs potassium and zinc.
- Do not drink alkaline water with your food (two hours before or after), as this dilutes the acid levels in the stomach needed for proper digestion.
- 87 percent of people have low HCL. After the age of 40, the HCL levels begin to decrease, and supplementing with HCL or enzymes may be beneficial.
- Eating an apple a day can help.

Acid Reflux Oil Remedy
- Peppermint oil 1 drop
- Lemon oil 1 drop

Mix with 1 Tbsp. of apple cider vinegar and a tsp of honey. Drink with 4 oz. of water

- Avoid caffeine, alcohol, nicotine & chocolate, which cause the sphincter muscle to relax, triggering reflux.
- Avoid carbonated drinks, artificial sweeteners, fried foods and trans fats. Sensitivities to citrus and tomatoes for some can cause heartburn.
- Eat vegetables, healthy fats and organic meats. Slow cooker meat and vegetables with bone broth is good. Fermented foods like homemade sauerkraut, kimchi & kombucha are good.
- Coffee depletes stomach acid (HCL), as do aspirin, tetracycline, prescription iron, smoking, steroids, beta blockers, Valium, nitrates & Demerol.
- HCL breaks proteins down into amino acids. Pepsin breaks amino acids into peptides, which are needed for neurotransmitters to keep us free from depression. Heartburn (indigestion) may be the true cause of depression for most people.
- Himalayan sea salt is a good source of chloride needed to manufacture HCL.
- Supplement your meals with potassium, zinc, and pepsin.
- Helicobacter pylori bacteria may be a factor. Kava Kalm eradicates H. pylori.
- Take 1 to 2 tablespoons of apple cider vinegar in 4 ounces of water 20 minutes before each meal. (You may add in a little honey if needed.) This increases the production of hydrochloric acid needed for digestion.
- Licorice root can help. Licro Plus is good.

Heartburn / Acid Reflux Support	
Alpha Gest	2 capsules with meals
Alpha Green II	2 capsules with meals
Hydrangea Plus	50 drops twice daily

- Fennel and ginger oil are good for digestion and ulcer prevention.
- A spoonful of buttermilk before meals can be beneficial.
- Tums and Rolaids coat the villi in the small intestine, so you don't absorb your nutrition as well. BR-SP Plus helps cleanse the sludge or coating of calcium from the villi.
- *I recommend Hydrangea Plus, Alpha Gest, Alpha Gest II or Alpha Gest III, Alpha Green II, Complete Probiotics & BR-SP Plus*

HEAVY METAL POISONING

- Trace amounts of heavy metals can build up in the body and cause health problems. Mercury binds to fatty tissues of the body like the brain.
- Turkey tail mushroom, according to Paul Stamets' research, rids the body of heavy metals.
- Cilantro, garlic, L-Glutamine, Glutathione, Selenium, Vitamin C, milk thistle, bentonite clay & Vitamin E are good.

Heavy Metals
Mercury
Aluminum
Lead
Arsenic
Cadmium
Nickel
Copper
Uranium
Thallium

- Intravenous chelation (EDTA) & DMPS-Glutathione therapies help remove metals from the body.
- *I suggest Metatox, KLS–Enviro, Kelp Complex, chlorella, Alpha Oxzyme & Hepachol*

Sources of Heavy Metals
- Vaccinations/Flu shot
- Silver dental fillings
- Fish (farmed)
- Household cleaners
- Insecticides
- Drinking water
- Tattoos
- Toothpaste
- Deodorants
- Antacids
- Metal pots/pans
- Cosmetics
- Coal power plants
- Automobile exhaust
- Cigarette smoke
- Floor polish/wax

HEMORRHOIDS

- Emotions: inability to let go, fear & tension, feeling burdened
- Hemorrhoids are swollen and inflamed veins in the rectum that form when we are constipated and strain when having a bowel movement. Like a rubber band that has the ability to expand and contract, so should your colon. When it balloons out, we call it a hemorrhoid. Copper is the mineral that allows it to expand and contract. Varicose veins and aneurysms are the next step if support isn't provided.
- Take natural laxatives and drink more water to keep the bowels moving easily so you don't have to strain.
- Prunes, prune juice, aloe vera juice, flaxseeds, chia seeds, lots of greens, apples, pears, berries, figs and fermented foods are good.
- Magnesium may help relax muscles so you're not so "uptight."
- Butcher's broom, horse chestnut and pygnogenol are good.
- Cypress oil mixed with olive oil applied topically can be soothing.
- *I recommend Chestnut Plus, Veno Plus & Vascutin*

HERPES (COLD SORES)

- Emotions: bitter words left unspoken, feelings of guilt, shame & anger
- Herpes Simplex I usually refers to fever blisters and cold sores.
- Herpes II Progenitalis usually refers to genital infections.
- L-Lysine at 3,000 mg daily, cat's claw, echinacea and golden seal can be very beneficial.
- Sangre de Drago is effective for healing cold sores.
- Garlic, aloe vera, echinacea, elderberry, astragalus, calendula and licorice root are beneficial.
- Vitamins C and E, zinc and B complex are good.
- *Recipe No. 1* Tea tree oil, myrrh, and clove oil mixed with some coconut oil and applied topically is good.
- *Recipe No. 2* Mixing some manuka honey with coconut oil, lavender oil and peppermint oil and applied topically helps clear up cold sores.
- Vitamin D at 50,000 IUs a day for 3 days will jump start the immune system.

- *I recommend Arco Plus, Camu Plus, Cat's Claw, Olive Leaf, Allibiotic, Alpha E Spleen, Immune Support & Alpha Flavin*

HIGH CHOLESTEROL

> "Sugar and refined carbs - not fat - are responsible for the epidemic of obesity, type 2 diabetes, and heart disease and the increased risk of dementia and premature deaths." Mark Hyman, M.D.

- 80 percent of all cholesterol is manufactured in your liver, regardless of what you eat. If you want healthy cholesterol levels, support your liver and your body will balance cholesterol levels just fine. Avoid falling into the pharmaceutical trap of taking dangerous statin drugs that do not reduce your risk of heart disease or stroke, but have dangerous side effects and rob you of one of the most important nutrients in the body for overall good health.
- Dietary fat and saturated fat do not raise saturated fats in your blood and cause heart disease.
- Carbohydrates — not dietary fats — cause heart disease.
- When you consume sugar and refined carbohydrates, you get more of the small LDL (bad cholesterol).
- When you eat saturated fat, you get more of the good, light, fluffy cholesterol.
- Essential fatty acids such as borage oil, fish oil & flaxseed oil are good for cholesterol.
- Niacin and garlic are good.
- Bergamot oil is good.

Cholesterol Is Needed For...
- Healthy brain function – memory & serotonin (feel good) receptors
- Manufacturing sex hormones: testosterone, estrogen, progesterone & DHEA
- Libido (A healthy sex drive)
- Healthy nerve function & myelin sheath
- Essential for building cell membranes
- Healthy immune system – production of lymphocytes, T-cells, helper T-cells
- LDL inactivates many strains of bacteria
- Helps liver produce bile acids for healthy digestion & waste removal
- Helps intestinal function, prevention of leaky gut & repairs damaged cells
- Helps mineral absorption, acts as a carrier for vitamins A, D, E & K

- I highly suggest reading the chapter on cholesterol so you understand that cholesterol is not your enemy. A healthy liver and gallbladder = healthy cholesterol.
- Eat vegetables, healthy fats, nuts, seeds, olive oil, avocados & salmon.
- Avoid trans fats, sugar and grains, the true culprits of heart disease.
- Eggs contain lecithin, which balances cholesterol levels in the body.
- *I suggest KLS Enviro, Omega Complete, Chola Plus, Hepachol & Beta Plus*

HIGH TRIGLYCERIDES

- Triglycerides are lipids or fat in your blood. When you eat more calories than you burn, the extras are converted into triglycerides and stored in your fat cells.

- Triglycerides are manufactured in our liver from the carbohydrates we consume.
- Avoid sugary foods, soft drinks, fruit juices and grains such as breads, pasta, crackers, rice, corn and oats. Eat lots of vegetables, healthy fats such as eggs, avocados, coconut oil, nuts and seeds. Wild-caught salmon, grass-fed beef, chicken & turkey are good.

Triglycerides	
Normal	150 or lower
Borderline High	150 - 199
High	200 - 499
Very High	500 or higher

- Garlic, fish oil, niacin, holy basil and alpha lipoic acid are good.
- *I suggest Ginger Plus II, Chola Plus, Diadren Forte, Diabetic Formula & Cinnamon 6*

HOT FLASHES

- Emotions: fear of aging, not feeling good enough, not being wanted
- The No. 1 cause of hormonal problems is stress. Hot flashes indicate that hormones are out of balance. Hormones are manufactured in the endocrine system. The adrenal glands manufacture sex hormones, and when we get stressed out (fight or flight), the adrenals can become exhausted. This will pull the thyroid out of balance as well. Supporting the adrenal glands through stressful times is important to keep hormones balanced. Adrenal support includes Licro Plus, Her Formula, Adrena Plus & MG/K Aspartate.

Hot Flash Oil Formula
▪ Clary Sage   5 drops
▪ Peppermint   5 drops
▪ Ylang Ylang 5 drops
▪ Chamomile   5 drops
Mix with 1 Tbsp. of carrier oil & massage onto skin or add oils to a warm bath.

- A toxic liver can cause hot flashes. KLS Enviro & Hepachol are good.
- *I suggest FHS Formula, Her Formula, Cohosh Plus, Female Formula, Female Balance, MB Builder, Endo Glan F, Evening primrose oil & Progesterone cream*

HYPERTENSION (HIGH BLOOD PRESSURE)

- We are all unique individuals, and some of us have higher or lower blood pressure than others. Healthy blood pressure levels can vary.
- The intersalt study compared 52 groups of people in 32 different countries and concluded that salt consumption has very little influence on blood pressure. According to Dr. David Watts, a high-salt diet causing high blood pressure is mostly a myth in most cases. Only about 10 to 15 percent may benefit from restricting salt. High amounts of sodium chloride and even potassium chloride have been shown to elevate blood pressure. Hormone (cortisol) levels are higher in the mornings than at night. This is evident with most men waking up with an

Normal Blood Pressure
Systolic **110-135**
Diastolic **65-85**

erection. This is also why blood pressure will usually be higher in the mornings than at night.
- Avoid coffee, alcohol and smoking, as they have been shown to raise blood pressure.
- High blood pressure is an emergency warning sign sent out by the cells when they are starving for oxygen and nutrition. The body increases blood pressure so more nutrition and oxygen can squeeze through clogged arteries and reach cells far away from the heart. We take blood pressure medication that acts as a dictator to force the body to reduce the pressure. The cells that screamed for nutritional support were told to "shut up" as the new high blood pressure dictator drug is now running the show. Eventually, those deprived cells become diseased, and then we ask for more drugs to deal with neuropathy, numbness, tingling, cold hands and feet and poor memory. Understand that the body is producing symptoms for a reason, and the purpose is to get our attention so that we fix the problem. Just as a smoke detector warns us of a fire, high blood pressure warns us of inflammation in the body, increasing pressure. Turning the smoke alarm off without finding the fire is as foolish as taking blood pressure medication without identifying why it is elevated.

Essential Oils For HBP
- Lavender   1 drop
- Frankincense 1 drop
- Clary Sage   1 drop
- Ylang Ylang 1 drop
Mix with steaming water and inhale for 5 minutes every night.

- Increased blood pressure can be caused from a calcium, magnesium & potassium deficiency. Magnesium helps dissolve calcium deposits, restricting blood flow in arteries.
- The adrenal glands help regulate blood pressure.
- Dr. Joseph Mercola explains that HBP is caused from a potassium deficiency.
- Potassium regulates heart muscle action and arterial blood pressure. Dulse, kelp, lima beans, bananas, apricots, prunes, almonds, avocados, spinach & walnuts are good potassium sources.
- Too much table salt and not enough organic sodium from vegetables may cause HBP. Eat celery, olives, beet greens, spinach, Swiss chard, dulse, kelp, Irish moss & dandelion.
- Pink Himalayan or sea salt is fine.

High Blood Pressure Lowering Foods
- Celery
- Olives
- Swiss Chard
- Beet Greens
- Avocados
- Dulse
- Spinach
- Kelp
- Broccoli
- Romaine lettuce

- Allergies can cause the arteries to swell up and narrow, thus causing increased pressure. Do an allergy test. Gluten and dairy are the usual offenders.
- Eat a no-grain, high-fat diet. Eliminate breads, pasta, corn, potatoes, rice & oats.
- Essential fatty acids and Vitamin C can help. Fish oil and flaxseed oil are good.
- Cadmium and lead poisoning from cigarette smoke, and even second-hand smoke, can cause elevated blood pressure. Mercury poisoning can be a culprit.
- Toxic liver or kidneys can cause fluid levels in the body to be high.
- Eat three cloves of garlic and lots of celery daily.
- Exercise is crucial for optimal blood pressure.
- Vitamin D is important.
- Garlic, cayenne, goldenseal, hawthorn and ginseng can help normalize blood pressure.
- Nattokinase dissolves fibrinogen, a component of blood clots and atherosclerotic plaque. It also lowers blood viscosity, which lowers systolic and diastolic blood pressure.
- Dr. Mark Hyman, as well as a friend of mine who is a cardiovascular surgeon, teaches that when the blood pressure runs high for a week, 150/100, it poses almost no danger, unless you are experiencing rapid drops.
- *I suggest Hawthorn Plus, Cal Lac Plus, MG/K Aspartate, Circu Plus, Alpha Green II & Rena Plus*

HYPOTENSION

- Low blood pressure many times is caused from weak adrenal glands. Stress exhausts the adrenals. Common symptoms are dizziness, fainting, blurred vision, fatigue, nausea and confusion.

ADRENAL TEST
- Take your blood pressure lying down
- Immediately stand up and take it again
- It should go up 5-10 points. If it does not, your adrenals are exhausted.

- Ginseng helps balance the body and regulate fluid levels. Licorice root is good.
- Eat salty foods like celery, okra, spinach, cucumbers, olives, parsley, apricots, strawberries, figs, collard greens, eggs and spirulina, and use pink Himalayan sea salt.
- Vitamins B12, D & C are important.
- Holy basil, bergamot and ginger oils can help regulate blood pressure. Take 2 drops of each oil twice daily in water or mix with 1 Tbsp. of coconut oil.
- *I recommend Licro Plus, Norepinephrine, Adrena Plus & MG/K Aspartate*

HYPOGLYCEMIA

- Blood sugar levels below 60 – 70 mg/dl indicate hypoglycemia. Low blood sugar can be caused from weak adrenal glands.
- Licorice, juniper berries, ginger, ginseng and cayenne can help.
- Chromium and vanadium are important for the pancreas to function correctly.
- The sycosis miasm can affect the pancreas.
- Eat green leafy vegetables, nuts, seeds, avocados, butter, coconut oil, olive oil, sweet potatoes, beans, wild-caught fish, eggs, buckwheat, grass-fed beef and chicken.
- *I recommend Diadren Forte, Ginger Plus I & Cinnamon 6*

HYPOTHYROIDISM

- Emotions: fears self-expression, not speaking up for what you think or feel. Feeling like a victim.
- The body will do everything in its power to keep the blood in homeostasis. So, before the blood chemistries change (showing abnormal T-3 or T-4 levels), the blood will rob from tissue to maintain homeostasis, thus showing normal thyroid levels in the bloodwork, when in actuality you may have hypothyroidism. Bloodwork is not always accurate.

Hypothyroid Symptoms
- Fatigue
- Weight gain
- Morning headaches
- Depression
- Constipation
- Cold body temperature
- Thinning hair
- Mental sluggishness

- Weak adrenal function, usually from stress, will pull the thyroid out of balance. So before jumping on thyroid medication, some adrenal support many times will balance the thyroid gland. Licro Plus and Adrena Plus are good.
- 90 percent of doctors test TSH (thyroid-stimulating hormone), which is produced in the pituitary gland and stimulates the thyroid to release T4 and T3 into the blood. This is only one part of the thyroid equation.
- The thyroid gland is only responsible for about 7 percent of your body's active thyroid hormone (T3). The other 93 percent thyroid hormone (T4) produced is inactive. The liver and kidneys are responsible for converting thyroid hormones. 60 percent of your total T3 occurs in the liver, so if you have a toxic liver (most Americans do), the conversion of thyroid hormones may not be occurring. Once again, like the adrenals, you may need liver support and not thyroid support to fix the problem. Liver support includes KLS Enviro, Hepachol or Beta Plus.
- Selenium is required to convert T-4 to T-3. Supplement with trace minerals.

- The PDR (Physicians Desk Reference) says, *"Do not take Synthroid if your adrenal glands are not making enough hormone."* Did your doctor check your adrenal hormones before prescribing thyroid medication? Oops!
- Sea vegetables like kelp are high in iodine, which nourishes the thyroid gland. A deficiency can cause goiters. When the thyroid is deficient in iodine, it will swell (goiter) in an attempt to pull iodine from the blood. Kelp Complex & Thyro Plus are good.
- Iodine must bind to a protein molecule to get to the thyroid. So, if you have indigestion, heartburn or are taking acid blockers and Tums, you are not digesting your foods and most likely not absorbing your nutrients adequately, thus iodine is not making it to the thyroid. Make sure your hydrochloric acid (HCL) levels are balanced and you are properly digesting your foods. Alpha Gest III or Alpha Zyme III are good.

Toxins Affecting Thyroid
- Heavy Metals
- Vaccines/Flu shots
- Silver fillings
- Soy
- Cosmetics
- Deodorants
- Chlorine/fluoride (water)
- Diet Drinks (Splenda)
- Lyme Disease
- Epstein-Barr (mono) virus
- Stress

- Avoid soy, as it is an endocrine gland disruptor. It can inactivate drugs like Synthroid, that's why the drug manufacturers tell you to avoid it. Many vegans eat soy and have thyroid issues.
- Avoid tap water containing chlorine and fluoride. Fluoride disrupts iodine in the thyroid.
- Chlorine is a toxic chemical to the thyroid.
- Splenda, the artificial sweetener with a chlorine molecule, is a neurotoxin that disrupts thyroid function. Avoid artificial sweeteners so your nerves, brain and endocrine system can function! They lead to intestinal cancer.
- Heavy metals, especially mercury, accumulate in the thyroid gland. High levels of copper can interfere with thyroid function and have an antagonistic effect upon iron. An iron deficiency can impair thyroid function. Iron is necessary for L-phenylalanine to convert to L-tyrosine, which is the precursor to the thyroid hormone thyroxine. Red meat and vegetables are high in iron. Dairy products (milk and cheese) can reduce iron absorption as much as 60 percent. Tannic acid in tea will reduce iron absorption as well. Antacids decrease stomach acids, which reduce iron availability as well.
- Too much lithium interferes with iodine uptake by the thyroid.
- Test for Epstein-Barr virus, which can sabotage healthy thyroid function.
- Radiation can affect the thyroid. Spirulina and dulse help remove radioactive iodine from the thyroid to bring it back into balance.
- If you have low ferritin (iron), the thyroid can't convert thyroid hormones.

- Avoid bromines found in flour to make breads and pastries (to keep them fresh) and Mountain Dew (brominated vegetable oil). They are endocrine disruptors, especially the thyroid. They displace iodine.
- Zinc is crucial to help the body absorb iodine. Pumpkin seeds are high in zinc.
- L-tyrosine is an important contributor to a healthy functioning thyroid.
- Ashwagandha helps balance thyroid hormones.
- Selenium is good, and medicinal mushrooms, nuts & seeds are good sources.
- Beets & goji berries are good.
- Vitamin B complex and probiotics are good.
- Pesticides, chemicals and heavy metals accumulate in the glands and need to be detoxified in order to achieve balance.
- Diadren Forte supports the liver, adrenals and enzymes to aid in the digestion of fats, carbs and proteins.
- Eat healthy fats like coconut oil, seaweeds, kefir, kombucha, sauerkraut, salmon, green leafy vegetables and bone broth. Slow cooker or steamed vegetables are good.
- Avoid gluten and dairy.
- Rubbing the essential oils lemongrass and myrrh on your neck (thyroid) area twice daily can help.
- *I suggest Kelp Complex, KLS Enviro, Thyro Plus, Endo Glan Plus, Omega Complete & Diadren Forte*

> "I believe iodine deficiency is the number one nutritional problem affecting a vast majority of Americans. Iodine deficiency is the main reason we are seeing such an epidemic of thyroid disorders including hypothyroidism, autoimmune thyroid disorders and thyroid cancer." David Brownstein, M.D.

IRRITABLE BOWEL SYNDROME

Gut Healers
Probiotics
Colostrum
Vitamin D
Glutamine
Fish oil
Turmeric

- Emotions: ugly, indigestible conflict, anger
- Check for parasites, as they can cause inflammation, infection and discomfort. Verma Plus, L/GB-AP Plus and Para Plus expel parasites.
- Test for food allergies, as gluten and dairy cause a lot of inflammation.
- Eat a gluten-free diet. No human can fully digest wheat, barley and rye.
- Take probiotics. Eating fermented foods is beneficial.
- Slow cooker vegetables with chicken or beef and bone broth is very healing for the gut. Avocados, salmon, eggs and coconut oil are good.

- Digestive enzymes are important. Alpha Gest III or Diadren Forte is good.
- Mix 1 drop of ginger oil with 1 drop of peppermint oil in 8 ounces of water and drink twice daily.
- *I suggest Immu C, Universal Complex, BR-SP, Alpha Gest III, Omega Complete, Colostrum & Complete Probiotics*

INCONTINENCE
- Muscle clenching or Kegel exercises, where you contract the floor of the pelvis as if trying to stop urine flow, can help strengthen the muscles that wrap around the urethra.
- Calcium, magnesium and selenium are important.
- *I suggest K/B Plus, Rena Plus & Cal Lac Plus*

IMPETIGO
- A highly contagious bacterial skin infection that usually affects infants and young children.
- Children need to wash their hands often and keep fingernails short. Adding some peppermint and tea tree oil in with a homemade soap or natural hand sanitizer is beneficial.
- Apple cider vinegar on a cotton ball, applied to the blisters on the skin, fights bacteria and eases inflammation.
- Coconut oil can be applied to the skin as well to help heal lesions. Manuka honey is beneficial.
- A few drops of tea tree oil mixed with 1 tsp. of coconut oil and applied topically is beneficial.
- Vitamins A & C are good, as are ginger, turmeric and grapefruit seed extract.
- *I suggest Echinacea & Goldenseal Formula, Red Clover Blend or Red Root Combination (for children)*

INDIGESTION
- Emotions: fear of losing job, losing security. Feeling everyone is against you.
- Dark circles under the eyes indicate problems in the small intestines, usually with the ileocecal valve. Supplement your diet with hydrochloric acid, pepsin and enzymes so you can break down your food. Alpha Gest III is good.
- If you experience bloating after every meal, you probably need more minerals, especially magnesium, potassium and zinc, which are needed for the stomach to manufacture hydrochloric acid. Alpha Zyme III is good.
- Chew your food 30 times before swallowing. Don't drink liquids with your meals. Wait 30 minutes before or after a meal to drink liquids.
- Support your adrenal glands with pantothenic acid. Diadren Forte is good.
- Follow proper food combining chart.

- Ginger can be beneficial, and peppermint oil is good. Probiotics can help.
- Basil is good for stomach cramps, nausea and gas.
- Don't eat late at night, no later than 6 p.m.
- 85 percent of adults have parasites. If you experience bloating after eating, you may need a parasite cleanse. Take EGA III, LG/B-AP & Para Plus.
- Bloating and burping after eating is usually a sign that the liver isn't producing enough bile to break down fats. Take Diadren Forte or Beta Plus.
- Take 2 tablespoons of apple cider vinegar in water with 1 teaspoon of honey before each meal. This increases the production of hydrochloric acid.
- *I recommend Hydrangea Plus, Universal Complex, Alpha Gest III, Alpha Green II & BR-SP Plus*

INFERTILITY / PREGNANCY

- Infertility can be caused from smoking, irregular periods and infections such as chlamydia.
- Suma and maca help nourish the reproductive organs and are high in amino acids, which play a big role in proper glandular function. Her Formula is good.
- Yarrow is good to balance the endocrine system, where hormones are manufactured.
- The adrenal glands contribute 35 percent of female hormones. After menopause, it's 50 percent, so if you have hormonal issues, support the adrenals. Licro Plus and Adrena Plus are good.
- Pregnancy cannot occur with improper adrenal function.

Low Cholesterol = Low Testosterone

- When people become acidic (acidosis), it can kill off sperm.

Herbs To Avoid During Pregnancy			
Aloe vera	Angelica	Arnica	Barberry
Black cohosh	Blue cohosh	Bloodroot	Cat's claw
Celandine	Dong quai	Feverfew	Ginseng
Goldenseal	Lobelia	Myrrh	Oregon grape
Pennyroyal	Rue	Sage	Saw palmetto
Tansy	Turmeric	Ephedra	Yohimbe

- Hormones need fats. Eat avocados, olives, eggs, butter, coconut oil, nuts & seeds. Use sea salt instead of regular iodized salt.
- Avoid soy, as it is an endocrine disruptor.
- Avoid drinking and eating out of plastic containers that have harmful PCBs in them.
- Avoid drinking public water. Public water contains estrogen hormones from all the women on birth control pills.

- Dong quai, wild yam, chaste tree berry, Schizandra, nettle, evening primrose oil, zinc, Vitamin E, Vitamin C, calcium and magnesium are all beneficial.
- CBD oil, lemon, ylang ylang and thyme oil are good.
- *I recommend Her Formula, MB Builder, Ovary Uterus Plus, Omega Complete & Endo Glan F*

INSECT BITES

- Poisonous snake and spider bites need immediate medical attention. Consult your doctor.
- Clean the area with warm, soapy water. Apply ice for 10 minutes to reduce swelling.
- A baking soda paste applied to wound helps. Simply mix some baking soda with a water and put on skin.
- Aloe vera is good for skin ailments.
- Do not scratch area, as this can worsen condition and spread infection.
- Echinacea, "king of the blood purifiers," will neutralize poisons in the blood. Take two dropperfuls every 15 minutes for several hours to help detoxify venom out of the body until you can get to the hospital.
- Black widow bite – Rub 1 drop of lavender oil over bite every 3 minutes until you reach the hospital.
- Brown recluse spider bite – Mix 1 drop lavender, 1 drop helichrysum & 1 drop Melrose together and apply to bite. Cover with oatmeal poultice.
- Lavender oil applied to spider bites can help relieve pain and inflammation and encourage healing.
- Lemon, peppermint, eucalyptus & lemongrass repels mosquitoes.
- Clove, thyme, oregano, citronella, vetiver, lemongrass & peppermint oils repel ticks. Apply thyme oil to tick to loosen from skin.
- Remove ticks from skin as soon as possible. Grab the tick as close to your skin with tweezers and pull out slowly with steady pressure, making sure to get its head. Once removed, wash the bite area with soap and water. Tick bites can

---

Essential Oil Bug Spray
- ½ cup Witch Hazel
- ½ cup Apple Cider Vinegar
- 40 drops Eucalyptus Oil
- 40 drops Lemongrass Oil
- 40 drops Citronella Oil
- 40 drops Tea tree Oil

Mix all ingredients in a spray bottle. Spray all over body, avoid mouth and eyes.

Mosquito, Tick & Ant Repellent
- 80% Water in 8 oz spray bottle
- 20% Isopropyl Alcohol
- 15 drops Rosemary
- 15 drops Peppermint
- 15 drops Lavender
- 15 drops Juniper (for ticks)

Tick Repellent
20 drops Lemongrass
20 drops Eucalyptus
4 oz. water

transmit: Lyme disease, Rocky Mountain spotted fever, Colorado tick fever, Tularemia & Ehrlichiosis.
- Neem oil can help. Raw honey on bites can help with pain and inflammation.
- Peppermint, tea tree, clove & lemon oils repel ants.
- Lavender, helichrysum, chamomile & birch oils are good for bee stings.
- *I recommend Echinacea Complex*

INSOMNIA
- Emotions: feelings of fear & anxiety. Deep-seated guilt. Not trusting the process of life.
- Your pineal gland, which secretes melatonin to help you sleep, needs 45 minutes of sunlight each day to be activated. This is why you sleep so good at night after spending a day swimming in the sun.
- Calcium, magnesium and potassium can help relax the body so that you can sleep.
- Valerian root, hops, lobelia, passionflower, chamomile and skullcap are good.
- Melatonin and serotonin can be beneficial.

Chinese Meridian Clock
11 p.m. – 1 a.m. Gallbladder
1 a.m. – 3 a.m. Liver
3 a.m. – 5 a.m. Adrenals (Lungs)

- Heavy metals can disrupt the nervous system, causing you not to be able to sleep.
- If you wake up from 11 p.m. to 1 a.m., that's usually an issue with the gallbladder. Take 2 capsules of Beta Plus with each meal and 50 drops of Hydrangea Plus twice daily.
- If you wake up from 1 a.m. to 3 a.m., the liver is most likely the problem. Take 2 capsules of Hepachol with each meal and 50 drops of KLS Enviro twice daily.
- If you wake up from 3 a.m. to 5 a.m., weak adrenal glands are usually the culprit. Take 3 capsules of Adrena Plus with each meal along with 2 MG/K capsules with meals, and see if you start sleeping better. Licro Plus at 50 drops twice daily supports the adrenals too. Other common symptoms associated with sluggish adrenals are fatigue (especially after lunch), low libido, depression and dizziness.
- Serotonin, L-tryptophan and 5 HTP before bed can help.
- GABA can help you relax and sleep.
- Nocturnal hypoglycemia (when your blood sugar drops while sleeping at night) causes you to wake up and have to get something to eat in order to get

Sleep Formula
- SLP Formula   25 drops before bed
- Valeri Plus   50 drops before bed
- MGK Aspartate   2 capsules before bed

back to sleep. The body produces cortisol (a hormone produced in the adrenal glands in response to stress and blood sugar regulation) from 3 to 4 a.m. When the blood sugar rises, it relaxes the nervous system and you can fall back asleep. Try eating a bedtime snack that's high in tryptophan (amino acid to help sleep). Foods high in tryptophan include eggs, nuts (almonds), chicken, turkey & cottage cheese.

- Vitamin B12 helps produce melatonin for sleep.
- Siberian ginseng is good for balancing rhythms in the body that may help with sleep.
- Remember, artificial sweeteners are excitotoxins that stimulate the brain. Avoid them.
- Do not take naps during the day. Work a job or stay busy with a hobby. Watching TV on the couch all day will cause you not to sleep well at night.
- A hot Epsom salt bath (2 cups) with 20 drops of lavender oil for 20 to 30 minutes can help you relax and sleep.
- Breathing in the essential oils chamomile, lavender, ylang ylang and clary sage can help you relax and sleep. Rub them on your temples, back of your neck, and bottom of your feet or diffuse them by your bed at nights.
- *I recommend Nerve Formula, Valeri Plus, MG/K Aspartate, Diadren Forte & SLP Formula*

> **Deep Breathing Exercise**
> - Breathe in deep and slow through your nose to the count of five, then breathe out for five. Repeat three times.
> - Doing this several times throughout the day is great for anxiety and relaxation.

KIDNEY DISEASE

- Emotions: criticism, being over-judgmental, shame.
- The kidneys filter toxins out of the blood and regulate fluid levels in the body.
- Goldenrod, uva ursi, parsley, corn silk, juniper berries, horsetail, burdock and gravel root are all good kidney flushers.
- Magnesium helps dissolve kidney stones.
- Alpha Ortho Phos (Orthophosphoric acid) can dissolve stones as well.

> **Kidney Stone Dissolver**
> - Alpha Ortho Phos 30 drops every hour for 2-3 days
> - Stonebreaker Plus 30 drops every hour for 2-3 days

> **Lemon Juice Kidney Stone Eliminator**
> 1. Mix 2 oz olive oil with 2 oz of lemon juice. Drink straight. Follow with 12 oz filtered water. Wait 30 minutes.
> 2. Juice half a lemon into 12 oz filtered water, add 1 tbsp apple cider vinegar. Drink.
> 3. Repeat the lemon juice/filtered water & apple cider vinegar every hour until symptoms are eliminated.

- Cranberries and celery juice are excellent. Blueberries, black cherries, beets, spirulina, spinach, and chlorella are good.
- Fear is the emotion that effects the kidneys. People get scared and wet their pants. When fear overtakes the body, the nerves corresponding to the muscles of the urinary tract short circuit. MG/K Aspartate & Kava Kalm are good.
- *I recommend Solidago Plus, K/B Plus, Stonebreaker Plus & Rena Plus*

LARYNGITIS (SEE SORE THROAT)
- Emotions: fear of speaking up, voicing opinions. Resentment of authority.
- Inflammation of the vocal cords.
- Ginger, garlic, echinacea, marshmallow root and Vitamin C are good.
- Lemon and peppermint oils are good. Add 2 drops of each to a warm glass of water with a little honey and apple cider vinegar.
- *I suggest Otalga Plus, Camu Plus, Allibiotic, Immune Formula & Alpha Flavin*

LEAKY GUT
- Leaky gut, also known as intestinal permeability syndrome, is when your intestinal lining becomes so porous that undigested foods, yeast, toxins and waste products absorb into the bloodstream because the "tight junctions" have now become "loose and porous."
- Food proteins that make their way into the bloodstream through the gut wall cause an inflammatory response (allergies) as the immune system reacts to them as foreign invaders.
- When you have leaky gut, typically whatever you are eating a lot of will show up as food allergies. Even healthy foods such as fruits and vegetables may show up as food allergies if they are passing through the intestinal wall into the blood and the body recognizes them as foreign toxins. After we heal and seal the gut, many food allergies/sensitivities are eliminated.

Causes Of Leaky Gut
- Prescription Drugs – antibiotics, birth control pills, steroids, pain medications, acid-blockers, statins & chemotherapy
- Heavy metals, fungus, candida yeast & mold
- Pesticides/Chemicals
- Gluten, Dairy, Sugar, GMO foods
- Parasites
- Low stomach acid, insufficient enzymes
- Food allergies
- Gallbladder, appendix removal
- H. Pylori bacterial infection
- Stress, high cortisol levels

Microbiome Healers
- Probiotics
- Vitamin D-3
- Glutamine
- Fish Oil
- Colostrum
- Licorice Root
- Frankincense
- Zinc Carnosine

- Chronic stress increases cortisol levels, which break down the protective lining of your intestinal wall, thus causing leaky gut. This leads to low libido, waking up still feeling tired in the mornings, anxiety, depression and belly fat.
- You have over 100 trillion microscopic organisms (bacteria) living in your gut and over 500 species. These 3 to 5 pounds of bacteria outnumber the cells in your body 10 to 1 and help aid in digestion and keep the gut wall healthy. This is your microbiome.
- Taking an antibiotic destroys your gut's microbiome.
- Birth control pills promote yeast infections.
- If you experience gas/bloating, food sensitivities, thyroid issues, chronic fatigue, skin issues, migraines and diabetes, you probably have leaky gut.

Gut Healing Foods
▪ Bone broth
▪ Kefir (from goat's milk)
▪ Fermented vegetables
▪ Steamed vegetables
▪ Omega 3s (salmon)
▪ Coconut oil

- Vaccinations are a major source of inflammation. They contain foreign proteins that can trigger leaky gut.
- Acid reflux medication contributes to inflammation and leaky gut.
- Probiotics, glutamine, colostrum, fish oil, Vitamin D, zinc carnosine, digestive enzymes, licorice root and frankincense oil are good to heal the gut.
- Epstein-Barr virus is almost always present with leaky gut.

Gut Healing Oils
▪ Peppermint 1 drop
▪ Lemon oil   1 drop
▪ Ginger oil   1 drop
▪ Chamomile 1 drop
Mix oils in 8 oz of water and drink 15 minutes before each meal.

- *I suggest Immu Boost, Immu C, Arco Plus, BR SP Plus, Alpha Green II, Colostrum & Complete Probiotics*

LICE

- Mix 1 Tbsp. tea tree oil with 3 Tbsp. of olive or coconut oil and cover your head with a shower cap. Leave on for ½ hour, then rinse.
- Lavender and eucalyptus oil can help.
- Wash all clothing and linens that may be infected in the hottest water possible. Dry in dryer at high temperature for at least 20 minutes.
- Another recipe that works well is 3 Tbsp. coconut oil, 1 tsp. ylang ylang, 1 tsp. anise and 1 tsp. tea tree oil. Blend all ingredients together and massage all over hair and scalp. Cover head in shower cap for 2 hours. Remove shower cap and comb hair. While hair is wet, combine 2 cups apple cider vinegar with 1 cup water in a spray bottle. Lean over sink and generously spray on hair and then comb hair out. Repeat this procedure until bottle is empty.

LIVER DISORDERS
- Emotions: Unresolved anger & resentment. Not forgiving, being judgmental.
- Your liver performs over 500 functions. Your health and vitality depend largely upon your liver. A well-functioning liver is a key to good health.
- Burning in the feet, allergies, headaches & arthritis can be caused from a toxic liver.
- Avoid alcohol, vaccines, coffee, tobacco, white bread, margarine, foods cooked in oils, drugs, chlorine and fluoride. These substances are very hard on the liver.
- Hepatitis – inflammation of the liver — is usually caused by a virus. Cat's claw and olive leaf are powerful anti-viral supplements.
- The best herbs for cleansing and strengthening the liver are milk thistle, dandelion, nettles, burdock, barberry, Oregon grape, holy basil, red root and yellow dock.
- For liver failure circumstances, take a high dose of Hepachol (5 capsules 3 times a day).
- *I recommend Dandi Plus, E Plus, KLS Enviro, Hepachol, Omega Complete & Beta Plus*

LOW SEX DRIVE (LIBIDO)
- It is estimated that 43 percent of women have sexual dysfunction.
- Both men and women need testosterone for healthy libido. The adrenal glands manufacture testosterone. Stress will exhaust the adrenals, leaving your sex drive weak. Adrena Plus & Licro Plus are good.
- Low libido in women is usually caused from low testosterone levels. The best essential oils for testosterone are sandalwood, cedarwood and rosemary.

Aphrodisiac Oil Blend
- 2 oz sweet almond oil
- 5 drops lavender oil
- 5 drops sandalwood
- 1 drop ylang-ylang
- 1 drop vanilla
- 1 drop cinnamon
- 1 drop jasmine

Massage on body

Low Cholesterol = Low Testosterone

- Testosterone promotes orgasm and is good for hot flashes.
- Cholesterol is necessary to produce sex hormones. Statin drugs are notorious for sabotaging a healthy sex life. Eat healthy fats (avocados, eggs, olives, butter, coconut oil, nuts and seeds) so your body has cholesterol to manufacture sex hormones.
- Avocados, figs and bananas help increase libido. Almonds, Brazil nuts, watermelon, sweet potatoes and dark chocolate may be beneficial.

- Too much estrogen can cause migraines, breast swelling and edema. Progesterone helps balance estrogen and acts as a mild sedative. It also helps prevent osteoporosis.
- Exercise is important for healthy blood flow. Balance is important. Too much exercise, like marathon runners, can over-stress the body, diminishing a healthy sex drive.
- Essential fatty acids like fish oil, borage, flax, krill and evening primrose oil are good.
- L-arginine, niacin, ginkgo, ginseng and ashwagandha are good.
- Licorice root is good for the adrenals and sexual function.
- Suma is female ginseng. Maca is Brazilian Viagra. It's very beneficial for menopause. It helps with female and male sex drive. Studies have shown that mice given maca reproduced 3 times as much as those who ate a normal diet. Suma and maca can help him and her get things rockin' and rollin' again.

  Maca – The Ultimate Female Aphrodisiac

- *I recommend Adrena Plus, Her or His Formula, Licro Plus, MB Builder, Endo Glan Plus, Omega Complete, FHS Formula or Testosterone*

LUPUS

- The question is, what toxin is in your cells causing the immune system to declare war on them? The body does not attack itself unless there's a toxicity issue. EDS will identify the culprit.

  Possible Toxins Causing Lupus

Heavy Metals	Mercury	Aluminum
Food Allergies	Gluten	Milk
GMOs	Mold	Parasites
Lyme Disease	Pesticides	Chlorine
Epstein-Barr virus	MSG	Fluoride

- Avoid gluten, sugar and trans fats.
- Eat vegetables, healthy fats such as avocados, bone broth, coconut oil, nuts and seeds, cucumbers and wild-caught fish.
- Sodium and potassium levels in the cells need balancing. Take alfalfa, chlorella, bee pollen and spirulina.
- Support the thymus gland.
- Essential fatty acids are important. Omega Complete is good.
- Drinking warm bone broth and supporting the gut is key.
- Lyme disease and heavy metals are common issues.
- Vitamin D, turmeric, holy basil, probiotics & MSM are good.
- Frankincense oil is king. Drink 3 drops in a glass of water twice daily.
- *I suggest Arco Plus, Immu C, KLS Enviro, Alpha Flavin, Omega Complete & Complete Probiotics*

LYME DISEASE

- Lyme disease is a bacteria transmitted from a tick or insect bite. Blood transfusions are another way of contracting Lyme disease.
- Borrelia burgdorferi bacteria is most common, and it can cause auto-immune-like reactions. Lyme is "the great imitator" because it mimics so many disorders such as arthritis, MS, ALS, fibromyalgia, etc.
- If you have aches and pains, burning sensations that jump around in your body, that come and go, then you may have Lyme Disease.
- Eat a gluten-free diet, as gluten adds to inflammation in the body. The Mediterranean or paleo diets are good.
- Lyme can have many co-infections. H pylori, Ehrlichia sennetsu, tularemia go along with Lyme. Bartonella, Borrelia burgdorferi and H pylori can become antibiotic resistance.

Overcoming Lyme Disease
- Cat's Claw   2 capsules 2 x a day
- Olive Leaf   2 capsules 2 x a day
- Ashwagandha   2 capsules 2 x a day
- Teasel Root   50 drops 2 x a day
- Colloidal Silver   2 tsp. 2 x day
- Digestive enzymes 2 with meals
- Protease 2 between meals 3 x a day

- Taking proteolytic enzymes on an empty stomach between meals to help break down the protein-based cell membranes helps expel bacteria and parasites.
- Drinking warm chicken or beef bone broth is good because it's anti-inflammatory and very healing to the gut. It's also anti-fungal.
- Eating fermented vegetables is good.
- Eat white or pale-yellow foods such as ginger, garlic and onions.
- Freeze-dried garlic, chlorella, cilantro & fish oil are good.
- Pau d'Arco, ginger, astragalus & ginseng are good.

Dr. Josh Axe's Lyme Disease Bath
- Chamomile oil   10 drops
- Frankincense oil   10 drops
- Lemongrass oil   10 drops
- Epsom Salt   1 cup

Mix in warm bath and soak for 20-30 minutes 3 times a week.

- Essential oils holy basil, myrrh, rosemary and thyme are good.
- Citronella, lemongrass, peppermint & clove oil repel ticks.
- Magnesium, Vitamins D & A, turmeric (curcumin), CoQ10, B complex, L-carnitine, Omega fatty acids, collagen type 2 and probiotics are beneficial.

> "We never had in the last five years a single MS patient, a single ALS patient, a single Parkinson's patient, who did not test positive for Borrelia Burgdorferi. Not a single one." Dietrich Klinghardt, M.D.

- Green tea extract, broccoli seed extract and resveratrol can be beneficial.
- Strengthening the immune system and improving gut health is the key to overcoming Lyme disease.
- *I suggest cat's claw, olive leaf, Arco plus, teasel root, colloidal silver, complete probiotics & protease*

MENIERE'S DISEASE
- Ringing in the ears, dizziness and nausea are symptoms usually caused from the lymphatic system not draining properly.
- Allergies, especially gluten and dairy, can trigger this. Do an EDS scan to check for allergies. Eat a gluten-free diet.
- Nettles, dandelion, solidago, echinacea, calendula, cat's claw, garlic and cayenne are good lymphatic drainers.
- Vitamin C (Citrus bioflavonoids) can help.
- Poor circulation may be a culprit. Ginkgo, butcher's broom and ginseng are good.
- *I suggest Circu Plus, Universal Complex, Licro Plus, Brain Formula, Alpha Flavin, Adrena Plus & Lymphatic Drainer*

MENOPAUSE
- Is not a disease but a natural process a woman's body goes through when the ovaries stop producing hormones and she no longer has a menstrual cycle, usually from age 45 to 55. Around age 35 your ovaries start (perimenopause) producing less estrogen and progesterone and fertility starts to decline.
- Support the endocrine system so that the glands can produce the hormones you need for balance. After the age of around 50, the adrenal glands become the supplier for estrogen instead of the ovaries.
- Exercise is important. Go for a 20-minute walk daily.
- Stress can deplete the body of hormones, causing imbalances. Adrena Plus, Licro Plus, Nerve Formula and MG/K are good.
- Eat healthy fats such as avocados, eggs, nuts, seeds, coconut oil, olive oil & olives. Cholesterol is needed to manufacture hormones. Stain drugs cause hormonal imbalances.
- Fish, flax and borage seed oils are good.
- Estrogen and testosterone are needed for vaginal lubrication.
- Natural progesterone cream containing wild yam is good.
- Black cohosh, chaste tree berry, angelica, dong quai, licorice, hops, vervain, damiana, ginseng, red raspberry leaves, St. John's wort, sarsaparilla, red clover, ashwagandha,

Hot Flash Eliminator	
FHS Formula	10 drops 3 x daily
Cohosh Plus	50 drops 3 x daily
Endo Glan Plus	2 capsules 3 x daily
Omega Complete	2 capsules 3 x daily

- holy basil, evening primrose & selenium are beneficial.
- Suma is female ginseng. Maca is very beneficial for menopause.
- Avoid synthetic estrogen formulas. Numerous studies show that hormone replacement therapy can increase your risk for breast cancer, blood clots, dementia, incontinence, heart disease and stroke. Only use bioidentical hormones as a last resort. Anytime we put extra hormones in the body, we are playing with fire.

Hot Flash Oil Formula	
Clary Sage	5 drops
Peppermint	5 drops
Ylang Ylang	5 drops
Chamomile	5 drops

Mix with 1 Tbsp. of carrier oil & massage onto skin or add oils to a warm bath.

- *I recommend Her Formula, Female Formula, Cohosh Plus, MB Builder, Omega Complete, Endo Glan Plus & F.H.S.*

MIGRAINE HEADACHE

- Emotions: resisting the flow of life, inability to handle pressure. Dislikes being pushed.
- Migraines can be caused from constipation, too many toxins in the blood stream. Get the bowels moving two to three times a day so toxins have a way out of your body instead of recirculating in the blood, putting pressure on the capillaries, thus causing a headache.
- A toxic liver can trigger headaches. Do a liver cleanse.
- The pituitary and thyroid glands can get knocked out of balance and create hormonal imbalances that trigger migraines. Manganese and kelp are good. Manganese is the mineral that nourishes the anterior pituitary, which can help relieve headaches. It also nourishes discs in the back. Many times, back pain and headaches are caused from a simple manganese deficiency, especially if chiropractic adjustments won't hold.

Migraine Triggers
Gluten
Aged cheese
Red wine (alcohol)
Fried foods
Nitrates in meats
MSG
Aspartame
Eggs
Chocolate
Peanuts
Caffeine
Stress

- Sodium deficiency can trigger headaches. Take spirulina and drink carrot and celery juice.
- Pain behind the left eye may be a zinc deficiency, while pain behind the right eye and the temple may be a cry for iron.
- Nettles, kelp, yellow dock, feverfew, beets and green vegetables are high in iron.
- Vitamin B6 and niacin can be beneficial.
- Tryptophan (amino acid), the precursor to serotonin, can help.
- Blood sugar issues can trigger headaches. Get off carbohydrates and sugars.
- Avoid gluten. No human can fully digest gluten, as it causes inflammation.

- Stop eating dairy. A specific protein called Tyramine in cheese can trigger migraines, as can the protein casein that comes from milk.
- Lectin sensitivity from legumes has been associated with migraines. Test for allergies to beans, peas, lentils & peanuts.
- Fish oil and magnesium can help.
- Exercise can make a difference, as can getting enough sleep.
- Drink plenty of clean, pure water. A 200-pound person needs 100 oz per day.
- Massaging some lavender and peppermint oils on the temples, behind the ears and on the neck can help. Try diffusing the oils or take 2 drops with water or coconut oil twice daily.
- *I recommend Pitui Plus, Endo Glan Plus, Circu Plus, Alpha Flavin, MG/K, Diadren Forte, Brain Formula, KLS Enviro & Gota Plus*

MITRAL VALVE PROLAPSE
- Improper closure of the valve between the heart's upper and lower left chambers.
- Minerals (magnesium, potassium and calcium) are needed for valves to open and close smoothly. MG/K is good.
- Like rust on metal pipes, calcium builds up on cartilage and can interfere with valves opening and closing smoothly. Taking Alpha Ortho Phos, 50 drops 3 times a day, dissolves calcium buildup, arthritis, bone spurs, kidney stones and cataracts which are indications of calcium plaquing occurring in the body. Eat a more alkaline diet (lots of vegetables) to reverse this process.
- CoQ10 and L-carnitine are good.
- *I suggest Heart Formula, Cardi Plus, MG/K & Alpha Ortho Phos*

MONONUCLEOSIS
- Emotions: anger at not receiving love and appreciation.
- Is called "the kissing disease" because it's a viral infection spread through bodily fluids, especially saliva, usually caused by the Epstein-Barr virus (EBV), that causes chronic fatigue. It can cause high fevers and swollen lymph nodes.
- Cat's claw, olive leaf, garlic, echinacea, pau d'arco, astragalus and licorice root are good for the immune system.
- Vitamin B12 and oregano oil are good.
- Homeopathic remedy "Infection EB" is good.
- *I recommend Infection EB, Arco Plus, Camu Plus, Lapacho Plus, Allibiotic, Complete Probiotics & Alpha E Spleen*

MORNING SICKNESS/NAUSEA
- Emotions: rejecting an idea or experience. Fear
- Pregnant women who experience morning sickness are usually suffering from a sodium deficiency. That fetus growing inside is robbing sodium from

the mother, leaving her depleted. Get your sodium levels up. Drinking freshly squeezed carrot and celery juice daily is very beneficial, ensuring that both mother and child get the nutrients they need. Dr. Oz's green drink is very beneficial as well.
- The best foods to replenish depleted sodium levels are spirulina, celery juice, alfalfa, okra (not fried), carrots, cabbage, spinach, strawberries, beets, cucumbers, plums, powdered whey, raw goat's milk, chicken and turkey gizzards.
- Consume soups and bone broth, fruits and vegetables, healthy fats and organic meats.
- Ginger can help with nausea. Peach leaves are good for morning sickness.
- Drink 1 to 2 drops of ginger oil in a glass of water and apply 2 drops of peppermint oil to the bottoms of your feet.
- Chamomile, lavender and lemon oils inhaled may be beneficial.
- Calcium, magnesium and Vitamins D and B6 can help.
- *I suggest homeopathic Morning Sickness, Nausea Relief, Nux Nausea, Alpha Green & intraMAX*

MULTIPLE SCLEROSIS
- Emotions: unwilling to be flexible, unforgiving of self & others, hard-heartedness.
- MS is an autoimmune disorder that affects the central nervous system, usually the myelin. Autoimmune disorders involve toxins causing the immune system to attack. EDS testing identifies the toxins.
- Heavy metals, especially mercury (a neurotoxin), many times is a culprit. The flu shot contains mercury! Stop poisoning your body and expecting it to function normally.
- Get silver dental fillings removed and replaced with composite materials. Locate a biological dentist for a safe extraction.
- Lyme disease and Epstein-Barr virus are involved in most cases. Measles virus may be a factor.
- Tetracycline for acne can cause MS.
- The chemicals xylene and Toluene accumulate in the muscles and can cause MS.
- Evening primrose oil, lipoic acid, Lion's Mane mushroom, magnesium, copper, potassium, B Vitamins, enzymes, fish oil, B12, turmeric and probiotics are beneficial.
- Malvin, pyrrole, serotonin, dopamine, and norepinephrine may help.
- The syphilinum miasm is usually present, affecting the nerves.
- Mold toxicity, food allergies and emotional stress can be contributors, damaging the nerves.

- Get off artificial sweeteners (aspartame) found in diet soft drinks. They are neurotoxins.
- Vitamin D is important. Sun exposure is the best source, at least 20 minutes a day.
- Soaking in a hot essential oil bath three times a week can help. Add 10 drops of rosemary oil, 10 drops of helichrysum oil and 10 drops of basil oil. Soak for 20 to 30 minutes.
- Rub helichrysum oil on your neck and temples daily.
- Taking 2 drops of Frankincense twice daily can help repair damaged nerves.
- Eat healthy fats such as coconut oil, avocados, olives, eggs, nuts, seeds, butter. Your nerves need cholesterol for health. Statin drugs deprive you of basic building blocks for a healthy nervous system.
- Eat a gluten- and dairy-free diet. Consume vegetables, berries, fruits, legumes, wild-caught fish (salmon) and fermented dairy.
- Exercise is important.
- *I suggest Nerve Formula, Gota Plus, Clear Mind, Brain Formula, KLS-Enviro, Arco Plus, Circu Plus, Evening primrose oil, Alpha Oxzyme & MG/K*

NARCOLEPSY
- Emotions: wanting to get away from it all, can't cope, extreme fear.
- Excessive daytime sleepiness that can lead to falling asleep unwillingly.
- Sunlight exposure is important for the pineal gland. Vitamin D is important.
- Exercise is important
- Ginkgo, gotu kola, 5-HTP, Vitamin B12 and fish oil are good.
- *I suggest Clear Mind, Brain Formula, Gota Plus, Circu Plus, Chola Plus, Omega Complete & Alpha Oxzyme*

NAUSEA
- Emotions: rejecting an idea, fear.
- 10 drops of Alpha Ortho Phos in a cup of water can help.
- Vitamin B6 may help.
- Digestive enzymes can help. Take Alpha Gest III or Diadren Forte.
- Massaging lavender, ginger and peppermint oils on your stomach can help. Rubbing them on your temples, behind the ears and on the bottoms of your feet can help.
- Drinking lemon water and inhaling lemon oil can help.
- Drinking chamomile tea is good.
- Cannabis (CBD) oil has proven very beneficial.
- *I suggest Nausea Relief, Nux Nausea, Black Radish Complex, Hydrangea, BR-SP & Alpha Gest III*

NEUROPATHY
- Heavy metals (mercury) can inflame the nerves.
- Epstein-Barr virus feeds off mercury and may be a culprit.
- Alpha lipoic acid, evening primrose oil, fish oil, Vitamin B12 and chromium are good.
- Alpha Ortho Phos dissolves blockages in the circulatory system, helping to alleviate numbness and tingling.
- Peppermint, helichrysum, lavender and frankincense are good to rub on topically.
- *I suggest Gota Plus, Heart Formula, Vascutin, Circu Plus, Alpha Lipoic Acid & Omega Complete*

NURSING COMPLICATIONS
- Herbs to help increase breast milk are alfalfa, blessed thistle, dandelion, fennel & red raspberry. Herbs that decrease milk supply and should be avoided are black walnut, sage & yarrow.
- *I suggest intraMAX, Alpha Green & Herbal Minerals II*

MUSCULAR DYSTROPHY
- Degeneration of the skeletal muscles.
- Heavy metals, pesticides & Lyme disease may be the cause.
- Selenium, CoQ10, Vitamins E and C, glutamic acid, L-glycine, carnitine, glucosamine & chondroitin may be beneficial.
- Exercise is important.
- *I suggest Gota Plus, Circu Plus, Immu C, Omega Complete, Alpha Oxzyme & Liga Plus*

NOSEBLEEDS
- A warning sign that the capillaries are weak and fragile.
- If you bruise easily and your gums bleed when brushing your teeth, this indicates that more Vitamin C (citrus bioflavonoids) is needed to strengthen tissue integrity.
- Camu camu from the Amazon rainforest is the world's highest concentration of Vitamin C. It contains 30 to 60 times more Vitamin C than an orange.
- Cayenne and yarrow can help. Calcium and magnesium levels may be low.
- Vitamin K is important for blood clotting. Eat green leafy vegetables, broccoli, cabbage, kale, cucumbers, fermented dairy and prunes.
- Allergies can be a cause.
- Don't blow your nose hard. A humidifier can sometimes help.
- *I recommend Camu Plus, Immu C, Alpha Flavin, Vascutin & Cal lac Plus*

OBESITY
- Emotions: fear, a need for protection. Using food as a substitute for affection. What are you trying to "protect" yourself from?

- So many people want to lose weight, but they are eating the wrong foods. Many will eat a cold cereal for breakfast and a pack of crackers for a lunch snack. These are two of the worst foods you can eat for weight loss. Flour, corn, rice, oats and wheat spike your blood sugar more than eating straight sugar. Avoid grains for weight loss.

Weight Loss Factors
1. Thyroid
2. Adrenals
3. Liver/Gallbladder
4. Pancreas (Enzymes)
5. Food Allergies
6. Grains & carbs
7. Exercise (Burst training)

- A sluggish thyroid is a common culprit when weight is an issue. Kelp is high in iodine, which nourishes the thyroid gland.
- Stress will put you in "fight-or-flight" mode and exhaust the adrenals. Sluggish adrenals and high cortisol levels then pull the thyroid out of balance. The reason you can't lose weight after eating a strict diet is because you have a hormone imbalance. Women are more affected by stress then men. Nerve Formula, Kava Kalm & MG/K are good for stress.
- Put down your phone, turn off the TV and get some sleep.
- Chickweed, Queen Anne's lace and apple cider vinegar can help.
- Drink lots of water, 16 ounces upon arising.
- Get the bowels moving two to three times a day.
- Stop consuming artificial sweeteners, especially diet soft drinks. They cause you to crave carbohydrates, retain fluids and spike insulin levels. They interfere with your metabolism, actually causing weight gain. Use stevia for a natural sweetener.

Foods That Cause Obesity	
Grains	Potatoes
Bread	Parsnips
Wheat	Cold Cereal
Flour	French fries
Corn	Soft drinks
Rice	Diet drinks
Oats	Fruit juices
Crackers	Sugar
Chips	Sports drinks
Pasta	Noodles

- Avoid "fat-free" products that are loaded with harmful chemicals.
- Certain medications like birth control, steroids and antidepressants can cause weight gain.
  Intermittent fasting is very beneficial. Skipping breakfast helps burn up glucose levels. Do not eat after 6 p.m. Read chapter on losing weight.
- A ketogenic diet is ideal to lose weight. Training the body to burn fat instead of carbs helps stabilize blood sugar levels and shed weight.

Foods For Weight Loss	
Vegetables	Berries
Coconut oil	Salmon
Olive oil	Tuna
Butter	Chicken
Ghee	Steak
Eggs	Beef
Avocados	Turkey
Olives	Peppers
Nuts	Cinnamon
Seeds	Kefir
Stevia	Buckwheat
Coconut flour	Bone broth
Almond flour	Arrow root

- Get plenty of sleep. A lack of sleep interferes with a healthy metabolism.
- If you carry most of your weight from the waist to the knees (big butt & thighs) you most likely need pituitary support. Pitui Plus is good. Manganese is the mineral that nourishes the anterior pituitary.
- If you carry most of your weight in the midsection and store belly fat or have a "beer belly," you probably need adrenal support to balance high cortisol levels, caused from stress. Adrena Plus, MG/K and Licro Plus are good.
- If you carry your weight mostly in the upper body and have thick shoulders, arms and neck, you most likely need thyroid support. If you carry your weight throughout the whole body you probably have a thyroid imbalance. Thyro Plus, Kelp Plus and Kelp Complex are good.
- Stop doing long cardio workouts for an hour a day.
- Burst training 3 times a week (20 minutes) is the most effective exercise to lose weight and stabilize blood sugar. Train smart, not long.
- Essential oils cinnamon, ginger and grapefruit are great for weight loss and cravings.
- Ashwagandha and holy basil are good.
- Eating hot peppers is thermogenic.
- Coconut oil is great for cravings and low energy.
- *I recommend Thyro Plus, Diadren Forte, Kelp Plus, Endo Glan Plus, MG/K, Kelp Complex & Her Formula*

OSTEOPOROSIS

- Emotions: feeling unsupported in life.
- Bone loss is usually caused by the sycosis miasm, which causes the parathyroid glands to be in a hyperactive state, signaling for more calcium in the blood. The body will then pull calcium from the bones, leaving them fragile.
- Calcium and magnesium in an absorbable form is important. Calcium carbonate comes from ground up egg and oyster shell and is not absorbed efficiently by most people. Plant-derived minerals are best, and then chelated minerals are next best. Calcium-rich foods are green vegetables such as broccoli, okra, spinach, kale, watercress, collard greens and kefir.
- Bisphosphonate drugs such as Fosamax and Boniva kill bone cells to produce denser bones so they look good on tests, but leave the bones weaker and brittle, so if you slip and fall, bones shatter easily. These drugs are harmful.
- Vitamins B12, D3 and K2 are important. Sun exposure on the skin for 20 minutes a day is good.
- See Arthritis section for more information on getting the body alkaline.
- Stop drinking fluoride in your water, as it has been linked to osteoporosis.

- Strength training with weights is good.
- Bone broth and collagen protein are good.
- *I recommend intraMAX, Alpha Green, Bone Health, Arnica Plus, Apizelen Plus & Alpha Gest III*

PAIN

- Emotions: feelings of guilt; guilt always seeks punishment. In a relationship that hurts.
- The prescription hydrocodone for pain is synthetic heroin and is very addictive. The brain and body react to it the same as heroin.
- Massage and chiropractic adjustments can greatly help.
- Acupuncture can be beneficial to move energy through the painful areas.
- Hydrotherapy — shower with hot water on painful area for 1 minute, then as cold as you can stand for 1 minute. Repeat this cycle six times. Always end with cold water.
- Stretching movements like yoga can be beneficial.
- A hot Epsom salt bath relaxes tight muscles and is anti-inflammatory.
- Bone broth is anti-inflammatory. Other foods that can help decrease pain are hot, spicy foods such as cayenne pepper (also very antifungal) & wasabi.
- Arnica, turmeric, chili peppers, evening primrose oil and holy basil are good.
- CBD or hemp oil has been shown to be nearly 100 times more potent than aspirin for pain.
- Wintergreen, lemongrass, rosemary and frankincense oil are very beneficial to rub on painful areas. Helichrysum is great for nerve pain.
- Sometimes a peppermint and lavender oil combination is very effective for pain, especially headaches.
- *I suggest Arnica Plus, R Plus, Liga Plus, Pain Relief Plus, Relieve Joint Pain & Alpha* Flavin

PARASITES

- 85 percent of adult Americans have parasites. Parasites are everywhere. We can get them from walking barefoot, swimming in lakes and rivers, drinking water and many foods, especially barbecue pork, sausage and animal meats. Raw seafood is sketchy. Traveling out of the country and ordering drinks with ice is risky. The water used to make ice is many times contaminated.
- Dogs and cats lick their anuses to clean themselves, and then lick you. Parasites can be transmitted through saliva.
- I suggest everyone do a parasite cleanse once a year. It's good to do a parasite cleanse for 8 weeks, to kill adults and

Parasite Cleanse
- Vermatox 5 drops twice daily
- L/GB-AP 50 drops twice daily
- Para Plus 2 capsules twice daily

- eggs that may hatch and re-infect the host.
- Garlic and onions are anti-parasitic.
- Black walnut (hull), wormwood, pink root, fennel, pumpkin seeds, male fern, hyssop, oregano oil, clove oil are anti-parasitic.
- A colonic can be beneficial. Make sure and keep your bowels moving while doing a parasite cleanse.
- *I suggest Vermatox, L/GB-AP, Verma Plus & Para Plus*

PARKINSON'S DISEASE
- Emotions: fears not being able to control.
- Test for the syphilinum miasm, as it can affect the nervous system.
- Test for Lyme disease (Borrelia Burgdorferi).
- Calcium, magnesium, copper and potassium deficiencies can be causes.
- Low dopamine levels are associated with Parkinson's. Copper is an essential element in dopamine metabolism. Copper is required for normal myelination (the fatty insulation) of nerves. Autopsies have shown that Parkinson's patients have increased iron levels, with low levels of copper in their brains.
- An out-of-balance parathyroid gland can trigger blood/calcium levels to be abnormal producing "the shakes."
- Bone meal and B vitamins can be beneficial.
- Eat fava beans, as they are rich in L-dopa.
- Phosphatidyl serine can help.
- Heavy metal poisoning is almost always a culprit. Get silver dental fillings removed and replaced with composite materials. Locate a biological dentist for a safe removal.
- Gingko, cayenne, valerian root, ginseng, passion flower, kola nut, rosemary, lobelia, L-dopa, dopamine, CoQ10 (Ubiquinol), Vitamins C and E, black currant oil, fish oil and hops can be beneficial.
- Turmeric, bee pollen, royal jelly, alfalfa and spirulina are good.
- CBD oil can be beneficial.
- Dopa Mucuna is a good nerve tonic which helps balance L-Dopa, which the body uses to make dopamine. It is used in India to treat Parkinson's.
- Intestinal gut health is crucial for reversing Parkinson's. Probiotics support a healthy microbiome.
- Low LDL cholesterol increases the risk of Parkinson's disease by 350 percent, according to the Journal Movement Disorders 23, No. 7 May 2008. The human brain is 60 percent fat. We need cholesterol for healthy

---

Parkinson's Support
- Lavender oil 2 drops
- Frankincense 2 drops
- Helichrysum 2 drops

Massage oils on your temples and behind ears twice daily.

Pesticides Linked To Parkinson's
- Rotenone
- Glyphosate
- Paraquat
- Maneb
- Benomyl
- 2,4-D
- Permethrin
- Beta HcH
- Atrazine

brain and nerve function. Stop robbing your brain of cholesterol by taking statin drugs. Eating a ketogenic diet is good.
- Avoid grains. Wheat (breads, crackers, cereals, pasta), barley, rye, corn, oats & rice cause inflammation in the body and lead to the deterioration of neurons in the brain.
- Eat healthy fats like avocados, eggs, coconut oil, olive oil, olives, real butter, raw nuts & seeds.
- Niacinamide 250 to 500 mg a day can help.
- *I suggest Nerve Formula, Brain Formula, Clear Mind, KLS Enviro, Circu Plus, Vitamin D, Omega Complete, Dopa Mucuna, L-dopa, Dopamine, Cal Lac Plus & Phosphatidyl Serine*

PICA
- An abnormal craving for substances other than food. Pica seems to be more prevalent in children and pregnant or nursing women.
- Children or adults who put strange objects, such as coins, paper clips, dirt, modeling clay, rubber, plastic straws, paper, crayons, laundry soap and boogers in their mouths are craving minerals, especially iron.
- Pagophagia is the compulsive desire to chew ice.
- Supplement with minerals, especially iron.
- *I suggest intraMAX, Herbal & Mineral Complete & Alpha Green*

PINK EYE (CONJUNCTIVITIS)
- Emotions: anger and frustration, what don't you want to see?
- Caused by the staphylococcus bacteria, it is very contagious. Sangre de Drago mixed in a saline solution and dropped in the eye will clear out infection and reduce inflamed membranes.
- Eyebright, goldenseal, echinacea, elderberry, holy basil, turmeric and colloidal silver may be beneficial.
- A freshly cut slice of tomato is very soothing and healing to the eye, as it contains a lectin that destroys the staphylococcus bacteria. Do not use canned tomato juice.
- Placing aloe vera gel all around the eye is anti-inflammatory.

Eye Drop Formula
- Take a saline bottle and empty ¼ of it
- Add 25% Immutox II (homeopathic formula)
- Shake well – Place 2 drops in both eyes
- Apply 2-3 times a day

- Take 2 drops of frankincense and chamomile oil with a glass of water twice daily for immune support.
- Rubbing neem oil all around the eyes before bed can help.
- *I recommend Echinacea Complex, Myrrh Plus, Camu Plus & Allibiotic*

PLANTAR FASCIITIS
- Inflammation of tissue that connects your heel bone to the toes.

- Rest or decreasing your exercise is a must. Icing the area several times a day for 20 minutes is good.
- Once inflammation subsides, stretching is very important.
- Wearing special shoes with arch support may be helpful.
- Magnesium, Vitamin C & turmeric are good.
- Mixing rosemary, lemongrass, wintergreen, peppermint and thyme oils with a spoonful of coconut oil and massaging it on your foot can help reduce inflammation and irritation.
- If you have heel spurs, Alpha Ortho Phos helps dissolve them.
- *I suggest Arnica Plus, R Plus, Alpha Flavin, Pain Relief Plus, Relieve Joint Pain & Liga Plus*

PNEUMONIA
- Emotions: tired of life, deep emotional wounds that have not healed.
- A respiratory infection (viral or bacterial) that affects the lungs.
- Weak adrenals always affect the lungs. Royal jelly is good for the adrenals.
- Mullein and lobelia are good for the lungs.
- Echinacea, elderberry, garlic, ginger and colloidal silver fight infection.
- Diffuse eucalyptus oil, as it helps loosen lung congestion. Mix eucalyptus oil and peppermint oil with coconut oil and rub on your chest before bed.
- Mold and fungus spores can cause lingering coughs. Mold X and 2 drops of oregano oil three times a day in water is good.
- Beryllium toxicity is associated with pneumonia and lung cancer.
- *I recommend Mullein Plus, Echinacea Plus, Camu Plus, Pneumo Plus, & Adrena Plus*

POISON IVY/OAK/SUMAC
- "Leaves of three, let it be," is wisdom for avoiding poisonous plants. Poison ivy contains an oil called urushiol that causes a rash with blisters. If you come in contact with poison ivy, wash your skin as soon as possible with hot, soapy water and scrub vigorously with friction, using a washcloth to ensure all the oil is washed off the skin. Wash and scrub with soap three times. Rinse with cold water, then rub some tea tree or lavender oil on skin. The ooze from the blisters is an allergic reaction from the body and does not contain urushiol oil, so therefore is not contagious.
- Wash all clothing and gloves after exposure because the urushiol oil can remain toxic for years.
- Homeopathic remedies clematis, graphite, mezereum, rhus tox and croton tiglium are effective.
- Burdock, jewelweed, nettle and aloe vera can help.

Poison Ivy Remedy
- 1 Tbsp. salt
- 1 Tbsp. baking soda
- 1 Tbsp. apple cider vinegar
Mix together and dip cotton ball or paper towel in solution and apply to skin

- Rubbing plantain leaves on the skin neutralizes the poison.
- Placing a cold compress over the blisters with lavender oil and ice in a cloth for 20 minutes at a time can help.
- Apple cider vinegar applied topically can be beneficial.
- Bentonite clay applied to rash and blisters helps the healing process.
- Essential oils tea tree, lavender, peppermint, chamomile & geranium oils are good.
- *I recommend Poison Ivy, Echinacea Plus, Camu Plus & Alpha E Spleen*

POLYCYSTIC OVARY SYNDROME

- Enlarged ovaries with cysts on them, producing higher than normal hormones, is the No. 1 cause of infertility.
- The sycosis miasm is usually the culprit causing the cysts. Detox the miasm.
- Chaste tree berry, suma, maca, dong quai, wild yam, damiana, black cohosh, licorice, hops, manganese and yarrow are good.
- Vitamin D, zinc, magnesium, calcium, chromium and evening primrose oil are good.
- A keto diet is very beneficial. Eat healthy fats. Hormones need cholesterol. Consume avocados, coconut oil, olive oil, nuts, seeds, eggs, butter and olives.
- Massage holy basil, geranium, clary sage and chamomile oils with coconut oil on your lower abdomen twice daily.
- *I suggest FHS Formula, Female Balance, Female Formula, KLS Enviro, Beta Plus, Endo Glan F & Ovary Uterus Plus*

PREMENSTRUAL SYNDROME (PMS)

- Emotions: giving power to others, rejecting the feminine process.
- Stress causes hormonal imbalances. Mental stress, emotional stress, physical stress and chemicals can all drain your hormones. Many of us worry about things we can't control and stay stressed. This is why there are so many hormonal imbalances.
- A woman's menstrual cycle has four phases it goes through each month and a normal cycle ranges from 26 to 32 days.
- *The first phase* is the construction phase when the cycle starts and will last four to seven days. This is when estrogens (seven of them) are elevated and the reproductive area is being rebuilt. It is important not to exercise during this phase (during your cycle) because you risk depleting your hormones. Exercising is stressful and can further deplete you of hormones. Women who exercise hard all the time, like marathon runners or CrossFit fanatics, sometimes will stop having a menstrual cycle. This is not good. It indicates your hormones are depleted and can lead to chronic fatigue syndrome.
- *The 2nd phase* (days 7 to 14) is when the cycle has stopped and your hormone levels are rising. If you are balanced, your sex drive should be at

its peak (like a man's). This is the ideal time for a woman to exercise. Most women will feel they can handle stress better at this time and things don't seem to bother them as much. This is also the phase where you metabolize your food better and don't gain weight as easily.

- *The 3rd phase* (days 14 to 21) is when your hormones change and it is easy to feel depressed, or on edge, because the hormone levels naturally decrease. This is the phase where the adrenals begin producing hormones instead of the ovaries. If you are emotionally stressed or have been exercising too hard, you can become very sick during this time. This is when you need to relax and take a break; otherwise, high cortisol levels will cause an imbalance in your progesterone levels. Progesterone is a calming hormone. It helps balance estrogen, but too much stress will leave you depleted. If estrogen levels aren't balanced (if too high), then you are at high risk for breast cancer.
- *The 4th phase* (days 21 to 28) is when the hormones are still decreasing but leveling back out. Usually the sex drive picks back up, but you may experience some mood changes depending on stress levels.
- During these 4 phases of a woman's menstrual cycle, it is normal for you to feel and experience different emotions as your hormones change. Nothing is wrong with you! You are not bipolar or in need of anti-depression medication! Your body is simply doing what God created it do, providing you with the opportunity and privilege of becoming pregnant and bearing children.
- Eat healthy fats to manufacture hormones and take time to relax and de-stress.
- Synthetic hormones and birth control increase your risk for cancer. Birth control is an endocrine disrupter. Women who take birth control will have the hormone in their bodily fluids (saliva) and can pass it to their partners when kissing and during sex. Men will get estrogens this way! There's a reason why some men don't want to be men anymore, or no longer want to be with a woman. These estrogens are abundant in our society, from foods and medications to plastics and clothing. They are femininizing agents, and this is why our young girls are starting to develop and go through puberty at age 8 instead of age 13.

Healthy Hormone Foods
- Coconut oil
- Avocados
- Walnuts
- Pecans
- Pumpkin seeds
- Eggs
- Olive oil
- Dates
- Maca
- Chocolate dark, cocoa

Endocrine Disruptors
- Birth control pills
- Dental fillings
- Plastic water bottles
- Plastic toys
- Plastic food containers
- Metal cans
- Flame retardant materials
- Vinyl products
- Fragrances
- Shampoos
- Household cleaners
- Soy (phytoestrogens)
- Processed meats & dairy

- Municipal city water is loaded with hormones. It is the No. 1 source of estrogen-causing hormonal imbalances. This is one reason we are seeing so many women diagnosed with breast cancer.
- Women who have pain on the right lower abdomen may think an ovary is causing it, but many times it is an irritated ileocecal valve caused by parasites. Para Plus expels parasites.
- PMS symptoms usually indicate that the endocrine system is out of balance. Supplementing with zinc, magnesium and Vitamin B6 can help (especially for frontal headaches).
- Too much copper and low zinc levels will cause PMS (headaches, depression, fatigue, emotional swings, weight gain, prolonged/heavy menstrual flow & food cravings). Estrogen is associated with copper. Birth control pills and intrauterine devices have a tendency to elevate copper levels, which prevent pregnancy. The excess copper creates an imbalance between estrogen and progesterone, as well as zinc and copper, which all lead to menstrual abnormalities.
- Zinc is required for progesterone, which is made in the ovaries and adrenal glands.
- The No. 1 cause of hormonal imbalances is stress. Once a woman gets stressed out and goes into fight-or-flight mode, the hormones are thrown out of balance. Magnesium helps us calm down after stressful situations. Nerve Formula, Kava Kalm and Valeri Plus are good.
- Chasteberry, dong quai, licorice, ashwagandha, holy basil, suma, maca, wild yam, damiana, black cohosh, hops, manganese, B vitamins and yarrow are good endocrine balancers.

PMS Oil Support
- Clary Sage   2 drops
- Holy Basil   2 drops
- Ylang Ylang   2 drops

Mix with 1 tsp coconut oil and massage on lower abdomen

- Testosterone helps increase sexual desire for both females and males.

80% of women who take birth control are deficient in vitamin B6.

- All hormones are made from cholesterol. If you take cholesterol-lowering drugs (statins) your hormones will be out of balance.
- *I recommend FHS Formula, Her Formula, Female Formula, Endo Glan F, Evening Primrose Oil & Ovary Uterus Plus*

PROSTATITIS
- Emotions: fear of aging, guilt, ugly conflict with sexual connections.
- The discoverer of the PSA test, Richard Ablin, Ph.D., in his book, *The Great Prostate Hoax*, explains how PSA screening causes serious harm to millions of men as they go through unnecessary and debilitating treatments and how

- it has become a public health disaster. Dr. Ablin informs that there is no reason for a healthy man to have a PSA test, because it doesn't work as a cancer indicator. Many factors other than cancer can cause prostate inflammation. See section on PSA test for more prostate information.
- When the prostate gland swells, it can cause pain, a constant need to urinate (especially at night) and a weak urine flow.
- Flaxseed oil, juniper berry, saw palmetto, ginseng, yohimbe, sarsaparilla, zinc, Vitamins A and E, lecithin, bee pollen, calcium and magnesium are all beneficial.
- According to the University of Arizona's medical school, (JAMA Dec. 25, 1996), selenium supplemented at 250 mcg/day will reduce one's risk of developing prostate cancer by 69 percent.
- Dr. Speckhart finds that gold crowns in the teeth can be a culprit for prostate cancer.
- Graviola is very effective for prostate cancer.
- Consuming frankincense, myrrh, oregano and rosemary oils, 1 drop of each with some water twice daily can be beneficial.
- Queen of the meadow is good for the prostate & diabetes according to Tommie Bass.

Prostate Support Oil Blend
▪ Frankincense 2 drops
▪ Oregano 2 drops
▪ Rosemary 2 drops
Mix with 1 tsp coconut oil & rub on skin below genitals twice daily

What To Do For A Healthy Prostate
1. Exercise regularly
2. Have 2-3 bowel movements daily
3. Avoid alcohol & caffeine
4. Avoid prolonged sitting
5. Enjoy a healthy sex life
6. Kegel exercises (stimulates blood flow)
7. Soak in warm Epsom salt baths
8. Take nutritional supplements
9. Get enough sleep (deep REM)
10. Eat cruciferous vegetables (broccoli)

- *I recommend, Juni Plus, Male Formula, His Formula, Flaxseed Oil, Prosta Plus Complete, Circu Plus & Endo Glan M*

PSORIASIS
- Emotions: fear of being hurt, emotional insecurity.
- An autoimmune skin disease causing inflammation and scaly skin.
- Leaky gut is almost always at the root. Rebuild the microbiome. Take probiotics to rebuild the microbiome. Fermented vegetables and dairy, like kefir, are good.
- Many types of skin conditions are caused from toxins built up in the liver and spleen. Flush the toxins out and the skin clears up. KLS Enviro, Alpha E Spleen & Hepachol are good.
- Check for food allergies, especially gluten. Eat a gluten-free diet. Avoid citrus and raw nuts and seeds.
- Digestive support with HCL acid and digestive enzymes can help.

- ½ cup apple cider vinegar in a warm bath can help.
- Vitamins D3 and K2 are important.
- Dandelion, burdock, milk thistle, echinacea, yellow dock and nettle are good.
- Turmeric, fish oil and evening primrose oil are good.
- Kelp is high in iodine, which keeps the skin from getting dry.
- Aloe vera, coconut oil and avocado oil-based creams can be beneficial.
- **SCABIES** – Use neem, turmeric, star anise oil, tea tree oil and homeopathic sulfur
- **RING WORM** – Use tea tree oil, garlic, olive leaf, cat's claw and pau d'arco.
- *I recommend KLS Enviro, Immu C, Trifolo Plus, Alpha E Spleen, Hepachol, Complete Probiotics & Omega Complete*

> **Psoriasis Oil Formula**
> - Tea Tree 5 drops
> - Myrrh 5 drops
> - Geranium 5 drops
> - Lavender 5 drops
>
> Mix with 1 Tbsp. coconut oil and rub on skin twice daily

RESTLESS LEGS SYNDROME
- Magnesium, potassium & calcium help relax muscles and the nervous system.
- Vitamin D3 is important
- Heavy metals can cause twitching in the muscles.
- Allergies, especially to gluten or dairy, can cause twitches.
- Digestive support to absorb minerals is important. Alpha Gest III or Alpha Zyme III is good.
- Taking a hot Epsom salt bath (2 cups) with lavender, chamomile and cedarwood oils, 10 drops each for 20 to 30 minutes before bed, can help calm and relax the muscles and nerves.
- *I suggest Nerve Formula, Kava Kalm, Valeri Plus, MG/K, Alpha Green II, intraMAX, Dopa Mucuna & Irie*

ROSACEA
- A skin condition with red, tiny bumps on face.
- Test for allergies, heavy metals, chemical & pesticide poisoning.
- Weak blood vessels can be an issue. Circu Plus or Veno Plus are good.
- Evening primrose oil is good.
- Vitamins C and D3 and turmeric can help.
- Mix 5 drops of lavender oil with 5 drops of geranium oil and 1 tsp. of coconut oil and rub on face.
- *I suggest Burdock Plus, KLS-Enviro, Alpha E Spleen, Evening primrose oil & Veno Plus*

SCAR TISSUE
- Can form after an injury or surgery.

- Enzymes break down proteins in the blood that cause inflammation.
- Serrapeptase is an enzyme derived from the silk worm that helps dissolve scar tissue, inflammation and arthritis. Take on an empty stomach.
- Frankincense, lavender, helichrysum, patchouli & tea tree are good for scar tissue. Mix with coconut or olive oil and massage on afflicted area twice a day.
- *I suggest Arnica Plus, R Plus, Vascutin, Alpha E Spleen & Alpha Flavin*

SCHIZOPHRENIA

- Zinc and Vitamin B6 are important.
- Hypoglycemia is almost always involved with schizophrenia. Support the adrenals, liver and pancreas. Diadren Forte is good.
- Schizophrenia is unknown in gluten-free societies. Avoid gluten. Eat a paleo or ketogenic diet. Celiac disease is common with schizophrenia.
- Eat healthy fats and low-glycemic foods to stabilize blood sugar levels. Drinking bone broth helps heal the gut.
- Exercising is important.
- Test for parasites. Certain parasites from cats (Toxoplasmosis Gondii) can be a factor.
- Dopamine can help. Vitamins D3 and C, L-lysine, ginkgo & ginseng are good.
- Niacin has been proven to be extremely beneficial by Dr. Abram Hoffer, who has treated over 5,000 cases with an 80 percent success rate. Usually 1,000 mg. to 3,000 mg. of niacin in the form of niacinamide given with each meal works well.
- *I suggest Brain Formula, Clear Mind, Evening Primrose Oil, Diadren Forte, Alpha Oxzyme & Chola Plus.*

SHINGLES

- Emotions: oversensitivity, fearing things won't work out the way you want.
- Shingles (Herpes Zoster) is caused by the varicella-zoster virus, the same virus that causes chickenpox.
- The chickenpox vaccine given to children reduces the amount of chickenpox cases, so adults are no longer being exposed. Being around young children with chickenpox gives your immune system a reminder/booster which helps prevent shingles.
- Take 50,000 IUs of Vitamin D3 a day for a week. K2 (MK7) is good to help absorb it.
- Vitamin C, Vitamin B12, garlic, onions & zinc are important.
- Manuka or local honey is good to put on topically.

Shingles Oil Remedy
- Tea tree 3 drops
- Helichrysum 3 drops
- Oregano 3 drops
- Peppermint 3 drops

Mix with ½ tsp coconut oil and rub on skin twice daily

- Cayenne, lobelia, echinacea, elderberry and cat's claw are good.
- Geranium oil applied topically helps relieve pain.
- *I recommend Camu Plus, Echinacea Complex, Immune Support, Allibiotic & Alpha E Spleen*

SINUSITIS

- Emotions: irritation by a person close to you. Trying to call the shots in someone else's life. Feeling sorry for yourself.
- More than 90 percent of sinus infections are fungal in origin. Mold can also be a cause. Antibiotics are useless against fungal infections and viruses.
- Oregano oil and garlic are great to clear up mold and fungal infections. Allibiotic and Mold X are good.
- Sinu Orega is a nasal spray containing oregano oil, bay leaf oil, sage oil and clove bud oil mixed with salt water. It's a great natural antibiotic/cleanser for the sinuses.
- Sinus problems are like a smoke alarm going off. We want to put the fire out, not treat the smoke. The liver & ileocecal valve are usually where the fire is, causing sinus issues and sounding the alarm. Toxins built up in the liver can trigger allergies and sinus issues. KLS Enviro & Ginger Plus I are good.
- If the gallbladder isn't secreting bile properly to break down fats, this can cause sinus trouble. Hydrangea Plus & Beta Plus are good.
- Parasites, causing an imbalance with the ileocecal valve, can trigger sinus issues. L/GB-AP, BR-SP Plus & Para Plus are good.
- If chiropractic adjustments don't hold, especially T-4, this could be a liver/gallbladder issue continuing to trip the circuit breaker since the nerves carry electricity.
- Sluggish thyroid and adrenal glands can be another factor. If the discharge from the nose is a thick green color, then the thyroid is usually sluggish. When the adrenal glands become exhausted, we are tired and may be allergic to citrus fruits.
- Gluten and dairy cause sinus congestion. Avoid grains, cereals, breads, milk and cheese, as they can trigger sinus congestion.

Sinus Congestion Neti Pot Cleanse
- 8 oz. water (if using tap water, boil for 5 minutes)
- 1 tsp. raw salt (do not use iodized salt)
- 1 tsp. baking soda (optional)
- 1 tsp. hydrogen peroxide (optional)
- Mix all ingredients in 8 oz. of warm (not too hot) water. Pour in neti pot or irrigation device.
- Tilt your head sideways over sink. Press the spout of your device into upper nostril and slowly begin to irrigate while breathing through your mouth and let water run out bottom nostril.
- Rotate your head and repeat on the other nostril.

- Vitamin B5 (pantothenic acid) is beneficial. Royal jelly is the best source.
- Stuffiness on the right side indicates the need for potassium, while stuffiness on the left side is usually a sodium deficiency.
- Alfalfa, bee pollen and spirulina are high in sodium and potassium. Echinacea and Vitamin B12 can help.
- For sinuses that continue to run, take Hista Plus, 3 with each meal, to dry up drippy sinuses.
- Cod liver oil, high in Vitamin A, can help.
- Serrapeptase, a proteolytic enzyme, can be beneficial to break up congestion.
- Nattokinase, made from fermented soybeans, relieves sinus inflammation and is good for lowering blood pressure.
- Bone broth is very anti-inflammatory and healing, especially with garlic, onions and other vegetables.
- Ginger tea with raw honey is good.
- Gotu kola and wood betony can help stop nasal drip.
- Peppermint, eucalyptus, melaleuca (tea tree oil), rosemary, and lemon oil can help open sinuses. Add 5 drops of peppermint and eucalyptus oil in hot water and breathe in steam.
- Rubbing 1 drop of peppermint or eucalyptus oil on the roof of your mouth and then drinking water can help open up the sinuses.
- The phenolic Rutin can help with pollen sensitivities, hay fever and nasal congestion.
- For tough guys, try a straight shot of ground horseradish with a shot of lemon.
- Quercetin can be beneficial.
- *I recommend Myrrh Plus, Licro Plus, Hista Plus, Mold X, Allibiotic, Adrena Plus & Royal Jelly*

Essential Oil Nose Spray
- 2 drops Tea Tree oil
- 2 drops Peppermint oil
- 2 drops Eucalyptus oil
- 2 drops Lavender oil

Boil ¼ cup distilled water for 1 minute with 1/16 teaspoon salt. Let cool & pour in 2 oz nasal spray bottle. Add oils & shake. Spray in nose as needed.

Sinus Cleanser Formula
- Eucalyptus   2 drops
- Peppermint 2 drops
- Lemon   2 drops
- Thyme   2 drops

Mix with water & drink twice daily

SKIN DISORDERS
- Emotions: Unresolved feelings of irritation, someone is irritating you.
- Test for allergies, fungal infections, heavy metals, parasites and Lyme disease.
- Many skin issues are caused from an overgrowth of candida yeast. See Candida protocol for eliminating yeast and fungus in the body. Heavy metals provide a favorable environment to feed yeast (candida). Until heavy

- metals are cleared out, yeast may continue to be a problem, causing skin rashes. Metatox, KLS Enviro & Chlorella are good.
- Avoid gluten, dairy and fried foods.
- Horses with beautiful, shiny hair are fed flaxseeds, which are high in omega-3 fats. If you have dry, itchy, flaky skin and dandruff, you may have an omega-3 deficiency. Eat healthy fats such as coconut oil, olive oil, ghee, butter, flaxseeds, fish oil, krill oil, borage oil and evening primrose oil.
- Aloe vera and bentonite clay can be applied topically,
- Vitamin C, zinc, garlic, turmeric and Vitamin D3 are important.
- Lavender and geranium oils mixed with coconut oil and rubbed on the skin can help heal rashes.
- *I suggest KLS Enviro, Nettle Plus, Lapacho Plus, Alpha E Spleen, Hepachol, Omega Complete, Complete Probiotics & Mold X*

SKIN TAGS (ACROCHORDONS)

- Are usually caused from the sycosis miasm, which causes warts, moles, cysts, tumors & skin tags. It causes excessive growth and hyperactivity in organs, glands and systems.
- Place a few drops of tea tree oil or oregano oil on a cotton ball and use a bandage or medical tape to cover skin tag. Repeat this procedure every night and morning until tag falls off. Do not use around eyes.
- Helichrysum oil may be beneficial as well.
- Apple cider vinegar may be just as effective as tea tree oil. Use the same application process as for tea tree oil.
- *I suggest homeopathic sycosis, Arco Plus, Camu Plus & KLS Enviro*

SMOKING (SEE ADDICTIONS)

- Eat healthy fats. A paleo or ketogenic diet, combined with proteins to help stabilize blood-sugar levels, is good.
- Niacin (Vitamin B-3) helps reduce nicotine cravings. If you experience flushing or tingling from taking niacin, switch to niacinamide.
- Supplement your diet with Vitamin C, chromium, lecithin, calcium, magnesium and a B complex.
- L-tryptophan at 50 mg a day can help.
- *I suggest Neuro Balance, Irie, Endo Glan Plus, Diadren Forte, Herbal & Mineral Complete*

Support To Quit Smoking
- Calcium/Magnesium – 600 mg
- Vitamin C – 1,000 mg
- Chromium – 100 mcg
- Niacin – 50 mg
- Soybean Lecithin
- 5-HTP – 200 mg

"One puff of a cigarette lets loose a trillion free radical molecules in the smoker." Hyla Cass, M.D. – UCLA School of Medicine

SORE THROAT/STREP

- Emotions: holding in angry words, feeling unable to express honest feelings.
- Most sore throats are caused from the streptococcus bacteria, rhinovirus or allergies.
- Tonsils are lymph glands and serve as filters for toxins. If they are swollen, there is a cause. Before letting a surgeon cut part of your God-given infection-fighting immune system out and throw it in the trash, test for allergies, infection and toxic irritations. Heal the cause.
- Gargle with warm salt water every hour. Salt kills bacteria. It is one of the oldest and least-expensive germ fighters around. Old-timers, before refrigeration, would cure their meat with salt to stave off bacteria and preserve it.
- Mixing a few drops of oregano oil with 3 drops of peppermint oil in warm salt water to gargle with for a couple of minutes is an excellent infection fighter. Spit out after gargling.
- Drink a hot lemonade. Squeeze the juice of a lemon in a glass of hot water and add 3 Tbsp. of apple cider vinegar and 1 Tbsp. of raw honey. Add 4 dropperfuls of una de gato (cat's claw), Arco Plus or Echinacea to make a powerful infection fighter. You may also add 20 drops of Sangre de Drago to "turbocharge" your immune system. Stir and sip. Gargle before swallowing.
- Drink warm bone broth. It's very anti-inflammatory and healing. Put a tablespoon of coconut oil in it for extra immune support.
- Making a slow cooker of homemade chicken vegetable soup with lots of onions and garlic is good.
- Eat three cloves of fresh garlic daily. Garlic is a natural antibiotic.
- Eat eggs, onions and apricots. They are high in sulfur. The tonsils are the sulfur sacks of the body. Tonsils help purify the blood and become inflamed when low in sulfur.
- Vitamins C, D, zinc, olive leaf, cat's claw, elderberry, licorice root, colloidal silver and probiotics are good.

Sore Throat Spray
- Colloidal Silver 1 Tbsp.
- Oregano Oil 2 drops
- Lemon Oil 2 drops
- Peppermint Oil 2 drops

Mix all ingredients in a spray bottle with 4 oz. of water and spray in throat every hour.

Master Tonic Immune Formula
- ¼ cup chopped garlic
- ¼ cup chopped white onions
- ¼ cup grated ginger
- 2 Tbsp. grated horseradish root
- 2 Tbsp. turmeric powder
- 1 habanero pepper or
- 1 tsp. cayenne (optional)
- 24 oz. apple cider vinegar (Organic Bragg)

Fill a 1-quart Mason jar with dry ingredients and mix well. Pour in vinegar and shake daily for 2 weeks. Strain, squeeze well and drink. Take 1 tbsp. up to 6 times a day. May consume immediately upon making recipe

- Probiotics are important to boost up immunity.
- Getting enough sleep is crucial for the immune system to be healthy.
- *I recommend Otalga Plus, Echinacea Plus, Arco Plus, Camu Plus, Immune Formula & Allibiotic*

STROKE
- Emotions: resistance, "I'd rather die than change." Feeling like giving up.
- Most strokes occur when an artery becomes blocked and oxygen and nutrients cannot circulate to the brain, thus causing the death of brain cells.
- Increase circulation to the brain. Circulation support includes; ginkgo biloba, ginseng, butcher's broom, cayenne, ginger, gotu kola, oat straw, rosemary, garlic and parsley.
- Avoid taking an aspirin a day to thin the blood, which causes blood vessels to break, which may lead to a stroke.
- A stroke on the right side of the body is usually caused from a potassium deficiency. Bee pollen, burdock and alfalfa are high in potassium.
- Strokes on the left side can be caused from a sodium deficiency. Spirulina, celery, watercress, Irish moss and dulse are high in sodium.
- Alpha Ortho Phos can dissolve calcium and arterial plaque buildup, which restricts blood flow.
- Soybean lecithin can help. Alpha lipoic acid is good.
- Niacin, Vitamin D3, and CoQ10 can help.
- Exercise is important as well as restful sleep.
- *I recommend Veno Plus, Gota Plus, Brain Formula, Chestnut Plus, Circu Plus, Omega Complete & Vascutin*

RECOGNIZING A STROKE
1. **Face drooping** – Ask them to smile. Does one side droop?
2. **Arm weakness** – Have them raise both arms. Does one arm drift downward?
3. **Speech Impairment** – Have them repeat a simple phrase. Is their speech slurred or sound strange?

*** *IF YOU SEE ANY OF THESE SIGNS CALL 911*

TEETH PROBLEMS & TEETHING
- For teething infants, mix 2 drops of clove oil with 1 tsp. of coconut oil and 1 tsp. of olive oil and rub on gums. Clove oil has a similar numbing effect as benzocaine.
- Homeopathic teething drops include: Chamomilla 30c, Belladonna 30c, Silicea 6x. Actaea 6c, Borax 6c for mouth ulcers, Kreosotum 6c for poor tooth enamel & decay, Mercurius 6c for sore gums & diarrhea, Aconite 30c for pain & fever, Colocynth 6c for sore gums & colicky & Nux 6c for teething symptoms with constipation.
- Catnip is good for teething pains and colic.

- Freezing a pacifier or wet washcloth and then letting the infant chew on it can be beneficial.
- For adult teeth problems, mix 2 drops each of clove, peppermint, myrrh and thyme oils with 1 Tbsp. of coconut oil and swish in mouth, then spit out.
- Avoid sugar and refined carbohydrates. Sugar causes cavities and infections.
- Eat vegetables, healthy fats, kefir, bone broth and organic meats.
- Use fluoride-free toothpaste. Fluoride is a deadly carcinogenic poison.
- Natural toothpaste consists of baking soda, coconut oil, peppermint oil, tea tree oil or clove oil.
- A molybdenum deficiency can cause cavities.
- Holy basil may be beneficial. Prickly ash bark tea is the best thing in the world for a toothache according to Tommie Bass.
- Calcium, magnesium, phosphorus, Vitamin D, K2 and collagen are important.
- Use 3 percent hydrogen peroxide (diluted from 35 percent food-grade hydrogen peroxide — made by adding 1 ounce to 11 ounces of distilled water) mixed with baking soda (1 teaspoon) to make a paste for brushing your teeth. This helps prevent cavities, whitens teeth and clears up gingivitis.
- To whiten your teeth and remove stains, dip a cotton ball into the 3 percent food-grade hydrogen peroxide solution and swab on teeth. Don't rinse the peroxide from your teeth and don't eat or drink for 30 minutes. Use a clean cotton ball each time so you don't contaminate your hydrogen peroxide solution.
- *I suggest Otalga Plus, swish in mouth for several minutes and then swallow*

TINNITUS
- Emotions: refusing to hear your inner voice, not wanting to listen to higher laws.
- Sluggish adrenal glands can trigger ringing in the ears. Licro Plus & Adrena Plus are good.
- Magnesium, calcium, manganese and Vitamin C (bioflavonoids) can help.
- Circulation support can be helpful. This includes ginkgo biloba, ginseng, butcher's broom, cayenne, ginger, gotu kola, oat straw and rosemary.
- *I recommend Gota Plus, Clear Mind, Immu C, Brain Formula, Alpha Flavin, Adrena Plus & Vascutin*

TOENAIL FUNGUS
- May be a sign of a weakened immune system and an overgrowth of candida yeast. See Candida protocol.
- Mix 10 drops of tea tree oil with 10 drops of oregano oil and 1 tsp. of coconut oil and apply to toes three times a day.

- Soak your feet in water mixed with 3 percent hydrogen peroxide 15 minutes a day.
- *I suggest Lapacho, Arco Plus, Candida Clear, Mold X, Allibiotic & Complete Probiotics*

ULCERS
- Emotions: what is eating at you? Seeking revenge. A belief that you are not good enough.
- Stress is a major source of ulcers. Kava Kalm & Irie are good to calm and relax.
- A simple ulcer test is performed by taking 2 capsules of protease on an empty stomach. If burning or discomfort occurs within 10 minutes, this is an indication of ulcers.
- Prescription pain medication will cause ulcers.
- Sangre de Drago is a powerful antioxidant that heals ulcers.
- Drinking raw, freshly made cabbage juice several times a day is beneficial for duodenal ulcers.
- Raw, freshly made potato juice is great for gastric (stomach) ulcers. Drink cabbage or potato juices immediately after juicing, because the medicinal value disappears the longer it sits.
- Check for H. pylori bacteria, as it can cause ulcers. Kava Kalm contains Holy Thorn (Espinheira Santa) herb, effective for eradicating H. Pylori bacteria.
- Licorice root is good for H. pylori as well. It helps heal intestinal inflammation & ulcers.
- Una de Gato (cat's claw) mixed with honey and vinegar in a little water helps heal ulcers.
- Wheatgrass, alfalfa, chlorophyll, spirulina, parsley, yellow root, cranesbill, camu, marshmallow root, gotu kola, papaya leaf, prickly ash bark, sage, goldenseal, meadowsweet, black seed, propolis, garlic and aloe vera will help heal ulcers.
- *I suggest Sangre de Drago, Licro Plus, Camu Plus, Alpha Green, Complete probiotics & BR SP Plus*

Ulcer Healing Formula
- Empty 4 capsules of Alpha Green in 2 oz. of water
- Add 25 drops of Sangre de Drago

Drink mixture 3 times a day

Essential Oils For Ulcers
- Peppermint 2 drops
- Chamomile 2 drops

Mix with water drink twice daily

URINARY TRACT INFECTIONS
- Emotions: feeling pissed off, usually at the opposite sex or your lover.

- Bladder or urinary tract infections are usually caused by E. coli infections, sexual intercourse, antibiotics and too much sugar. Usually the body is too acidic. Get the pH more alkaline by eating plenty of vegetables.
- Drink lots of lemon water to flush out the urinary tract and alkalize pH.
- Magnesium is good to help pass any gravel or stones.
- Organic, unsweetened cranberry juice is good to drink.
- Probiotics help build up the immune system.
- Solidago (goldenrod), corn silk, uva ursi, juniper, goldenseal, garlic and parsley are good.
- Add 2 drops of lemon oil with a glass of water and drink twice daily.
- *I suggest K/B Plus, Solidago, KLS Enviro, Echinacea Complex, Alpha Green II & Rena Plus*

Urinary Support
- Oregano oil 2 drops
- Clove oil 2 drops
- Myrrh oil 2 drops

Mix with 1 Tbsp. of coconut oil and consume twice daily

VARICOSE VEINS
- Emotions: wanting to run away, standing in a situation you hate. Feeling overburdened.
- Varicose veins are many times caused from a copper deficiency. Copper is the mineral that allows tubing in the body to stay pliable.
- Horse chestnut and butcher's broom are good.
- Exercise is important. Compression socks can help.
- Massaging essential oils cypress, geranium, fir needle and thyme with some coconut oil on your legs twice daily is beneficial. Start at the ankles and move up the legs, but avoid pressing directly over veins. Once finished, lie on your back with legs elevated on pillows for 10 minutes.
- *I recommend Veno Plus, Chestnut Plus, Vascutin, Alpha Flavin & intraMAX*

VERTIGO
- Emotions: refusing to look, not wanting to accept things as they are.
- Dizziness occurs many times because of sluggish adrenal glands. Licorice, kelp and ginger support the adrenals.
- Royal jelly is high in pantothenic acid, which is good for the adrenals.
- Vitamin C from citrus bioflavonoids can be beneficial for chronic fatigue and vertigo.
- B vitamins are important.
- Increasing circulation can help. Support includes ginkgo biloba, ginseng, butcher's broom, cayenne, ginger, gotu kola, oat straw, rosemary, garlic and parsley.
- *I recommend Adrena Plus, Alpha Flavin, Circu Plus, Gota Plus, Clear Mind & Brain Formula*

VITILIGO
- Emotions: feeling like you don't belong, not one of the group.
- A disorder that affects pigmentation of the skin, causing white, blotchy patches.
- Autoimmune issues may be a factor.
- Vitamins A, B12, D, C, folic acid, zinc, copper & beta carotene can help.
- L-phenylalanine 100 mg a day can help.
- Gingko biloba & evening primrose oil are good.
- *I suggest KLS Enviro, Burdock Plus, Alpha E Spleen, Evening Primrose oil & Probiotics*

WARTS
- Emotions: expressing hate, refusing to see the beauty in life. Belief in ugliness.
- Warts are caused from the human papillomavirus (HPV). There are more than 100 types.
- Apple cider vinegar applied twice daily and then covered with a bandage is a simple remedy that has proven effective. May take 8 weeks to kill the wart.
- Thuja occidentalis 30x helps eliminate warts.
- Salted onion is good to put on warts.
- Echinacea, olive leaf, garlic, selenium & zinc are good. The sap from dandelions or fig trees will eliminate warts.
- Lemongrass has been proven to eliminate the herpes simplex type 1 virus (cold sores). It's very anti-viral.
- *I suggest Arco Plus, Immu C, Olive leaf & Allibiotic*

Wart Remover Formula
- Lemongrass oil   10 drops
- Tea Tree oil   10 drops
- Oregano oil   10 drops
- Mix in 1 oz glass dropper bottle
- Add 1 tsp. coconut oil

Fill remainder of bottle with organic apple cider vinegar. Apply to warts twice daily, covering with bandage.

> **"Many of life's failures are people who did not realize how close they were to success when they gave up."** Thomas Edison

Health Tips

- Pain and symptoms occurring on the left side of the body are usually an indication of a sodium deficiency. The best foods to replenish depleted sodium levels are spirulina, celery juice, alfalfa, okra (not fried), carrots, cabbage, spinach, strawberries, beets, cucumbers, plums, powdered whey, raw goat's milk, chicken and turkey gizzards.

    > **Carrier Oils for Essential Oils**
    > - Coconut oil
    > - Olive oil
    > - Jojoba oil
    > - Almond oil
    > - Avocado oil
    > - Apricot Kernel oil
    >
    > When using essential oils, they are very powerful and can burn. Many need to be diluted with a carrier oil.

    When talking about sodium, I don't mean the junk you buy from the store to sprinkle on French fries. I'm talking about organic sodium that Mother Nature puts in plant foods. Sodium found in fruits, vegetables and herbs are absorbable at the cellular level. It is the fuel your body needs.

    Table salt is produced by heating sodium chloride up to about 1500 degrees to solidify the salt crystals. Additives are used as anticoagulants so the salt will pour under moist conditions. This man-made product is not completely soluble in water or the blood stream and it can adhere to the arteries.

- Problems manifesting on the right side of the body are warning signals that you are in desperate need of potassium. The best sources of potassium are bee pollen, alfalfa, burdock, potatoes, oranges, tomatoes, bananas, kelp, apricots and dates.

- Be aware that conventional methods of checking the blood for nutritional deficiencies are many times inaccurate. The body does everything in its power to keep the blood in homeostasis. When the blood chemistry changes, we have very serious deficiencies and we are way late to the rescue.

> "The journey of a thousand miles begins and ends with one step." Lao Tsu

Herbal Formulas For Children

For children, we use herbal formulas by Nutritional Resources, containing glycerin instead of an alcohol base. These are some of our best formulas, and great for adults too.

HERBAL FORMULA	USE FOR	INGREDIENTS
Breeze Blend	Respiratory issues, coughs	Astragalus, chamomile, horehound, licorice, lobelia, mullein, Oregon grape & sage
Calming Chamomile	To calm & relax	Catnip, chamomile, passion flower, spearmint, rose bud, hops, shavegrass & essential oils
Candosolve Blend	Antibacterial & antifungal	Chaparral, bayberry, pau d'arco, black walnut & olive leaf
Cedar Berry Blend	Blood sugar balancing	Alfalfa, burdock, cedar berry, dandelion, elderberry, fenugreek, juniper berry, uva ursi, goldenseal & essential oils

Children's Composition Plus	Colds, fevers & flu	Chamomile, elder flowers, peppermint, yarrow, lemon balm & essential oils
Digestive Bitters	Expels parasites	Gentian, myrrh, orange peel, peppermint, wormwood & essential oils
Echinacea & Elderberry	Immune/lymph support	Echinacea & elderberry
Echinacea For Health	Immune support	Echinacea, Oregon grape, black walnut, lemon balm, thyme & essential oils
Herbal Minerals II	Mineral support, pica	Alfalfa, chamomile, dill, nettle, oatstraw, peppermint, red raspberry, shavegrass & yarrow
Herbs Achoo	Allergies	Boneset, dandelion, fennel, fenugreek, marshmallow, mullein, Oregon grape & slippery elm
Iodine Combination	Thyroid support	Black walnut, bladderwrack, dulse, Irish moss, kelp & essential oils
Kids Cascara Blend	Healthy bowels, laxative	Catnip, elderberry, licorice, cascara sagrada, anise, black walnut, fennel & essential oils
Magnificent Mullein	Dry cough	Marshmallow, mullein, angelica, calendula, elderberry, orange peel, lobelia & essential oils
Night Night Combo	Calms the nerves for sleep	Catnip, chamomile, hops, skullcap & valerian
Pau d'Arco Plus	Candida yeast/Immune	Pau d'arco, reishi mushrooms, usnea, burdock, echinacea, red clover, thyme & essential oils
Red Clover Blend	Skin problems	Burdock, chaparral & red clover
Red Root Combination	Immune/lymph	Red root, echinacea, elderberry, blue vervain, yarrow, myrrh, thyme & essential oils
Schizandra Nectar	Helps with stress	Ginkgo, gotu kola, schizandra berry, Siberian ginseng, stevia & essential oils
Super Catnip & Fennel	Indigestion & colic	Catnip, fennel, meadowsweet, licorice & essential oils
Sweet Tooth	Deters cravings for sweets	Gymnema, licorice, burdock, dandelion, Siberian ginseng, stevia & essential oils
White Willow Plus	Headache & pain reliever	White willow, meadowsweet, wild lettuce & essential oils
Wonderful Wild Cherry	Wet cough & respiratory	White pine, wild cherry, elderberry, elecampane, licorice, spikenard, cinnamon & essential oils

Dr. Sainsbury's Health Plan

1. 50 to 75 percent of your diet should consist of nature's food from the garden
Vegetables (green, crunchy & organic if possible) should be the staple of your diet. If it grows in the garden, it's usually OK to eat with the exception of corn and potatoes. Potatoes are high glycemic foods and should be consumed sparingly. Sweet potatoes are a healthier choice when consumed in moderation. Fresh berries and fruits in moderation are good. If it won't spoil, nature didn't make it. Living foods contain enzymes. Cooking over 118 degrees destroys nutritional value and enzymes needed for digestion.

2. Eat healthy fats & avoid grains Eat avocados, olives, eggs, coconut oil, butter, nuts and seeds. The ketogenic diet is good as well as the paleo diet. Gluten-free breads made from almond or coconut flour are OK. Ezekiel bread (from sprouted grains) is a healthier choice than regular wheat bread but still elevates blood-sugar levels and may contain gluten depending upon harvest dates. Gluten-free grains such as brown or black rice, quinoa or buckwheat may be used sparingly.

Dairy products are mucus-forming. Try eliminating all dairy for a week and see if you feel better. Goat's milk is better than cow's milk. If you can't get milk from a farmer in its natural raw state, leave it alone. Homogenized and pasteurized dairy products are big culprits for respiratory illnesses and allergies, especially for children. They can cause arthritis too.

- Substitute your table salt with sea salt.
- Cook with ghee, coconut oil or butter. Eat olive oil raw.
- Eat meat in moderation. Fish (that have scales and fins), chicken, turkey, steak and beef from organic sources are best. Wild-caught Alaskan salmon is good (canned Alaskan salmon is OK).
- Organic eggs are good, they don't cause high cholesterol.
- Beans, lentils and peas are healthy but may be an issue for diabetics. Use sparingly.
- Raw honey, molasses and stevia are good sweeteners. Use stevia if you have blood sugar issues.

> "…White sugar, white bread, pasta, and pastry that Americans eat have given them more chronic diseases than any other nation in the world. The reason they don't spoil is that they are so doped up with potentially hazardous artificial chemicals that they are virtually embalmed. One of the characteristics of wholesome food is that if it gets old, it spoils, so you won't hurt yourself by eating it." Dr. David Reuben

3. **Keep your pH (saliva) balanced** Your body functions best when the pH of the saliva is 6.8 to 7.0. Eating raw fruits and vegetables will help you achieve this. All herbs are alkaline-forming foods. Freshly-squeezed lemon in your water is alkalizing. The body needs water, but we want healthy, chemical-free water. Most bottled water is acidic.

4. **Two to three bowel movements a day is healthy** The body will become diseased if it doesn't eliminate wastes regularly. Prunes are natural laxatives. All fresh fruit helps the bowels move, especially when consumed in the morning for breakfast; however, if you have blood-sugar issues, skip most fruits, especially the sweet ones like bananas and watermelon.

Eating heavy cooked foods like biscuits, muffins, pancakes, French toast and milk with cereal causes the bowels to become sluggish. Cooked foods cause constipation. Chronic diarrhea is often constipation in disguise. Aloe vera juice, cascara sagrada, senna, magnesium and psyllium husk powder are good natural laxatives.

5. **Avoid soft drinks & artificial sweeteners** If you have diabetes or blood sugar issues, use stevia for a sweetener. Stevia is an herb from South America that is 200 times sweeter than sugar with 0 calories. It actually helps regulate the blood sugar. Artificial sweeteners cause cancer by interfering with cellular activity. They also cause blood sugar disturbances. Carbonated drinks block calcium absorption in the body and are very acidic with a pH of 2.

6. **Avoid radiation - microwave ovens & airport full-body scanners** Radiation causes cancer. Warning signs "CAUTION RADIATION," are there to protect us. Pregnant women are told to avoid X-rays because radiation can harm the fetus. What else do you think it may cause to delicate cells? Researchers believe that 50 percent of America's cancers are radiation-induced. Every time you go through an airport scanner, you are being exposed to radiation, increasing your risk of cancer and possibly causing infertility. Avoid these at all costs. Let them do a pat down.

    Microwaves are radiation ovens that destroy nutritional value of food. Research has proven that microwaving food kills 98 percent of cancer-fighting nutrients in broccoli. Eating microwaved food has been shown to alter your blood chemistry by creating unnatural radiolytic compounds favoring cancer. Dr. Hans Hertel has proven microwaving food to be dangerous and a risk for cancer. Do not radiate your food and then ask God to bless it to nourish and strengthen your body. You might as well set a gallon of gasoline on the table and ask him to turn it into grape juice, as long as you have that kind of faith! Think before you swallow. We can't make foolish decisions like jumping off the roof of a building and then praying to God to save us. We live in a world of cause and effect. The way your food is prepared affects your health. Be responsible, not unreasonable. Yes, I know we all are going to die eventually, but the goal is to stay healthy by avoiding those things we know to be harmful. Ignorance is not bliss. It may cost you a lot of unnecessary pain and suffering.

7. **Drink clean, purified water** Avoid drinking tap water containing chlorine and fluoride. Natural spring water is good, if the spring is a clean source. A water purifier like the Berkey www.berkeyfilters.com is good. Reverse osmosis is good. Structured water is good. Distilled water is good; add a pinch of sea salt to provide minerals. Plastic bottled water leaches chemicals (xenoestrogens) into the water and is usually acidic. Get a filtration system for your house. It will pay for itself in less than a year. A wise person drinks clean, chemical-free, healthy water.

8. **Limit your consumption of sugar & processed food** Read labels and stay away from ingredients you can't pronounce. These chemicals were never meant to be put in the body. After years of consumption, they accumulate in the body and interfere with cellular activity. Remember, respect the temple God has given you. There are no trade–ins, like we are privileged of doing with automobiles, when they begin to fall apart. Be wise, live long and prosper!

9. **Cook with garlic, ginger, turmeric & onions often** These foods are powerful immune supporters, Mother Nature's superior antibiotics, without the adverse side effects. They have been proven to be antiviral, antibacterial and antifungal. In parts of Russia where people can't afford medicine, garlic is referred to as "Russian Penicillin." Eating a couple of cloves a day keeps the doctor away. Eat it liberally when cold and flu season hits. A soup with lots of garlic and bone broth keeps the armed forces of your immune system stocked with ammunition to protect against viruses, bacteria and cancer.

10. **Eat meat sparingly** Meat takes a lot of energy to break down, and it produces uric acid. Every case of gout/arthritis I have ever seen comes from heavy meat eaters. Eat it in moderation. Eat lots of vegetables, especially fresh cherries. Uric acid can accumulate in the joints and cause inflammation and pain. Many Americans get up in the morning and have a sausage biscuit for breakfast, a hamburger for lunch, and spaghetti and meatballs for dinner. They eat meat three times a day and their bodies are flooded with acids, causing inflammation and zapping energy.

11. **Breathe deeply** Oxygenate the cells in your body. Breathe in through your nose as deeply as you can 50 times a day. Dr. Otto Warburg won the Nobel Prize for discovering that cancer cells can't survive where there is oxygen. Diffusing essential oils or rubbing some lavender, peppermint or eucalyptus under the nose is beneficial.

> "All chronic pain, suffering and diseases are caused from a lack of oxygen at the cell level." Arthur C. Guyton, M.D.

12. **Avoid drinking a lot of liquids with meals** Drinking water, juice or soft drinks with meals dilutes digestive juices. With the exception of a few sips here and there, wait 30 minutes before or after a meal to drink liquids. Chew each bite of food at least 30 times before swallowing. Chewing your food and mixing it with enzymes in your saliva is the first step in digestion.

13. **Get enough sleep** Most people need eight hours every night. Some need 10 and others only need six. Give your body what it needs. We are all different. Children need 12 hours each night for their growing bodies. Remember, sleep is when your body heals, so don't cut yourself short. Most people catch colds after a lot of stress and not enough sleep. Get up when you are rested and go to bed when you are tired.

    Exercise and hard labor make you sleep well at night. Some Americans don't sleep well because they don't do anything all day. Sorry, but watching TV is in the same category of not doing anything. Usually, the earlier you go to bed, the better. The body rests best before midnight and this is also when hormones are manufactured. Sleep studies indicate that every hour you sleep before midnight is equivalent to two hours of sleep after midnight. Remember, early to bed and early to rise makes one wise.

14. **Avoid aluminum cookware** Aluminum is linked to Alzheimer's and nervous system disorders. Most restaurants cook with aluminum pots and pans. Use stainless steel, glass or earthen cookware. Cast iron is OK.

15. **Do a liver, kidney, gallbladder & spleen cleanse once a year** You take your car in and change the oil every 3,000 miles and tune it up, right? How about giving your body a tune-up? Dandelion, nettles, goldenrod, milk thistle, artichoke leaf, boldo, uva ursi, juniper, corn silk, burdock and parsley are good for these organs. A 30-day cleanse, taking 50 drops 3 times a day with our KLS-Enviro formula, provides a good tune-up. This is preventive medicine.

16. **Fast once a month (no food for 24 hours, water only)** After God created the earth in six days, He then rested of His labors. Sunday is a good day to let your digestive system rest from laboring by fasting for 24 hours. Control the desires of the flesh by giving up food for a day and be spiritually enlightened. This keeps your priorities in check and realigns what your goals are in life. Give your body a break from working so hard all the time. If your cells could talk, they would tell you they are overworked and underpaid. They need a break occasionally, just like you do. Fasting helps you appreciate food and creates gratitude.

17. **Fast and do a colon cleanse every year** It is believed that all disease starts in the colon. Eat only fresh fruits and vegetables while doing a cleanse. Juicing is very healthy. Dr. Richard Anderson's Arise & Shine Cleansing Program is very effective for cleansing the body. It consists of taking psyllium husk and bentonite clay shakes several times a day along with Chomper and Herbal Nutrition herbal formulas. Most of us do well to cleanse for 21 days, with the last 3 days having water only, no food. This takes self-discipline, but you reap

what you sow. This is a good insurance policy for the body. It's a great way to lose a few extra pounds put on over the holidays and boost up your immune system, so you don't catch the next onslaught of cold viruses that come your way.

When I did my first cleanse, I had eight large bowel movements every day. The old fecal matter (mucoid plaque) that came out looked like black strips of tire off the highway. I thought I was healthy and in good shape, but little did I know my intestinal tract was way overdue for a cleanse. See ariseandshine.com for more information.

18. **Do a parasite cleanse every year** Microscopic parasites are everywhere. These little guys set up shop in your body and steal your nutrition. They can interfere with the functions of organs and glands, especially the liver, gallbladder, ileocecal valve, intestinal tract and appendix. We de-worm our pets and animals, but somehow think we humans are immune. Microscopic parasites are everywhere. No one is 100 percent immune to parasites. Anywhere your blood goes, parasites can go. If you have pets, you are at high risk. Pets lick their hind ends to clean themselves, then you come home from work and they lick you. The bottom line is, animals and humans get parasites. Do a parasite cleanse once a year.

19. **Get chiropractic adjustments regularly** Adjustments keep your spine aligned. Life is traumatic, and a good adjustment keeps pressure off nerves that correspond to every organ and gland in the body. Headaches can be triggered by pinched nerves as well as every other symptom you can name. If you have back or neck pain, go get an adjustment, not a prescription for pain medication.

20. **Get a massage periodically** Massage is a great stress reliever. Most of us need stress release, and a massage can help you relax. It is very effective for helping the lymphatic system drain toxins as well. Some headaches and joint pains are caused by tight muscles. Relaxing those muscles with massage can sometimes be the magic touch that heals. The laying on of hands is healing. A good massage and chiropractic adjustment can make you feel like a new person. When tight muscles relax then vertebrae can line up and pain disappears.

21. **Use real butter, not margarine** Avoid artificial man-made chemicals that the body can't metabolize. Margarine is one molecule away from plastic and probably just as toxic. Read the ingredients on what you buy. If it says hydrogenated oil or partially hydrogenated oil, avoid it. Artificial fats and oils are what block arteries and cause heart disease. They cause an immune response that leads to arteriosclerosis and plaque build-up. Use real butter — organic, of course, is better. Cook with coconut butter (oil), and use olive oil raw.

22. **Drink 16 ounces of water upon arising every morning** Hydrate your 100 trillion cells after sleeping all night. They need water to function and cleanse out toxins. Try washing your car or the dishes without water, it doesn't work. Water is a cleanser, and most Americans are severely dehydrated. If you wait until you are thirsty to drink water, you are way too late. You can't flush a toilet without water, and your bowels will have a difficult time moving when they are dried up from a lack of water.

23. **Avoid cooking with nonstick cookware** These chemicals absorb into your food from the pan and cause health problems. Use stainless steel, glass or earthen cookware.

24. **Stay away from "fat free" products** "Fat free" usually means "loaded with chemicals." There's a price to be paid for everything you choose to put in your mouth. What you don't know may kill you, if you keep doing it ignorantly. Cook with coconut oil, ghee or butter.

25. **Forgive those who have trespassed you** By holding on to anger, resentment, bitterness, hurt or a grudge of any sort, you are not hurting the other person, you are only hurting yourself. We are commanded to forgive so we can set ourselves free. It is good to forgive others and be kind for their benefit. However, it is more important to forgive so that we liberate ourselves from negative emotions. By holding onto negativity, we usually hurt ourselves the most. Quit worrying about what others say and do and release your own trash. Or better said, take the beam out of your own eye first and stop making others wrong.

26. **Laugh often** It has been said, "Laughter is the best medicine." Laughing has been shown scientifically to increase B-cells, which help fight infections. Laughing dilates blood vessels, which increases blood flow to all areas of the body and helps pump the lymphatic system. A good belly laugh helps you relax. A laugh and even a smile eases tension so things flow easier. No one enjoys being around someone who is serious all the time and never laughs. Laughing often is a key to stress reduction and good health. Find the little things in life that make you smile and laugh. It's a wise investment.

> **"Approach impossible goals by breaking them down into possible increments. Or, to put it another way: how do you move a mountain? One rock at a time."**
> John W. Travis, M.D.

HEALTH EVALUATION

Place number next to the symptoms which apply to you:
Use (1) for MILD symptoms (2) for MODERATE symptoms (3) for SEVERE symptoms

GROUP ONE

___ "Nervous" Stomach
___ Dry mouth, eyes, nose
___ Pulse speeds after meals
___ Keyed-up – fail to calm
___ Mentally alert, quick
___ Extremities cold, clammy
___ Heart pounds after retiring
___ Acid foods upset
___ Cold sweats often
___ Fever easily raised
___ Neuralgia-like pains

___ Are your symptoms made worse by emotional stress?

GROUP TWO

___ Perspire easily
___ Muscle-leg-toe cramps
___ Eyelids swollen, puffy
___ Indigestion soon after meals
___ Digestion rapid
___ Vomiting frequent
___ Difficulty swallowing
___ Constipation, diarrhea
___ Joint stiffness after rising
___ Circulation poor, sensitive to cold
___ Subject to colds, asthma, bronchitis
___ Are your symptoms made worse by physical stress?

GROUP THREE

___ Afternoon headaches
___ Get "shaky" if hungry
___ Faintness if meals delayed
___ Heart palpitates if meals Missed or delayed
___ Awaken after few hours can't get back to sleep
___ Crave candy or coffee in afternoons
___ Abnormal craving for sweets or snacks

GROUP FOUR

___ Bruise easily
___ Sigh frequently
___ Breath heavily
___ Opens window in rooms
___ Susceptible to colds/fever
___ Swollen ankles
___ Muscle cramps
___ Shortness of breath
___ Dull pain in chest or radiating into left arm
___ Hands & feet go to sleep easily, numbness
___ Tendency to anemia
___ Tension under breastbone or feeling of "tightness"

GROUP FIVE

___ Dry skin
___ Skin rashes frequent
___ Bitter metallic taste in mouth in mornings
___ Bowel movements painful or difficult
___ Biliousness (constipation, headaches)
___ Greasy foods upset
___ Stools light colored
___ Pain between shoulder blades
___ Laxatives used often
___ History of gallbladder attacks or gallstones
___ Sneezing attacks

GROUP SIX

___ Lower bowel gas several hours after eating
___ Burning stomach sensations, eating relieves
___ Coated tongue
___ Indigestion ½ - 1 hour after
___ Gas shortly after eating
___ Stomach "bloating" after eating; may continue for 3-4 hours

GROUP SEVEN

(A)

___ Pulse fast at rest
___ Nervousness
___ Can't gain weight
___ Intolerance to heat
___ Highly emotional

(C)

___ Low blood pressure
___ Failing memory
___ Increased sex desire
___ Headaches
___ Decreased sugar tolerance

(E)

___ Hot flashes
___ Headaches
___ Dizziness
___ Increased blood pressure
___ Sugar in urine (not diabetes)

___ Flush easily
___ Night sweats
___ Inward trembling
___ Heart palpitates
___ Insomnia

___ Masculine tendencies-female

(B)

___ Impaired hearing
___ Decrease in appetite
___ Ringing in ears
___ Constipation
___ Mental sluggishness
___ Headaches upon arising wear off during day
___ Slow pulse, below 65
___ Increase in weight

(D)

___ Bloating of intestines
___ Abnormal thirst
___ Weight gain around hips or waist
___ Sex desire reduced or lacking
___ Tendency to ulcers, colitis
___ Increased sugar tolerance
___ Menstrual disorders
___ Delayed menstruation

(F)

___ Low blood pressure
___ Chronic fatigue
___ Weakness, dizziness
___ Tendency to hives
___ Arthritic tendencies
___ Perspiration
___ Crave salt
___ Brown spots on skin
___ Allergies – asthma
___ Exhaustion
___ Respiratory disorders

GROUP EIGHT

(Female Only)

___ Painful menses
___ Premenstrual tension
___ Very easily fatigued
___ Depressed feeling

___ Menstruation excessive prolonged
___ Painful breasts
___ Menstruate too frequently

___ Vaginal discharge
___ Menopause, hot flashes, etc.
___ Menses scanty
___ Acne, worse at menses

(Male Only)

___ Tire too easily
___ Urination difficult
___ Night urination frequent

___ Pain on inside of legs or heel
___ Feeling of incomplete bowel evacuation

___ Prostate trouble
___ Leg nervousness at nights
___ Diminished sex desire

GROUP NINE

___ Chronic cough
___ Pain around ribs
___ Shortness of breath
___ Chest pain

___ Difficulty breathing
___ Coughing up phlegm
___ Coughing up blood

___ Bronchitis (frequent)
___ Infections settle in lungs
___ Sensitive to smog

GROUP TEN

___ Frequent urination
___ Rose colored (bloody)
___ Dripping after urination
___ Difficulty passing urine

___ Cloudy urine
___ Rarely need to urinate
___ Strong smelling urine
___ Frequent bladder infections

___ Painful/burning when passing urine
___ Urination when you cough or sneeze

GROUP ELEVEN

___ Throat infections
___ Poor wound healing
___ Slow to recover from colds or flu
___ Chronic lung congestion
___ Post nasal drip

___ Gets boils or styes
___ Swollen lymph glands
___ Catch colds or flu easily
___ Breathe through mouth
___ Swollen tongue

___ Bumpy skin on back of arms
___ Inflamed or bleeding gums
___ Hyperactivity
___ Food sensitivity or allergies

KEY

Group One **Sympathetic Nervous System** – People who are Sympathetic Dominance are in high gear. They burn up their mineral reserves, especially magnesium and potassium. Many of these people are on diuretics, which flush out minerals, thus worsening the condition.

Group Two **Parasympathetic Nervous System** – Those who are Parasympathetic Dominance are usually always in slow gear and have difficulty "getting in gear." They need extra phosphorus. Lecithin is high in phosphorus.

- Understand that the sympathetic and parasympathetic nervous systems need to be balanced like a teeter-totter for optimum health.

Group Three **Pancreas** – Regulates sugar metabolism. Diabetes and (hyper) or hypoglycemia are common symptoms. Normal glucose levels are 70 to 110. Stay off dairy products and red meat. Supplement your diet with enzymes. Ginger and licorice can help.

Group Four **Cardiovascular System** – If you experience pain, you may need heart support. Magnesium, L-carnitine and L-taurine are good for the heart. If there is no pain, then you probably need circulatory support. Ginkgo biloba, ginseng, butcher's broom and flaxseed oil are good for circulation.

Group Five **Liver and Gallbladder** – Relates to digestion and the breakdown of fats. Parasites can be a factor causing symptoms. Stones can form and cause symptoms. The best herbs are dandelion, milk thistle, globe artichoke, turmeric, boldo and Oregon grape.

Group Six **Digestion (Gastro-Intestinal Tract)** – Gas and bloating usually indicates the need for more enzymes. Heartburn and burning in the stomach indicate the need for more hydrochloric acid. For ulcers, we use wheatgrass, barley greens, alfalfa, chlorophyll, spirulina, parsley and marshmallow root. An intestinal cleanse may be needed to blast through built-up fecal matter.

Group Seven
A **Hyper-thyroid** – Need more calcium.
B **Hypo-thyroid** – These people usually carry most of their weight from the waist up. Kelp is needed. Check body temperature. Temperature should be between 97.8 and 98.2.
C **Hyper-Pituitary** – Manganese and yarrow are good.
D **Hypo-Pituitary** – Weight gain from the waist to the knees. These people have a tendency to carry their weight in the buttocks, hips and thighs. Manganese and yarrow are beneficial.
E **Hyper-Adrenal** – Pantothenic acid found in Royal Jelly, bovine adrenal concentrate and licorice can help.
F **Hypo-Adrenal** – These individuals usually experience fatigue and dizziness when standing up too quickly and have respiratory issues. They have a tendency to gain weight in the midsection or belly. Support includes pantothenic acid, adrenal concentrate, licorice and ginger.

Group Eight   **Reproductive System (Female)** - Yarrow, black cohosh, blue cohosh, dong quai, zinc and amino acids can help.

                       Reproductive System (Male) – Flaxseed oil, juniper berries, saw palmetto, ginseng and yohimbe are good.

Group Nine   **Respiratory System** – Respiratory symptoms may be caused from weak adrenal glands. Mullein, myrrh, ginger, althea and nutmeg are good.

Group Ten   **Kidneys and Bladder** – Golden rod, uva ursi, juniper berry, corn silk, parsley and horsetail are good. Orthophosphoric acid dissolves kidney and bladder stones.

Group Eleven   **Immune System** – Echinacea, una de gato (cat's claw), elderberry and garlic are good.

Homemade Natural Remedies

ALL PURPOSE CLEANER
¼ teaspoon organic liquid dishwashing soap
1 tablespoon baking soda
½ teaspoon borax
Mix in spray bottle with 1 cup water

ALL PURPOSE DISINFECTANT
1 cup water
2 tablespoons Castile soap
1 teaspoon tea tree oil
10 drops eucalyptus oil
Mix together in a spray bottle

DETOX BATH
Fill bathtub with hot water
2 cups Epsom salts
½ cup Baking Soda
10 drops lavender oil
Soak for 30 minutes
Dim the lights or use candles
Put on favorite relaxing music

NATURAL DEODORANT
1 cup coconut oil
1 cup baking soda
100 drops of favorite essential oil.
Females – lavender or lemon
Male – bergamot or cypress
Mix all ingredients in a bowl. Put mixture in empty deodorant container or store in glass jar.

HOMEMADE TOOTHPASTE
½ cup baking soda
½ cup coconut oil
15 drops Peppermint Oil or (clove, lemon or myrrh)
Mix to form a thick paste. Store in a glass container with lid. Adding Hydrogen Peroxide will help whiten teeth.

Natural Weed Killer
1 gallon vinegar
2 cups Epsom salt
¼ cup Dawn dish soap

The Chinese Meridian Clock

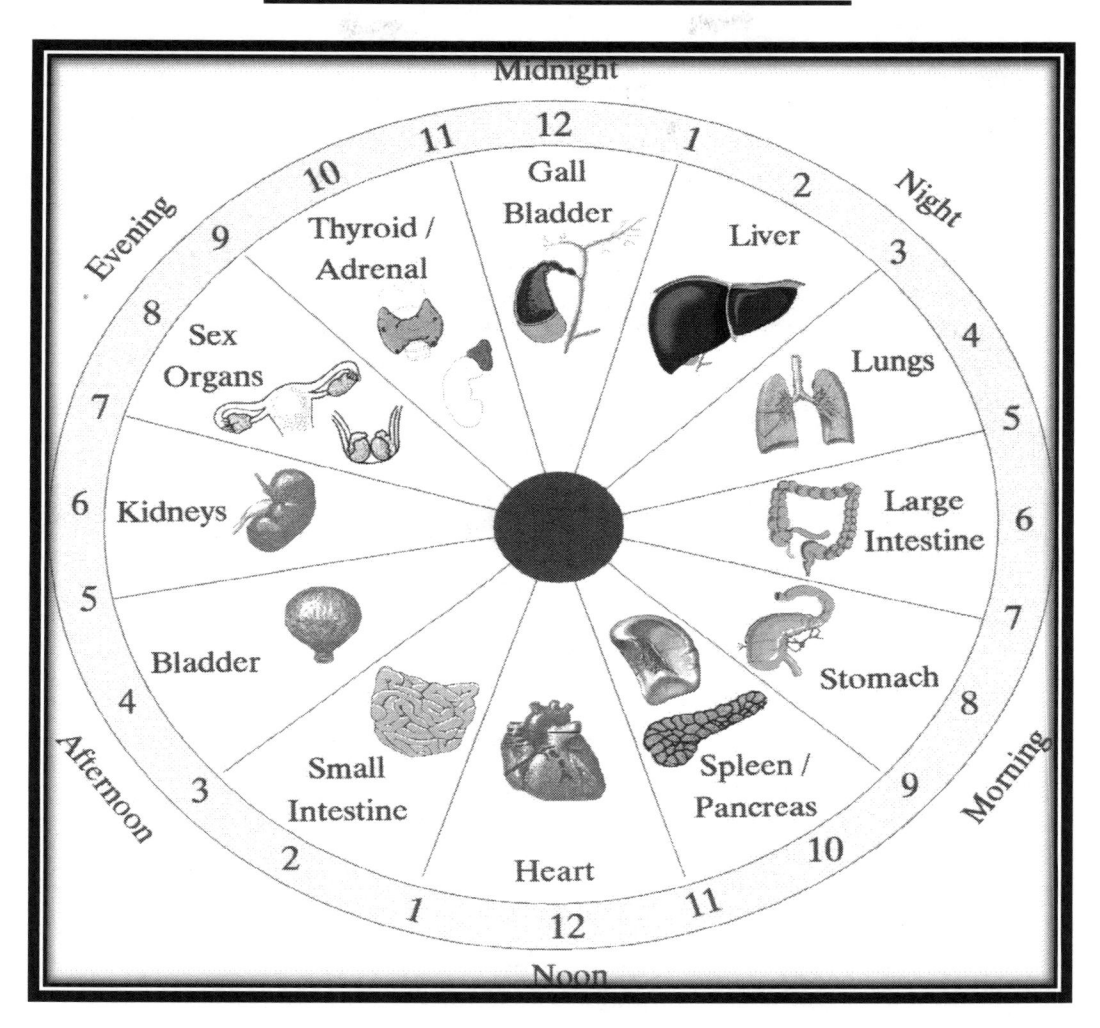

	Meridian Clock Sleep Solutions	
Time	*Organ/Gland*	*Remedy*
11pm – 1am	Gallbladder	Hydrangea, Diadren Forte
1am – 3am	Liver	KLS Enviro, Beta Plus
3am – 5am	Lungs (Adrenals)	Adrena Plus, MG/K Aspartate

    The human body has 12 meridians, and energy moves through these meridians in a 24-hour cycle. Every two hours, the energy is strongest within a specific organ or gland at certain times indicated on the clock. So, if you wake up every night from 11 p.m. to 1 a.m., you may have an issue with your gallbladder. If you wake up from 1 a.m. to 3 a.m., you may have an imbalance with your liver. If you have to get something to eat in order to get back to sleep, that's usually an indication that your blood sugar has dropped. After eating, your blood sugar rises, your nervous system relaxes and you can fall back to sleep. Diadren Forte is a good blood-sugar-stabilizing formula. If you wake up from 3 a.m. to 5 a.m., you may have an issue with the lungs or adrenal glands (the adrenals control the lungs). Many report that they are wide awake at 3 or 4 a.m., but then when it's time to get up at 7 a.m., that's when they are finally sleeping well. This is usually caused from sluggish adrenal glands caused from stress and possibly blood-sugar issues. If you don't sleep well and you wake up at different times, I would suggest taking MG/K, Diadren Forte and KLS Enviro. This supports healthy blood-sugar levels, the nervous system, liver, gallbladder and adrenal glands. Eating a high-fat, high-protein dinner and avoiding carbohydrates can help, such as baked salmon or chicken with steamed vegetables. A couple of boiled eggs, avocado or handful of nuts like almonds, pecans and walnuts are beneficial to help stabilize blood-sugar levels throughout the night.

> **"We who have no time for our health today, may have no health for our time tomorrow."** Anonymous

Stress – Fight Or Flight

About 86 percent of all illnesses and doctor visits are stress-related. Dr. Bruce Lipton, researcher at Stanford University, claims that up to 95 percent of all physical and nonphysical health problems are stress related. Many experts, along with the CDC, state that stress is the No. 1 killer on the planet. Dr. Lipton explains that stress is caused from wrong beliefs, and the wrong belief is an interpretation of destructive cellular memories.

Symptoms of Stress	
Fatigue	Allergies
Insomnia	Indigestion
Headaches	Irritability
Muscle pain	Belly fat
High BP	Diabetes

Stressful situations, when you are in danger, like a bear chasing you in the woods, cause you to go into fight-or-flight mode. Hormones relay messages from the brain to tell the rest of the body what to do, so when we are stressed, signals from the brain tell the adrenal glands to pump out hormones like epinephrine (adrenalin) and cortisol along with some 50 other hormones. This mashes the gas pedal of the sympathetic nervous system to the floor, signaling for the heart to beat faster, increasing blood pressure to rush blood to the muscles, preparing you to run for your life or stay and fight. Noradrenalin stops digestion (there's no time for a bowel movement when a bear is chasing you), and hormones necessary for you to feel sexual desire (and there's no time to make love when a bear is threatening you) are reassigned to your survival system instead of relaxation and enjoyment.

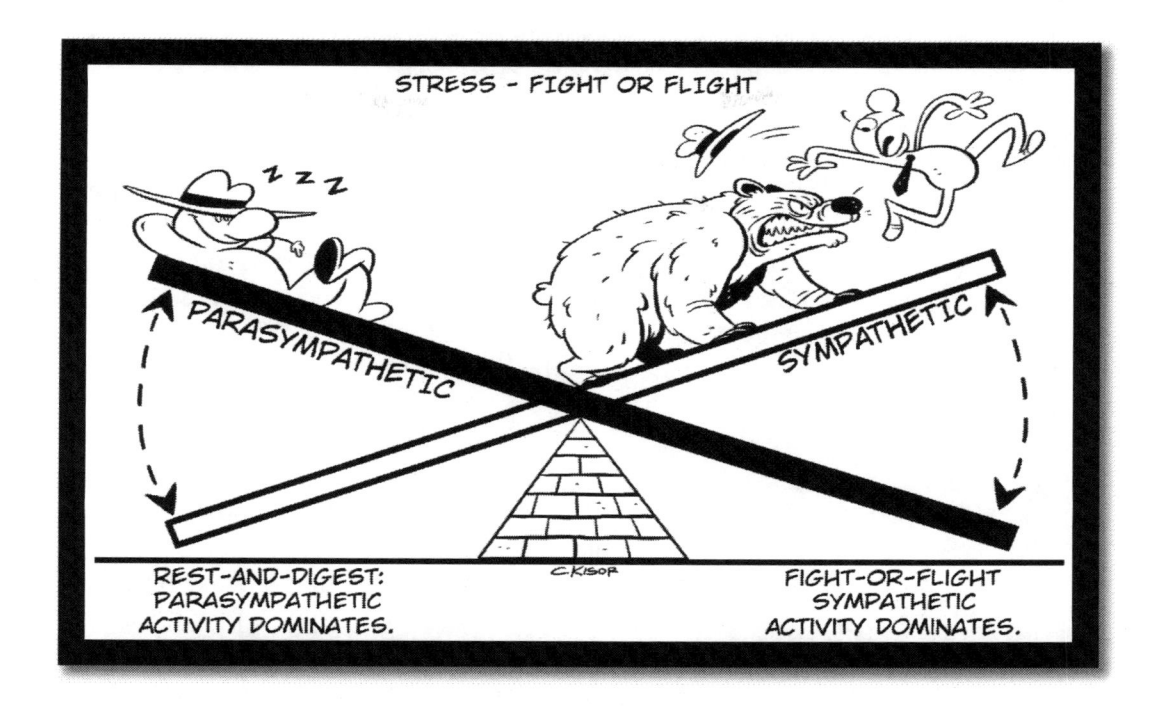

STRESS – FIGHT OR FLIGHT

REST-AND-DIGEST: PARASYMPATHETIC ACTIVITY DOMINATES.

FIGHT-OR-FLIGHT SYMPATHETIC ACTIVITY DOMINATES.

The adrenals secrete cortisol, which breaks down fat into sugar, giving you energy for the perceived threat (bear chasing you), but when we stay keyed up in fight-or-flight mode (and there's no bear chasing you, but you keep rethinking it or fearing it will happen again), this hormone causes you to become fatigued, gain weight (belly fat) and have insomnia. Too much cortisol constantly being pumped out because you chronically feel threatened and in danger will start to break down tissue and organs, causing joint pains and inflammation. Cortisol breaks down the protective lining of your intestinal wall, causing leaky gut. High cortisol levels slow down your immune system, leaving you susceptible to infections and cancer. This is why stress kills. When we are in a relaxed state and cortisol levels are balanced, it helps control blood sugar levels, balance out blood pressure along with regulating fluid levels, so we wake up in the mornings feeling refreshed with a sharp mind and memory and a healthy sex drive.

So, how do we reduce our stress levels to achieve optimal health so we can rest and digest? The problem is, many times there is no physical threat (no bear chasing us), the stress is only us perceiving something bad happening, such as worrying about all the things that could go wrong. In other words, most of our perceptions are "what ifs," fearing the worst, keying us up into fight-or-flight mode, when there is no real danger. This mental stress affects the

Perceived Stress – Mental Bears Chasing You
▪ What ifs???
▪ Worrying about things you can't control
▪ Fearing the worst will happen

physical body. This is why Dr. Lipton teaches that stress is caused from wrong beliefs.

It's not what happens that creates your emotional experiences in life, it's how you react to them. We all have stress, but to continue to worry about things that we can't control will cause exhaustion and zap your vitality. Also, your body can't tell the difference between running for pleasure and running from danger. So, if you are stressed to the max with exhausted adrenals, but you are forcing yourself to go the gym and work out for an hour every night, what message is your body getting? Is the bear chasing you again? More stress, regardless of the motivation, causes the same physiological changes within the body. Be smart and give your body what it needs.

Stress Support To Calm & Relax
- Irie 10 drops 3 x daily
- Kava Kalm 50 drops 3 x daily
- Valeri Plus 50 drops 3 x daily
- MGK 2 capsules with meals
- Adrena Plus 2 capsules with meals

It has been said that for every five minutes you are emotionally upset, it takes up to eight hours for your body to recover and come back to balance. This is why you seldom get sick when things are going well. A cold usually hits when you are stressed out and emotionally upset.

> "One minute of anger weakens the immune system for four to five hours. One minute of laughing boosts your immune system for 24 hours." Les Brown

Having fun, laughing more and going for a 20-minute walk every day has tremendous health benefits, including altering your mood and decreasing stress. It has been noted that small children laugh about 300 times a day, whereas adults only laugh about 17 times a day. Understanding how the brain works and healing unresolved emotional traumas can also help us destress, relax and experience a healthier, balanced state of living.

4-7-8 Breathing Technique For Anxiety, Stress, Cravings & Sleep

Deep breathing exercises are simple to do and can help calm and relax you when feeling stressed. When you become stressed, your breathing becomes shallow, creating a state of mild hypoxia, or oxygen deprivation. A lack of oxygen allows carbon dioxide to build up, creating oxidative stress and inflammation.
1. Place tongue on the roof of your mouth, right behind your front teeth.
2. Breathe in through your nose for a count of 4.
3. Hold your breath for a count of 7.
4. Release your breath from your mouth with a whooshing sound for a count of 8.
5. Without a break, breathe in again for a count of 4, repeating the entire technique 3 to 4 times in a row.

Chapter 10
EMOTIONS - ENERGY IN MOTION

> "Life is not a dress rehearsal. This is it. RIGHT NOW. You can choose to live it to the fullest or sit on the sidelines and watch it go by." Dr. Richard Schulze

Every problem in your life has a cause. What the body creates, it can take away. Your body communicates to you through pain and discomfort so you will make a change. When people do all the right things to get well but the body does not respond, there are usually emotions causing inflammation and preventing a healing response. Emotions play a huge part in a person's ability to heal, especially cancer.

Vultures and hummingbirds both fly over the same valley. Ones sees death, the other sees flowers and life. What do you see in the world? What do you want to see? Do you find people in your world with smiles and laughter, or are you the Grinch stealing the Who Hash, the pessimist always pointing out the problems in life? We usually find what we are looking for. That way, we get to be right.

> "The wound is the place where the light enters you." Rumi

Healing The Cause Of Cancer

A few years ago, 55-year-old Jan came to our clinic. She had multiple myeloma, cancer of the bone marrow plasma cells. After spending over $300,000 on chemotherapy treatments, her insurance maxed out and refused to pay for more treatments. She began to worry about how she was going to afford further treatments, because her oncologist told her the chemotherapy was the only thing keeping the cancer from spreading. On the other hand, it was leaving her exhausted and unable to work.

The first thing we did was an EDS exam. The evidence of why cells were mutating pieced together like a puzzle. As with most cancer patients, we found poor circulation, heavy metals, her pH was very acidic, a miasm (inherited glitch in the DNA) and emotional trauma from many years ago. We put her on a program to detoxify her for the miasm and heavy metal poisoning. We also put her on circulation support, pH alkalizing green cell foods, herbal drainer formulas to support her liver, and Graviola and cat's claw for her immune system. All of these supplements are important, but they do not work effectively until we remove the mental/emotional cactuses growing inside that feed cancer subconsciously. Yes, subconsciously, meaning you are not even aware of them most of the time. Weeding your garden requires pulling the weeds out by the roots, so they won't grow back. Only a fool clips the tops off with scissors. Just as weeds will grow right back if the roots are left, so will cancer come back if the mental/emotional blueprint is not healed that nourished it to grow in the first place. We suggest all cancer patients have an RFA (Relaxed Focused Attention) emotional release session to heal emotional traumas from the past, whether you are aware of them or not. Some individuals claim that they have near perfect relationships with love and forgiveness for everyone but remember, "Denile" is more than just a river in Egypt.

> **"All disease originates in the mind. Nothing appears on the body unless there is a mental pattern corresponding to it."** Joseph Murphy, Ph.D.

Jan came back to do an emotional release session. What we found feeding her cancer occurred when she was 19 years old, while attending college. Jan got pregnant, and she wasn't married. She came from a very religious family, and getting pregnant outside of marriage was frowned upon, to say the least, especially with her father, who was a pastor at church. To escape her father's wrath, and the embarrassment and shame of having an illegitimate child, she chose to have an abortion and never told a soul. Roughly, 36 years later, Jan was fighting cancer and this emotion of "guilt" was eating her alive, literally. Deep down inside, she felt guilty and unworthy of God's blessings, especially good health. Cancer was the way, she subconsciously felt, that she could bear the cross of her guilt and pay the price.

> **"From the bitterness of disease, man learns the sweetness of health."** Catalan Proverb

Almost everyone with cancer has emotional conflicts from the past impairing their immune system. If you are a Christian, then you believe that Christ already paid the price for our sins, but most people do not know how to let go and accept the Savior's atonement. They like to say and think they do, but subconsciously they hang on, and punish themselves, instead of allowing the blood of Christ to truly set them free. To tell someone to "just forgive," is like telling someone who is fighting mad to "just calm down and relax." It doesn't work, and may actually make them worse, because now they are mad at you for telling them not to feel how they feel.

> **"Releasing resentment will dissolve even cancer."** Louise L. Hay

We went through the RFA (Relaxed, Focused Attention) process and Jan came to understand more about her feelings and what decision she made subconsciously about life. She was then able to forgive herself fully, just as an adult forgives an innocent child. Guilt can dissolve into nothing through the power of love. Love resonates at 528 Hz frequency, and according to Dr. Len Horowitz, can repair damaged DNA. Once Jan felt that God had forgiven her, and yes, she had to forgive herself too, then she no longer needed to carry the cross of guilt, and her body chemistry changed. As she released the need to feel guilty and punish herself, an enormous amount of life-force energy (love and light) healed her. She walked out of our office that day healed emotionally, mentally and spiritually. The chains of guilt no longer held her in bondage, and with that freedom, her immune system was balanced and charged, strong enough to eradicate the abnormal cells we call cancer.

> **"I am convinced that unconditional love is the most powerful known stimulant of the immune system. If I told patients to raise their blood levels of immune globulins or killer T cells, no one would know how. But if I can teach them to love themselves and others fully, the same changes happen automatically. The truth is: love heals."** Bernie Siegel, M.D., Author of *Love Medicine & Miracles*

Now Jan works 12 hours a day, six days a week, and her co-workers can't believe it. She went from being diagnosed with cancer to chemotherapy treatments and was given a 6-month death sentence by her oncologist if she quit her treatments. When she announced that she was stopping the chemotherapy, everyone expected her to die, especially her doctor. Obviously, he didn't understand what was causing her cancer, and what was needed to turn her immune system back on the way God created it. This is true for most cancer patients.

Jan believes that had she chosen to continue to follow her oncologist's program, to kill, kill, kill cancer with poisonous chemotherapy, without ever addressing the cause of it, then she would have died. The body can only tolerate so much poison before it gives up, especially when there are unhealed emotional issues feeding it on the subconscious level. So, remember, cancer is not caused from a deficiency of poisonous chemotherapy. Lack of forgiveness, guilt and resentment are usually at its roots, if you want to dig down to the cause.

> **"I feel that all disease is ultimately related to a lack of love, or to love that is only conditional, for the exhaustion and depression of the immune system thus created leads to physical vulnerability. I also feel that all healing is related to the ability to give and accept unconditional love."** Bernie Siegel, M.D.

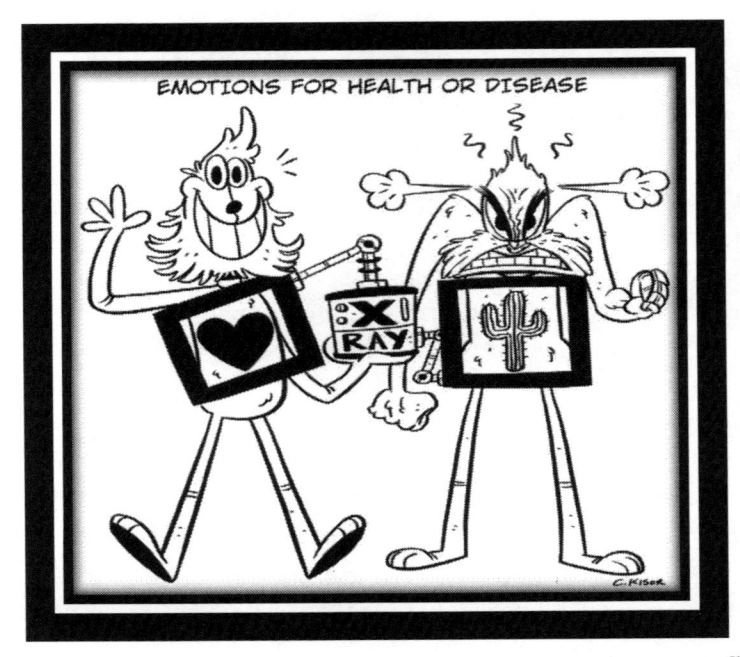

Tears of joy are considered nontoxic, but tears of anger are loaded with proteins and are said to be more poisonous than snake venom. You can't expect healing to occur on the physical level when on the emotional level you are filled with thorns of anger, guilt, resentment, hate and fear. When these dark, dis-ease producing emotions are resonating within, healing is blocked. The intelligence that instructs the cells of your body cannot send out healthy, energetic frequencies if negative feelings are flowing through you.

Most cancer patients struggle with the inability to forgive. Unresolved emotional friction causes anxiety and depression. It is interesting to note that one out of every five Americans takes antidepressant drugs, and one out of five Americans also dies of cancer. Is this coincidence? A lack of forgiveness may be the chief cause of most cancers. Most women with breast cancer have usually had a broken heart sometime in their life. When cancer shows up in the left breast of right-handed women, that usually represents a conflict with child, your home or mother. If cancer manifests in the right breast, that usually involves a conflict with your spouse or significant other.

> "If cancer or any other illness returns, I do not believe it is because they did not 'get it all out,' but rather that the patient has made no mental change."
> Louise L. Hay

Healing My Allergies

When I was 21 years old, I developed terrible allergies. My nose was constantly stopped up, and having to breathe through my mouth was sheer misery. The only time I got relief is when I would work out. I went to see a medical doctor and explained how I was miserable from not being able to breathe through my nose. He asked if I had any nasal discharge. I replied, "No, it's like someone poured cement in my sinuses, and it's totally sealed off." He immediately wrote a prescription for two drugs. I took the drugs and experienced fatigue, constipation and headaches, and still got no relief from my allergies. Three weeks later, I went back to tell him that it wasn't working, so we went through the same procedure again, and he prescribed some different drugs.

The second round of drugs also failed to clear up my sinus problem, so this time my doctor referred me to an ear, nose and throat specialist. He X-rayed my nose. We looked at the X-ray together and he pointed out that my left nostril was smaller than the right. He told me, "we could do surgery and widen the nasal passage of the left nostril, but there's no guarantee that it will help clear up your nose." That was completely ridiculous to me. I wanted to know what was causing my allergies and how to heal them, not just a guess as to what might help.

I realized then that the guessing games doctors play with their drugs isn't health care. No testing is done to find what is wrong, or how it got that way. They simply are suppressing symptoms with harmful chemical-drugs, and if that doesn't work, they suggest surgery. That is not health! I wanted to heal my stopped-up nose, and I knew there was a cause. The doctors failed miserably in even attempting to find it, let alone eliminating it. Common sense kept badgering me with the question, *"If you don't find the cause, how are you going to cure it?"*

After the drugs failed to clear my sinuses, I tried visiting health food stores. I talked to nutritionists and bought a lot of herbs and supplements for colon and liver cleanses, but once again to no avail. I was still unable to breathe through my nose and finally declared to my mom one night that I would pay anything if I could just breathe. In that moment of misery, I vowed to myself that I would find the cause and cure for my allergies. I had no idea how, but I knew I had to study health, not disease, drugs and surgery, to find the solution.

> **"When you are sick of sickness, you are no longer sick."** Old Chinese Proverb

Divine Guidance – When The Student Is Ready, The Teacher Appears

One cold, snowy day in the winter, I was studying for a college algebra exam. As I sat there studying, something within told me to turn on the radio, but I ignored it. I had another strong premonition to turn the radio on, but rationalized that I couldn't, I had to study or else I would flunk my test. On the third time, I finally turned the radio on to hear Dr. Jack Stalkwell's K-Talk program with his guest, Max Skousen, talking about how to heal allergies. It's amazing what happens in life when you listen and act upon those quiet whispers from within. I immediately knew that the teacher had appeared if I, the student, was ready.

It is important to understand that everything in life is resonating energy. We resonate at specific frequencies and attract or repel certain people to us. Have you ever had good or bad vibes about someone? A great book to explain how we attract certain people and things into our lives, including

> Watch
> **"The Secret"**
> The Law Of Attraction

success and failures, and even bad or good relationships, is the documentary "The Secret," by Rhonda Byrne. It teaches you how to stop being a victim and start attracting what you want and choose into your life.

> **"With everything that has happened to you, you can either feel sorry for yourself or treat what has happened as a gift. Everything is either an opportunity to grow or an obstacle to keep you from growing. You get to choose."** Dr. Wayne Dyer

Max announced that he would be speaking at a local hotel on how to heal allergies, and I made it a priority to attend. We do that in life, make things that are important to us top priority. So, I went and learned what causes allergies, and it was one of the most profound lectures I have ever heard. Max explained how the RFA process works. After listening to his amazing presentation on how powerful the subconscious mind is, I went and had an RFA (emotional release) session, and it was incredible. After one session, my stopped-up nose was completely healed. We addressed the root cause, fixed the problem, and my allergies were healed.

> **"The visible world is the invisible organization of energy."** Dr. Heinz Pagels, 1939-1988

Kinesiology

Kinesiology, or muscle testing, received scientific attention through the works of Dr. George Goodheart and later Dr. John Diamond. How does kinesiology work? Our body sends out very minute electrical currents, which flow from the brain to all of the muscles. If the mind is speaking truth, it is in harmony and the electrical signal goes out unimpaired. But if the mind is not telling the truth, it creates conflict, creating some degree of static and confusion, so that the electrical current is not sent out with the same strength and therefore causes a weakness in muscular response. If doing a muscle test with an arm, the muscles become weaker to some degree when making a false statement, as opposed to being strong when stating something that is true.

Through muscle testing, we can identify what is causing a person's illness, who was involved, and the time it occurred. Health practitioners use this technique to determine which supplements are good for your body and which ones are not by holding a supplement in one hand and muscle testing the opposite arm. A strong response indicates that the product is strengthening you and therefore good for you. A weak response indicates that the supplement is weakening you and therefore is not good for you. Muscle testing acts as a human lie detector. Your body will give answers when asked. For more information on how kinesiology works, and especially for the skeptics who feel they need a medical doctor to tell them what to do, I recommend reading *Power vs. Force* by David R. Hawkins, M.D., Ph.D.

> **"Your subconscious mind is all-wise. It knows the answers to all questions. However, it does not know that it knows."** Joseph Murphy, Ph.D.

Many allergies are caused by traumatic experiences that have occurred in life. Through the RFA process, I learned that my allergies were caused by something that happened when I was in the second month of my mother's womb. Since a baby in the womb is a magnet to mother's feelings, he or she feels everything mother does, and those feelings are permanently recorded in the subconscious mind. Once we make a decision about those feelings, subconsciously, then a story is created that usually forms a concrete belief, which becomes our law of truth. It is interesting to note that the ear of the fetus in the womb is the first part of the physical body to fully develop, so before you were born, you were hearing what was going on in the world of your mother, and all of her conversations.

> **Once We Make A Decision With Intense Emotion, It Becomes Our Truth.**

The RFA process takes about one hour. My allergies were not caused from a physical problem, they were caused from an emotional trauma from the past, and once we released the negativity programmed in my subconscious, healing occurred. I can now breathe through my nose. I didn't need a bunch of drugs or surgery. I didn't need a neti-pot, enema, herbs, minerals or any other natural supplement. What I needed was an emotional release, a subconscious detox to heal the cause.

> **"Disease will never be cured or eradicated by present materialistic methods, for the simple reason that disease in its origin is not material. Disease is in essence the result of conflict between soul and mind, and will never be eradicated except by spiritual and mental effort."** Edward Bach, M.B., B.S., D.P.H., Creator of Bach Flower Remedies

The Power Of The Mind

All the religious books ever written from the beginning of time state over and over again that the greatest force in human existence is the power of belief, or faith. So much of our life hinges on what we believe and what we don't believe. William James, the father of American psychology, taught that the subconscious mind has the power to move the world, and that it is one with infinite intelligence and boundless wisdom. Think back on a time when you experienced being freezing cold, the coldest you have ever been in your life. Now imagine yourself being very cold again, in that same situation. If you concentrate hard enough, you can actually decrease your body temperature enough to produce goose bumps. Tibetan monks in China can spend the night meditating in the high mountains, where the temperature drops below freezing, wearing only a sheet, and stay perfectly warm, whereas normal Americans would go into shock within four hours and die. The monks have mastered the art of meditation, and what the mind instructs the body to do, it obeys. In this situation, it is instructed to keep a certain temperature.

> **"The mind is so powerful that it can create an experience to support any belief. Then we believe the experience proves the belief, not knowing that the belief created the experience."** Krishnamurti

The power of suggestion is real. The right brain does not know the difference between real life and the imagined. Under hypnosis, a person can become so rigid that a 200-pound weight can rest on his stomach while his body is suspended between two chairs. Take another person and hand him an onion and tell him it is an apple, and he enjoys eating it with no watering of the eyes or burning of the mouth. Just thinking about something that you know you are allergic to can actually cause allergy symptoms to appear. Suggest to someone that they are allergic to dust and you are now going to hold some in front of them. Instead, you hold a cup full of paper clips, and they begin sneezing uncontrollably. What do you think caused the individual to sneeze? Was it the paper clips or the suggestion? The cause of many dis-eases (something is out of ease) is a belief in the subconscious mind.

The brain has two parts, the conscious and subconscious. The left brain is the conscious, rational, thinking side, and the subconscious is the right brain, where all of our feelings and skills come from. Since our right brain (subconscious) has total recall of every feeling we have ever felt, many of us have issues from the womb, birth and early childhood. The left brain, the one we rationally think with, forgets all the time, but the right brain never forgets. And once we make a decision with feeling, subconsciously, it becomes our reality or our law of truth.

LEFT BRAIN	**RIGHT BRAIN**
Conscious Mind	Subconscious Mind
Thoughts	Feelings
Logical	Heart

> **"The miracle-working powers of your subconscious mind existed before you and I were born, before any church or world existed."** Joseph Murphy, Ph.D.

The RFA process gets a person relaxed and focused. Our subconscious mind is like a large library of feelings and information, so it can be accessed at any time. When I went through the RFA process, we found the cause of my allergies was a feeling of not being wanted and loved by my mother. The reality is, most of us have unresolved issues with feeling unloved or unwanted subconsciously, which means you are probably not aware of them.

> **"What we believe is the truth is only our perception of what is, not necessarily what is."** Max Skousen

Muscle testing revealed that something traumatic occurred in the second month, when I was just a fetus in mother's womb. During the RFA process, we discovered that I felt that my mother, who already had four children, didn't really want me, and therefore didn't love me. I made a subconscious decision that I was right: "My mom doesn't love me." So, 22 years later, I was venting the hurt of not being wanted and loved through the form of an allergy (stopped-up nose). The mind is so powerful that

> **The Right Brain (Subconscious) Cannot Tell The Difference Between Real Life And Imagination**

it will vent the hurt or pain through a physical symptom such as an allergy rather than feeling it in the heart. The amazing thing about this whole ordeal was that it was a made-up story I created based upon a feeling and assumption that wasn't true, but I was believing it subconsciously to be true, so it became my reality. That is how powerful the subconscious brain is! We make up stories based upon feelings, assuming things to be true. And once you create the story, you will defend it, because it's your new truth. And the subconscious always gets to be right about your beliefs. You will go through life creating situations to prove to yourself how right you are about your story!

> **"...the emotion that has the greatest impact on the physical health, are the emotions that we experience in the womb. So before we are even born we are picking up on mom's emotion and dad's emotion and carrying those forward into our life."** Dr. W. Lee Cowden

The truth is, my mother did love me and wanted me, but I made a decision subconsciously based upon a feeling that she didn't, and it was affecting my health. **It doesn't matter what is real; it only matters what you believe,** because that is what becomes your reality. To help you understand, answer the following question.

> **Is Cinderella a real story?   ___YES or ___NO**

If you answered "YES" you are correct. It is a real story. You can go to any library or bookstore and get the book or movie and read or watch it. It is a real story written in 1697 by Charles Perrault. It is told throughout the world in many countries and languages and people have loved and embraced it.

Now, if you answered "NO," Cinderella is not a real story, you are right too. Of course, it's not true. There never was a lady named Cinderella who lost her slipper at the ball. It was a fictitious story, all made up. Perrault wrote the story in a book and published it. Millions of people have read the made-up fairy tale and enjoyed it.

> **"Everything you can imagine is real."** Pablo Picasso, Spanish Artist, 1881-1973

My made-up Cinderella story was that my mother didn't love me. That became my reality. Was it a true story? Yes and no. It was true to me because I made it up, and what you make, you will love and defend at all costs. I was playing this tape or movie subconsciously for 22 years that I was unloved and unwanted. Now consciously, I knew and felt that my mother loved me. We always had a great relationship; however, my subconscious mind had been made up, and no matter how great and loving she was, subconsciously, I was unloved because that is what I created, and the subconscious mind always gets to be right. The tricky part about this is we are not aware of the feelings and decisions that have been made in the subconscious mind. This is why we use the RFA process. It identifies the feelings, decisions and story we have made about life so we can heal it and create a new story of something positive to play in place of the negative one.

> **"Many illnesses which are manifestations of chakra imbalances are the results of faulty data on old memory tapes which have been recorded and programmed into the unconscious mind during early portions of the individual's life. These tapes have been unconsciously playing back messages told to them by others or falsely thought by themselves, which are no longer appropriate to present-day circumstances."** Richard Gerber, M.D.

After healing my allergies, I spoke to my mother and asked her if anything traumatic happened when she was pregnant with me. She paused for a moment and then nodded her head and said, "Yes, when I was about 2 months pregnant with you, I went to my doctor and he said that since the world was overpopulated and that I already had four children, he suggested considering having an abortion, and this made me so mad!" This infuriated my mother to know that she had trusted this doctor to deliver her babies. She was angry and frustrated and felt compelled to find a new doctor. So, here I was, the baby in mom's womb, feeling her anger and frustration when her doctor suggested an abortion. In that moment, I made a subconscious decision that, *"My mom was upset and that it was all my fault. She doesn't love me. She doesn't want me."*

This is how powerful our minds are at taking a feeling and making an assumption, and then creating a story subconsciously. And since we create the story, we always get to be right about it. In other words, we will create situations to prove how right we are about them, until we heal it and create something different.

> "Since the brain has no way of telling the difference between a real event or an imagined one, you can live or relive everything in your mind, and program, delete or program everything you want. We are built out of atoms, which means pure energy, and energy does not need time to change. …Tumors the size of a fist can disappear in seconds through this conditioning." Dr. Leonard Coldwell

RFA CHECKLIST – HEALING THE CAUSE OF DIS-EASE

_____Easily embarrassed and self consciousness
_____A feeling of shame about hidden secrets
_____Fear of abandonment
_____Intense fear of speaking before a group
_____Irrational fear, such as height, water, freeways, germs, untidiness, claustrophobia, flying or others
_____Chronic depression
_____Tendency toward extreme gullibility
_____General lack of ambition
_____Difficulty in knowing or asking for what you want
_____Fear of intimacy
_____Deep hurt because of having been molested or raped
_____Deep distrust of the opposite sex
_____Insatiable need of approval
_____Difficulty in making up your mind
_____A need to control or manipulate others
_____Constant procrastination
_____Dyslexia
_____Physical conditions, such as asthma, hay fever, migraine headaches, frequent colds, arthritis, etc.
_____Hypertension, chronic pain, etc.
_____Sexual impotence (male)
_____Sexual frigidity (female)
_____Uncontrollable, spontaneous body movements (ticks)
_____Deep sense of unworthiness
_____Feeling of financial insecurity or bondage
_____Persistent jealousy
_____Addictions to alcohol or drugs
_____Compulsive over-eating
_____Feeling of being too fat
_____Sleeping problems
_____Sensitivity to certain foods
_____Intolerance to certain people, music, subjects, situations, places, sounds
_____Times of severe loneliness
_____Chronic fatigue
_____Deep resentment for having been offended, exploited or misunderstood
_____Feelings of being overwhelmed
_____Persistent feelings of being unloved or unappreciated
_____Deep dissatisfaction with your job, career, home, spouse, church, etc.
_____Frustration in not having a meaningful life, not doing what you want to do
_____Difficulty with remembering or concentration
_____Constantly comparing yourself to others

_____ Feeling like a victim of other people or circumstances
_____ Others

> **"All that we are is the result of what we have thought."** Buddha 563-483 B.C.

Allergies – Caused By A Traumatic Emotional Event

Many allergies are the result of incorrect neurological programming caused from a traumatic emotional event. We find that the body is not allergic to any non-poisonous thing. When any kind of threat is programmed in the mind, while in the presence of a specific food or smell, an allergy may develop. The right brain cannot differentiate between a real threat and the circumstance (food). All gets programmed in the right brain as part of the problem. For example, Sharon and her husband were at a restaurant eating shrimp one night when he announced that he had a new lover and that he wanted a divorce. In that traumatic moment of feeling hurt, rejected and betrayed, her mind associated the smell and taste of shrimp with hurt, rejection and betrayal. So now, every time she smells shrimp, her throat begins to swell shut, because she is venting the hurt, rejection and betrayal through the form of an allergy, instead of feeling it in her broken heart. It is easier for us to feel discomfort in the form of an allergy than it is in the heart that has already been broken.

> **"We are the only creatures on earth who can change our biology by what we think and feel."** Deepak Chopra, M.D.

Case study

For most of my adult life I suffered with terrible allergies: dust, pollen, animals, etc. I was particularly sensitive to cats, which was a nightmare for me because I love cats. And yet I could not get near them without a full-blown allergy attack, with red, itchy, watery eyes, constant sneezing, severely runny nose, and difficulty breathing. If you have ever suffered from severe allergies, you know that it affects your whole life.

Over the years, I have tried almost every allergy medication there is, prescription and over-the-counter. They would relieve the symptoms for a little while, but they never went totally away and I didn't like the way they made me feel. Natural remedies and homeopathic formulas made me feel better without the side effects, but nothing ever worked long.

Then one day I found the most adorable little gray kitten that had been abandoned. Even though I knew it would trigger an allergy attack, I had to bring it home anyway. I started on herbal remedies and supplements right away, hoping that this time it would be okay. But it wasn't. The attack was so severe that I could barely even breathe.

I didn't know what to do. I know it sounds silly, but I really, really wanted this kitten. So, in desperation, I asked Dr. Sainsbury to help me.

I went in for an appointment, and through the use of a method called RFA, he used guided imagery to help me get to the emotional root of my condition and figure out the cause of my allergies. Once the cause was discovered, he helped me release the negative emotions I was holding on to that kept causing the allergies, and he gave me some mental tools to use to help keep me from slipping back into old patterns.

The whole process took about an hour, and when I came out of his office, my allergies were completely gone! Sounds crazy, I know! But I literally went into his office sick as a dog and left feeling completely well.

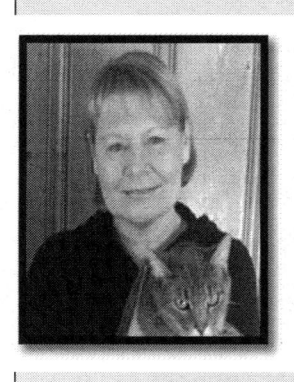

However, the real test came when I went home and let my kitten sleep in my lap. I had absolutely no symptoms at all!!! None! From that moment on, I have never had any allergy problems at all. There was a time or two that I was afraid they might be coming back, but I used the techniques that Dr. Sainsbury showed me and it has never happened.

That was about 3 years ago, and I am still allergy-free. I have a cat that stays in the house all of the time, and I never have any symptoms at all.

Thank you, Dr. Sainsbury, for giving me my life back!

Karen Carswell
Rainbow City, Alabama

"I believe we create every so-called illness in our body. The body, like everything else in life, is a mirror of our inner thoughts and beliefs. The body is always talking to us, if we will only take the time to listen. Every cell within your body responds to every single thought you think and every word you speak." Louise L. Hay

The Subconscious (Right Brain)

1. The right brain (subconscious) has total recall of every feeling we have ever felt.
2. It is not logical; instead, it just knows – right or wrong.
3. The subconscious brain cannot tell the difference between real life and imagination. That is what has got us into trouble, but it is also the way we can heal through imagined, positive experiences (new movies).
4. Once a decision is made with feeling, it becomes the law or "your truth" from then on until it is recognized and changed.
5. All of our feelings, including our upsets, come from our right brain.
6. We are never upset for the reason we think. The immediate problem is almost always coming from a deeper issue from the past. Many issues are traced back to early childhood.

"The mind is a complete library of everything that has ever happened to us. This library is called programming." Valerie Seeman Moreton, N.D.

The Five Lies of Your Mind

1. It claims to know why others are doing what they are doing.
2. It claims to know what is happening at a distance.
3. It claims to know what is going to happen in the future.
4. It claims to know what is to your advantage.
5. It claims to know what ought to be different than what is right now.

Dr. Bruce Lipton explains that the subconscious mind is 90 percent programmed by the time we are 7 or 8 years old, and that most of your life's script has been written by that time. In order to understand why people behave the way they do, it is crucial to understand that your mind is programmed for survival. Its job is to protect you, and it does this through three crucial decisions. The first decision is to always keep you safe. Second, the mind works to protect you, by always being right, and last, it works so that you will be accepted by others. So, next time you have a misunderstanding or argument, remember that the mind of that individual is working perfectly to keep him or her safe, right and accepted.

Your Mind Is Programmed For Survival
1. To keep you **SAFE**
2. To always being **RIGHT**
3. To be **ACCEPTED** by others

Your mind is not you; it's just a servant. At any given moment when the brain instructs your body to move, it obeys. Your body has form like the hardware of a computer. The mind is like the software, containing all the information you have ever programmed into it. But the computer (hardware and software) is useless until you plug it into the wall to receive the electricity that brings it to life. Even though you cannot see electricity, it is very real, and the part it plays is paramount. Your spirit is the energy (electricity) that brings your body and mind to life. It is connected to source, the infinite Life Force — God.

> **"The universe simply gives us whatever we believe."** Carol Tuttle, Author of *Remembering Wholeness*

You have a body and you have a mind, but you are not what you have. You have a house, a car, socks and shoes, but that is not who you are. You are spirit, an eternal spiritual being, whole, complete and perfect; however, most people don't know it or believe it.

> **"... Is it not written in your law, I said, Ye are Gods?"** Jesus Christ, St. John 10:34

Before birth, we existed as a fetus in mother's womb and enjoyed a peaceful, loving place, symbolic of the Garden of Eden. When it came time for delivery and we had to leave the comfort of mother's womb and enter the lone and dreary world, we began to experience a world filled with opposition. Instead of being in a peaceful, comfortable state, we began experiencing pain and discomfort. We got hungry, sick, too hot and too cold. Some of us may have even been given up for adoption and felt rejected and unloved. Shortly after birth, our minds began to be programmed, and we made subconscious decisions about life based upon our experiences and feelings:

1. **Pain is bad, comfort is good.** For the rest of our lives we strive to regain the non-disturbed state we once knew in the womb. How many of us were an accident? In other words, was the pregnancy planned or even wanted? Was mom ready to have a baby? So many of us started our life off feeling unwanted. And did they want a boy or a girl?
2. In order to be non-disturbed, **I must have my own way**. And this is when we learn that by complaining, we get it. When I cry, mom will feed me, change my diaper or hold me.
3. The third decision is, **it's important to please others**. Sometime around the age of 2, a child begins to learn the word, "No!" No, you can't touch that, it will burn you. No, don't throw your toys in the toilet. No, don't bite! The child must choose to have his own way or please others.
4. The fourth decision is made about the age of 5, to **obey my authorities** and do as I'm told, to stay out of trouble and be non-disturbed.
5. The fifth decision comes sometime around age 10, when a child realizes he or she **must be different in order to be accepted**. Changing is required to fit in with friends by wearing certain clothes or listening to certain music. It's not safe to be just me.
6. The sixth decision comes after realizing that I can't be different, I have to be me. So, **it's YOU that needs to be different**. You will have to change for us to get along.

7. The seventh decision comes around age 12, when a child proclaims that he or she is important and **You better listen to me**. This is when healthy self-esteem and the ego are being formed.

> "If you want to know what your beliefs are, look at what you have in your life. Life always reflects our beliefs." Colin Tipping, Radical Forgiveness

The Now

It is important to remember that your mind functions in the past, from past experiences, or in the future, in made-up possibilities. Both are illusions. Who you really are, is spirit, and spirit functions in the moment, or the now. Now is an eternal place, outside time. That is why now is called the present, because it is a gift. Now in this present moment, we are free to choose who we want to be, and what we want to create. When we live in the present moment, we cannot feel resentment, because resentment only lives in the past. We also can't feel fear, because fear only exists in the future. When we live in the now, we have full power to live fully as a child, coming from our spiritual self, love. Christ said, "…Except ye be converted, and become as little children, ye shall not enter into the kingdom of heaven." Matthew 18:3 Small children live in the now, that is why it is so easy to love them.

> "If you are depressed, you are living in the past. If you are anxious, you are living in the future. If you are at peace, you are living in the present." Lao Tzu 601-533 BC

Fear-Based Questions
1. Did I do the right thing?
2. Am I doing the right thing?
3. Will I do the right thing?

Most fears are illusions created by the mind to keep you safe and comfortable. However, this can also cause our lives to be dominated by fear. The RFA process has been created to heal our negative programming. RFA is not hypnosis, it is an emotional release, created to understand, forgive, love and heal, by identifying the illusions of your conclusions. Many of those conclusions are in the subconscious, creating negative feelings so you don't even know they exist. My illusion of conclusion was that my mom didn't love me. People who have everything going for them, but for some strange reason, suffer from depression or anxiety, usually have an unresolved issue in the subconscious.

Most of us are walking around in adult bodies, but the fears and subconscious decisions from childhood keep us trapped from being truly free, and we don't even realize it. We are still playing out traumatic experiences from when we were younger, and they are very much affecting our lives. For example, people who never have enough money, many times are being controlled by a deeper subconscious belief from childhood programming that money is the root of all evil, or it's easier for a camel to go through the eye of a needle, than a rich man to enter the kingdom of God. Some have the belief that struggling financially keeps a person humble; therefore, you stay close to God as opposed to those who are rich, who tend to become ungrateful and prideful, thus losing favor in God's eyes and heaven. These types of beliefs will cause you to struggle financially, just as someone who has made a subconscious decision that they are unlovable. The right brain always gets to be right about your belief. You will then create experiences to prove yourself right.

> **"All dissatisfaction with your life can be attributed to the difference between what is true and what you believe to be true."** Max Skousen

Anxiety & Panic Attacks – Caused From Childhood Trauma

Maria came to see me with severe panic attacks. After testing her, we discovered there was an emotional trauma from childhood causing the anxiety attacks. When she was 5 years old, she watched her mother be burned alive. They lived in a poverty-stricken area of Cuba, in an adobe house, where they cooked on a stove made of clay bricks. Her mother was wearing a dress with an apron, making tortillas. She unknowingly had spilled oil on it, and being around the hot stove, her clothing became engulfed in flames. She rolled on the ground screaming, trying to put the fire out. Little 5-year-old Maria and her sister tried to help, but by the time they could get a bucket of water to put the fire out, their mother was so badly burned she passed way in the hospital. In that moment, Maria subconsciously made the decision that she was "powerless." Now, 35 years later, Maria keeps having panic attacks. Her mind keeps taking her back to when she was 5, and she went into "fight-or-flight" mode, re-experiencing panicking, trying to help her mother. Now, when she gets in a situation and feels powerless, or unable to control a situation or another person, her mind immediately goes into panic mode, the same feeling she felt when she saw her mother being burned.

Once we took Maria through the RFA process and healed the panic-stricken, 5-year-old Maria (inner child), so she no longer had to play that old traumatic movie, the panic attacks ceased. From an adult perspective, we created a new tape or movie to play in place of the old one. We imagined 40-year-old Maria coming back from the future in the form of an angel to comfort and love 5-year-old Maria and reassure her that everything was going to be OK. Remember, the subconscious cannot tell the difference between real life and imagination. Once the inner child is comforted and feels that she is loved and safe, then we have them make a new decision about life.

Obviously coming from a place of love and safety, the individual can make a positive decision about how life will be, and this becomes the new movie for them to play. So now, when she gets in situations that she can't control, and she feels powerless, her mind doesn't start playing the old panic movie of feeling powerless. Instead, she plays a new movie of 40-year-old Maria coming as a beautiful angel to rescue little Maria so she feels safe, loved and comforted. Being empowered with this love, she now can relax and do her best in each situation, without having a panic attack.

> **"Everyone you meet is fighting a battle you know nothing about. Be kind always."** Ian Maclaren

It is estimated that 1 in 4 people have been sexually abused. People who find it difficult to express their feelings usually have had deep emotional trauma before the age of speech. The reality is, we all have scars from the past in some form or fashion. Healing the inner child, or traumas from the past, can dissolve allergies, fears, phobias, dyslexia, ADD, OCD and many other illnesses. We have witnessed amazing healing experiences. Once you release the negative belief and heal it, then proper energy flow is re-established, and organs, glands and systems are restored to health.

> **The Battle Within**
> 1. I am not loved or accepted
> 2. I am not good enough

As a parent, can you stop loving your child? No. What about if they are disobedient to your commandments? Most parents have unconditional love for their children. That doesn't mean that you necessarily like and approve of all their decisions, but regardless of what they choose, you love them. You love them because love is the very essence of who you are. Your spirit or electrical energy of your aliveness is made of love. You have been created in the image of God, but your mind works out of fear, opposite to who you really are.

> **"Your spirit is so large and powerful energetically that it won't fully fit into your physical body at this point in time. If your entire Spirit moved into your physical, your body would literally explode. This is because your physical body is resonating at a very low vibration relative to your spirit."** James Malcolm

The Needy Mind – Always Wanting Things To Be More, Better & Different

Our minds function on need, and they are greedy and needy. Many of us allow our minds to play out this need for things to be more, better or different. We do this by changing jobs, relationships, homes, hobbies, automobiles or friends, but we never quite get complete satisfaction. Once we change something, it's just a matter of time before the need compels us to change again. The dilemma is, the mind would rather be safe and right than happy. As we continue our search for happiness, we never find it because happiness can never be found outside of one's self. Happiness is only found within, so the sooner you choose to love yourself, the person God created, the closer you come to experiencing peace and happiness. Another key to happiness is understanding that you cannot make everyone like you. When you let go of the need to be a people-pleaser, you step closer to experiencing peace. Remember, co-dependency is a roller coaster of emotional slavery.

> "...for, behold, the kingdom of God is within you." Luke 17:21

Your brain is so powerful that you will find what you are looking for, consciously or subconsciously. If you are looking for sadness, you will find it. If you are looking for rejection, you will get it. If you are looking for joy or love, you will get it. God or the universe, whatever you call source, always answers the prayer of the heart, not the prayer of the mind.

> **The Universal Law of Life: WE LIVE IN WHAT WE SEND OUT**

The greatest way to experience love is to give it away. We cannot feel love coming to us. True love is only experienced as we give it away and send it out. *"It is more blessed to give than to receive."* Acts 20:35 **The greatest mystery of life is, "getting" destroys, and "giving," gives life.** We never have what we get; we only have what we give away. Give suffering to others, and it eats at your own heart and you suffer. Give happiness to others, and it fills you with joy and happiness. When you give up the need to feel sorry for yourself and let go of your own problems and serve others, then you become what you give. This is a magic success formula for depression. What we give comes back to us like a boomerang. It seems like a paradox, but the more you give, the more you have, and you only have what you give. This is why people who volunteer with church groups and charitable organizations to help those in need are usually some of the happiest people you'll ever meet, because they are living in what they are giving.

> "A candle loses nothing of its light by lighting another candle." James Keller

If you want to be miserable, hate everyone and everything. Dwell

> **If you want to know what you have a problem with, look at what bothers you the most in your family.**

upon all the times you felt others did you wrong. If you hold a grudge and seek revenge, it won't affect the other person one bit, but you'll be as miserable as you can be. Why? Because you get what you give. This is called the law of attraction.

The first step in healing is to love yourself. Some people are sick because deep down inside, they hate themselves. When we fully accept ourselves, just the way we are and just the way we are not, imperfections and all, then we come closer to fully loving and accepting the person we are, the awesome and unique person God created, warts and all. God could have made you different, but He didn't. You are who you are.

> "Most people are searching for happiness. They're looking for it. They're trying to find it in someone or something outside of themselves. That's a fundamental mistake. Happiness is something that you are, and it comes from the way you think." Wayne Dyer, Ph.D.

The reality is, we all have the same personality traits, we just manifest them differently as we journey through life. Given the right circumstances, we can all be mean, stubborn, greedy, impatient, angry, vengeful and mad. We can also be loving, kind, sweet, patient, forgiving, compassionate and happy, depending upon the day, place and circumstance. In other words, we all have our own version of Dr. Jekyll and Mr. Hyde syndrome, to some degree, because we all have wants, needs and desires. We have a good side and a bad side. Part of me is good, loving, kind and peaceful on most days. The other side of me, especially on a bad day, can be angry and mean.

Healing comes from the word whole, just as the word holy. To be healed or as Christ said, "Be made whole," is to come back to who you really are – wholeness.

THE TWO FACES OF MAN

OUR GOOD SIDE	OUR BAD SIDE
Christ	Satan
Good	Evil
Light	Darkness
Love/Trust	Fear/Hate
Acceptance	Judgment
Peace/Calm	War/Chaos/Worry
Joy	Sadness
Happiness	Anger/Resentment
Forgiveness	Grudge/Revenge
Gratitude	Greed
Innocent	Guilty
Honorable	Shameful
Honesty/Truth	Deceit/Lies/False
Responsible	Blamer/Accuser
Strong	Weak
Loyal	Unfaithful/Cheater
Giving	Selfish
Confident	Low Self-Esteem
Productive	Lazy/Apathetic
Wisdom	Foolishness
Healthy	Diseased
Life	Death

> **Indian Tale of Two Wolves**
> An old Cherokee told his grandson, "My son, there is a battle between two wolves inside us all. One is evil. It is anger, jealousy, greed, resentment, inferiority, lies and ego. The other is good. It is joy, peace, love, hope, humility, kindness, empathy and truth." The boy thought about it, and asked, "Grandfather, which wolf wins?" The old man quietly replied, "The one you feed."
> Author Unknown

> "The universe is an illusion — not that it isn't real, but that it is totally different than it appears." Max Skousen

What We Hate In Others Is What We Condemn In Ourselves

When someone does or says something that irritates you, usually it is the very thing you are guilty of doing also, but at a deeper level. In this sense, people we dislike mirror what is going on within us. We attract people

> **What you sow, you reap.**
> **What you give, you get.**
> **What you see in others, exists in you.**
> **What you send out, comes back.**

who resonate with our own issues, so we can heal them. For example, if you believe you can't trust people, you will attract people to you who will betray you. If you have a pattern of attracting relationships to you that never seem to work out, examine your beliefs about being worthy of people's love and being safe with members of the opposite sex. If rejection is your issue, you will attract people to you who reject you. In this sense, they serve as your teachers. Then you get to choose if you want to heal or be right about your beliefs. There is always a payoff for you getting to be right, a confirmation about your own belief that you authored subconsciously, and so you unconsciously create all sorts of ways to prove yourself right. This is how powerful and intelligent your mind is, and consciously you don't even know it!

Remember, you can only see in others what you can relate to inside yourself. The reality is, nothing is happening to you, everything is happening for you. When you change yourself and your beliefs, then the world reflects back to you the change, and you no longer attract those people or situations to you.

> **"Everyone is doing the best he or she can under the circumstances. If you don't understand how they could do this, then you don't understand their circumstances."** Virginia Satir

Most people believe God is the creator of all. If He creates all, then he created you, me and the person you dislike just the way He did, and just the way He didn't. To say you hate someone is, in a sense, a way to hate God's creations. Whatever you resist, persists. Wouldn't life be boring if we were all the same?

Peace comes when we accept everyone and everything just the way they are, and just the way they aren't. That doesn't mean you condone everything you believe is wrong, like prostitution, drug abuse and murder. What that means is, you step back and give others the space they need to be who they choose to be and stop resisting what is, by making them wrong. By allowing them to be who they want to be and giving up your need to control, you begin to flow with the process of life and enter a peaceful state. Christ taught, take the beam out of your own eye before judging others. In other words, let others be who they choose to be. Are you going to allow your brain to run you, or are you going to run your brain?

> "In my counseling I have found that practically everyone (on a subconscious level), does not love themselves. They do not accept themselves nor trust themselves. Most of these same people don't even like themselves. Interestingly enough, they all think they like, love, accept and trust themselves. But subconsciously, they do not feel it." Karol K. Truman, Author of *Feelings Buried Alive Never Die*

Most Of Us Would Rather Be Right Than Happy

> Every problem has a cause. Every cause has a cure. Most of the time there is a major belief at the core of your problem. Your brain keeps playing the same old movie, repeating the same pattern.

Most of us would rather be right than happy, even if it means being miserable. The survival mechanism of the mind is a need to be right. The majority of us pay that price to be right. We may be miserable and unhappy in our relationships, but at least we get to be right.

> "If you were taught that having enough faith that God will heal you, and you feel chronically sick, do you then judge yourself as unfaithful? What did your religious tradition say about the unfaithful? Did they inherit the Kingdom of Heaven? ... Do you believe yourself abandoned by God?" Dr. Keesha Ewers

Double-Minded – Thinking One Way & Feeling The Other

"Draw nigh to God, and he will draw nigh to you. Cleanse your hands, ye sinners; and purify your hearts, ye double minded." James 4:8 We all process information in two ways: how we think about it and how we feel about it. Many times, we think consciously one way, but subconsciously (our heart) feel differently. The people we are closest to in our families are usually the ones we have issues with. The reason is, at some point, someone usually says or does something to upset us. Remember, once we make a decision with feeling subconsciously, that becomes our truth from here on out. So, many of us think we love mom and dad and family members, but subconsciously or in our heart, we may have been upset in the past and made a decision about them that may be disrupting our peace. This is called being double-minded. Muscle testing reveals if a person is double-minded. Simply ask, "Do you think you love (*say his or her name*)," and then muscle test to see if they are strong or weak. Most people will test strong. Then ask, "Do you really love (*say his or her name*) with all of your heart?" and muscle test. Many times, the individual will go weak because of an emotional upset from the past that is causing them not to love the person with all of their heart.

> **"A double-minded man is unstable in all his ways."** James 1:8

Sometimes spouses are double-minded about their partners. They think they love their mate, but subconsciously or in their heart, they don't fully. Often, there has been a fight, disagreement or upset in the past that caused hurt feelings, and a conclusion was made such as, "Well, if he or she really loved me, they wouldn't have said or done that." Remember, the right brain has total recall of every feeling we have ever felt. It never forgets. And the reality is, almost everyone has a quarrel now and then.

> **"An angry man is full of poison."** Confucius

Many dis-eases in the reproductive organs such as cancer in the breast, cervix, ovaries, uterus, prostate or testicles are a result of unforgiveness with a spouse or intimate partner. It is a fact that more murders are committed within families, especially spouses, than strangers. If we want to experience vibrant health, integrating the left and right brain and healing traumatic experiences from the past are key elements to living a healthy, loving, peaceful life. When you give up blaming others and look within and find the real cause, then you can own your dis-ease and heal it. The problem is, most people are enjoying being a poor victim and playing the blame game because their ego is addicted to being right. By letting go of the need for someone or something having to be at fault, then we create a shift for healing miracles.

> **"The doctor who can cure one disease by knowledge of its principles may, by the same means, cure all the diseases of the human body; for their causes are the same."** Benjamin Rush, M.D.

Many Christians believe that if they had enough faith, they can move mountains or at least be healed. So, if you are sick, does that mean you lack faith in God's ability to heal you? Some believe that they must be perfect or "keep the commandments" to be worthy of blessings of health. Some children feel that the only time mom and dad ever showed them love and affection is when they were hurt or sick. So, fast-forward 30 years, and here you are, sick with cancer. Do loved ones shower you with love and affection, so you finally get what you've wanted, to feel loved? Never underestimate how powerful the subconscious mind is at getting what it wants.

Dyslexia

Dyslexia is the result of the mind working opposite to its normal function, causing both hemispheres, the right and left brain, not to function at the same time.

This switching off of one side of the brain is usually caused from emotional trauma or severe injury and illness. Dr. Gordon Sherman explains that dyslexia is not a disease (a problem with hardware) but distorted neuron patterns (mental software problem) that can be reprogrammed. People who are dyslexic will become, in certain situations, either right- or left-brain dominant. If they are right-brain dominant, they will be very emotional and illogical. Someone who is left-brain dominant will be very logical with no emotion. We all know the family member who never shows any emotion, even at a funeral (left-brain dominant), and then there's aunt Betty, who is constantly crying over everything, to the point that she can't make reasonable decisions (right-brain dominant).

You can muscle test to identify if a person has dyslexia. An **X** symbol is used to represent the left and right brain integration. Two parallel lines **II** is the symbol that represents separateness or that the left and right brain are not integrated.

Draw a large (**X**) on a piece of paper and have the person focus on it while you muscle test them. Now draw two parallel lines (**II**) on a piece of paper and have the individual focus on the two lines while you muscle test. If they are strong on the **X**, that indicates both the left and right brain are integrated. If they test strong on the **II** two parallel lines, then the left and right brain are not integrated, indicating dyslexia. The RFA emotional release process integrates the left and right brain to heal dyslexia.

Healing Our Emotional Conflicts

> **"All disease is provoked by unexpected trauma caused by a shock event."** Ryke Geerd Hamer, M.D.

After his son was shot and killed, Dr. Ryke Geerd Hamer developed testicular cancer, which initiated an investigation on what part emotional trauma plays in the development of disease, especially cancer. He developed "The German New Medicine," a cancer therapy

Emotional Release - Healing Therapies
- RFA (Relaxed Focused Attention)
- EFT (Emotional Freedom Technique)
- B.E.S.T. (Bio Energetic Synchronization Technique)
- RET (Rapid Eye Technology)
- BodyTalk Therapy
- Radical Forgiveness
- The German New Medicine
- The Landmark Forum

that explains that every cancer and related disease is provoked by unexpected psychic conflict-shock experience which manifests in the psyche, brain and corresponding organ. At the time of conflict, a short circuit occurs in the brain, which can be photographed by computed-tomography (CT), which looks like rings on a shooting target.

> "Through the millennia, humanity has more or less consciously known that all diseases ultimately have a psychic origin…; it is only modern medicine that has turned our animated beings into a bag full of chemical formulas." Ryke Geerd Hamer, M.D. (1935-2017)

Placebos: A Factor In Your Healing

Your mind has the power to make you sick or well, and when patients get better from ingesting a sugar pill that they believe is medicine, that is called the placebo effect.

Everyone knows that surgery either helps or it doesn't, right? An interesting study was published in the 2002 New England Journal of Medicine on patients who had severe, debilitating knee pain. At Baylor School of Medicine, Dr. Bruce Moseley knew that knee surgery was beneficial for his patients. Dr. Moseley wanted to investigate his surgeries to identify which part of the surgery was giving his patients the most relief. He divided his patients into three groups. In group number one, he shaved the damaged cartilage. In the next group, he flushed out the knee joint, removing anything thought to be causing inflammation. Both of these two groups received standard procedures. In the last group, he performed "fake" surgery. He sedated the patients, made three standard incisions and behaved exactly as if he were doing a real surgery, but did not shave or flush anything out of the knee. After about 40 minutes, the time the normal procedure takes, Dr. Moseley sewed up the incisions just the same as a real knee surgery. All three groups were then given the same postoperative care, including an exercise rehabilitation program.

The results left Dr. Moseley baffled. All three groups improved. The real head-scratcher was that the placebo group that received fake surgery, improved just as much as the other two groups! Dr. Moseley concluded, *"My skill as a surgeon had no benefit on these patients. The entire benefit of surgery for osteoarthritis of the knee was the placebo effect."* Members of the placebo group were seen playing basketball and other athletic activities that they were unable to do before their "fake surgery." Two years went by before the placebo patients were finally told the truth. Tim Perez was a placebo surgery patient who used a cane before the surgery and is now able to play basketball. His response was, *"In this world, anything is possible when you put your mind to it. I know that your mind can work miracles."*

> "Doctors should not dismiss the power of the mind as something inferior to the power of chemicals and the scalpel. They should let go of their conviction that the body and its parts are essentially stupid and that we need outside intervention to maintain our health." Bruce Lipton, Ph.D.

What Are You Getting To Be Right About In Life?

Are you ready to heal, or do you subconsciously like the payoff you receive by being sick? Does the thought of family, work and friends expecting too much from you, if you were healthy, fill you with fear? Would more responsibility be heaped upon your shoulders than you feel you could bear? Does the thought of being perfectly healthy have you scared stiff with arthritis? Does your need to control a child who is choosing to do things that you perceive to be bad or wrong have you all uptight and constipated? Are your allergies flaring up because your kids won't do what you think is right, or best for them? Do you sometimes feel they are a pain in the neck or keister? Maybe there's more truth to those thoughts than you know. Perhaps if you were healthy, there would be no excuse for failure in certain areas of your life? Fear is a disease that manifests itself with physical symptoms. Why? Because we have a need to control.

> **"Lack of self-love can lead to attention seeking. Some people get sick because they are used to getting attention when they are sick. If they want a lot of attention, they get seriously sick! Some even die for revenge. Death is a way of saying, 'See what you did to me!'"** Dr. Leonard Coldwell

A 42-year-old disabled and severely arthritic male came into the office and pleaded for help. He was in so much pain he could hardly walk. In our first appointment, we found out why he was sick. Addressing the cause of his arthritic state, we found it to be an emotional/mental issue. Subconsciously, he was afraid to face the world as a healthy, able man, fully responsible and capable to earn a living for his family. His only skills were in construction, and he hated construction work. The thought of sweating in the summer heat every day to earn a living, not to mention a few traumatic experiences he had in the past with co-workers, plagued him with overwhelming fear. After feeling persecuted and rejected by them, he made a subconscious decision that he never wanted to be in that type of situation again. Subconsciously, he figured out a way to escape the misery of having to go to work every day. His arthritis gave him a scapegoat, a way out, so his wife had to work. By him staying home, he did not have to face a bitter and cruel world, as he perceived it. This fear was the real cause of his arthritis. Sure, his body was malnourished and toxic, but his mind and emotions had him scared stiff.

> **"The greatest wrong as a counselor or friend is to tell a person they are not responsible for their problem or circumstance. ...People create their experience of life, yet when they have a problem, they commonly believe that someone or something 'did it to them.' Blame is a way of escaping responsibility."** Valerie Seeman Moreton, N.D.

Statistically speaking, more people die from heart attacks on Mondays than any other day of the week. Why? Because they hate their jobs. The subconscious mind figures out a way to get out of work, a way to escape the hell that they perceive has them trapped.

> **"Whether you think you can or think you can't; either way, you're right."**
> Henry Ford, 1863-1947

Writing A Letter To Bring Closure & Healing

Something very powerful to help resolve emotional conflicts is to write a letter to the person you are upset with, and yes, you can write a letter to God. If the person is deceased, that is fine too. If you have unresolved emotional baggage with a loved one who has died, and you never got to say goodbye or apologize for any hard feelings, then writing a letter can be powerful. Some people are angry with God for allowing a loved one to die, or mad at the person for dying and leaving them all alone.

> **"There is no death. Only a change of worlds."** Chief Seattle, 1786-1866

Write your letter and pour out your heart and feelings, and say exactly what you think and feel. Don't hold anything back. You want all those bottled-up emotions to come out in your writing. Once you've finished your letter, put an empty chair in the room and close your eyes and invite the person you are upset with to come and sit. Imagine them sitting there. Remember, your subconscious cannot tell the difference between real life and imagination. Now open your eyes and read the letter to them. After you finish, you can either mail the letter to them if you choose, or take it outside and light it on fire, and watch it burn and completely dissolve. It's symbolic of us dissolving the trapped emotions within. This is crucial, so we can let go and move forward. This helps bring closure to the situation. Do not keep the letter! The purpose is to dissolve the emotions associated with the conflict. Remember, energy is neither created nor destroyed, so we want to transform it. By burning all those vented hurts and pains, you are able to move through those feelings and bring closure to the event.

> **"Feelings control our glands. Glands control DNA. Anything less than feelings of love depresses all body functions, propelling us towards death. Calm, vibrant, joyful love vitalizes all body functions, propelling us towards unending life and health."** Richard Anderson, N.M.D.

Resolving Conflicts

Colin Tipping, founder of the Radical Forgiveness workshops, had a simple but profound formula that works in any situation where you find yourself upset and falling into the victim consciousness role (usually blaming someone). By using this formula, the situation can easily be defused, by simply taking a minute and saying:

> **FOUR STEPS TO RESOLVING CONFLICTS**
> 1. Look what I created.
> 2. I notice my judgments and I love and accept myself for having them.
> 3. I am willing to see the perfection in this.
> 4. I choose peace now.

Using these four steps to resolve conflicts puts the power back into your hands, being a co-creator with Source, rather than being a powerless victim. Every negative emotion begins with a feeling that was judged and then suppressed. When an upsetting problem arises, if you will go through these four steps, many upsets can easily be diffused. By stating out loud, "Look what I created," we are acknowledging the fact that we create our reality, and we also create the opportunity to heal. There is a divine purpose involved, regardless of you understanding or believing how. It's important not to play the blame game by criticizing, complaining and condemning. Simply take ownership of what you created, how you feel, and allow yourself to feel it fully, and then let it dissolve naturally, so you move past it. Next, acknowledge your judgments and express love for yourself and for everything your judgmental mind has judged. The third step is to see the perfection in this, realizing that your soul created this experience for you to learn and grow. Remember, there are no mistakes, just opportunities to heal. And last, simply stop resisting what is and flow with the process of life by choosing peace.

> "**Happiness is like a butterfly, the more you chase it, the more it will evade you, but if you notice the other things around you, it will gently come and sit on your shoulder**." Henry David Thoreau

In order to resolve a conflict where you have been upset, here is a step-by-step formula to help transform it. To download a free copy of the three-page Radical Forgiveness Worksheet, go online to www.radicalforgiveness.com. These are the basic steps of the worksheet. Fill out the worksheet and do not discuss it with anyone. This is part of transforming it.

Radical Forgiveness

1. **Tell your story**. Explain why you are upset. Having your story heard and being validated is the first step to letting it go.
2. **Feel your feelings fully**. Accept your feelings and stop judging them. You cannot heal what you don't feel. Own your feelings and realize that no one can make you feel anything, they are a reflection of how you view the situation.
3. **Collapse the story**. Even though you may not know how or why, your soul created this situation in order for you to learn and grow. This takes the power out of the victim story you made up.
4. Recognize that you get upset when someone resonates in you those parts of yourself that you have disowned, denied, repressed and projected on to them.
5. Understand that (the person you're upset with) is reflecting what you need to love and accept in yourself.
6. By forgiving this person, you heal yourself.
7. Realize that nothing anyone has done is either right or wrong. It just is. Drop all judgment now.
8. Release the need to blame them and your need to be right. Now you are willing to see the perfection in this situation.
9. Even though you may not understand how you subconsciously chose to do this dance, you now thank and bless them, for being willing to play the role they played in your healing.
10. **Reframe the story** by releasing all the feelings you had consciously at the beginning.
11. Express appreciation for the person's willingness to mirror your misperceptions.
12. Realize that you were experiencing your own victim story and framing the situation. You can now change your reality by reframing your story and being willing to see the perfection in the situation.
13. Completely forgive yourself and accept yourself as a loving and creative being. Release the need to hold onto emotions and ideas connected to the past.
14. Surrender to God or the universe and trust that this situation will continue to unfold perfectly according to divine guidance and spiritual law. Acknowledge your Oneness with Source and allow perfect light and love to flow through you.
15. **Integrate the shift** by completely forgiving the other person as you realize that they did nothing wrong and that everything is in divine order. Acknowledge, accept and love the person unconditionally, just the way they are and just the way they are not.
16. Recognize that you are a spiritual being having a human experience and love and support yourself in every aspect of being human.
17. Choose peace now.

"**Not forgiving is like you drinking poison and expecting the other guy to die.**"
Mark Twain

The World We Create With Thoughts

> **"Many of my patients have nothing wrong with them except their thoughts."**
> Greek Physician

The average human has about 60,000 thoughts a day, and of those thoughts, 94 percent are recycled, meaning you have thought them before. A thought has a frequency that can be measured. Fear activates 1,400 physical and chemical responses and can trigger a response from 30 different hormones. Toxic thoughts make you sick. We choose the thoughts that we dwell upon, which form our feelings, which lead to our beliefs. Then, we make decisions based upon our feelings and beliefs, and then act upon them. This creates our experiences, which becomes our reality.

> **"A thought held long enough and repeated enough becomes a belief. The belief then becomes biology."** Christiane Northrup, M.D.

Whatever you think, you become. Whatever you dwell upon is where you direct your energy. If you spend your time thinking about how lonely you are and how you'll never meet anyone to connect with, you're probably not going to meet that certain someone special. Just as water will take the shape of any object you pour it into, so will the direction of your life flow, according to the guidance of your thoughts. The dilemma is, most people focus on what they don't want out of fear, and then wonder why it keeps showing up in life. The person who wants to lose weight, usually focuses on losing weight, which perpetuates the problem. Shifting your focus on what you want, instead of not what you want, makes all the difference. For example, instead of focusing on losing weight, try focusing on being fit and healthy. Start focusing on what you want, not what you don't want, because what you feed grows. Act as if you already have it, and it just may manifest in your life — if you believe it.

> **"In our laboratory experiments, we have found that the act of thinking releases an energy which we can store in the lattice system of a cut quartz crystal. These patterns of thought vibrations are stored and oscillate like a magnetic field.... When one pulses one's thought, that energy... has the power of a laser."** Marcel Vogel, Ph.D., IBM Scientist for 27 years (1917-1991)

When we break down feelings, we have a tendency to categorize them into positive and negative feelings. The reality is, **there is no such thing as a negative feeling**. The truth is, they only become negative or bad when they are suppressed and denied. We are human and we are meant to feel our feelings. This is why antidepressant drugs can be dangerous. They put us in zombie mode so we don't feel our feelings fully, we just exist with no great sadness nor joy. No thanks, I don't want to live like that. If something sad happens, I will mourn and cry and feel my feelings and express them fully. If something funny occurs, I will laugh until my ribs hurt and if it's joyful, I will smile and beam with light and love, like I do when I hear my children laugh and we are manifesting happiness, living life to the fullest.

> **"What we sow or plant in the soil will come back to us in exact kind. It's impossible to sow corn and get a crop of wheat, but we entirely disregard this law when it comes to mental sowing."** Orison Swett Marden

Being Grateful

When you choose to fill your mind with thoughts of appreciation, it fosters love. Throughout the world, there are people less fortunate, suffering from all manner of pain and inflictions. Some are paralyzed and confined to wheelchairs; others are blind or deaf. As you read these words, some are in extreme agony, vomiting or coughing so hard they can hardly breathe. If you are able to read this book, then most likely you aren't experiencing any of those terrible things at the present time. Most of us have a lot to be thankful for and are blessed. Realize that your situation could always be worse. An attitude of gratitude produces health. Be grateful. You don't appreciate what you have until it is gone.

> **"We become that upon which we put our attention. God if thou seest God, dust if thou seest dust."** Anonymous

Weight Gain – Self Protection

Amy came to see us because she couldn't lose weight, no matter what she did. She weighed over 300 pounds. When we did an EDS test, we found an emotion, rape, showed up as the root cause of her weight gain. Amy protested, saying, "I've never been raped." Further testing revealed a traumatic experience occurred when she was 20 years old in college. She nodded her head and proceeded to tell me about a time a football player took her out on a date. After dinner, they drove up to a secluded place in the woods. He had one thing on his mind, and when he started getting forceful, Amy jumped out of his pickup, and he chased her. In that moment of running from her date, Amy made two decisions subconsciously with intense feelings about life. The first decision was, "I can't trust men," and the second was, "If I'm fat and ugly, no one will ever try to hurt me again." So, do you think any of her marriages will ever work? Of course not, because the right brain always gets to be right. Amy had been married five times and was currently divorced. When she showed me a picture of what she looked like in college, I was stunned. She was a drop-dead gorgeous, 5-foot-9, 120-pound perfect model. It is interesting to note that she never was raped, but just the fear and emotion of being raped, was resonating in her subconscious as if she had. Remember, the right brain cannot tell the difference between real life and imagination. After healing this traumatic event through the RFA emotional release, and making new decisions with feelings of love, safety and trust, Amy was able to lose over 100 pounds.

> "We must take responsibility for the way we feel. The notion that others can make us feel good or bad is untrue. Consciously or, more frequently, unconsciously, we are choosing how we feel at every single moment." Candace B. Pert, Ph.D.

Common Subconscious Decisions & Beliefs That Keep Us Stuck

DECISION	BELIEF
Nobody loves me	It's not safe to be me
I'm not good enough	Nobody likes me & I'm all alone
I am unimportant	The world is unsafe
I can't trust men/women	They are out to hurt me & then leave
I'm unwanted	Nobody cares about me
God doesn't love me	If He did, He wouldn't let me suffer like this
I'm a failure, a sinner	I'm not worthy of love/peace/happiness/health
To be humble I must be poor	A rich man cannot enter the kingdom of God
Nothing ever goes my way	Life isn't fair, I always have bad luck
If _____ really loved me	He or she would know what I need

We all know someone who has "a button" that can be pushed. The button triggers a memory from an earlier upsetting experience, thus beginning a cascade of hormones being released, believing you are in danger and under attack. When this button keeps getting pushed, and you go into fight-or-flight mode, as if a bear is chasing you, cortisol floods the bloodstream so you have energy to run or fight. The dilemma is, there is no bear chasing you, but all of that extra cortisol breaks down your gut wall, and the body will store it in the form of belly fat, so you can survive when a bear begins to chase you and you can't stop to eat. This continuous stress relays the message to the body to store fat, so you have plenty of energy for future emergency situations. Over time, extra hormones (progesterone) are stored in the adrenals for survival mode, putting you in estrogen dominance, thus leaving you at high risk for breast cancer.

> "The power of the visible is the invisible." Marianne Moore, American Poet

Just as tomato seeds fail to germinate on a tar-paved highway, neither does health flourish in a body riddled with fear, hate and anger. Dark emotions resonating within only produce chaos and dis-ease. You can't sit on the couch all day watching soap operas where people are lying, cheating, manipulating, seeking revenge and expect to go out and have awesome relationships. Feeding your mind images of guilt, hate and revenge feeds your shadow side. Get out in the community, church, school, etc., and make a difference by doing something good and start be-ing someone who makes a difference. Live your life to the fullest. Be anxiously engaged in a good cause. Stop complaining and be part of the solution, not part of the problem. Give up playing the blame game. Let go of the need to make someone else wrong and start taking responsibility for the part you have played. Be the source of whatever you choose to create.

> "You are far greater than you think you are, but what you think, you are!"
> Max Skousen

Letting Go

To let go doesn't mean to stop caring; it means I can't do it for someone else.
To let go is not to cut myself off; it's the realization that I can't control another.
To let go is not to enable, but to allow learning from natural consequences.
To let go is to give others the space to choose what they want, which means the outcome is not in my hands.
To let go is to release the need to change or blame another; I can only change myself.
To let go is not to care for, but to care about.
To let go is not to fix, but to be supportive.
To let go is not to judge, but to allow another to be a human being.
To let go is not to be in the middle arranging all the outcomes, but to allow others to affect their own outcomes.
To let go is not to be protective; it is to permit another to face reality.
To let go is not to deny, but to accept.
To let go is to release the need to be right and stop making others wrong.
To let go is not to nag, scold, or argue, but instead to search out my own shortcomings and correct them.
To let go is not to adjust everything to my desires, but to take each day as it comes and cherish myself in it.
To let go is not to criticize and regulate anyone, but to try to become what I dream I can be.
To let go is to stop playing small and start making a difference.
To let go is to be part of the solution, not part of the problem.
To let go is not to regret the past, but to grow and live for today, right now in the present.
To let go is to fear less and love more.

> "You constantly tear down or build up your health according to the nature of your thinking." Catherine Ponder

Love

Love is the light and energy in all creation. Love is the magnetism that holds every atom together in the universe. Love is what heals illness. Love is the most powerful force in the universe. When you fully trust God with all of your heart and mind, then you come to understand that everyone in life is doing the very best they can with what they have at this time. Divine healing occurs when you understand that your soul has created every situation that you judged to be a disaster as a loving opportunity to heal and grow. The truth is, there are no mistakes. Everything is happening according to a divine plan.

> **"Don't pass judgment on me until you've walked a mile in my moccasins."**
> Navajo Indian Proverb

Trusting God is when you trust that everything works for your greatest good. When you reach this level of trust, then there is nothing to fear. The war is over, you win. You come home to perfect balance, love and peace.

> **"Faith is not our ability to believe, but trusting God's ability to deliver."**

Your spirit or Higher Self understands your ego, subconscious decisions, and all the negative programming you have dealt with throughout your life. Since spirit gives us free will, it cannot intervene in our made-up stories and illusions of conclusions. However, it will bring people into your life who will act out parts of your story over and over again until you see the light, the truth that will set you free.

> **"Reasons aren't real; people make them up to justify what they want to do."**
> Adelaide Bry, Author of *est 60 hours that transform your life*

True love is not a feeling. It is an understanding. When you understand why people do and say the things they do, then you can forgive and healing takes place. This is love. This is what the RFA process allows you to experience. You cannot take an individual who has had something terrible happen like murder or rape, and then force them to forgive the perpetrator. Without understanding why they did what they did, true forgiveness is difficult. They can say that they forgive with their conscious mind, because they believe that's what they should do, but most likely, buried deep down in the heart, there's hurt, anger and revenge. Understanding is the key to forgiveness and forgiveness is the key that unlocks the hurt in the heart, so healing takes place.

> **"He who cannot forgive others, breaks the bridge over which he himself must pass."** William Thackery

Emotions – Energy In Motion			
Abandoned	Abused	Affair	Anger
Anxiety	Apathy	Argumentative	Bitterness
Boredom	Compulsive	Contradict	Critical
Cynical	Death	Demanding	Depression
Despair	Destruction	Dishonest	Dominating
Doubtful	Dread	Embarrassment	Envy
Fear	Fight	Frustrated	Worried
Greedy	Grief	Grudge	Guilt
Hateful	Hunger	Hurt	Immoral
Impatience	Inadequacy	Indecisive	Infidelity
Irritation	Jealousy	Judgment	Kill
Loneliness	Obsessive	Paranoia	Persecuted
Powerlessness	Pride	Rape	Regret
Rejection	Remorse	Repulsive	Resentment
Resigned	Ridicule	Ruthless	Self Pity
Selfish	Shame	Spiteful	Submissive
Suspicion	Unloved	Upset	Vulnerable

Every emotion resonates at a specific frequency that can be measured. Which emotions are resonating in your body, compromising your health? An EDS scan can identify emotions resonating in the body.

Agape Love

The ancient Greek language had eight different ways to express love. In English we just have one word – love.

> "Here is where it is. Now is when it is. You are what it is." Werner Erhard

8 Ancient Greek Words For Love

1. **Eros**: Sexual or passionate love, as in the word erotic.
2. **Pragma**: Longstanding love, such as two people in a lengthy marriage.
3. **Storge**: Parental & family love, such as love of a parent for a child.
4. **Philia**: Deep friendship or brotherly love, as in the city of Philadelphia. Loyalty.
5. **Philautia**: Self love or love for one's own self & wants.
6. **Ludus**: Playful love, such as flirting & teasing between two new lovers.
7. **Mania**: Obsessive love, neglecting yourself in order to win someone's affection.
8. **Agape**: Selfless, unconditional love, charity, understanding & comprehending our oneness.

The first seven types of love; eros, pragma, storge, philia, philiautia, ludus and mania are feelings that happen to us. They all have to do with a feeling of warmth, attachment, enjoyment and being comfortable. Through these we obtain our greatest pleasures, but also experience our greatest emotional pains when the objects of these affections are taken away from us.

The eighth type of love is Agape. Agape is understanding, light and compassion. It is a way of seeing rather than feeling. It is understanding that we (spiritually) are one with our source, just as the Father and Son are one. *"(There is) One God and Father of all, who is above all, and through all, and in you all." Ephesians 4:6* Quantum physics helps us understand scripture. All matter consists of energy resonating in specific patterns. Quantum physicists state that the universe is a hologram and everything in it, including each one of us, is a hologram too. In other words, one cell in my body contains all the information in the DNA to reproduce a whole new me.

> **"While our bodies and our senses tell us we are separate individuals, we are all one. We all individually vibrate as part of a single whole."** Colin Tipping – Radical Forgiveness

Just as the sun cannot obtain light from an outside source, neither can you obtain love by getting it from something outside of you. All things come from within. We have all the attributes of love, just as a ray of sunlight contains all the attributes of the sun.

> **"In the deeper reality beyond space and time, we may be all members of one body."** Sir James Jeans, 1877- 1946, Physicist, Astronomer, Mathematician

> ## EGO
> ♦ Your ego is what you think you are. It is not the reality of what you are, but everything you have come to believe is true about you.
> ♦ Your reality is not the reality. If it were, it would remain constant and would be the same for everyone.
> ♦ You made up this reality, and it changes every moment of every day, so in this way it is a fantasy or an illusion.
> ♦ Because you created your reality, you love it and must defend it at all costs.

> **"What you make, you love, and must protect and defend with everything you have."** Max Skousen, 1921-2002

EGO	HIGHER SELF
I am a poor victim, life isn't fair	I am free to create my own reality & I choose peace
There is never enough	There is plenty for everyone, including me
I could get sick & die	I am safe, one with my Creator, part of a perfect divine plan
I get all I can get	I flow peacefully with the process of life
Every day is a struggle	I surrender to Spirit; everything works for my greatest good

True love is giving someone the space for him or her to choose to be just the way they are and just the way they are not. Love is never in competition with anything, even hate. When someone or something attempts to enforce authority to protect them or the institution and all is done in the name of what is "good and right," then we have conflict. Being good and right always co-exists with fear. Anxiety and worry are other names for fear. Agape love is the Greek word explaining the type of love Jesus Christ taught. It does not exist with fear. As John the Beloved proclaimed, *"Perfect love (Agape) casts out fear because fear is torment and he that feareth is not yet made perfect in love." 1 John 4:18*

"I used to be a truth seeker until I realized I AM that which I AM seeking."
James Chappell D.C., N.D., Ph.D.

Why Relationships Fail

A sparkle in the eye and there's something magic about that person that just makes you want to be with them. Conversation leads to a date, and after spending time together, you "fall in love." Many get married to whom they think they love. Their partner seems to fill all of their needs, and when they are apart, they count down the minutes until they can be together again.

After a while of being together and fulfilling each other's needs, stored in our powerful subconscious mind is a mountain of guilt and troubled feelings from childhood programming. After suppressing these feelings and beliefs most or our life, we look for someone to blame them on when our buttons are pushed, and it's usually our spouse or a family member. By projecting our issues onto others, we get to blame them and escape responsibility for being the source of our problems. When the excitement and newness of marriage wears off, and each partner begins to run their pattern of blame, it's easy to become annoyed with them, because it's usually easy to spot. And the typical blamer's projection may sound something like this. "It's not my fault we aren't close anymore, you don't treat me like you used to when we were dating, and I don't feel you love me anymore."

> **"What comes out when life squeezes you? When someone hurts or offends you? If anger, pain and fear come out of you, it's because that's what's inside."**
> Dr. Wayne Dyer

When we enter a relationship to get something out of it, which most of us do, then we feed each other by repressing guilt and doing and saying the little things to make each other feel good. Over time, usually, we get tired of playing the "give to get game." Once a partner concludes that the other can no longer give all that is needed to feed the greed of the ego and keep saying and doing nice things, then the ego says, "This just isn't working out or another can be found," and the relationship ends. Usually with time, a new partner is found to fulfill our needs. Eventually, as the excitement of a new relationship dwindles, your old programmed subconscious beliefs begin to manifest once again and the projection of blaming your partner for problems repeats another cycle, because you have never healed what destroyed your first relationship. In time, the stagnant relationship is no longer fun, happy and "in love," because both partners were expecting the other one to "make them feel loved." Your partner will never be enough if, subconsciously, you have a belief that you are unloved, not good enough or can't trust men or women. Could this possibly be why half of all marriages end in divorce? It's difficult to be healthy when we are involved in tumultuous relationships.

> **"All it takes to make a difference is the courage to stop proving I was right in being unable to make a difference, to stop assigning cause for my inability to the circumstances outside myself, and to be willing to have been that way, and to see that the fear of being a failure is a lot less important than the unique opportunity I have to make a difference."** Werner Erhard – Founder of Est, now The Landmark Forum

Are there beliefs from childhood you are projecting onto your spouse so you can be right instead of happy? Our subconscious beliefs are what sabotage true love and interfere with having extraordinary relationships. Once you are healed and you no longer have the need to play the blame game with each other, then each partner is free to be their true self and loved for who they are and who they are not, whole, complete and perfect, warts and all.

> **"Fear defeats more people than any other thing, and it is the fear, not the thing we fear, that causes failure. Face the thing you fear and death of fear is certain."** Ralph Waldo Emerson

Validating Children's Feelings

When children misbehave and a parent chooses to scream and yell at them to shape up, most of the time, it only complicates the problem. Usually, a more effective and peaceful route to take is to stop resisting them for being upset and validate their feelings. Try putting yourself in their shoes and simply explain that you know they are upset and that it's OK to be upset. Everyone gets upset occasionally. We are all human. Many times, kids act up because they are starving for attention and they think no one cares about them. They may get a spanking, yelled at or grounded, but nonetheless, they got what they wanted, your undivided attention.

> **"Parents misuse power every time their requests evoke guilt."** Dr. Keesha Ewers

When children are upset, their feelings need to be validated, not condemned. To simply hold an upset child in your arms and tell him or her how much you love them and that it's all right to feel the way they feel, creates a safe environment. This works for adults too. Ask them to explain why they are upset, and many times they have valid reasons and we adults are the ones to blame for something we did or said. Keep in mind that when children feel unloved, they misbehave. What are we creating by how we choose to interact with our children?

> **"Your children will see what you're all about by what you live rather than what you say."** Dr. Wayne Dyer

I remember a time my 4-year-old daughter was in a terrible mood and everything I asked her to do she replied with a sharp, rebellious, "No!" In that moment I had choices. I could have chosen to spank her and demand for her to pick up the toys. I could have threatened to punish her such as no TV, but I didn't. Instead I walked over to her. She had a mean scowl on her face with her bottom lip curled up. I picked her up in my arms and in a soft, loving voice asked her what was wrong. She started crying and said, "Nobody likes me." She proceeded to name a few previous events that I was familiar with, but had shrugged off as no big deal. To me, the incidents weren't a big deal, but to little 4-year-old Brooky, it was as if the world was coming to an end. Her reason for being upset was perfectly legitimate when I understood how she saw it. I told her that I would like to be her friend and asked her if she would help me fix lunch, because I needed a good helper to put the vegetables in and stir the soup. I knew she liked to help cook and that brought a smile back to her sweet face. After lunch, I asked if she could help me out and pick the toys up in the living room. She replied, "Sure Daddy, I can do that." Our attitudes, tone of voice and the way we choose to approach each situation with children and adults can have the same consequences as throwing water or gasoline on a fire. Are we being part of the problem by throwing gas on the fire with how we choose to interact by blaming, accusing and condemning, or are we part of the solution?

> **"...that which cometh out of the mouth, this defileth a man."** Matthew 15:11

Accepting God's creations just how He created them is the first step toward peace. The need to make others wrong so we can be right creates conflict. Attempting to change things without first accepting them as they are, just how God made them, is like wearing Chinese handcuffs. The harder you try, the more resistance you create. What you resist, persists.

> **"Conflict cannot survive without your participation."** Wayne W. Dyer, Ph.D.

In order to completely heal something, we must take responsibility for it. So many of us are addicted to the drama of being poor victims and unlucky in life. We can play the blame game all we want, but remember, when you blame someone, you are escaping responsibility. As long as you see the problem as an outward force, you are unable to affect it, and therefore not responsible, but the second you own it, become responsible for it, you can do what you choose with it. This is living powerfully.

> **"To transform anything, we must experience it fully and love it just the way it is."** Colin Tipping

Transforming Your Life – The Landmark Forum

> First I was dying to finish high school and start college.
> And then I was dying to finish college and start working.
> And then I was dying to marry and have children.
> And then, I was dying for my children to grow old enough so I could return to work. And then, I was dying to retire.
> And now, I am dying...And suddenly realize I forgot to live.

The Landmark Forum is a three-day transformational seminar taught all over the world to help you understand why you are the way you are. Most of us have some pretty good reasons as to why we don't have what we want. The Landmark Forum opens your mind so that you can see why you are the way you are and that the world you live in doesn't have to be the way it is right now. You have the power to create something different, if you choose.

> **"Everything you teach you are learning."** A Course in Miracles

> **The Mind Judges Everything To Be:**
> 1. Right or Wrong
> 2. True or False
> 3. Good or Bad

Everything we experience in life can be summed up by, "It Is." However, our minds work in opposition to who we really are. So instead of just experiencing life for what it is, we judge everything to be either right or wrong, true or false, good or bad. We attach beliefs and ideals to everything. Then we create stories about everyone and everything in our life. These stories prove our beliefs to be right and usually clutter our lives so much that we no longer are free to experience the experience of life.

> **"One creates from nothing. If you try to create from something, you're just changing something. So, in order to create something, you first have to be able to create nothing."** Werner Erhard

The Landmark Forum is not about change. It is transformation with the emphasis put on accepting yourself as you really are. It is not something to make your life more, better or different, but to transform the way you experience life, so that the problems and situations you have been trying to change just clear up in the process of living.

Instead of trying to change things by making them different, nothing really changes because the source is still the same. When we try to fix things, we are only rearranging what is. In other words, one can't create from something. You can only change it by making it more, better or different. But, when you create nothing, then you are free to create something.

Many of us have created a destructive way of being from a traumatic experience of the past. We are not free. Our life is a living testimony of a vicious cycle of mistakes made over and over that causes failure and misery. Some people always have money problems, others attract liars or cheaters to them, and some attract abusive partners. How many women hated their fathers while growing up because they were abusive alcoholics? Then, they grow up and foolishly marry an abusive alcoholic, someone just like their dad, because they are subconsciously programmed to attract that type of person to them, even though they hate and despise abusive alcoholics? No one in their right mind would consciously choose that, but most of us know people who are caught in these destructive patterns and can't seem to get out. What are they getting to be right about?

> **"Nothing ever goes away until it teaches us what we need to know."** Pema Chodron

I remember a conversation I had with a lady who moved into town several years ago. She was a nice person, but her daughter had made some unwise choices that resulted in painful consequences. When people started gossiping, a vicious war broke out and feelings were hurt. I'll never forget what she said to me. "Everywhere we go, people are out to get us." She was caught in the matrix and couldn't see that it wasn't the fact that people were mean and out to get her, but that she obviously had a subconscious belief about life that kept her attracting these types of situations and people to her, so she could prove herself right. What was she proving? She was proving to herself that the world is filled with mean and hurtful people who were out to get them. And guess what? She got to be right. The subconscious always gets to be right. As a consequence, she and her family would pack up and move to a new city every five years or so because the nice people turned out to be mean and hurtful backstabbers. That's her story.

Is that a great story or what? It's a real story for her, but 100 percent made up in the confines of her own mind, and now they go out, city to city, and prove their story right, without ever having the slightest clue as to how they are creating it subconsciously. These people are not free. The past is creating their future. The Landmark education helps us see the traps we are caught in, the rackets we run, in order to be right and blame someone else for our problems. These destructive, stressful dramas create disease, especially cancer.

> **"Loving people live in a loving world. Hostile people live in a hostile world. Same world."** Wayne W. Dyer, Ph.D.

Most of us have an X, Y and Z, where something traumatic happened to us that caused us to be a certain way. For most of us, usually something happened when we were 3 to 9 years old that made us feel that **"something is wrong (I'm not good enough)."** Somewhere between the ages of 9 to 16, something occurred that made us feel like **"I don't belong."** Usually around high school graduation or age 16 to 21, most of us had another trauma knock us off balance that made us feel that **"I'm all alone and on my own."** Most people connect these three dots perfectly when they go through the Landmark, and it becomes apparent why we are the way we are. Our X + Y + Z creates OUR IDENTITY.

Traumatic Events = Our Identity
X = (age 3- 9)   I'm not good enough
Y = (age 9-16)   I don't belong
Z = (age 16-21) I'm all alone, on my own

What the forum does is clear our minds long enough so that we can experience directly, just "being." This amazing awakening is called, "getting it." Through this experience, we realize that anything we call a problem is a barrier we have created that keeps us stuck in our preconceived opinions, judgments, fears and needs. This gives us the space and ability to experience living so that the situations we have been attempting to change clear up just in the process of life itself. If you have a problem in life, you can either choose to have it and take responsibility for it, or choose to be a poor, helpless victim and resist it.

If you desire to know the truth that will set you free, then start taking responsibility for how your life is and isn't. If you have relationships that stink, it is because you caused them to be that way. This is empowerment. To point the finger and play the blame game gives your power away and makes you a victim. Living a powerful life means that you are the source of the quality of all your relationships.

> "All anger is nothing more than an attempt to make someone feel guilty…" A Course in Miracles

Pain is a given in this life, but suffering is an option. There is no suffering in reality, only in your story. Once we stop blaming people and things for our problems, and start taking responsibility and realize that we are source, then we shift our energy and begin to live the life we love and love the life we live. The Landmark Forum opens our eyes to see how our past has been creating our future. Once we transform our way of be-ing, then we become empowered to create something we choose instead of past programming. For more information about seminar locations and dates, go to www.landmarkworldwide.com.

The Power Of The Spoken Word

> "In the beginning was the Word and the Word was with God, and the Word was God." St. John 1:1

God created the world and the world was in darkness. He created light by the power of the spoken word. He commanded, "Let there be light," and there was light. As a child of God, YOU have been given dominion and authority over the elements of the earth.

Thoughts are energy. The words we speak are energy. Whenever you speak something, you give it power. Words have tremendous energy behind them, especially if they are intermingled with strong emotions. Understand that every single "I'm not …" is a creation. The power of the spoken word can create health or illness. Always put affirmations in the present tense such as "I am" or "I have." Never use "I am not." Speaking positive affirmations with feeling can be a powerful way to start each day.

> "We can easily forgive a child who is afraid of the dark; the real tragedy of life is when men are afraid of the light." Plato

Positive Affirmations

1. I let go of fear, anger and the need to be right.
2. I let go of struggle, friction and contention.
3. I am willing to change. I let go of the past now.
4. I give up the need to be right.
5. I give up being a failure. I am alivement, empowerment, success & fulfilled in all that I do.
6. I am calm, relaxed and harmonized with everyone and everything.
7. I accept everyone just the way they are and just the way they are not.
8. I give and I receive. I flow peacefully with the process of life.
9. I love myself and I love others.
10. I am happy, healthy, wealthy and successful.
11. I am a magnet to success. Everything I touch is a success.
12. I attract wonderful people into my life who I can serve and who can serve me.
13. I am worthy and deserving of God's greatest blessings and choose to receive them now.
14. Golden opportunities are everywhere and I attract them to me now.
15. I am loving, lovable and loved.
16. I can do all things through Christ who strengthens me now.
17. I am worthy and deserving of the very best and I receive it now.
18. Divine intelligence gives me all the ideas I can use.
19. Infinite wisdom fills my mind with brilliant ideas & motivation to reach my goals.
20. I touch, move and inspire others.
21. I make a difference in all that I do.
22. Every day, in every way, I am getting better and better and better.
23. All things work for my greatest good and I trust God completely.
24. I am eternally grateful for the abundance that is mine.
25. My life is fun and fulfilling.
26. Nothing has the power to irritate me.
27. I am powerful beyond measure.
28. God blesses me beyond my fondest dreams.
29. I am safe because I am one with the Creator.
30. I am whole, complete and perfect.
31. My life is a beautiful manifestation of the glory of God.

Read these affirmations every morning and before bed. This gives your mind a blueprint. By saying these affirmations daily, with emotion, you program yourself to receive rich blessings. Spending 20 minutes every morning on a rebounder (mini-trampoline), saying them out loud, with sunshine on your face, breathing fresh air, sets your intentions of what you are creating and attracting into your life.

"Far better it is to dare mighty things, to win glorious triumphs even though checkered by failure, than to rank with those poor spirits who neither enjoy nor suffer much because they live in the gray twilight that knows neither victory nor defeat." Theodore Roosevelt

Winning

> "Reality" is what we take to be true.
> What we take to be true is what we believe.
> What we believe is based upon our perceptions.
> What we perceive depends upon what we look for.
> What we look for depends upon what we think.
> What we think depends upon what we perceive.
> What we perceive determines what we believe.
> What we believe determines what we take to be true.
> What we take to be true is our reality.
> — Max B. Skousen, The Hidden Key to Inner Peace

Many depressed people walk around with their head hung down, chin on chest, which is a sign that they are trying to protect their hurt heart. They have a look on their face that says, "Poor me, my life is hard." They have given up, thrown in the towel and are just trudging along. It reminds me of the handful of kids I went to school with who quit football and wrestling every season because, "it's too hard." They weren't willing to pay the price, and that is fine, everyone deserves to choose what they want. But, with no guts, there is no glory and what a shame to waste your precious life and God-given talents like that. So much potential is waiting like a seed in your garden to spring to life, because our potential is truly limitless, if we will put forth an honest effort.

> **"I'd rather be a failure at something I enjoy than be a success at something I hate."** George Burns

The definition of hell is not wanting what you have. The definition of heaven is wanting what you have. Live your life to the fullest. Be your dreams. Life goes by too fast not to have what you truly want. The only difference between a diamond and a piece of coal is time and pressure. Has the diamond always been there, just needing the right environment to transform from coal to a beautiful shiny diamond?

> **"You are here to enable the divine purpose of the universe to unfold. That is how important you are!"** Eckhart Tolle

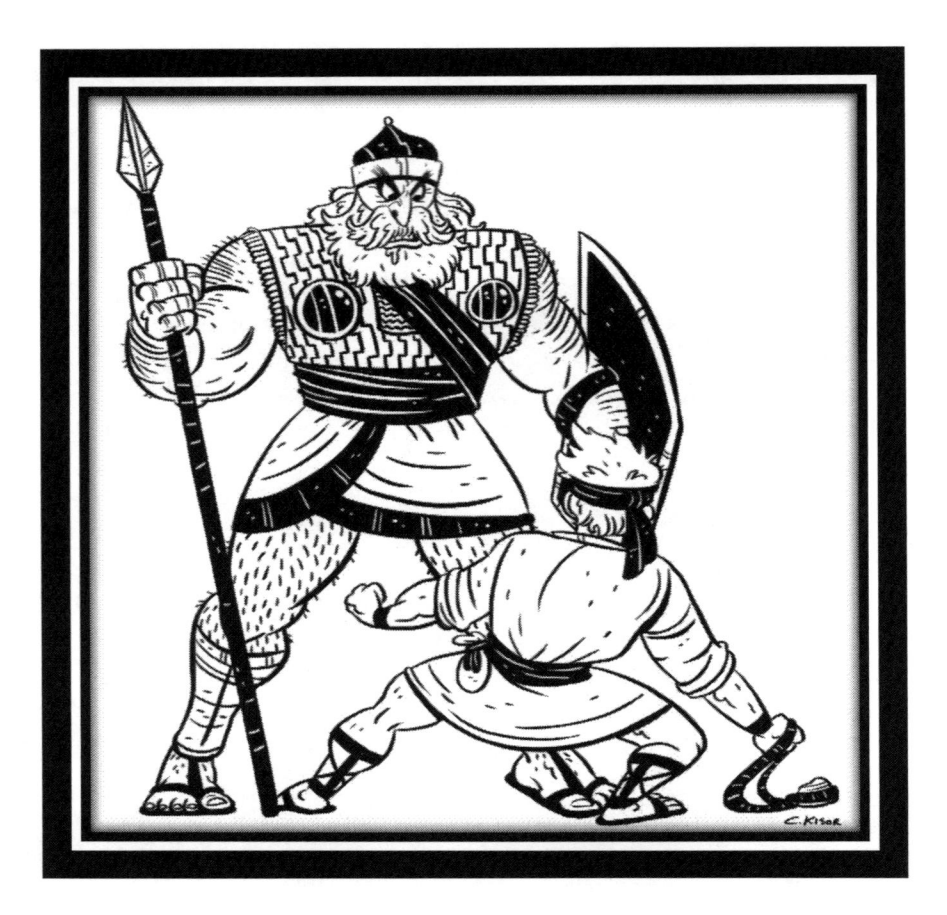

When Goliath came to fight the Israelites, everyone cried out in fear, "He is so big we'll never win." David looked at the same obstacle, grabbed his sling, picked up a rock and said, "He is so big, how can I miss?"

> "Our deepest fear is that we are powerful beyond measure. It is our light, not our darkness, that most frightens us. We ask ourselves, who am I to be brilliant, gorgeous, talented, and fabulous? Actually, who are you NOT to be? You are a child of God. Your playing small doesn't serve the world. There's nothing enlightened about shrinking so that other people won't feel insecure around you. We are all meant to shine, as children do. We were born to make manifest the glory of God that is within us. It's not just in some of us; it's in everyone. And as we let our own light shine, we unconsciously give other people permission to do the same. As we're liberated from our own fear, our presence automatically liberates others." Marianne Williamson

All of us have talents bestowed upon us from on high. To find and magnify those talents is a key to health, happiness and fulfillment. You can't wake up every morning and hate your job and expect to be healthy. Find what you enjoy doing and then find a way to get paid for doing it. This brings fulfillment into your life. This is the secret to good health and a great life. Set that intention for yourself and attract it to you.

> **"There is an aspect of human physiology that physicians have not yet understood and only reluctantly acknowledge. This dimension of human physiology is the domain of Spirit as it relates to the physical body. The spiritual dimension is the energetic basis of all life, because it is the energy of spirit which animates the physical framework. The unseen connection between the physical body and the subtle forces of spirit holds the key to understanding the inner relationship between matter and energy. When scientists begin to comprehend the true relationship between matter and energy, they will come closer to understanding the relationship between humanity and God."** Richard Gerber, M.D. - Author of Vibrational Medicine

Every thought you think creates your future. What you feed grows. Choose your thoughts carefully, because what you dwell upon has a magical way of manifesting itself in life. Act as if you already have what you want and give thanks for it, and then it will manifest in your life.

> **"The last suit that you wear, you don't need any pockets."** Wayne W. Dyer, Ph.D.

Conclusion

Two forces exist in this world. One is light and the other is darkness. May God bless you abundantly as you walk through this journey we call life. And may greatness be the result of your involvement with humanity as you live your life to the fullest, making the world a better place with your unique, one-of-a-kind spirit.

> **"Goodbyes are only for those who love with their eyes. Because for those who love with heart and soul, there is no such thing as separation."** Rumi

The great mystery of life is to experience transformation. Does a lowly caterpillar comprehend that the day soon cometh when he gives up crawling on his belly only to receive his wings to soar through the sky as a butterfly? Transformation is discovering what you already are.

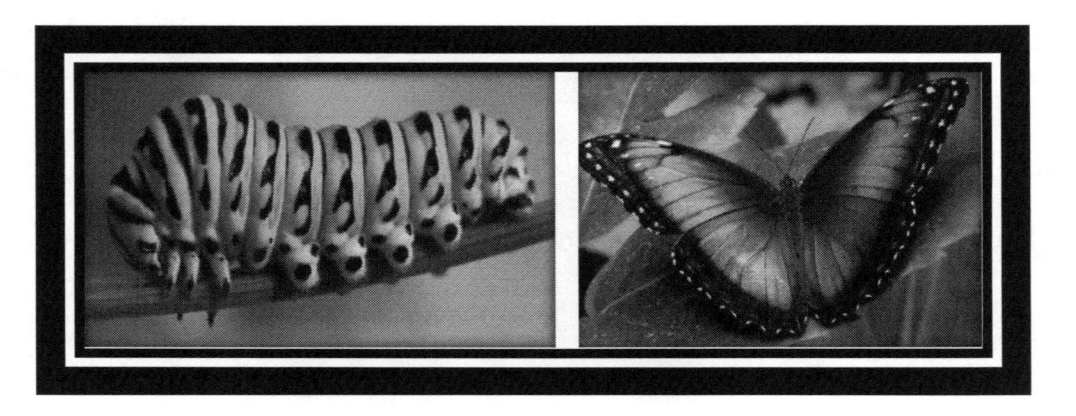

> **"May we all stand firm in the knowledge and comfort that all things are now, have always been and forever will be, in Divine order, unfolding according to a Divine plan. And may we truly surrender to this truth, whether we understand it or not. May we also ask for support in consciousness in feeling our connection with the Divine part of us, with everyone and with everything — so that we can truly say and feel — we are One."** Radical Forgiveness, Colin Tipping

Remember, YOU cannot become what you already are.

www.healingthecause.com

Index

A

A1C, 143, 414
Acetylcholine, 382, 385, 411
Acidosis, 90, 400
Acne, 161, 380, 486
Acupuncture, 3, 37, 458
ADD/ADHD, 140, 380, 382
Addictions, 503
Agape love, 529
Alfalfa, 354, 389, 391, 397, 469, 477, 478
Allergies, 4, 6, 8, 42, 131, 267, 284, 295, 298, 417, 436, 450, 455, 466, 478, 486, 496, 504
Aloe vera, 416, 442, 466, 470, 479
Aluminum, 6, 32, 158, 298, 304, 306, 329, 383, 482
Amygdalin, 23, 401
Anemia, 387
Antibiotics, 5, 138, 218, 219, 220, 402, 409, 427, 468
Antimony, 32
Anxiety, 7, 8, 509, 529
Apple cider vinegar, 440, 462, 470, 476
Arsenic, 32, 34, 42
Arthritis, 5, 227, 390, 457
Ashwagandha, 414, 422, 427, 439, 457
Aspartame, 4, 155, 156, 157, 167, 426
Aspirin, 7, 365
Asthma, 308, 392
Astragalus, 477
Autism, 5, 6, 248, 249, 254, 293, 313, 315, 327, 335
Autoimmune disorders, 311, 453

B

Back pain, 136
Basil, 422, 441
Bee pollen, 354, 384, 391, 472
Bentonite clay, 403, 462
Bergamot, 433
Beryllium, 32, 401, 461
Bilberry, 421
Black cohosh, 386, 450
Black walnut, 425, 459, 478
Blood sugar, 380, 428, 437, 451, 477
Blood type, 212, 230, 231
Bone broth, 154, 403, 408, 416, 427, 458, 469
Bread, 144
Breastfeeding, 367
Bronchitis, 486
Burdock, 426, 461, 466, 476, 478
Burns, 537
Burst training, 122, 123, 457

C

Cadmium, 32, 418, 436
Caffeine, 4, 158
Calcium, 133, 360, 387, 390, 392, 395, 396, 404, 406, 409, 419, 422, 429, 440, 443, 453, 455, 457, 459, 473
Calendula, 42
Cancer, 3, 4, 5, 6, 8, 19, 23, 24, 25, 31, 50, 52, 58, 61, 78, 79, 80, 81, 82, 83, 84, 88, 89, 90, 91, 92, 93, 94, 95, 96, 97, 98, 113, 126, 179, 234, 246, 265, 273, 275, 320, 321, 323, 324, 355, 358, 360, 362, 363, 373, 379, 399, 400, 401, 493, 494
Candida, 39, 221, 391, 404, 469, 473, 474, 478
Cascara sagrada, 380
Cataracts, 420
Cayenne, 410, 455, 468
CDC, 6, 25, 53, 58, 218, 238, 242, 251, 252, 255, 259, 266, 268, 273, 274, 275, 278, 279, 282, 283, 284, 289, 290, 292, 293, 295, 296, 299, 300, 301, 302, 303, 304, 306, 307, 309, 312, 313, 314, 315, 316, 317, 319, 324, 325, 328, 341, 342, 343, 345, 346, 405, 490
Celiac disease, 467
Chakras, 5, 232
Chamomile, 42, 453, 477, 478
Chelation, 23
Chemicals, 5, 173
Chemotherapy, 4, 88, 96, 97, 98, 224, 333
Chickenpox, 6, 318, 320, 329
Chickweed, 456
Chiropractic, 7, 223, 347, 395
Chlorella, 393, 470
Chlorine, 7, 358, 438
Cholesterol, 5, 161, 199, 200, 201, 202, 203, 204, 205, 206, 207, 208, 211, 412, 420, 447, 450
Choline, 210
Chromium, 148, 381, 414, 415, 437
Chronic fatigue, 486, 503
Cilantro, 431
Cinnamon, 148, 333, 403, 415, 424, 434, 437
Circulation, 215, 419, 472, 473, 485
Citronella, 449
Clove, 442, 472
Coconut oil, 125, 396, 403, 440, 457
Cod liver oil, 390, 469
Coffee, 158, 431
Colds, 4, 115, 408, 478
Colloidal silver, 408
Colostrum, 367, 380, 395, 405, 410, 440, 446
Constipation, 64, 87, 107, 161, 429, 485, 486
Copper, 33, 432, 459, 475
CoQ10, 210, 386, 392, 412, 449, 452, 455, 459, 472
Corn, 144, 158
Coughs, 409
Cravings, 7
Crohn's disease, 23, 410

D

Dandelion, 380, 415, 466, 482
DDT, 6, 174, 213, 275, 276, 280, 315, 324
Deep breathing, 400
Dehydration, 165, 428
Depression, 139, 161, 377
Diabetes, 4, 5, 6, 58, 140, 142, 157, 218, 319, 335, 379, 385, 487
Diarrhea, 6, 137, 169, 336, 416
Diet drinks, 154
Digestive enzymes, 440, 454
Distilled water, 166, 480
Dizziness, 475, 485
DNA, 5, 79, 88, 95, 96, 112, 157, 172, 188, 189, 213, 234, 236, 242, 245, 284, 290, 305, 311, 327, 329, 338, 356, 358, 360, 362, 378, 493, 495, 519, 528
Dong quai, 442
Dopamine, 381, 382, 386, 393, 412, 460, 467
Drugs, 3, 4, 7, 20, 21, 25, 58, 68, 75, 108, 112, 170, 172, 175, 208, 209, 319, 363, 369
Dry skin, 485
Dyslexia, 8, 503, 515

E

Echinacea, 38, 116, 333, 405, 408, 409, 416, 422, 424, 440, 442, 443, 460, 461, 462, 468, 469, 471, 472, 475, 476, 478, 488
Eczema, 295
Edema, 169
Eggs, 5, 144, 210, 211, 419, 433
Ego, 233
Elderberry, 478
Electro Dermal Screening, 3, 37, 38
Emotional stress, 410
Enzymes, 398, 403, 467
Epilepsy, 5, 171
Epsom salt, 118, 158, 198, 391, 410, 444, 458, 466
Epstein-Barr virus, 39, 394, 405, 426, 427, 438, 446, 452, 453, 455
Estrogen, 61, 399, 450, 464
Evening primrose oil, 63, 380, 386, 398, 417, 419, 423, 427, 434, 453, 454, 466
Exercise, 4, 107, 121, 122, 385, 396, 409, 411, 412, 418, 429, 436, 448, 450, 452, 454, 455, 472, 475, 482

F

Fasting, 4, 91, 125, 126, 134, 414, 482
Fatigue, 161, 178, 327
Fats, 4, 123, 124, 127, 348, 385, 419
FDA, 3, 7, 23, 24, 48, 50, 52, 58, 67, 68, 69, 72, 74, 155, 156, 175, 209, 211, 236, 252, 254, 274, 275, 299, 301, 302, 303, 306, 315, 324, 325, 357, 360, 364, 365, 373, 374
Fear, 233, 288, 331, 445, 452, 503, 518, 522, 530
Fennel, 431, 478
Fenugreek, 149
Fermented vegetables, 104, 403, 465
Fever, 4, 6, 113, 287, 334, 485
Fish oil, 381, 385, 395, 398, 418, 436, 452
Flaxseed oil, 380, 424, 465, 488
Flu, 6, 307, 334, 424
Fluoride, 7, 358, 359, 360, 361, 362, 363, 438, 473
Food poisoning, 42
Forgiveness, 508, 520, 528, 540
Frankincense, 385, 391, 395, 448, 454, 467
Frequent urination, 486
Fungus, 4, 92, 392

G

GABA, 122, 381, 382, 388, 412, 443
Gallbladder, 5, 190, 196, 487
Gallstones, 191, 198, 425
Gardasil, 6, 256, 306, 311, 312, 313, 328
Garlic, 114, 118, 333, 400, 408, 416, 424, 432, 434, 436, 459, 471
Gas, 4, 96, 361, 485, 487
Geranium, 468
Germs, 112, 222
Ginger, 87, 415, 434, 437, 441, 445, 453, 468, 469, 487
Ginkgo biloba, 385, 399, 406, 487
Ginseng, 149, 406, 422, 427, 436
Glutamine, 431
Glutathione, 385, 393, 412, 431, 432
Gluten, 4, 127, 129, 381, 384, 394, 404, 413, 428, 436, 468, 478
Glyphosate, 305
Goat's milk, 212, 479
Goiters, 4, 162
Goldenseal, 440
Gota kola, 408
Graviola, 3, 25, 84, 401, 465, 493
Gymnema sylvestre, 148

H

Hashimoto's disease, 32, 130, 297
Hawthorn, 387, 392, 397, 430, 436
Headaches, 7, 161, 169, 233, 365, 483, 485, 486
Heartburn, 134, 431, 487
Heavy metals, 31, 164, 384, 402, 410, 415, 418, 421, 438, 443, 453, 455, 466, 469
Helichrysum, 458, 470
Hemorrhoids, 432
Hepatitis, 250, 306, 329, 340, 447

Herpes, 39, 432, 467
High blood pressure, 411, 435
Holy basil, 380, 422, 429, 436, 473
Homeopathy, 3, 6, 41, 43, 333, 405
Hormones, 364, 434, 441, 462, 490
Horse chestnut, 475
Hot flashes, 434, 485
Hydrangea, 425, 429, 431, 441, 443, 454, 468
Hydrogen peroxide, 410
Hyperactivity, 379, 486
Hypertension, 379, 503
Hypoglycemia, 467
Hypothyroidism, 178, 427

I

Indigestion, 134, 478, 485
Infertility, 161, 441
Inflammation, 103, 194, 398, 445, 460
Insomnia, 486
Insulin, 4, 87, 140, 143, 319
Intermittent fasting, 456
Iodine, 390, 420, 423, 438, 439, 478
Iron, 6, 270, 386, 387, 403, 438

J

Juicing, 389, 390, 482

K

Kava, 388, 414, 431, 445, 456, 464, 466, 474
Kelp, 381, 386, 405, 411, 412, 414, 421, 423, 426, 427, 432, 438, 439, 456, 457, 466, 487
Ketones, 123, 126
Kidney stones, 212, 425
Kinesiology, 8, 498
Kirlian photography, 35, 36

L

Laetrile (Vitamin B17), 23, 373
L-Arginine, 387
Laughter, 484
Lavender, 414, 417, 442, 443, 446, 470
L-Carnitine, 387, 392
Lead, 33, 249, 261, 312
Leaky gut, 417, 445, 465
Lecithin, 384, 390, 425, 487
Lemon, 408, 442, 445
Lemongrass, 476
Leukemia, 321
Leukocytosis, 4, 113, 422
Licorice, 391, 431, 436, 437, 448, 474, 475
Lion's mane, 423
Liver, 95, 196, 198, 406, 437, 487
L-lysine, 408, 467
Lobelia, 392
Love, 8, 233, 495, 525, 527, 529
Low blood sugar, 437
Lyme Disease, 384, 449
Lymphatic, 4, 101, 105, 418, 450

M

Magnesium, 42, 159, 162, 387, 393, 405, 406, 409, 419, 421, 428, 432, 435, 444, 449, 461, 464, 466, 473, 475, 487
Malaria, 6, 334, 336
Mammograms, 3, 81, 83
Manganese, 395, 451, 457, 487
Manuka honey, 440
Massage, 395, 458, 462, 483
Measles, 6, 281, 282, 285, 320, 321, 334, 453
Melatonin, 362, 443
Memory, 161, 206
Menopause, 61, 486
Mercury, 6, 33, 164, 171, 236, 237, 238, 239, 241, 242, 248, 249, 298, 299, 300, 303, 316, 329, 385, 419, 431, 436

Meridians, 3, 37
Miasms, 7, 88, 90, 378
Microbiome, 4, 137, 152
Microwaves, 480
Milk, 4, 126, 144, 355, 383, 390, 425
Minerals, 131, 133, 452, 455, 478
Mold, 392, 398, 404, 409, 453, 461, 468, 469, 470, 474
MSG, 298, 329, 413
Mucus, 329, 383
Mullein, 391, 392, 398, 409, 461, 478, 488
Multiple sclerosis, 155, 379
Mumps, 6, 320, 334
Muscle cramps, 409, 485
Muscle testing, 498, 501, 514
Muscular dystrophy, 379
Myrrh, 384, 424, 460, 469

N

Nattokinase, 397, 436, 469
Nausea, 453, 454
Nervous, 485, 487
Nettle, 470
Neurological, 234
Neurotransmitters, **204**
Nickel, 33
Nopal cactus, 149
NutraSweet, 154, 155, 156, 157
Nuts, 144

O

Olive leaf, 408, 476
Olive oil, 87, 196
Orange, 144, 213, 233
Oregano, 398, 468
Oregon grape, 447, 477, 478, 487
Ornithine, 196, 197
Oxygen, 90

P

Pain, 170, 391, 395, 396, 404, 451, 458, 461, 477, 485, 486, 507, 535

543

Parasites, 336, 409, 416, 425, 458, 468, 487
Parkinson's disease, 155, 204, 303, 385, 459
Parsley, 400
Patchouli, 420
Peanuts, 144
Peppermint, 423, 424, 443, 455, 469
Pertussis, 6, 285, 286, 287, 294
Pesticides, 32, 34, 439
Phosphorus, 388
Pica, 460
Pineal, 233
Pituitary, 233, 487
Placebos, 8, 517
PMS, 93, 161, 462, 464
Pneumonia, 58
Polio, 6, 267, 268, 271, 272, 273, 275, 277, 278, 280, 329
Postpartum depression, 413
Potassium, 435
Pregnancy, 441
Probiotics, 381, 382, 385, 387, 392, 393, 394, 395, 403, 404, 405, 408, 409, 410, 414, 415, 416, 417, 426, 428, 431, 440, 441, 446, 448, 452, 459, 466, 470, 472, 474, 475, 476
Prostate, 4, 84, 85, 464, 486
Prostatitis, 424
Protein, 7, 309, 351
PSA test, 84, 85, 464
Psorinum, 379, 392, 398, 417
Psyllium, 409, 416
Pubmed.com, 318

R

Radiation, 427, 438, 480
Rebounding, 4, 107, 108, 400
Resentment, 389, 445
Rheumatoid arthritis, 389
Rhodiola, 382, 413, 422, 427
Rife, 50, 51, 52
Rose, 486
Rosemary, 427
Royal jelly, 391, 398, 405, 461, 469, 475

S

Salt, 5, 191, 192, 471
Saturated fats, 127, 210
Saw palmetto, 426
Scarlet fever, 287
Schizophrenia, 467
Seizures, 379
Selenium, 427, 431, 437, 439, 455
Serotonin, 388, 419, 443
Sex, 87, 161, 486
Shingles, 6, 318, 467
SIDS, 241, 251, 256, 261, 287, 290, 291, 344
Silver dental fillings, 236
Sleep, 7, 118, 407, 482
Smoking, 315
Sodium, 5, 191, 192, 229, 359, 383, 390, 391, 405, 420, 448, 451, 477
Soy, 419
Spirulina, 228, 383, 438, 472
Staphylococcus, 39, 333
Statin drugs, 86, 203, 207, 386, 411, 412, 414, 420, 447, 454
Stevia, 4, 167, 480
Stress, 7, 160, 164, 406, 420, 421, 426, 436, 447, 450, 456, 462, 474, 490
Stroke, 58
Subconscious, 506
Sugar, 4, 5, 90, 121, 127, 143, 144, 167, 210, 348, 392, 393, 402, 433, 473, 485
Sulfur, 419
Suma, 419, 441, 448, 451
Sweating, 292
Sycosis, 379, 411
Syphilinum, 379
Syphilis, 379

T

Testosterone, 405, 447, 448, 464
Tetanus, 6, 302, 322, 323, 334
Thyme, 392
Thymus, 233
Thyroid, 161, 233, 381, 478
Tin, 33
TMJ, 178
Tonsils, 471
Toxins, 38, 136, 429, 468
Toxline, 242
Tuberculosis, 378
Turkey tail, 403, 431
Turmeric, 391, 400, 406, 423, 459, 466

U

Uranium, 33
Uric acid, 149, 481
Uva ursi, 541

V

Vaccines, 6, 7, 32, 254, 255, 260, 263, 277, 284, 293, 296, 297, 298, 300, 302, 304, 308, 309, 310, 311, 320, 323, 324, 325, 326, 333, 343, 345
VAERS, 6, 254, 258, 279, 284, 312, 319, 342
Valerian, 388, 419, 443
Varicose veins, 432, 475
Virus, 6, 39, 163, 271, 273, 329
Vitamin A, 22, 162, 196, 281, 282, 318, 332, 367, 380, 421, 469
Vitamin B, 393, 408, 419, 430, 439, 470
Vitamin B17 (Laetrile), 23
Vitamin C, 84, 117, 129, 158, 196, 210, 245, 280, 332, 382, 391, 405, 408, 409, 421, 424, 426, 430, 431, 436, 442, 445, 450, 455, 461, 467, 470, 473, 475
Vitamin D, 110, 117, 204, 205, 332, 380, 381, 382, 386, 390, 391, 392, 398, 399, 406, 410, 412, 414, 421, 422, 432, 436, 446, 448, 454, 460, 462, 473
Vitamin E, 125, 387, 397, 398, 419, 421, 427, 430, 431, 442
Vitamin K, 455
Vomiting, 485

W

Warts, 379, 476
Water, 4, 7, 106, 134, 165, 166, 241, 357, 358, 363, 417, 484
Weight gain, 486, 487
Whey, 349
Willow, 478
Wintergreen, 398, 458

X

Xenoestrogens, 150

Y

Yarrow, 441, 488
Yeast, 221, 402, 406, 415

Z

Zinc, 395, 396, 439, 464, 467, 541

Made in the USA
Columbia, SC
06 January 2025